Nausea & vomiting

Parenteral drugs likely to be essential

*Consider reversible cause:
  Urinary tract infection
  Constipation
  Superimposed anxiety (use benzodiazepine)

*Assess likeliest cause:

Drugs (opioids, chemo.)—	1st line Haloperidol
/Metabolic (urea, calcium)—	2nd line Levomepromazine
Gastric stasis—	1st line Metoclopramide
	2nd line Cyclizine
Intestinal obstruction	
No colic—	Metoclopramide + Dexamethasone
With colic pain	1st line Hyoscine butylbrornide + haloperidol
	2nd line Add in Levomepromazine
Raised ICP	1st line Dexamethasone + Cyclizine
	2nd line Levomepromazine

(Beware that levomepromazine can reduce the fit threshold)

Uncertain cause	Levomepromazine

** Please note that 33% of patients may require two drugs **

Drug doses

Metoclopramide	10–20mg q.d.s. p.r.n. SC (po for nausea alone)
Cyclizine	50mg t.d.s. p.r.n. SC (po for nausea alone)
Levomepromazine	6–12.5mg b.d. p.r.n. SC (po for nausea alone)
	5–12.5mg/24h SC infusion
Haloperidol	1.5mg b.d. p.r.n. SC (po for nausea alone)

OXFORD MEDICAL PUBLICATIONS

Oxford Handbook of
Palliative Care

Oxford Handbook of
Palliative Care

Max S. Watson

Locum Consultant in Palliative Medicine,
Northern Ireland Hospice,
Research Fellow,
Belfast City Hospital,
Belfast, UK

Caroline F. Lucas

Deputy Medical Director,
Princess Alice Hospice, Esher, Surrey;
Clinical Director,
North Surrey Primary Care NHS Trust;
Honorary Consultant in Palliative Medicine,
St Peter's Hospital, Chertsey, Surrey, UK

Andrew M. Hoy

Medical Director,
Princess Alice Hospice, Esher, Surrey;
Consultant in Palliative Medicine, Epsom and
St Helier NHS Trust, UK

Ian N. Back

Consultant in Palliative Medicine,
Holme Tower Marie Curie Centre, Penarth;
Consultant in Palliative Medicine,
Pontypridd and Rhonda NHS Trust,
Mid Glamorgan, UK

OXFORD
UNIVERSITY PRESS

OXFORD

UNIVERSITY PRESS

Great Clarendon Street, Oxford OX2 6DP

Oxford University Press is a department of the University of Oxford.
It furthers the University's objective of excellence in research, scholarship,
and education by publishing worldwide in

Oxford New York

Auckland Cape Town Dar es Salaam Hong Kong Karachi
Kuala Lumpur Madrid Melbourne Mexico City Nairobi
New Delhi Shanghai Taipei Toronto

With offices in

Argentina Austria Brazil Chile Czech Republic France Greece
Guatemala Hungary Italy Japan Poland Portugal Singapore
South Korea Switzerland Thailand Turkey Ukraine Vietnam

Oxford is a registered trade mark of Oxford University Press
in the UK and in certain other countries

Published in the United States
by Oxford University Press Inc., New York

British Library Cataloguing in Publication Data
Data available

Library of Congress Cataloging in Publication Data
Data available

Typeset by Newgen Imaging Systems (P) Ltd., Chennai, India
Printed in Italy
on acid-free paper by Legoprint S.p.A

ISBN 0-19-850897-2

10 9 8 7 6 5 4 3 2 1

This book is dedicated to computer-abandoned families in Dungannon, Esher, Epsom, and Cardiff. Without their patience and understanding support, this project could never have been completed.

MW, CL, AH, IB

You matter because you are you. You matter to the last moment of your life and we will do all we can not only to help you die peacefully but to live until you die.

(Dame Cicely Saunders)

Foreword

Derek Doyle
President Emeritus of the International Association for Hospice and Palliative Care,
Vice President of the National Council for Hospice and Specialist Palliative Care Services,
Medical Director/Consultant Physician St Columba's Hospice, Edinburgh, UK (retired)

Before his Cubist phase Picasso painted a moving scene, one that he had perhaps witnessed as a boy. He entitled it *Science and Charity* (words that will remind some readers of the motto of the Royal College of General Practitioners). An old doctor, in what is clearly a poor home, is sitting by the bedside of a dying patient. His expression is one of compassion and deep thought as he leans on the bed looking at the patient he has perhaps known for many years. It is impossible not to be moved by this image of a general practitioner in 'the old days' and tempting to compare him with us who care for the dying in a very different world.

Some will look at the painting and sigh with nostalgia for far-off days when, as young GPs, they too made time to sit by a bedside. Today, even if they wanted to, there is seldom sufficient time. They might smile to see so few pieces of equipment—no syringe drivers and drips, nebulisers or suction machines, or even catheter bags. Neither are there any nurses. Many might be surprised to see someone who looks so young dying at home—something that is getting less common in today's world in spite of the expressed wishes of so many patients and the personnel and resources being poured into community care.

Others will wonder if that old doctor ever felt as they often do today when caring for the dying; lonely, sometimes a little frightened, less confident and competent than at any other time in their work, and, in our secularized society, often at a loss to help with existential questions.

Junior hospital doctors (and, one would like to think, some consultants) will perhaps look at the painting and give a wry smile. The old man may have felt inadequate, poorly trained, and lonely but, they will ask themselves, is that any different from what they feel day in day out, caring for the dying in the wards of our hospitals? Yes, they have had a few lectures on palliative care and communication skills but their sense of inadequacy in the face of a spectrum of suffering is little assuaged. They have had tutorials on ethical decision-making but in today's real world most responses seem to be knee-jerk reactions made under pressure, not decisions talked through with colleagues in the luxury of a mutually supportive team.

It is tempting to wonder what Picasso's doctor would have thought about today's palliative care and this new book. We can be sure he would have smiled with disbelief at something so much a part and parcel of every doctor's life being glorified with a name like *palliative care*. After all, he might have asked, is that not what good care is all about; comforting, explaining, and listening, being there when needed and especially when the days of further tests and new therapies have long passed; sharing one's humanity with all its frailties with someone on the loneliest journey of life. He might be shocked to learn why 'the principles of all clinical care' as he knew them, had to be dignified with such a title in the last decades of the 20th century.

Given a copy of this new *Handbook* he would have been amazed and, hopefully, a little envious. Amazed at the cornucopia of drugs and formulations available to today's doctors to ease suffering. Amazed at how much scientific research has uncovered and made possible. Amazed at how many, other than doctors, now share in this ministry of caring and in doing so bring a richness of skills and compassion. Envious that, to his surprise, it is now possible to have so much information and guidance at one's finger tips, in a book small enough for his desk or his bag. Surprised and thrilled, one hopes, that underpinning this handbook is a yet more comprehensive *Oxford Textbook of Palliative Medicine*, the resource for the specialists in palliative medicine—the specialists across the country, eager to take away some of the loneliness and sense of inadequacy our old doctor felt at that bedside.

No, there is nothing new about the principles of palliative care. They are the age-old principles of all good care but, as this *Handbook* so beautifully illustrates, now enhanced by new knowledge, new drugs, new approaches, new insights—all available to every doctor, nurse, chaplain, professional allied to medicine privileged to share themselves with someone on their final journey. What a challenge but what a privilege, as Picasso's doctor would surely have reminded us. Picasso seems to have chosen the right words for us—palliative care is, before all else, science and charity in action.

Edinburgh, September 2004

Preface

Most clinical professionals have been affected by caring for patients with palliative care needs. Such patients may challenge us at both a professional and at a personal level in areas where we feel our confidence or competence are challenged.

'I wanted to help her, but I just didn't know what to do or say'

As in every other branch of medicine, knowledge and training can help us extend our comfort zone, so that we can better respond to such patients in a caring and professional manner. However, in picking up this handbook and reading thus far you have already demonstrated a motivation that is just as important as a thirst for knowledge, the central desire to improve the care of your patients.

It was out of just such a motivation that the modern hospice movement began 40 years ago, and it is that same motivation that has fuelled the spread of the principles of palliative care—in fact the principles of ALL good care—across the globe: respect for the person, attention to detail, scrupulous honesty and integrity, holistic care, team caring, and consummate communications (often more about listening than telling and talking).

'I knew we couldn't cure him, but didn't know when or how to start palliative care'

Increasingly it is being recognized that every person has the right to receive high quality palliative care whatever the illness, whatever its stage, regardless of whether potentially curable or not. The artificial distinction between curative and palliative treatments has rightly been recognized as an unnecessary divide, with a consequent loss of the border crossings that previously signified a complete change in clinical emphasis and tempo.

Medical knowledge is developing rapidly, with ever more opportunities for and emphasis on curative treatment, to the point when any talk of palliative care can sometimes be interpreted as 'defeatist'.

Today the principles of palliative care interventions may be employed from the first when a patient's illness is diagnosed. Conversely, a patient with predominantly palliative care needs, late in their disease journey, may benefit from energetic treatments more usually regarded as 'curative'.

'I just felt so helpless watching him die. Surely it could have been better?'

Governments and professional bodies now recognize that every nurse and doctor has a duty to provide palliative care and, increasingly, the public and the media have come to expect—as of right—high quality palliative care from their healthcare professionals irrespective of the clinical setting.

Many of these palliative care demands can best be met, as in the past, by the health care professionals who already know their patients and families well. This handbook is aimed at such hospital or community-based professionals, and recognizes that the great majority of patients with palliative needs are looked after by doctors and nurses who have not been trained in specialist palliative care but who are often specialist in the knowledge of their patients.

'Even though I knew she had had every treatment possible, still, when she died I really felt that we had failed her and let her family down.'

Junior healthcare staff throughout the world have used the Oxford Handbook series as their own specialist pocket companion through the lonely hours of on-call life. The format, concise (topic-a-page), complete and sensible, teaches not just clinical facts but a way of thinking. Yet for all the preoccupation with cure, no healthcare professional will ever experience greater satisfaction or confirmation of their choice of profession, than by bringing comfort and dignity to someone at the end-of-life.

'I had never seen anyone with that type of pain before and just wished I could get advice from someone who knew what to do.'

The demands on inexperienced and hard-pressed doctors or nurses in looking after patients with palliative care needs can be particularly stressful. It is our hope that this text, ideally complemented by the support and teaching of specialist palliative care teams, will reduce the often-expressed sense of helplessness, a sense of helplessness made all the more poignant by the disproportionate gratitude expressed by patients and families for any attempts at trying to listen, understand and care.

'It was strange, but I felt he was helping me much more than I was helping him'

While it is our hope that the handbook will help the reader to access important information quickly and succinctly, we hope it will not replace the main source of palliative care knowledge: the bedside contact with the patient.

It is easier to learn from books than patients, yet what our patients teach us is often of more abiding significance: empathy, listening, caring, existential questions of our own belief systems and the limitations of medicine. It is at the bedside that we learn to be of practical help to people who are struggling to come to terms with their own mortality and face our own mortality in the process.

Readers may notice some repetition of topics in the handbook. This is not due to weariness or oversight on the part of the editors, but is an attempt to keep relevant material grouped together—to make it easier for those needing to look up information quickly.

It is inevitable that in a text of this size some will be disappointed at the way we have left out, or skimped, on a favourite area of palliative care interest. To these readers we offer our apologies and two routes of redress: almost 200 blank pages to correct the imbalances, and the OUP website, http://www.oup.co.uk/isbn/0-19-850897-2, where your suggestions for how the next edition could be improved would be gratefully received.

Acknowledgements

This Handbook could not have been completed without the whole-hearted involvement of a team of healthcare professionals who freely shared of their time and expertise in advising, editing and contributing various chapters or sections.

That such writing was completed on top of existing heavy clinical work loads is a testimony to these advisors, their capacity for hard work and commitment to sharing knowledge and expertise.

The costs of such extracurricular activities as contributing to handbooks like this is ususally also paid for by the families and partners of those whom we have trapped in their studies—thank you.

We particularly thank Catherine Barnes and Georgia Pinteau at Oxford University Press for their patience through the long birthing process of the handbook, and their ready supply of encouragement.

We are indebted to Ian Back both for permission to use some of the material contained in his excellent *Palliative Medicine Handbook* and for his input into the project despite several other major commitments.

The South West London and The Surrey, West Sussex and Hampshire Cancer Networks gave permission to use material contained in their Adult and Paediatric palliative care guidelines.

Jan Brooman at the Princess Alice Hospice Library was an invaluable help in the painstaking task of checking through the references.

The management and colleagues at the Princess Alice Hospice and the Northern Ireland Palliative Medicine Training Scheme have been very supportive of this project.

Handbooks, by their very nature, are distillations of accumulated and shared clinical knowledge. There is no claim to originality in these pages. We must accredit the hundreds of palliative care professionals who have observed, researched, recorded and written in journals and textbooks, to create the palliative care knowledge base which has been our primary text—a text which, almost unbelievably, did not exist in medical literature only 40 years ago.

MW
CL
AH
IB

We are indebted for permission to reproduce material within the Handbook from the following sources.

I. Back (2001) *Palliative Medicine Handbook*, 3rd edition. Cardiff: BPM Books.

E. Bruera and I. Higginson (1996) *Cachexia-Anorexia in Cancer Patients*. Oxford: Oxford University Press.

D. Doyle, N. Hanks, and N. Cherny (eds.) (2004) *Oxford Textbook of Palliative Medicine*, 3rd edition. Oxford: Oxford University Press.

J-H. R. Ramsay (1994) A King, a doctor and a convenient death. *BMJ*, **308**: 1445.

The South West London and the Survey West Sussex and Hampshire Cancer Networks. M. Watson and C. Lucas (2003) *Adult Palliative Care Guidelines*.

K. Thomas (2003) *Caring for the Dying at Home: companions on the journey*. Oxford: Radcliffe Medical Press.

R. Twycross, A. Wilcock, S. Charlesworth, and A. Dickman (2002) *Palliative Care Formulary*, 2nd edition. Oxford: Radcliffe Medical Press.

Winston's Wish: supporting bereaved children and young people. www.winstonswish.org.uk.

www.rch.org.au/rch_palliative; www.rch.org.au.

Contents

Advisors and contributors

Jennifer Barraclough
Former Consultant in Psychological Medicine
Sobell House
Churchill Hospital
Oxford

Pauline Beldon
Nurse Consultant Tissue Viability
Epsom and St Helier NHS Trust
Surrey

Jo Bray
Former Occupational Therapist
Project Director
Royal Marsden Hospital
Chelsea

Jan Brooman
Librarian
Princess Alice Hospice
Esher

David Cameron
Associate Professor of Family Medicine
University of Pretoria
South Africa

Beverly Castleton
Medical Director for Specialist Services and Consultant Physician
Care of the Elderly and the Young Physically Disabled
Surrey Heath and Woking NHS PCT
Chertsey

Robin Cole
Consultant Urological Surgeon
St Peter's Hospital
Chertsey

David Conkey
Clinical Oncology Department
Belvoir Park Hospital
Belfast

Simon Coulter
Specialist Registrar
Palliative Medicine Training Scheme
Belfast

Jill Cooper
Head Occupational Therapist
Royal Marsden Hospital
Sutton

Elizabeth Cruickshank
Speech and Language Therapist
South Glasgow University Hospitals
NHS Trust
Glasgow

Dwipaj Datta
Specialist Registrar
Palliative Medicine Training Scheme
South Thames
London

Judith Delaney
Haematology/Oncology Senior Pharmacist
Great Ormond Street Hospital for Children NHS Trust
London

Julie Doyle
Consultant in Palliative Medicine
Northern Ireland Hospice and Mater Hospital
Belfast

Martin Eatock
Consultant Medical Oncologist
Belfast City Hospital
Belfast

Patricia Enes
Formerly Research Nurse
Princess Alice Hospice
Esher

Gill Eyers
Senior Principal Pharmacist
Princess Alice Hospice, Esher
Kingston Hospital NHS Trust
Surrey

Craig Gannon
Consultant in Palliative Medicine
Princess Alice Hospice
Ashford and St Peter's Hospitals NHS Trust
Surrey

Louise Gibbs
Consultant in Palliative Medicine
St Christopher's Hospice
Lawrie Park Road
Sydenham, London

J. Simon Gibbs
Senior Lecturer in Cardiology
National Heart and Lung Institute at
Imperial College London, and
Honorary Consultant Cardiologist
Hammersmith Hospital, London

David Head
Former Chaplain
Princess Alice Hospice
Esher

Irene Higginson
Professor of Palliative Care and Policy
King's College School of Medicine and Dentistry
London

Jenny Hynson
Consultant Paediatrician
Victorian Paediatric Palliative Care Program
Royal Children's Hospital
Melbourne
Australia

David Hill
Consultant in Anaesthesia and Pain Management
Ulster Hospital
Honorary Senior Lecturer
Queen's University
Belfast

Allan Irvine
Consultant Radiologist
Ashford and St Peter's Hospitals NHS Trust
Surrey

Aleen Jones
Consultant Physician
Care of the Elderly
South Tyrone and Craigavon Area Hospitals
Craigavon

Emma Jones
Consultant in Palliative Medicine
Phyllis Tuckwell Hospice
Farnham

Carol Katté
Stoma Care Specialist Nurse
Ashford and St Peter's Hospitals NHS Trust
Surrey

Sian Lewis
Senior Dietician
Velindre Hospital
Cardiff

Victoria Lidstone
Specialist Registrar
Palliative Medicine Training Schemes
South Thames/South Wales
Cardiff

Mari Lloyd-Williams
Professor, Honorary Consultant in Palliative Medicine
Director of Primary Care
University of Liverpool
Liverpool

Jayne Macauley
Consultant in Palliative Medicine
Antrim Area Hospital and Northern Health Board
Antrim

Sarah McKenna
Consultant Medical Oncologist
Belfast City Hospital Trust
Belfast

Pamela MacKinnon
Formerly at the Department of Human Anatomy and Genetics
University of Oxford
Oxford

Sarah MacLaran
Specialist Registrar
Palliative Medicine Training Scheme
Myton Hamlet Hospice, Warwick

Dorry McLaughlin
Lecturer in Palliative Care
Northern Ireland Hospice Care
Belfast

Penny McNamara
Consultant in Palliative Medicine
Sue Ryder Care—St John's
Bedford

Elaine McWilliams
Clinical Psychologist
Harrow Primary Care Trust
Harrow

Anne Miller
Consultant Haematologist
Ashford and St Peter's Hospitals NHS Trust
Surrey

Dan Munday
Consultant in Palliative Medicine
Honorary Senior Lecturer Warwick University
Coventry Primary Care Trust
Warwick

Simon Noble
Specialist Registrar Palliative Medicine
All Wales Higher Training Programme
Cardiff

Victor Pace
Consultant in Palliative Medicine
St Christopher's Hospice
Lawrie Park Road
Sydenham, London

Sheila Payne
Professor in Palliative Care
Sheffield Palliative Care Studies Group
University of Sheffield
Sheffield

Margaret Reith
Social Worker Team Manager
Princess Alice Hospice
Esher

Joan Regan
Specialist Registrar
Palliative Medicine Training Scheme
Belfast

Patti Stevely
Day Hospice Manager
Senior Physiotherapist
Princess Alice Hospice
Esher

Robert Sudderick
Consultant in Otolaryngology and Head
and Neck surgery
Royal Surrey County Hospital
Guildford

Keri Thomas
GP, National Clinical Lead Palliative Care
Cancer Services Collaborative of NHS Modernisation Agency
Macmillan Gold Standards Framework Programme
Associate Clinical Director Community Palliative Care, Birmingham
Senior Clinical Lecturer, Warwick University

Patrick Trend
Consultant Neurologist
Royal Surrey County Hospital
Guildford

Jo Wells
Nurse Consultant in Palliative Care
Princess Alice Hospice
Kingston Hospital NHS Trust
Surrey

Andrew Wilcock
Macmillan Clinical Leader in Palliative Medicine and Medical Oncology
Nottingham University
Consultant Physician, Hayward House Macmillan
Specialist Palliative Care Unit
Nottingham City Hospital
Nottingham

Abbreviations

AF	atrial fibrillation
AIDS	acquired immune deficiency syndrome
Amp.	ampoule
b.d.	twice daily
BNF	British National Formulary
BP	blood pressure
Caps.	capsules
CD	controlled drug
CHF	congestive heart failure
CMV	cytomegalovirus
CNS	central nervous system
CO_2	carbon dioxide
COPD	chronic obstructive pulmonary disease
COX	cyclo-oxygenase
CSCI	continuous subcutaneous infusion
C/T	chemotherapy
CT	computerized tomography
CTZ	chemoreceptor trigger zone
CVA	cerebrovascular accident
DIC	disseminated intravascular coagulation
DN	District Nurse
DVT	deep vein thrombosis
ECG	electrocardiogram
EDDM	Equivalent Daily Dose of Morphine
FBC	full blood count
FEV_1	forced expiratory volume in one second
FNA	fine needle aspiration
g	gram
GERD	gastro-oesophageal reflux disease
GI	gastrointestinal
GP	General Practitioner
Gy	Gray(s) a measure of radiation
h	hour or hourly
HAART	highly active anti-retroviral therapy
HIV	human immunodeficiency virus
HNSCC	head and neck squamous cell carcinoma

ICP	intracranial pressure
i/m	intramuscular
Inj.	injection
i/r	immediate release
i/t	intrathecal
i/v	intravenous
IVI	intravenous infusion
IVU	intravenous urogram
KS	Kaposi's sarcoma
kV	kilovolt
l	litre
L/A	local anaesthetic
LFT	liver function tests
LVF	left ventricular failure
MAI	Mycobacterium avium intracellulare
MAOI	monoamine oxidase inhibitor(s)
max.	maximum
MeV	mega electronvolt
mcg	microgram
MND	motor neurone disease
m/r	modified release
MRI	Magnetic Resonance Imaging
MUPS	multiple unit pellet system
MV	megavolt
m/w	mouthwash
NASSA	noradrenergic and specific serotoninergic antidepressant
neb	nebuliser
NG	naso-gastric
NMDA	N-methyl-D-aspartate
nocte	at night
NSAID	non-steroidal anti-inflammatory drug
NSCLC	non small cell lung carcinoma
NYHA	New York Heart Association
o.d.	daily
o.m.	in the morning
OTFC	oral transmucosal fentanyl citrate
PCA	Patient Controlled Analgesia
PCF	Palliative Care Formulary
PCT	Palliative care team
PE	pulmonary embolism
PEG	percutaneous endoscopic gastrostomy

PET	positron emission tomography
PHCT	primary healthcare team
p.o.	by mouth
PPI	proton pump inhibitor
PR	per rectum
p.r.n.	when required
PSA	prostate-specific antigen
PV	per vagina
q.d.s.	four times daily
QoL	quality of life
RBL	renal bone liver (investigations)
RCT	randomized controlled trial
RT	radiotherapy
SALT	speech and language therapy
SC	subcutaneous
SCLC	small cell lung carcinoma
S/D	syringe driver (CSCI)
SE	side-effects
SERMs	selective oestrogen receptor modulators
SL	sublingual
soln.	solution
SPC	specialist palliative care
SR	slow or modified release
SSRI	selective serotonin reuptake inhibitor
stat	immediately
Supps.	suppositories
Susp.	suspension
SVC	superior vena cava
SVCO	superior vena cava obstruction
Tabs.	tablets
TB	tuberculosis
TBM	tubercular meningitis
t.d.s.	three times daily
TENS	transcutaneous electrical nerve stimulation
TIA	transient ischaemic attack
TSD	therapeutic standard dose
U&E	urea and electrolytes
URTI	upper respiratory tract infection
UTI	urinary tract infection
VTE	venous thromboembolism
WHO	World Health Organization

Introduction

Palliative care definitions

Palliative care is the active, holistic care of patients with advanced, progressive illness. Management of pain and other symptoms and provision of psychological, social and spiritual support is paramount. The goal of palliative care is achievement of the best quality of life for patients and their families. Many aspects of palliative care are also applicable earlier in the course of the illness in conjunction with other treatments.[1]

Palliative care:
- Affirms life and regards dying as a normal process
- Provides relief from pain and other symptoms
- Integrates the psychological and spiritual aspects of patient care
- Offers a support system to help patients live as actively as possible until death
- Offers a support system to help the family cope during the patient's illness and in their own environment.

Principles of palliative care

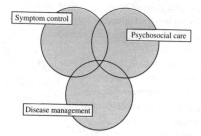

No single sphere of concern is adequate without considering the relationship with the other two. This usually requires genuine interdisciplinary collaboration.[2]

General palliative care is provided by the usual professional carers of the patient and family with low to moderate complexity of palliative care need. Palliative care is a vital and integral part of their routine clinical practice which is underpinned by the following principles:
- Focus on quality of life which includes good symptom control
- Whole person approach taking into account the person's past life experience and current situation

- Care which encompasses both the person with life-threatening illness and those that matter to the person
- Respect for patient autonomy and choice (e.g. over place of care, treatment options)
- Emphasis on open and sensitive communication, which extends to patients, informal carers and professional colleagues

Specialist palliative care

These services are provided for patients and their families with moderate to high complexity of palliative care need. The core service components are provided by a range of NHS, voluntary and independent providers staffed by a multidisciplinary team whose core work is palliative care.[2]

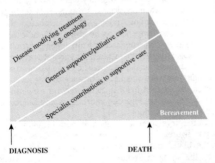

Supportive care is that which helps the patient and their family to cope with cancer and treatment of it—from pre-diagnosis, through the process of diagnosis and treatment, to cure, continuing illness or death and into bereavement. It helps the patient to maximize the benefits of treatment and to live as well as possible with the effects of the disease. It is given equal priority alongside diagnosis and treatment.

The principles that underpin supportive and palliative care are broadly the same.

Hospice and hospice care refer to a philosophy of care rather than a specific building or service and may encompass a programme of care and array of skills deliverable in a wide range of settings.

Terminal care is an important part of palliative care and usually refers to the management of patients during their last few days, weeks or months of life from a point at which it becomes clear that the patient is in a progressive state of decline.

1 World Health Organization (1990) *Cancer Pain Relief and Palliative Care*. Geneva: WHO: 11 (World Health Organization technical report series: 804)

2 National Council for Hospice and Specialist Palliative Care Services (2002) *Definitions of Supportive and Palliative Care*. London: NCHSPCS (Briefing Bulletin 11)

History of palliative medicine as a specialty

The specialty of palliative medicine as a specific entity dates from the mid 1980s. However, medical activity related to terminal care, care of the dying, hospice care and end-stage cancer is of course as old as medical practice itself.[1] Palliative medicine is the medical component of what has become known as palliative care.

The history of the hospice movement during the nineteenth and twentieth centuries demonstrates the innovations of several charismatic leaders. These practitioners were enthusiasts for their own particular contribution to care of the dying, and they were also the teachers of the next generation of palliative physicians. Although they were products of their original background and training, they all shared the vision of regarding patients who happened to be dying as 'whole people'. They naturally brought their own approaches from specific disciplines of pharmacology, oncology, surgery, anaesthetics or general practice. This whole person attitude has been labelled as 'holistic care'. Comfort and freedom from pain and distress were of equal importance to diagnostic acumen and cure. However, rather than being a completely new philosophy of care, palliative medicine can be regarded more as a codification of existing practices from past generations.

Histories of the development of palliative medicine illustrate the thread of ideas from figures such as Snow, who developed the Brompton Cocktail in the 1890s, to Barrett who developed the regular giving of oral morphine to the dying at St Luke's, West London, to Saunders who expanded these ideas at St Joseph's and St Christopher's Hospices. Worcester, in Boston, was promoting the multidisciplinary care of whole patients in lectures to medical students at a time when intense disease specialization was very much the fashion as it was yielding great therapeutic advances.[2] Winner and Amulree, in the UK in the 1960s, were promoting whole person care particularly for the elderly, first challenging and then re-establishing the ethical basis for palliative medicine.

The early hospice movement was primarily concerned with the care of patients with cancer who, in the surge of post-war medical innovation, had missed out on the windfall of the new confident and increasingly optimistic medical world.

That this movement was responding to a need perceived across the world, has been evidenced by the exponential growth in palliative care services throughout the UK and across the globe since the opening of St Christopher's hospice in south-east London in 1967.

The expansion is set to increase further, as the point has now been reached where patients, doctors and governments alike are calling for the same level of care to be made available to patients suffering from non-malignant conditions as for those with cancer.

If this new challenge is to be met, healthcare professionals from early in their training will need to be exposed to palliative care learning which can be applied across the range of medical specialities.

The essence of such palliative medicine learning both for generalists and specialists remains that of clinical apprenticeship. Alfred Worcester, in the preface to his lectures, notes that:

The younger members of the profession, although having enormously greater knowledge of the science of medicine, have less acquaintance than many of their elders with the art of medical practice. This like every other art can of course be learned only by imitation, that is, by practice under masters of the art. Primarily, it depends upon devotion to the patient rather than to his disease.[2]

1 Saunders C. (1993). Introduction—history and challenge. In C. Saunders, N. Sykes (eds) *The Management of Terminal Malignant Disease. 3rd edition*, pp. 1–14. London: Edward Arnold.

2 Worcester A. (1935) *The Care of the Aged the Dying and the Dead*. London: Bailliere & Co.

The death of Harold Shipman

> Dr Harold Shipman died on 13 January in Wakefield Prison. He hanged himself on the day before his 58th birthday. He was convicted in January 2000 of the murder of 15 people. However, it is estimated that he killed at least 215 mainly elderly people. As well as being the UK's most prolific serial killer, what is most shocking is that his victims were his patients. They looked up to him as a trusted GP and friend. What significance does this have for those concerned with palliative care in both the UK and beyond?

All medical practice, but particularly palliative care, relies on the establishment of a relationship of trust between patients and their healthcare professional advisors. This trust is threatened by dishonesty on the part of doctors or nurses. For this reason, the palliative care movement has embraced the philosophy of truthful disclosure of clinical information to patients if that is what is asked for. This philosophy is sometimes confused with total disclosure of every last documented outcome and complication of a proposed management plan, whether or not the recipient of the information is in an emotional or intellectual state to process it. This offloading of detail may be advocated as part of the process of obtaining informed consent, or it may be the result of defensive practice to protect against future litigation. Neither is in the patient's best interest. Furthermore, frank disclosure does not imply brutal use of stark prognostic details, without first listening carefully to the patient's informational requests. So honesty and truthfulness are prerequisites for trust. Trust in turn is essential to prevent advice from becoming paternalistic.

Harold Shipman used opioids to kill his victims. We will never know the details of dose and methods, but it is safe to assume that he gave very large doses to opioid-naïve patients. This fact has not always been reported to the public, with the unfortunate consequence that there is now increasing suspicion of strong opioids even when such drugs would relieve severe pain. This makes palliative care more difficult and results in increased suffering especially for the vulnerable.

Although Shipman showed no remorse or inclination to collaborate in establishing his motives, while he was still alive there was still the chance that we might eventually have gained some insight into his psychopathology. Now he has killed himself, we are simply left to speculate that in death as in life his motive was the need to exert control over all those around him.

The popular press has named his activity as 'euthanasia without consent'. This term is unfortunate for several reasons. We do not have evidence that all his victims died peacefully and without anguish. They were certainly not given any opportunity to complete unfinished business with family and friends. In the immediate aftermath of Shipman's death, anger and resentment among relatives has increased not diminished. There would seem to be no sense of closure which either understanding or remorse might have brought. The use of the word euthanasia only muddies the water in a debate which is difficult in any event. Finally, although death can be viewed as the inevitable relinquishment of autonomy, at least in a physical sense, choices can be exercised before such relinquishment. Shipman removed consent, choices and therefore all autonomy and self-determination. His activity was murder with or without an understandable motive.

Since the conviction four years ago, there has been an exhaustive judicial inquiry of current law and regulations relating to death registration, monitoring of single-handed general practice, prescription, availability and supply of controlled drugs. The Prime Minister has already said that the recommendations of this review will be implemented in full. There is, however, considerable anxiety that this may result in a straitjacket for sensible community palliative care. It would be doubly tragic if Shipman's legacy of murder resulted in the frustration of good palliative care. An exceptional case makes for bad law.

Reproduced with kind permission from the *European Journal of Palliative Care*.

Communication

Effective symptom control is impossible without effective communication

Buckman 2000

Communication is fundamental to good palliative care, but difficulties can arise that need to be understood and addressed.

Society's attitudes towards death and dying can hinder open communication. Health professionals may be uneasy with issues of death and dying: they may wish to protect themselves and others, and feel a sense of discomfort with strong emotions.

It is easy for the busy health professional to use a variety of blocking tactics which inhibit communication, such as hiding behind task-focused practice. An additional hazard may arise if the setting is not conducive to privacy with space and time to listen.

Information-giving can take the place of hearing the underlying feelings and emotions. The essence of good communication is not what we say, but how we listen. The quality of listening empathically to patients should not be underestimated if patients are to feel understood and cared for.

Communication in palliative care is necessary to achieve accurate assessment of patients' physical, emotional and psychosocial needs. If we are to be able to find ways of supporting patients and families facing change and uncertainty, we as health professional needs to find out about the patient's expectations and goals.

Enabling people to make informed choices and to make future plans involves careful listening and sensitive responses. Attending to cultural and language issues, and helping people face some of the strong emotions aroused by their situation such as anger, denial, depression and fear, are essential in providing holistic PALLIATIVE CARE.

Buckman, R. (2000) Communication in palliative care: a practical guide.
In D. Dickenson, M. Johnson and J. S. Katz (eds.) *Death, Dying and Bereavement*, 2nd edn.
pp 146–73. London: Sage.

Prognostication in end-of-life care

The natural history of disease has been documented over many years. This has become increasingly less relevant as successful therapies have developed. In present day palliative medicine, prognosis frequently relates to chronic progressive disease in patients with multiple co-morbidities, and not to the recovery prediction of a young adult with an acute illness, as was more common in the nineteenth century.

The reasons for making an attempt at predicting how long a patient with incurable disease might live include:

- Providing information about the future to patients and families so that they can set goals, priorities and expectations of care
- Helping patients develop insight into their dying
- Assisting clinicians in decision-making
- Comparing like patients with regard to outcomes
- Establishing the patient's eligibility for care programmes (e.g. hospice) and for recruitment to research trials
- Policy-making regarding appropriate use and allocation of resources and support services
- Providing a common language for healthcare professionals involved in end-of-life care.

Prognostic factors in cancer

There is a good literature on the probability of cure for the different cancers.

- Although individual cancers behave differently, as a generalization, predictions relate to tumour size, grade and stage
- Other factors include hormonal status (for hormone-dependent tumours such as cancer of the breast and prostate)
- Age
- Biochemical or other markers
- The length of time taken for the disease to recur.

In palliative care such prognostic indices may not be so relevant.

Factors such as physical dependency (due to e.g. weakness, low blood pressure), cognitive dysfunction, paraneoplastic phenomena (e.g. anorexia–cachexia, cytokine production), certain symptoms (weight loss, anorexia, dysphagia, breathlessness), lymphopaenia, poor quality of life and existential factors (either 'giving up' or 'hanging on' for symbolically important times) may be more important.

Some patients may survive for a long time (months and years) with a seemingly high tumour load, while others succumb within a short time (days) for no obviously identifiable reasons.

Several scores have been developed to aid prediction of survival. The Palliative Prognostic (PaP) score is predictive of short term survival and summarizes scores for dyspnoea, anorexia, Karnovsky performance status, the clinician's estimate of survival (in weeks), total white count, and percentage of lymphocytes.

Oncologists rely on prognosis assessments in order to predict which patients are likely to benefit from oncological interventions. Many of their decisions are based on the patient's functional status.

Patients with an ECOG score greater than two are usually deemed unsuitable for most chemotherapy interventions.

Eastern Co-operative Oncology Group (ECOG)

Fully active; able to carry on all activities without restriction	0
Restricted in physically strenuous activity but ambulatory and able to carry out work of a light or sedentary nature	1
Ambulatory and capable of all self care; confined to bed or chair 50% of waking hours	2
Capable of only limited self-care; confined to bed or chair 50% or more of waking hours	3
Completely disabled; cannot carry on any self care; totally confined to bed or chair	4

Prognostic factors in non-malignant disease

Predicting prognosis in patients with a non-cancer diagnosis is very difficult. These patients often remain relatively stable, albeit at a low level, only to deteriorate acutely and unpredictably. They are usually then treated acutely in hospital, and the disease course may consist of acute exacerbations from which recovery may take place.

One study showed that even in the last 2–3 days of life patients with congestive heart failure (CHF) or COPD were given a 80 per cent and 50 per cent chance respectively of living six months.

There are, however, general and specific indicators of the terminal stage approaching.

General predictors

Those predicting poorer prognosis include reduced performance status, impaired nutritional status (greater than 10 per cent weight loss over six months) and a low albumin.

Specific predictors

Congestive heart failure (CHF)
- More than 64 years old
- Left ventricular ejection fraction less than 20 per cent
- Dilated cardiomyopathy
- Uncontrolled arrhythmias
- Systolic hypotension
- CXR signs of left heart failure
- A prognosis of less than six months is associated with NYHA Class IV (chest pain and/or breathless at rest/minmal exertion) and already optimally treated with diuretics and vasodilators

Chronic obstructive pulmonary disease (COPD)
- Advanced age
- FEV_1 less than 30 per cent
- Pulmonary hypertension with cor pulmonale/right heart failure
- Other factors NHO sob at rest
- On 24 hour home O_2 with pO_2 less than 50 mm Hg and/or pCO_2 more than 55 mm Hg and documented evidence of cor pulmonale

Cortical dementias (Alzheimer's disease)
- Functional status—the onset of being unable to walk unaided
- Unable to swallow
- Unable to hold a meaningful conversation
- Increasing frequency of medical complications, e.g. aspiration pneumonia, urinary tract infections, decubitus ulcers

Stroke
- Impaired consciousness
- Lack of improvement within three months of onset
- Age
- Incontinence
- Cognitive impairment
- Dense paralysis

Communicating prognosis

Prognostication is a notoriously difficult task to perform accurately. The world abounds with stories of patients who have been told by their physicians that they have only a matter of months to live who twenty years later can recount in vivid detail the day they were given the news.

One of the reasons that prognostication is so difficult is that it is fraught with uncertainty and also with opportunities for misunderstandings between doctors and patients, who often have very different agendas as to what they want to get out of the interview.

> Mr. Jones listened carefully as the consultant went into great detail about the nature and the extensive spread of his metastatic prostate tumour. The explanations were detailed and scientific and long. Eventually the consultant stopped. 'Now Mr. Jones, do you have any more questions'
>
> 'Well, I didn't like to interrupt you but I was only asking how long I had before I needed to go down to get my X-Ray.'

Over the past 20 years there has been a huge shift in attitudes regarding disclosure of information to patents, and a culture of complete disclosure has now become the norm. Yet prognostication does not just involve passing on clinical details and predictions of disease progression; it also involves assessing:
- What does the patient actually want to know? (Giving too much information to a patient who does not want to have the exact details spelt out is as unprofessional as the patronising attitudes of 'best not to trouble the patient'
- How is the patient dealing with the information that is being given?

- How can the patient be helped to deal with the implications
  of the news?

To pass on facts without regard for the implications of those facts is to increase the risk of dysfunctional communication taking place. (📖 See Chapter 2)

Risk and chance

While doctors are used to describing risk in terms of percentages, when such percentages are measuring out your own longevity it is hard to translate the mathematical chances into personal experience.

A doctor may feel that he has provided the patient with the clear facts when he states that in 100 patients with the particular malignancy, 36 will be alive after five years following treatment. Such sentences can be easily misunderstood, and the patient may hear something very different from what the doctor is saying.

Professional discomfort

Doctors are also particularly vulnerable to miscommunication at the time of passing on prognostic information.

- Society in the west is now death-denying, and if the prognosis is
  poor it can be uncomfortable for the doctor to pass on the
  information and confront the patent with their imminent death
- There is increasing fear of litigation, particularly if disease is not
  responsive to treatment, and any admission of failure may come
  across as an admission of guilt
- Doctors may feel uncomfortable in dealing with the emotional impact
  that their news may have on the patient, and develop techniques to
  protect themselves from this discomfort

Prognostic information can be extremely important to patients as it allows them to focus on tasks and goals which they want to achieve before their disease takes over: communicating such information effectively is a skill which all healthcare professionals should covet.

Ethical issues

An ethical framework
- Respect for autonomy (self-determination)
- Beneficence (do good)
- Non-maleficence (do no harm)
- Justice (fairness)

The concept of exploring end-of-life issues is inherent to palliative care. With good communication and trust in the patient/professional relationship, patients' attitudes and concerns can be discussed sensitively, confusion unravelled and fears dispelled. Some patients like to consider writing a formal Advance Directive or 'living will', which should give a more formative clearly defined record of patients' wishes in order to facilitate more informed decision-making. In practice, when patients ask for euthanasia there may be areas of 'unfinished business', fear, guilt or other issues that need to be explored. After sensitive and open communication, most patients feel a sense of relief and their need to press for a deliberate ending of their life diminishes.

We live in a world which has become increasingly complex. Ethical issues that arise towards the end-of-life are often fraught with difficulty in an increasingly technological age in which the process of dying may be prolonged. In healthcare, there is often no right or wrong decision, but only a consensus view of a clear aim, considered on the basis of ethical principles. The most widely used ethical framework in health issues in the West comprises:

- **Autonomy** (the patient should be informed and involved in decision-making)
- **Beneficence** (do good)
- **Non-maleficence** (do no harm)
- **Justice** (balancing the needs of individuals with those of society)

In the abstract, these principles can seem straightforward; in the heat of a clinical situation their application can be anything but clear. It is, however, very useful to have a framework with which to deal with ethical crises.

The following clinical scenarios are examples which occur commonly. Applying the principles of ethics in order to reach a balanced compromise can help provide a path through uncertainty.

Example 1: 'My father is not drinking adequately. Why are you not giving him extra fluids?'

Ethical issues
- **Beneficence**: Will artificial fluids help the patient?
- **Non-maleficence**: Will giving or not giving artificial fluids cause the patient harm?
- **Autonomy**: Does the patient want a drip?

It is instilled in all of us, from childhood years onwards, that food and drink are essential for life. There are clinical situations in palliative care when extra systemic fluids might be useful, for instance in hypercalcaemia or profuse diarrhoea and vomiting. These may be salvageable clinical situations where we are expecting the patient to return to his 'normal', albeit generally deteriorating, state of health.

Artificial hydration
- A blanket policy of artificial hydration, or of no artificial hydration, is ethically indefensible
- If dehydration is thought to be due to a potentially correctable cause, the option of artificial hydration should be considered
- The appropriateness of artificial hydration should be weighed up in terms of harm and benefit on a day-to-day basis

When someone is considered to be dying irreversibly, however, the routine of giving systemic fluids may not be in the patient's best interests.

Background information
There are a few studies addressing this issue, but there is no proof that either the giving or withholding of fluids interferes with the length of remaining life or affects comfort.
- Biochemical parameters show that only 50 per cent of patients have any evidence of dehydration within the final 48 h of life and, even then, only in mild to moderate degree
- There is no evidence that thirst or dry mouth (particularly) improve with artificial hydration
- The extensive experience of nurses working in hospices suggest that systemic fluids at best make no difference and, at worst, may actually contribute to suffering at the end-of-life
- The more fluid available, the more likely it is that it will gather in lungs and dependent parts of the body particularly in the presence of hypoalbuminaemia, which is common in advanced malignancy
- Artificially increasing fluids at the end-of-life, when the body physiology is winding down, may lead to worsening respiratory secretions, increased vomiting, raised intracranial pressure in the presence of intracerebral disease, and an uncomfortable urinary output

- Families can spend precious time worrying about intravenous infusions running out or plastic cannulae being displaced and causing discomfort, instead of concentrating on quality time with the patient

Discussion

Withholding systemic fluids is inevitably a very emotive issue signifying finally and clearly, perhaps for the first time to the family, that their loved one is now entering the final stages of their life. In practice, patients are often able to take small amounts of fluids until shortly before death. It should be explained to families that the body is gradually shutting down and is unable to handle an extra fluid load. They need to be aware that the patient will not be allowed to suffer from pain or other discomfort and they will need explanations of the measures that will be taken to avoid discomfort. These will include medication where necessary and most importantly meticulous mouthcare to prevent the common symptom of a dry mouth.

Palliative care is neither about shortening life nor prolonging the dying period.

Occasionally, families cannot bring themselves to accept the inevitability of death and insist on artificial hydration. Although healthcare professionals must act only in the best interests of the patient, it would be unwise to ignore the views of the family, who have to go on surviving with vivid memories of the dying phase. On occasion, if it is felt that extra fluids will not adversely affect comfort, it is sometimes helpful to have a contract with the family for a relatively small volume of fluid to be used subcutaneously or intravenously for a defined short period, on the understanding that it would be discontinued at any time if it was thought to be causing the patient distress.

As in most ethical crises, a balance has to be made—in this situation, between the harm caused by withholding or giving artificial hydration.

- Acknowledge family distress
- Explore concerns
- Discuss the above points
- Reassure the family that the patient will be looked after and kept comfortable whether fluids are given artificially or not

Example 2: 'How long have I got left?'

Ethical issue

- **Autonomy**: Is every attempt beng made to inform the patient adequately?

This type of question usually relates to prognosis. As ever, however, it is always important to make sure that the question has been entirely understood, since to enter into a conversation about how long a patient has to live when all they want to know is when they are going to leave hospital can cause unnecessary distress.

> Centuries of systematic insensitive deception cannot be instantly remedied by a new routine of systematic insensitive truth telling.
>
> Buckman

When it is certain that the patient is talking about prognosis, first find out what they already know, how they see the situation, why they are asking the question and how much they really want to know.

The following questions can be useful:

- 'What have the doctors told you so far?'
- 'What has prompted you to ask this question now?'
- 'How do *you* see the situation?'
- 'Are there other specific issues, related to how long there is left, on your mind that you would like to talk about?'
- 'Are you the kind of person who likes to know everything?'

In practice, patients often say that they have not been told anything by the doctors: this may be true, or they may have inadvertently used denial mechanisms to 'forget' the bad news. The patient may also deny knowledge in an attempt to find out more information. It is important to explore what they understand accurately thus far. Patients often want to achieve goals such as writing a will, attending a family wedding, reaching a wedding anniversary, being reunited with old friends and family who they have not seen for a long time or seeing their religious adviser. Patients may not find it easy to discuss these issues, with even close family members, and may need help to facilitate discussions. They may need help in setting realistic and achievable goals while planning their limited future.

Before addressing prognosis directly, it is important to be aware of the full medical history and to build up a picture of the pace of clinical deterioration. Questions such as 'I believe you have not been feeling so well recently' or 'the doctors/your medical notes tell me that you feel that life has become more difficult over the past few weeks' open up these issues, giving you and the patient a chance to estimate prognosis. Remember that studies show that health professionals tend to overestimate prognosis.

Background

Literature on determining prognosis is available, especially for patients with cancer. For a population presenting with a defined stage, grade, cancer type and histology, five year survival rates are available and often quoted to families. Many other factors have been studied singly and in combination in an attempt to categorize patients into prognostic groups, and this can be helpful in broad terms. In practice, however, it is not possible to predict prognosis for an individual accurately, because there are so many different influencing factors—including psychosocial, emotional and existential issues—all of which defy measurement of any kind.

- Make sure that you are answering what the patient wants to know
- Stress that you are not evading the question but that is is difficult to answer
- Find out specific issues that should be addressed e.g. weddings, wills etc.
- Do not be specific but use weeks/months, etc.

Despite all these pitfalls, it is still important to answer the patient's question. It is still relatively common for a precise prognosis, for example 'six months', to be given and this is invariably inaccurate. If the patient dies before the due date, the family feel cheated of time that they would otherwise have spent differently had they known that time was so short. If the patient survives longer than the due date, both patient and family may feel proud that they have defeated the odds and take comfort from this; on the other hand, if the family have altered their lifestyles including giving up work (and salary) to look after a patient who has not significantly deteriorated by the due date, family tensions inevitably build up alongside all the normal feelings of guilt and anger.

It is not helpful to give a precise date, which patients and families often take literally, but to talk in terms of days/weeks, weeks/months and months/years. It is also important to say that even within these broad terms we may still be innacurate.

It is also useful to talk about the pace of deterioration and to say that the pace may continue at the same rate but it may also either stabilize for a while or speed up.

Example 3: 'Don't tell my mother the diagnosis. I know her better than you.'

Ethical issues

- **Autonomy**: Does Granny not need to be told regardless of what the family think?
- **Benificence**: Would it help Granny to know her diagnosis?
- **Non-malevolence**: Would it harm Granny to know her diagnosis?

It is common to be caught in the hospital or health practice corridor by anxious relatives who (possibly wrongly) have been told that their relative has cancer, before this information has been given to the patient. There is increasing evidence that patients want to know what is wrong with them and to be involved in decisions. Generally speaking, we have moved away from a paternalistic approach in truth-telling whereby doctors often avoided telling patients they had cancer, to a more open approach, respecting the principle of autonomy.

However, the family have known the patient over many years and are aware of how she has responded to bad news in the past. They may feel that there is no point in discussing the diagnosis, particularly if the patient is very elderly and there is no available treatment.

- For understandable reasons the family want to protect the patient from bad news, but very often they want to protect themselves from further hurt and the reality that the patient may now be entering the last stages of life
- It needs to be acknowledged with the family that this is a difficult area but that the patient may have important things to say or do (financial, wills, gifts etc.) or opinions to voice (regarding both medical and after-death decisions)
- The family also need to know that patients pick up non-verbal clues from professionals and relatives; they are often aware of the diagnosis and are not unduly surprised if it is confirmed
- Patients often want to protect the family, denying that they know anything
- The family need to be aware that patients are often comforted by a 'label' to their illness, even if it is cancer, because it explains why they have been feeling so unwell. This gives them a genuine reason for feeling so wretched
- Families need to know that it becomes more difficult to conceal the truth from the patient as time goes on and as more professionals, family members and friends share the secret. There are increasing opportunities for the truth to slip out and for the patient to lose trust in and be angry with the family for not having been more honest in the first place
- Families also need to know that patients are not always frightened of death but of the process of leading up to it, over which they may want some control
- It is very important not to lie to the patient as this breaks all communication and confidence

- Acknowledge family anxiety
- Inform family of the issues as above
- Stress that it is important for neither professionals nor family to lie if the patient starts asking direct questions

If there are no particular decisions to be made, the patient has dealt with his or her affairs and is living with the family, there may be no pressing need to try to discuss the issue and invite family disquiet. However, if the patient begins to ask direct questions, the family should be advised not to lie. The family also needs to be aware that family tensions reduce considerably when there are open discussions about diagnosis.

The professional is able to override family views if it is clearly in the interests of the patient to do so, but it is also always advisable and prudent to listen to and take account of the views of the family. If it is felt important to discuss the diagnosis, it is usually acceptable to families to say that we will try to find out what the patient understands by their illness and whether or not they would like more information.

Example 4: 'I want full resuscitation if my heart or lungs fail.'[1]

Ethical issues

- **Autonomy**: Does the patient have the right to demand treatments from nursing and medical staff?
- **Beneficence**: Would it be in the patient's best interests to initiate resuscitation?
- **Non-malevolence**: Would it do the patient any harm to initiate resuscitation?
- **Justice**: Would it be an appropriate use of resources to initiate resuscitation measures and appropriate a bed in ITU?

Background

Patients and families are increasingly aware of the many ethical issues surrounding cardiopulmonary resuscitation. These have been highlighted recently with 'DNR' (Do Not Resuscitate) notices being recorded in patients' notes without the patients being aware that they had been thus assigned. This has caused much concern, particularly among the weakest and most vulnerable sections of the community.

The issues have caused marked unease within hospices where, until very recently, resuscitation was regarded as an unacceptable practice. Patients with non-malignant disease and patients with cancer in the early stages, however, are increasingly requiring specialist palliative care. Such patients may feel very strongly that, in the event of a sudden cardiac or respiratory collapse, they want full resuscitation.

Litigation anxiety can cause a dilemma and increase the strain on staff to make the right decision. The need to document the resuscitation status of patients, following full discussion, can of itself lead to increased stress for all involved in handling what can be a very distressing issue.

- **Autonomy**: Patients have the right to ask for whatever treatment they choose. Medical and nursing staff are not obliged to comply with such expressed wishes if:
  - they feel it would not be in the patient's best interests
  - the intervention is deemed to be futile

Good practice would dictate that such matters are addressed by the whole multiprofessional team, though the senior doctor has ultimate responsibility for the decision.[2]

Achievement of success from CPR in any setting:	
In hospital	15%
In community	1–5%
In hospices	1%

1 Willard C. (2000) Cardiopulmonary resuscitation for palliative care patients: a discussion of ethical issues. *Palliat Med* **14**: 308–12.

2 National Council for Hospice and Specialist Palliative Care Services. *Ethical decision-making in palliative care. Cardiopulmonary Resuscitation (CPR) for people who are terminally ill.* London: NCHSPCS.

A king, a doctor, and a convenient death

Lord Dawson of Penn was the most admired and respected doctor of his generation. The skill with which he managed King George V's respiratory illness in 1928 undoubtedly saved the king's life and made Dawson a national celebrity. He was also respected within the medical profession. He was president of the Royal College of Physicians, elected twice president of the BMA, and honoured with a viscountcy.

His reputation would have been considerably diminished, however, had it been known that when the king was suffering from cardiorespiratory failure in January 1936 he administered a lethal combination of morphine and cocaine at a time when the king was already comatose and close to death. His action remained a well kept secret and the truth came to light only 50 years later when his private diary was opened, Dawson having died in 1945.

The king had been in failing health for several weeks when Queen Mary summoned Dawson to Sandringham on 17 January. Contemporary accounts of the king's last days given by the Archbishop of Canterbury and others tell of days that were tranquil and pain free with the king sitting in an armchair before a log fire for much of the time but becoming steadily weaker and with consciousness gradually slipping away.

At 9:25 pm on 20 January Dawson issued the memorable bulletin stating that the king's life was moving peacefully towards its close. The action which he took one and a half hour later is described in his diary thus:

'At about 11 o'clock it was evident that the last stage might endure for many hours, unknown to the patient but little comporting with the dignity and serenity which he so richly merited and which demanded a brief final scene. Hours of waiting just for the mechanical end when all that is really life has departed only exhausts the onlookers and keeps them so strained that they cannot avail themselves of the solace of thought, communion or prayer. I therefore decided to determine the end and injected (myself) morphia gr.3/4 and shortly afterwards cocaine gr. 1 into the distended jugular vein.'

Dawson did not consult the other two doctors in the case, and his diary indicated that he was acting entirely on his own. To her credit, Sister Catherine Black of the London Hospital, who was present and who had nursed the king since the 1928 illness, refused to give the lethal injection, which is why Dawson had to give it himself. Nevertheless, faced with conflicting loyalties, she kept quiet about what had been done and her autobiography published in 1939 made no mention of what must have been the most poignant and unforgettable episode in her long and distinguished career.

The reason for his action, which Dawson frankly admits in his diary, was to ensure that the announcement of the king's death should appear first in the morning edition of the Times and not in some lesser publication later in the day. To make doubly sure that this would happen Dawson telephoned his wife in London asking her to let the Times know when the announcement was imminent.

Nevertheless, it was surely special pleading to claim that he also acted to reduce the strain on the royal family. Apart from the Prince of Wales, who was unhappy at being separated from his mistress Mrs Wallis Simpson, there was no evidence of such strain and in particular, as Dawson noted in his diary, Queen Mary remained calm and kindly throughout. The earlier death suited Dawson. Having issued his famous bulletin he had a vested interest in ensuring that death occurred sooner rather than later. At the same time it allowed him to get back to his busy private practice in London.

1 grain ≡ 65mg

Although Dawson spoke against euthanasia when it was debated in the House of Lords in December 1936, he clearly felt that it or something similar might sometimes be appropriate for his own patients and there is no reason to think that King George V was the only patient he treated in this way. He described his management of the king's final illness as 'a facet of euthanasia or so called mercy killing.' But even the most ardent supporter of euthanasia would hesitate to describe the killing of an unconscious patient, without the patient's prior knowledge or consent, as mercy killing. Indeed, when examined closely this and almost all similar cases turn out in the end to be examples, not of mercy killing but of convenience killing. This was so in this case and the person most convenienced was Dawson.

The ethical line which separates acceptable from unacceptable conduct is sometimes a narrow one. What caused Dawson to stray across the line is a matter of speculation but the likely answer is that he was guilty of the besetting sin of doctors and that is of arrogance. Although in daily contact with the great and good of the land, including the Archbishop of Canterbury who was living at Sandringham at the time, he arrogantly assumed that he, and he alone, had the special insight to appreciate the importance of the timing of the king's death. It was also unfeeling of Dawson to involve Sister Black in his plan and arrogant to assume that her conscience was as elastic as his own.

This whole episode seems a piece of pointless folly which Dawson was wise to conceal at the time. The emergence of the truth 50 years later did nothing to enhance his reputation nor did his half hearted espousal of euthanasia do anything to diminish the opprobrium which rightly attaches to doctors who break the sixth commandment.

J H R Ramsay

BMJ (1994); **308**: 1445, permission from the BMJ Publishing Group.

Consent and competence

A patient is able to give *valid consent* to a procedure if he is *informed, uncoerced,* and *competent*.

'Informed' means that a patient has all the relevant information, given in an appropriate form, with which to make a decision.

'Uncoerced' means that the person is free to make decisions without any undue influence or pressure from any other person.

'Competence' (the medical term) or 'capacity' (the legal term) may conveniently be considered in five sections:
1 The patient must be able to understand the issue in question
2 The patient needs to be able to retain the information in memory for long enough to use it in making a decision
3 The patient needs to be able to *believe* the information given
4 The patient needs to be able to weigh the information in the balance and aggregate arguments for and against in order to reach a decision
5 The patient must be able to express the decision in some form

If a patient is not competent to be involved in discussions regarding medical care, in England a medical decision should be taken in the 'best interests' of the patient. It is best practice for the multidisciplinary team and the family to be involved in these discussions. The family cannot make decisions for incompetent patients but, where possible, they should be consulted to find out what the patient would have wanted. It often focuses the minds of a distressed family to ask questions such as 'What do you think your mother would want, given this situation?'

Points to :
- It is perfectly in order to provide all measures to enhance competence by managing the environment e.g. optimize the senses (glasses/hearing aids), comfortable familiar environment with good lighting and heating, and bringing an advocate to the meeting, writing materials, interpreter etc.
- Patients are entitled to make seemingly illogical decisions provided they are made with competence
- Patients may be competent even if they are mentally ill
- Patients may have lucid intervals

Specific situations

In palliative medicine we may be asked to assess competence in order that a patient can, for instance, make a will, change a codicil to a will, execute an Enduring Power of Attorney or write an Advance Directive. All the above points apply.

Making a will

Clinical staff are generally advised not to witness the signing of a will for fear of legal complications. In palliative care, however, we are endeavouring to support patients and their families through a very difficult time and it may be helpful for us to assist. In this situation, a senior doctor, if witnessing a signature, would be advised to do this only if they have assessed competency. The competency then needs to be documented.

Enduring Power of Attorney

As above, doctors witnessing the signing of these documents should ensure and document that the patient is fully competent. (📖 See also Chapter 16.)

Advance Directives (Living Wills)

Again, doctors need to assess and document competency. (📖 See also Chapter 16.)

Euthanasia

He jests at scars, that never felt a wound.

Shakespeare, *Romeo and Juliet*

Etymologically, the term euthanasia derives from the ancient Greek, '*Eu*', meaning good and '*thanatos*', meaning death, thus a 'good death'. Today, the term euthanasia refers to the administration of death, the active intentional ending of life. It is a final and irreversible step and the subject of great debate, engendering on one hand strong feelings about the right to demand death and, on the other, strong feelings that life is so precious that we have a duty to preserve it at all costs. It must not be forgotten that patients are often making decisions regarding euthanasia on the basis of inadequate prognostic information, since medical advances will never be able to identify accurately when an individual patient will die naturally.

Proponents of euthanasia feel that

Euthanasia is the only alternative to avoiding a painful death

Comment: Although the control of pain is not perfect, patients can usually achieve a degree of relief acceptable to them. Public education has started to erode the myth that all patients with cancer inevitably die in considerable pain, although this fear is still held strongly by some.

In practice, even patients with distressing symptoms and an apparent high level of suffering rarely request euthanasia consistently.

Euthanasia is the only answer to the fear of being kept alive at all costs

Comment: Extraordinary advances in medicine over the last few centuries have pushed forward the frontiers, extending the quantity of life and potentially, therefore, the extension of an 'unacceptable' poor quality of life. Medical ethics, however, has also advanced, allowing competent patients to refuse treatment and supporting the concept that burdensome, futile treatment is bad medicine. Assuming that healthcare professionals act with multidisciplinary support within an ethical framework, the fear of being kept alive at all costs should be minimized.

Euthanasia is the only way to die with dignity

Comment: Families are torn between not wanting to see their loved ones deteriorate and wanting them to survive as long as possible to nurture precious time. A natural death and all the potential healing and strengthening of family unity that so often occurs during the final days is often worthwhile and dignified, a sentiment supported by most healthcare professionals experienced in the care of the dying. Furthermore, the efficacy of drugs used to carry out euthanasia is unpredictable. There are literature reports of failure to achieve coma and patients reawakening in considerable discomfort, which can hardly be described as dignified.

Euthanasia should be legalized to uphold the principle of autonomy

Comment: In the West, individual rights have been elevated to a central tenet of society, implying that the individual has the right to control their own destiny. In society, however, others also have rights and the concept of a healthcare professional delivering euthanasia as a technical act may not be in the best interests of individuals or society.

Euthanasia, if carried out, should rightly occur only when the patient is fully competent and consistently requests it. However, patients who are ill, often bed-bound, unable to care for themselves and wholly reliant on others for care may feel a burden and under pressure to acquiesce.

A diagnosis of a reversible clinical depression may be missed if families and healthcare professionals are slow to recognize it. The concept of the 'slippery slope' argument, in which patients may be subjected to euthanasia without their expressed consent and within a short time of having had the discussions, has already been reported in the literature.

Whatever the arguments, the fundamental principles are that life is infinitely precious and that the vulnerable deserve protection. We should always consider the views of our competent patients and act in the best interests of those who are not able to give consent.

It is also fundamentally important to recognize what is *not* euthanasia, which includes the following, where the primary intention is to prevent suffering.

Euthanasia is not
- Witholding or withdrawing futile, burdensome treatment including nutrition and hydration if the patient is dying and is unable to swallow
- Giving opioids, or any other medications, to control symptoms including pain, fear, and overwhelming distress
- Sedating a patient in the terminal stages if all other practical methods of controlling symptoms have failed
- Issuing a *Do Not Resuscitate* order

The Royal Dutch Medical Association has formulated five requirements that must be fulfilled for euthanasia to be acceptable or legally excusable. These are:
1 There is voluntary, competent and durable request on the part of the patient
2 The request is based on full information
3 The patient is in a situation of intolerable and hopeless suffering (physical or mental)
4 There are no acceptable alternatives
5 The physician has consulted another physician before performing euthanasia

The physician has to notify the local medical examiner and complete an extensive questionnaire. It is then reported to the public prosecutor who decides if prosecution is necessary. This notification procedure has formal legal status and also covers cases involving euthanasia without the patient's explicit request.

In some States in the USA, physicians are allowed to prescribe medication to hasten death in terminally ill adults.

A Time to Go

Doctor you must help me,
And there's something you must know,
My mind's made up I'm certain,
It's time for me to go.

I'm old and tired and weary,
I've lived a life first rate,
But there's just no denying,
I'm well past my sell-by date.
Just give me the tablet,
Just send me off to sleep
For I don't want to go on living
And I want to 'shut-eye' for keeps.

Now Doctor I've been thinking,
How I'd like it all to be.
Vivaldi in the background
Test Match special on TV.
With the smell of cut grass wafting
And a cup of Earl Grey tea,
Doctor you've got to help,
You've got to help poor me.

Now Doctor please, please listen.
I know you think euthanasia's wrong,
But just between ourselves
How d'you expect me to carry on?
My bridge partners just left me.
My son's off in Ceylon,
English cricket's just appalling
And my get up and go has gone.
To crown it all last Thursday,
A lady from meals on wheels,
Came offering gammon and pineapple,
I mean Doc, how would *you* feel?

So pronto I called my GP
Something must be done no doubt
And I was sent to Hospice,
As he said 'To get sorted out'.

So Doctor I am waiting
I don't want this to drag on and on
I've made up my will, killed the cat,
And my mind is set upon,
A peaceful departure from this long dark vale of tears
And just in case you'll ask me,
I've no doubts, no bills, no fears.

Doctor you've got to help me.
Last night I couldn't sleep.
There was such an infernal racket
And I thought I heard someone weep.

And then again this morning,
That nice woman in number nine?
She wasn't there to talk to
About her illness which was a bit like mine.
I glimpsed a hearse pass by the window
Please tell me it's not true
Are people here really dying?
O what am I to do?

Doctor you've got to help me
I've got to get out of here.
Though you're all most pleasant
This is just not for me I fear.
My pains have eased
My mind is clear
Doctor,
Why on earth are you keeping me here?

Doctor you must help me,
And there's something you must know
My mind's made up I'm certain
It's time for me to go.

M. Watson
2002

Chapter 2

Breaking bad news

I have received two wonderful graces. First, I have been given time to prepare for a new future. Secondly, I find myself—uncharacteristically—calm and at peace.

Cardinal Basil Hume, breaking the news of his imminent death from cancer to the priests of Westminster diocese, 16 April 1999

Patients and relatives need time to absorb information and to adapt to bad news. Health professionals need good communication skills, including sensitivity and empathic active listening.

Breaking bad news takes time, and issues often need to be discussed further and clarified as more information is imparted.

There is increasing evidence that most patients want to know about their illness. Many patients who have been denied this knowledge have difficulty in understanding why they are becoming weaker and are then relieved and grateful to be told the truth. They may be angry with the family who have known about the illness all along and have not thought it right to tell them.

Professionals often become involved unwittingly in a potential conspiracy of silence when the family demand information before the patient has been appraised of the situation. The family might say, 'Do not tell him the diagnosis/prognosis because he will not be able to cope with it. We know him better than you do.' The family needs to know that their concerns, of not wanting to cause any more hurt to the patient, have been heard. They also need to be aware that the bad news may be more painful for themselves than for the patient. The family also need to know that it would be unwise for clinical staff to be untruthful if the patient appeared to want to know the truth and was asking direct questions, because of the inevitable breakdown in trust that this could cause.

Advising patients and families with regard to prognosis is important since they may want (and often need) to organize their affairs and plan for the time that is left. However, it is *not possible to be accurate with prognosis*. Overestimating or underestimating the time that someone has to live can cause untold anguish. It is therefore more sensible to talk in terms of days/weeks, weeks/months, and months/years as appropriate.

There is a balance to be made between fully informing the patient about their disease and prognosis, completely overwhelming them with facts and figures, or providing only minimal and inadequate information.

While it is important to avoid being patronizing, it is also important not to cause distress by 'information overload'.

It is important to be aware that people have divergent attitudes to receiving bad news and that this needs sensitive handling. Patients and families respond badly to being told bad news in a hurried, brusque and unsympathetic manner with no time to collect their thoughts and ask questions. However sensitively bad news is imparted, patients and families are naturally devastated and the impact of the news can obliterate a great deal of the communication that took place. Patients may either not remember or misinterpret what has been said, particularly if they use denial as a coping technique.

A strategy for breaking bad news

> Nothing in all the world is more dangerous than sincere ignorance and conscientious stupidity.
>
> Martin Luther King 1929–68: *Strength to love (1963)*

Outlining a strategy for breaking bad news is difficult because it turns a process which should be natural and unforced into something which seems constrained and awkward. The following advice encompasses the techniques that health professionals have found, through trial and error, to be helpful. It can be used as a guide to develop an individual's personal confidence and skills in breaking bad news.

The goals of breaking bad news

The process of breaking bad news needs to be specifically tailored to the needs of the individual concerned, for every human being will have a different history and collection of fears and concerns. The goal of breaking bad news is to do so in a way that facilitates acceptance and understanding and reduces the risk of destructive responses.

The ability to break bad news well involves skills which need to be coveted and trained for, audited and kept up to date with as much objective determination as that shown by a surgeon in acquiring and maintaining surgical skills. The consequences of performing the process badly may have immediate and long term damaging effects for all involved, every bit as catastrophic as surgery going wrong. For example, patients and families may lose trust. Having awareness of strategies to complete the process well is vital, but breaking bad news must never become so routinized that patients, or their families, detect little individual caring compassion.

Break bad news well and you will always be remembered, break bad news badly and you will never be forgotten.

Preparing to tell bad news

Acquire all the information possible about the patient and their family. (A genogram is particularly useful in quickly assimilating the important people in the patient's life, and the web of relationships within the family.)

Read the patient's notes for

- Diagnostic information
- Test results
- Understanding of the patient's clinical history
- The support system for the individual
- Background knowledge of the patient's life—making basic mistakes will undermine the patient's confidence)
- Understanding of spoken language, e.g. English. If not, arrange for an interpreter to be present

Discuss with other members of the team, and then select the most appropriate team member to break the bad news. Decide which other member of the team should be present during the interview. Ensure there is an interpreter or advocate present for those with special needs or language difficulties.

Check that you have
- A place of privacy where there will be no interruptions. Unplug the telephone and switch off the mobile phone etc.
- Tissues, a jug of water, and drinking glasses
- Time to carry out the process
- Your own emotional energy to do so—this job is better done earlier in the day than late
- Pressing tasks are completed so that there will be minimal interruptions

Plan
Prepare a rough plan in your mind of what you want to achieve in the communication, and what you want to avoid communicating. Having a rough goal will bring structure to the communication, though it is important to avoid imposing your agenda on the patient's agenda.

Setting the context
- Invite the patient to the place of privacy
- Introduce yourself clearly
- Let the patient know that they have your attention and how long you have got
- Ensure that the patient is comfortable and not distracted by pain or a full bladder etc.
- Give a 'warning shot' indication that this is not a social or routine encounter
- Sit at the same eye level as each other within easy reach

A *warning shot* is concerned with preparing a patient that bad news is coming. This allows them to be more receptive than if it comes 'out of the blue'. An example would be, 'I'm sorry to say that the results were not as good as we had hoped.'

Assess
- How much the patient knows already
- How much the patient wants to know
- How the patient expresses him/herself and what words and ways he/she uses to understand the situation

'Are you the sort of person that likes to know everything?'

Acquire empathy with the patient
- What would it be like to be the patient?
- How is the patient feeling?
- Is there anything that is concerning the patient which he or she is not verbalizing?
- What mechanisms has the patient used in the past to deal with bad news?
- Does the patient have a particular outlook on life or cultural understanding which underpins his or her approach to dealing with the situation?

- Who are the important people in the patient's life?
  Respond to *non-verbal* as well as *verbal* clues

Encourage the patient to speak by listening carefully and responding appropriately.

Sharing information

- Having spent time listening, use the patient's words to recap the story of the journey so far, checking regularly with the patient that you have heard the story correctly

> 'Would you mind if I repeated back to you what I have heard you tell me to make sure I have understood things correctly?'

- Slowly and gradually draw out the information from the patient while regularly checking that they are not misunderstanding what you are saying
- Use the 'warning shot' technique to preface bad news to help the patient prepare themself
- Use diagrams to help understanding and retention of information if appropriate and acceptable to the patient
- Avoid jargon and acronyms which are easily misunderstood
- Do not bluff. It is acceptable to say 'I do not know, and I will try to get an answer for you for our next meeting'

Remember to ensure that

- The patient understands the implications of what you are saying
- The patient is in control of the speed at which information is being imparted
- The patient can see that you are being empathic to their emotional response. It can be very appropriate to say something like 'Being told something like this can seem overwhelming'
- You address the patient's real concerns, which may be very different from what you expect them to be
- You offer a record of the consultation, for example a tape recording or short written notes if appropriate

Response

- You should respond to the patient's feelings and response to the news
- You should acknowledge the patient's feelings
- You should be prepared to work through the patient's emotional response to the bad news with them

> 'It can be very distressing to get such news, and it is not unusual to feel very angry, or lonely or sad on hearing such news.'

Let the patient speak first

Use open questions, such as:-
'How are you feeling today?'
'Can you tell me how this all came about?'
'How do you see things going from here?'

Make concrete plans for the next step

'Your appointment to see Dr. Brown the oncologist is provisionally booked for next Thursday at 2 o'clock. How would that fit in with your other arrangements?'

Immediate plans
'What are you doing now?' 'How are you getting home?' 'Who will you tell?' 'How will you tell them?' 'What will you say?' 'How will they cope?'
   Such questions can help the patient to start formulating the answers that they will need for their family or friends.

Summarize
For the patient
● Try to get the patient to repeat the key points to ensure they have understood

For other healthcare professionals
● Record details of the conversation in the patient's notes clearly
● Convey information quickly to those who need to know, most importantly the GP

Deception is not as creative as truth. We do best in life if we look at it with clear eyes, and I think that applies to coming up to death as well.

Cicely Saunders, in *Time* 5 September 1988

Deal with questions
● 'Are there any questions which you would like me to deal with at this point?'

Contract for the future

'I know the news today was not what you were hoping for but you are not going to go through this on your own. We are there for you, your family is there for you and we are going to go through this together. Dr. Brown will be seeing you next Thursday and I'll see you back here on Monday morning.'

● Closing remarks should identify support networks, including contact telephone numbers and times of easy access. Be fairly concrete about the next meeting but also allow the patient the option to postpone if they do not feel able to attend

10 Steps to breaking bad news (Adapted from Peter Kaye, 1996)

1 Preparation
Know all the facts before the meeting. READ THE MEDICAL RECORDS. Find out who the patient wants to be present. Ensure comfort and privacy. Minimize the risk of interruptions.

2 What does the patient know?
Ask the patient for a brief narrative of events (e.g. 'how did it all start?').

3 Give a warning shot
e.g. 'I am afraid it looks rather serious'—then allow a pause for the patient to respond.

4 Allow denial
Allow the patient to control the amount of information and to proceed at his/her own pace.

5 Explain (if requested) and check understanding
Narrow the information gap step-by-step. Use diagrams if the patient thinks it would be helpful. Use simple language.

6 Is more information wanted?
It can be very frightening to ask for more information and the patient may not want to know any more. Inquire gently, by asking if they would like further information.

7 Listen to concerns
Ask, 'what are the things that bother you most at the moment?'. This could be to do with their physical or emotional health or relate to social or spiritual issues.

8 Encourage ventilation of feelings
This conveys empathy and may be the key phase in terms of patient satisfaction with the interview. Check that there is nothing else that the patient wants to talk about.

9 Summary and plan
Summarize concerns, plan treatment, and foster hope. Check with the patient that he/she would have no objection to your talking with the family either alone or together.

10 Offer availability
Most patients need further explanation (the details will not have been remembered) and support (adjustment takes weeks or months), and benefit greatly from a family meeting.

Further reading

Books

Bacon F. (1912) *Of Death*. In *Essays*, London: Black.

Heaven C. and Maguire P. (2003) Communication issues. In M. Lloyd Williams (ed.) *Psychosocial Issues in Palliative Care*. pp. 13–34. Oxford: Oxford University Press.

Kaye P. (1996) *Breaking bad news. A 10 step approach*. Northampton: EPL Publications.

Wilkes E. (1982) *The Dying Patient: The medical management of incurable and terminal illness*. Lancaster: MTP Press.

Worden J. W. (2002) *Grief Counseling and Grief Therapy*, 3rd edn. London: Routledge.

Reviews

Saunderson E. M., Ridsdale L. (1999) General Practitioners' beliefs and attitudes about how to respond to death and bereavement: qualitative study. *BMJ*, **319**: 293–6.

Articles

Charlton R. and Dolamn E. (1995) Bereavement: a protocol for primary care. *British Journal of General Practice*, **45**: 427–30.

Jewell D. (1999) Commentary: Use of personal experience should be legitimized. *BMJ*, **319**: 296.

Raphael B. (1977) Preventive intervention with the recently bereaved. *Archives of General Psychiatry*, **34**: 1450–4.

Chapter 3

Research in palliative care

In the culture I grew up in you did your work and you did not put your arm around it to stop people from looking—you took the earliest opportunity to make knowledge available.

James Black, On modern medical research, *Daily Telegraph*, 11 December 1995

Good medical practice requires evidence of effectiveness to address deficits in care, strive for further improvements, and justly apportion finite resources.

The Declaration of Helsinki was drawn up by the World Medical Association in 1964 in response to the need for a code of ethics on human experimentation. This is particularly pertinent in the field of palliative care, where the core practice is looking after the dying. It acknowledges the need for guidance for the physician caught in the conflict between patients' own best interests and the necessity to advance knowledge for society as a whole. Research must conform to strict ethical principles and be scrutinized by independent assessors.

The origins of palliative care research in the modern UK Hospice movement date from the founding of St Christopher's Hospice in 1967. Dame Cicely Saunders advocated scientific observation and systematic research as an essential component of the specialty. The burgeoning interest in the provision of palliative care services and the national agenda for practising evidence-based care has stimulated the development of collaborative, often multidisciplinary, research committees between clinical units and academic institutions.

The Palliative Care Research Forum of Britain and Ireland developed in 1991; the science committee for the Association for Palliative Medicine and the Palliative Care Forum of the Royal Society of Medicine were created in 1996 and 1997 respectively. On a local palliative care network level, there are numerous research committees which are either self standing or have grouped in response to the initiatives of the Supportive and Palliative care remit of the National Cancer Plan. The importance and principle of research is now inherent in specialist training.

Palliative care research largely encompasses: the control of symptoms, ethical issues, clinical decision making, communication, family and carer issues, interdisciplinary team issues, health systems and services and existential and spiritual concerns both before and after death.

Evidence-based medicine

Evidence-based practice is the conscious, explicit and judicious use of current best evidence in making decisions about the care of individual patients.

The gold standard of evidence for the harm or efficiency of an intervention is the randomized controlled trial (RCT), though RCTs are not the only method of such assessment. There are many factors apart from the results of RCTs which must be accorded due weight in decisions affecting the care of patients. The key element of evidence-based medicine is to integrate the best available evidence with patient preference. The nature of palliative care lends itself more readily to investigation by those methods which are considered by some to hold less weight such as the descriptive study. An overview of quantitative and qualitative research methodology and the difficulties encountered in palliative care research will be outlined.

Table 3.1 The five strengths of research evidence

Type	Strength of evidence
I	Strong evidence from at least one systematic review of multiple well-designed randomized controlled trials
II	Strong evidence from at least one properly designed randomized controlled trial of appropriate size
III	Evidence for well designed trials without randomization, single group pre-post, cohort, time series or matched case-control studies
IV	Evidence from well-designed non-experimental studies from more than one centre or research group
V	Opinions of respected authorities, based on clinical evidence, descriptive studies or reports of expert committees

The Agency for Health Care Policy and Research (AHCPR) 1997

Quantitative methodology

The biomedical model of scientific research aims to define objective reality which can be discovered, measured and understood through scientific method. Rigorous, systematic examination allows the identification and assessment of the probability of causal relationships between variables through statistical analysis. Quantitative researchers are rigid in adhering to the original focus of the research question and maintain an objective distance from the research itself. Quantitative research is *deductive* and based on questions/hypotheses of existing theory and knowledge. Examples of quantitative designed research include RCTs, experiments and surveys on representative samples.

Arguments against over reliance on quantitative trials in palliative care include the following:

1 Quantitative trials should not be considered as the only method of assessing scientific validity.
2 Quantitative trials do not lend themselves to issues such as quality of life, emotional distress, and other domains of the patient's experience.
3 It would be impractical and unethical to engender doubt on the efficacy of almost all already widely-used treatments in palliative care solely on the basis that they had not been submitted to quantitative trials.
4 It is almost impossible to isolate a single variable and watch the effect of it changing, particularly in the frail, elderly, clinically deteriorating and dying. A variety of methods is needed to assess the usefulness of interventions.
5 It is frequently not possible to recruit the number of patients that are required for statistical significance to a quantitative trial.
6 Quantitative research, while extremely important, is not suited to answering all types of research question, particularly those relating to patient experience.
7 It could be considered as unethical to subject patients to a trial with a placebo arm—i.e. a trial arm with no active treatment—especially in dying patients.

In order to encompass these difficulties in palliative care, research methods other than purely quantitative must be used.

Systematic reviews

These aim to locate and appraise research evidence to provide informative empirical answers to scientific research questions. They adhere to strict scientific design to make them more comprehensive, to minimize bias and to ensure reliability. The protocol defines a clear question and the methodology is explicit. Research from all sources is obtained and this may involve the use of electronic databases as well as personal searches according to a pre-defined protocol. Systematic reviews can be regarded as reliable summaries of research evidence.

Qualitative research

> He uses statistics as a drunken man uses lampposts—for support rather than for illumination
>
> Andrew Lang, 1844–1912, attributed

'Quantitative' research uses often uncritically respected, 'tried and tested' techniques of measurement, data collection and analysis. 'Qualitative' research techniques, which are often more suited to palliative care, incorporate the subjective experience, which cannot be measured so easily within a mathematical framework. Evidence from qualitative research studies has not been bestowed with the weight of evidence attributed to quantitative research, although the techniques are rigorous and are gradually becoming more accepted. Qualitative research can be extremely demanding if carried out well, with major time and cost implications, especially for the process of analysis. Specific aims (generic goals) and objectives (specific ends or outcomes) and precision and clarity are important whether or not the methodology, data collection and analysis is qualitative or quantitative.

Qualitative research takes account of ways in which the research subject makes sense of their individual experience. There is interaction between the researcher and the subject. Ideas and concepts develop as the research progresses and these may then be redirected back to further inform the research findings. Words are used as opposed to numerical data. The method is *inductive*, to discover new knowledge and to ground it in the subjective experience. Qualitative research has the power to disrupt existing assumptions and to challenge what has been considered as reliable, factual material. It also lends itself to the imaginative expression of language, making research findings more widely interesting and relevant to those accustomed to the more precise biomedical model of research reporting.

Qualitative and quantitative research methods can be combined to offer a different perspective and to enhance knowledge in a more holistic way.

A range of techniques, guided by set principles, exist. Examples of such techniques include:

1 Observation—Researchers are involved in a field work setting within, for instance a ward, recording conversations, encounters, non-verbal communication, spatial arrangements and physical environment. Aspects such as the quality of care of patients can be explored in this way.

2 Participant observation—Researchers become an active subject within the study group. For instance, they may join in with practical tasks in a ward or day hospice setting with the sole purpose of observing and not influencing.

3 Interviews—This is the most widely adopted method within qualitative research. Interviews may be interactive, with opportunities to develop or deepen the discussion according to the subject in question. Bereavement issues may usefully be conducted in this way.

4 Focus groups—Group interviews have the capacity to generate large amounts of data. Tape-recorded transcripts may be analysed. A number of computer packages exist to sort and code items for analysis, which facilitates the handling of large volumes of data. The researcher acts as the facilitator, usually for a group of about eight people. Ideas and experiences can be explored. For instance, a multidisciplinary group of healthcare professionals might explore issues surrounding the attitudes to such issues as organ donation at the end-of-life.

5 Documentary analysis.

6 Case studies—Case studies serve to structure research problems and can involve observation, interviewing and the analysis of documentary sources. Detailed explanation of a single case can accrue data from a variety of perspectives, using different qualitative methods to focus on a common issue or research question. The particular case can then be understood in its wider context. For instance, a case study of a single hospice might look at defined aspects of care and how they interrelate across different care settings to provide consistent, holistic care for patients.

Quantitative and Qualitative Research Differences

QUANTITATIVE RESEARCH	QUALITATIVE RESEARCH
Tests theories	Develops theories
Rigid methods	Flexible methods
Experiments	In depth interviews
Surveys	Observation
Large samples	Small samples
Numbers	Words
Statistics	Meaning

Argument for palliative care research

Basic research is what I am doing when I don't know what I am doing.
Wernher von Braun, A Random Walk in Silence, 1973

Research is an unavoidable imperative if progress is to be made.
- The terminally ill should not be considered as 'special' and shielded from studies (although there should be stringent criteria for the research design and ethical scrutiny)
- Patients receive considerable attention which they may appreciate
- A new treatment might benefit the patient
- Autonomy—patients should be given the chance to be involved in studies
- Patients and families often genuinely want to 'give' in order that others can get better care

Difficulties in palliative care research

Practical considerations

- Attrition of patients from studies leading to difficulties in recruiting adequate numbers of patients, particularly to quantitative studies
- Eligibility criteria for inclusion into studies, particularly if the patient is deteriorating, restricts the inclusion of adequate numbers
- Measures of end points and outcomes are often complicated in an already complex clinical scenario
- Funding has been limited
- Compliance of deteriorating patients may be difficult to sustain

Ethical and emotional considerations

- Patients are often considered too unwell, with distressing symptoms, to be asked to partake in research
- Some professionals feel that patients with a short prognosis should not have extra burdens placed on them
- Patients are vulnerable and may be exploited
- The research may be of no benefit to the patient taking part
- Questionnaires if used may be painful and intrusive either for patients, families or in bereavement
- Fully informed consent may be difficult to obtain; patients may try to please researchers by agreeing to take part without really wanting to; some patients feel that they may be punished or ignored if they do not take part; acute symptoms do not allow for adequate time for patients to decide whether or not they want to be involved; patients are not infrequently cognitively impaired
- Trying a new treatment may engender false hope
- Research may encourage the patient to focus on their illness instead of enjoying precious time
- Information given by the patient's proxy may be misleading

There is limited evidence based in the delivery of palliative care, thus potentially exposing patients to toxic treatment of unknown benefit. We have an ethical imperative to provide the best care for our patients. Although research in palliative care is fraught with practical, ethical and emotional issues, we can only improve care by carrying out studies; these must be carefully designed to be of minimal burden and to provide maximum use of precious research opportunities.

Despite the difficulties, an evidence base is forming in such areas as ethical issues, control of symptoms, palliative rehabilitation, clinical decision-making, communication, family and caregiving issues, interdisciplinary team working, health systems and existential and spiritual issues.

Provided that palliative care investigators compassionately apply ethical principles to their research, there is no justification for not endeavouring to improve the standards of palliation.

Further reading

Dollery C. T. (1979) A bleak outlook for placebos (and for science). *European Journal of Clinical Pharmacology*, **15**: 219–21.

Greenhalgh T. and Donald A. (2000) Evidence based healthcare workbook: understanding research: for individual and group learning. London: BMJ Books.

Jones B., Jarvis P. Trials to assess equivalence: the importance of rigorous methods. *BMJ*, **313**: 36–9.

Rothman K. J. and Michels K. B. (1994) Sounding board: the continuing unethical use of placebo controls. *NEJM*, **331**: 394–8.

Further reading

Principles of drug use in palliative medicine[1]

> We can no more hope to end drug abuse by eliminating heroin and cocaine than we could alter the suicide rate by outlawing high buildings or the sale of rope.
>
> Ben Whittaker, *The global fix*, 1987

Drugs are not the total answer for the relief of pain and other symptoms. For many symptoms, the concurrent use of non-drug measures is equally important, and sometimes more so. Further, drugs must always be used within the context of a systematic approach to symptom management, namely:

- evaluation
- explanation
- individualized treatment
- attention to detail

In palliative care, the axiom 'diagnosis before treatment' still holds true. Even when the cancer is responsible, a particular symptom may have different causes, e.g. in lung cancer vomiting may be caused by hypercalcaemia or by raised intracranial pressure—to name but two out of many possible causes. Clearly, treatment will vary according to the cause.

Attention to detail includes *precision in taking a drug history*. It is important to ascertain, as precisely as possible, the drug being taken, the dose and the frequency and to confirm that the drug alleviates the symptom throughout the day and night. It is very common for patients to be non-compliant with medication for many different reasons. In palliative care, patients may not have understood the reason for taking medication regularly to prevent symptoms. The medication consequently may not help adequately, leaving him/her either to suffer in pain, thinking that the drug does not work, or to take inappropriately large extra doses which cause side-effects. Patients may also stop taking the drugs because of the side-effects. Vicious circles may develop, adding to patient and family despair. As the patient becomes weaker and less well they may become less able to swallow large numbers of tablets, leading again to less than optimal symptom control.

Attention to detail also means *providing clear instructions for drug regimens*. 'Take as much as you like, as often as you like', is a recipe for anxiety and poor symptom relief. The drug regimen should be written out in full for the patient and his family to work from (Figure 4.1). This should be in an ordered and logical way, e.g. analgesics, antiemetics, laxatives, followed by other drugs. The drug name, times to be taken, reason for use ('for pain', 'for bowels' etc.) and dose (x ml, y tablets) should all be stated. The patient should also be advised how to obtain further supplies e.g. from the General Practitioner.

[1] General guidance about the use of drugs in palliative care (www.palliativedrugs.com).

When prescribing an additional drug, it is important to ask:
- What is the treatment goal?
- How can it be monitored?
- What is the risk of adverse effects?
- What is the risk of drug interactions?
- Is it possible to stop any of the current medications?

Good prescribing is a skill, and makes the difference between poor and excellent symptom control. It extends to considering size, shape and taste of tablets and solutions; and avoiding awkward doses which force:
- patients to take more tablets than would be the case if doses were 'rounded up' to a more convenient tablet size. For example, it is better to prescribe m/r morphine 60mg (a single tablet) rather than 50mg (3 tablets: 30mg + 10mg + 10mg)
- nurses to spend more time refilling syringes for 24h infusions. For example, in the UK, it might be appropriate to prescribe diamorphine 100mg (a single ampoule) instead of 95mg (60mg ampoule + 30mg ampoule + 5mg ampoule)

It is necessary to be equally thorough when re-evaluating a patient and supervising treatment, because it is often difficult to predict the optimum dose of a symptom relief drug, particularly opioids, laxatives and psychotropic drugs. Some drugs, e.g. steroids, may be given as a trial only and continued or stopped as appropriate after a certain time. Arrangements must be made, therefore, for continuing supervision and adjustment of medication.

Finally, it may be necessary to compromise on complete symptom relief in order to avoid unacceptable adverse effects. For example, the sedative side-effects of levomepromazine or the dry mouth caused by octreotide may limit dose escalation in inoperable bowel obstruction. The patient may prefer to reduce the frequency of nausea or vomiting to an acceptable level (i.e. vomit once a day) rather than to tolerate side-effects of higher doses of effective medication.

The drugs mentioned in this text are listed alphabetically in the formulary and are based on as robust evidence as is currently available. Many of these drugs are used outside their current product licences.

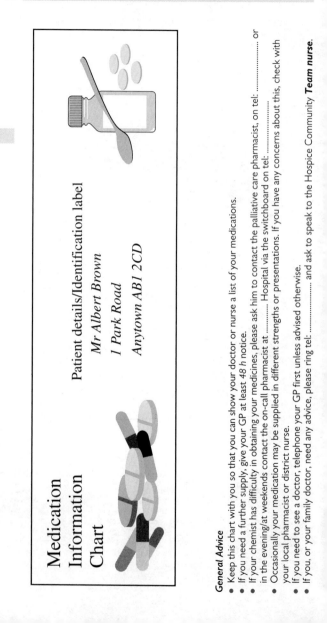

Medication
Information
Chart

Patient details/Identification label

Mr Albert Brown
1 Park Road
Anytown AB1 2CD

General Advice

- Keep this chart with you so that you can show your doctor or nurse a list of your medications.
- If you need a further supply, give your GP at least *48 h* notice.
- If your chemist has difficulty in obtaining your medicines, please ask him to contact the palliative care pharmacist, on tel: .... or in the evening/at weekends contact the on-call pharmacist at .... Hospital via the switchboard on tel: ....
- Occasionally your medication may be supplied in different strengths or presentations. If you have any concerns about this, check with your local pharmacist or district nurse.
- If you need to see a doctor, telephone your GP first unless advised otherwise.
- If you, or your family doctor, need any advice, please ring tel: .... and ask to speak to the Hospice Community *Team nurse.*

Regular Medication	STRENGTH	REASON	WHEN TO TAKE				
Description (Trade Name)			ON WAKING	LUNCH 2pm	TEA 6pm	BED TIME	
Morphine Sulphate MR (MST) Purple tablet	30mg	Pain Relief * take 12 h apart *	1			1	
Diclofenac Round brown tablet	50mg	Bone Pain	1		1	1	
Sodium Valproate (Epilim) Lilac tablet	200mg	Nerve Pain				2	
Codanthramer Orange liquid	Strong	For Bowels			TWO 5ml spoons		
Domperidone (Motilium) Small white tablet	10mg	Stop Sickness	2	2	2	2	
As Needed							
Morphine Solution (Oramorph) Clear liquid	10mg in 5ml	Breakthrough Pain	Take ONE 5ml spoon every 2–4 h if needed				
Asilone suspension White liquid		Indigestion	Take TWO 5ml spoonfuls QDS/PRN times a day				

Completed by: _S Thorp_   Nurse/Pharmacist   Checked by _M Smith_   On: _24.2.05_

Fig. 4.1 Sample Medication Information Chart. Adapted with permission from HAYWARD HOUSE Macmillan Specialist Palliative Care Unit, City Hospital NHS Trust Nottingham.

The use of drugs beyond licence

If a lot of cures are suggested for a disease, it means that the disease is incurable.
Anton Chekov, *The cherry orchard*, 1904

The Medicines and Healthcare Products regulatory Agency in the UK grants a product licence for a medical drug. The purpose of the drug licence is to regulate the activity of the pharmaceutical company when marketing the drug. The licence does not restrict the prescription of the drug by properly qualified medical practitioners. Licenced drugs can be used legally in clinical situations that fall outside the remit of the licence (referred to as 'off-label'), for example a different age group, a different indication, a different dose or route or method of administration. Use of unlicenced drugs refers to those products that have no licence for any clinical situation or may be in the process of evaluation leading to such a licence.

A recent audit in palliative care found that 'off-label' use is common (around 25 per cent of prescriptions affecting 66 per cent of patients in one specialist palliative care unit), but the use of unlicenced drugs is rare. Recommendations from bodies such as the General Medical Council and the medical defence organizations place a duty on doctors to act responsibly and to provide information to patients on the nature and associated risks of any treatment, including 'off-label' and unlicenced drugs.

Guidance also recommends that such drugs are prescribed by a consultant or GP, following informed consent by the patient, and that this decision is recorded in the patient's notes. This may not be practical in palliative care where the use of 'off-label' medication is routine.

Prescribing outside the licence

In the UK, a doctor may legally:
- prescribe unlicenced medicines
- in a named patient, use unlicenced products specially prepared, imported, or supplied
- supply another doctor with an unlicenced medicine
- with appropriate safeguards, use unlicenced drugs in clinical trials
- use or advise the use of licenced medicines for indications or in doses or by routes of administration outside the licenced recommendations
- override the warnings and precautions given in the licence

The responsibility for the consequences of these actions lies with the prescribing doctor.[2,3]

It has been recommended that when prescribing a drug outside its licence, a doctor should:[4,5]
- record in the patient's notes the reasons for the decision to prescribe outside the licenced indications
- where possible explain the position to the patient (and family as appropriate) in sufficient detail to allow them to give informed consent (the Patient Information Leaflet obviously does not contain information about unlicenced indications)

- inform other professionals, e.g. pharmacist, nurses, general practitioner, involved in the care of the patient to avoid misunderstandings

In addition to clinical trials, prescriptions beyond licence may be justified:
- when prescribing generic formulations (for which indications are not described)
- with established drugs for proven but unlicenced indications
- with drugs for conditions for which there are no other treatments (even in the absence of strong evidence)
- when using drugs in individuals not covered by licenced indications, e.g. children

2 Anonymous (1992) Prescribing unlicensed drugs or using drugs for unlicensed applications. *Drug and Therapeutics Bulletin* **30**: 97–9.

3 Cohen P. J. (1997) Off-label use of prescription drugs: legal, clinical and policy considerations. *European Journal of Anaesthesiology* **14**: 231–50.

4 Atkinson C. V. and Kirkham S. R. (1999) Unlicensed uses for medication in a palliative care unit. *Palliative Medicine* **13**: 145–52.

5 Association of Palliative Medicine, Pain Society (2002) *The use of drugs beyond licence in palliaitive care and pain management.* Southampton and London: APM and Pain Society.

Drug interactions in palliative care

> It may seem a strange principle to enunciate as the very first requirement in a hospital that it should do the sick no harm.
>
> Florence Nightingale, *Notes on Hospitals*, 1863

The potential for drug interactions is high in palliative care due to polypharmacy. The following are some selected drug interactions which are pertinent to palliative care prescribing:

Warfarin

The anticoagulation effect of warfarin can be affected by many drugs. Anticoagulation may increase with:

- amiodarone
- erythromycin, clarithromycin
- cranberry juice
- dextropropoxyphene (co-proxamol)
- fluconazole, itraconazole, miconazole, ketoconazole
- metronidazole
- NSAIDs
- paracetamol
- quinolone antibiotics (e.g. ciprofloxacin)
- St. John's Wort
- testosterone

Amiodarone

A number of drugs used concomitantly with amiodarone increase the risk of ventricular arrhythmias and the advice is to avoid them:

- tricyclic antidepressants (amitriptyline etc.)
- phenothiazines, haloperidol
- flecainide
- quinine
- erythromycin (parenteral)

The low doses of haloperidol as an antiemetic, and tricyclic antidepressants used for neuropathic pain, used in palliative care, probably carry a reduced risk, but one that cannot be completely dismissed.

MAOIs (antidepressants) and selegiline

There is a serious and potentially fatal interaction (serotonin syndrome) between pethidine and MAOIs. A similar reaction is seen with selegiline, an MAO-B inhibitor.

No adverse interaction normally occurs in patients on MAOIs given morphine, but there are isolated and unexplained reports of patients who became hypotensive and subsequently unconsciousness and who rapidly improved with naloxone. Some very limited evidence also suggests that no interaction occurs with methadone.

The concurrent use of MAOIs and phenothiazines is usually safe and effective. The exception appears to be levomepromazine (methotrimeprazine) which has been implicated in two fatal reactions with pargyline and tranylcypromine.

Anticonvulsants

Carbamazepine levels are increased (risk of toxicity) with:

- clarithromycin
- dextropropoxyphene (co-proxamol)
- erythromycin
- fluoxetine
- fluvoxamine

Phenytoin levels are increased (toxicity) by:

- amiodarone
- aspirin
- clarithromycin
- diltiazem
- fluconazole
- fluoxetine
- fluvoxamine
- metronidazole
- miconazole
- nifedipine
- omeprazole
- trimethoprim

Carbamazepine and phenytoin levels are decreased (risk of fits) by corticosteroids.

Carbamazepine, phenytoin and phenobarbital can reduce the efficacy of corticosteroids. This two-way interaction is common when managing patients with cerebral tumours.

Antifungal drugs

- fluconazole, miconazole increase phenytoin levels
- fluconazole and miconazole increase the effect of sulphonylureas e.g. gliclazide, glibenclamide (risk of hypoglycaemia)
- fluconazole increases celecoxib levels—halve celecoxib dose
- itraconazole, ketoconazole and possibly fluconazole increase sedation with midazolam
- fluconazole, miconazole, itraconazole, and ketoconazole all enhance warfarin anticoagulation

Proton pump inhibitors (PPIs)

- omeprazole increases blood diazepam levels (increase in sedation)
- omeprazole enhances anticoagulation effect of warfarin

Metronidazole

- disulfiram-like reaction with alcohol
- enhances anticoagulation with warfarin
- increases phenytoin blood levels (toxicity)
- increases blood levels of fluoruracil increasing toxicity

SSRI antidepressants

- fluoxetine and fluvoxamine increase carbamazepine and phenytoin blood levels (toxicity)
- fluoxetine increases plasma levels of flecainide
- serious reaction with MAOIs, selegiline (serotonin syndrome)
- increased serotonergic effects with St. John's Wort (avoid)

St. John's Wort

- increased serotonergic effects with SSRIs (avoid)
- reduced anticoagulant effect of warfarin
- reduced plasma levels of carbamazepine, phenytoin, phenobarbital (risk of fits)
- reduced plasma levels of digoxin

Dextropropoxyphene (in co-proxamol)

- increases blood levels of carbamazepine up to sixfold (toxicity)
- enhanced anticoagulation effect of warfarin

Regular paracetamol may also affect warfarin anticoagulation.

Torsades de pointes

An increasing number of drugs have been recognized to prolong the QT interval and potentially cause torsades de pointes, a serious cardiac arrhythmia. A register of drugs that cause QT prolongation is available on the internet at http://www.torsades.org

Corticosteroids

The use of corticosteroids in palliative care varies considerably from unit to unit and physician to physician. Traditionally they have been used to reduce oedema, to promote appetite and well-being; and for their specific use in disease processes such as asthma, or chronic lymphatic leukaemia or in emergency situations where their use can buy time until a more definitive treatment can be instituted.

Corticosteroids are produced by the adrenal gland and have a number of physiological rôles including catabolic effects on protein, carbohydrate and fat metabolism, and anti-inflammatory effects. They influence water and electrolyte balance and suppress immunity.

Dexamethascne is the corticosteroid of choice in palliative care.

Indication for use	Daily dose of dexamethasone
Anorexia	2–4mg
Weakness	
Pain (where caused by tumoral oedema)	
Improvement in well being/mood	
Nerve compression pain	4–8mg
Liver capsule pain	
Nausea	
Bowel obstruction	
Post-radiation inflammation	
Raised intracranial pressure	12–16mg
Superior vena caval obstruction	
Carcinomatosa lymphangitis	
Malignant spinal cord compression	

Side-effects of corticosteroids include a rise in blood glucose, increased susceptibility to infection (especially oral thrush) fluid retention and additive insult to the gastrointestinal mucosa with NSAIDs. Insomnia and agitation sometimes lead to a disturbed mental state.

Steroids may also give rise to proximal myopathy often manifesting as difficulty in standing from a sitting position. Classical Cushingoid effects may develop including a very frail skin which bleeds easily on contact. If patients are expected to be on long term steroids (longer than 6 months or so) such as patients with cerebral tumours, consideration may need to be given to prophylaxis for osteoporosis.

Equivalent anti-inflammatory effects of steroids
- Prednisolone   5mg
- Hydrocortisone   20mg
- Methylprednisolone   4mg
- Dexamethasone   750mcg
- Cortisone acetate   25mg
- Betamethasone   750mcg
- Triamcinolone   4mg

Reducing steroids

Dexamethasone above 2mg daily—reduce by 2mg every 5–7 days (and check for symptoms before the next dose reduction), until reaching 2mg

Dexamethasone doses of 2mg or less—reduce by 0.5mg every 5–7 days or on alternative days for a more conservative approach.

Consider:
- Doubling the dose for patients on phenytoin, carbamazepine or phenobarbital
- Giving steroids before midday since they may disturb sleep
- Prophylactic gastric mucosal protection if also taking NSAIDs
- Switching from dexamethasone to prednisolone if myopathy develops
- The possibility that steroids may be masking the clinical signs of perforation of an abdominal viscus or sepsis
- Carefully weigh up the burden/benefit of continuing steroids subcutaneously should the patient become unable to swallow
- Checking blood glucose if any relevant symptoms occur

Always:
- Reduce dose of steroids to the minimum possible
- Review treatment every week, stopping after one week if no benefit
- Reduce dose slowly every few days if the patient has taken steroids for longer than two weeks or has been taking a relatively large dose

In the terminal care situation the patient's inability to swallow oral medication is often the provoking factor which leads to stopping steroids. The continuing of steroids by injection should be considered on an individual basis.

Side-effect risks of steroids

Doses of dexamethasone >4mg o.d. are likely to lead to significant side-effects after several weeks

Doses <4mg o.d. are often tolerated in patients with a prognosis of months

Doses <4mg can be stopped abruptly IF used for less than three weeks

Further reading

Book

Back I (2001) *Palliative Medicine Handbook*. 3rd edn. Cardiff: BPM Books pp. 126–9.

Formulary

Drugs in **bold** can be given in a syringe driver

Drug	Route	Dose	Frequency	Indications/Side-effects/Remarks
Alfentanil	CSCI	Titrate	24h	Synthetic opioid working on similar opioid receptors to fentanyl. Alternative CSCI-delivered opioid for patients unable to tolerate diamorphine. e.g. in renal failure Alfentanil 1mg = diamorphine 10mg
Aminophylline				Theophylline
i/r	p.o.	100–300mg	t.d.s.	Reversible airways obstruction
m/r	p.o.	225–450mg	b.d.	Theophylline concentration for optimal response is 55–110micromol/l Narrow therapeutic/toxicity margin Half life increased in heart failure, the elderly, and with drugs such as erythromycin and ciprofloxacin. SE: Tachycardia, palpitations, nausea, CNS stimulation.
Amitriptyline	p.o.	10–50mg	nocte	Neuropathic pain. Start at 10–25mg. Faster effect at lower doses than for depression. Salivary dribbling in MND. SE: Blurred vision, dry mouth, hypotension. Caution if cardiac disease, or history of urinary retention
Artificial saliva	Spray, gel, pastilles		As required	Contains mucin, an animal product not suitable for some religions
Arthrotec (see also	p.o. p.o. (m/r)	50mg 75mg	t.d.s. b.d.	Contains diclofenac + misoprostol (for prophylaxis against NSAID gastro-duodenal ulceration).

Baclofen	p.o.	5–10mg max. 100mg/day	t.d.s.	Spasticity i.e. in MND Increase dose slowly SE: sedation and weakness
Benzydamine	0.15% oral rinse spray	15ml 4–8 puffs	1.5–3h p.r.n.	Local analgesic spray Dilute with water if stings
Bethanecol	p.o.	25mg	t.d.s.	Dry mouth
Bicalutamide (Casodex)	p.o. p.o.	50mg 150mg	o.d. o.d.	Anti-androgen With orchidectomy or gonadorelin therapy start three days beforehand Prostate cancer SE: GI upsets, nausea, vomiting, depression, loss of libido
Bisacodyl	p.o. PR	5–20mg 10mg	nocte— b.d. o.d.	Stimulant laxative. 5mg Tabs—action 10–12h. 10mg Supps.—action 20–60 mins. Avoid in bowel obstruction
Bupivacaine	neb.	5ml 0.25%	6 h	Useful for persistent dry cough, not breathlessness. Beware reflex bronchospasm. (Pretreat with nebulised salbutamol.) No food for one hour after treatment because of pharyngeal anaesthesia
Buprenorphine	SL	0.2–0.4mg	t.d.s.	0.4mg t.d.s. Equivalent to 10–15mg morphine 4 h **Beware use in palliative care as it is a partial agonist, i.e. it can displace more effective opioids from their receptor sites**
Buprenorphine	Transdermal matrix patch	35, 52.5, 70 mcg/h	Every three days	Maximum dose = 140mcg/h For breakthrough buprenorphine SL or other opioids can be used
Buscopan see Hyoscine butylbromide				

Drug	Route	Dose	Frequency	Indications/Side-effects/Remarks
Capsaicin	topical	0.075% cream	q.d.s.	Neuropathic pain/post herpetic neuralgia. May cause stinging. Wear gloves to administer. Avoid contact to sensitive areas
Carbamazepine	p.o.	100–200mg (max. 1.2g)	b.d.	Tonic-clonic/partial seizures; neuropathic pain. Build up dose slowly. Check serum levels. Watch drug interactions. Tabs./chewtab/Supps. SE: Ataxia and blood, hepatic and skin disorders
Carbenoxolone	m/w	1% sachet	q.d.s.	Mild oral and perioral ulcers
Carbocisteine	p.o.	750–1500mg	t.d.s.	Reduces sputum viscosity and increases expectoration. SE: Gastric irritant. Avoid if peptic ulceration
Celecoxib	p.o.	100–200mg	o.d.–b.d.	Cyclo-oxygenase-2 inhibitor. Pain and inflammation with reduced gastric side-effects
Chlorphenamine	p.o.	4mg	4–6h	Sedating antihistamine. Allergic reactions SE: Sedation
Chlorpromazine	p.o. PR	25–50mg 100mg	o.d.–t.d.s.	Severe agitation. Tenesmus (low dose). Hiccup (low dose). SE: sedative/hypotensive. Half dose in elderly. Supps. available by special order

Clonazepam	p.o.	0.5–2mg	nocte or b.d.	Neuropathic pain, anticonvulsant, sedative.
	CSCI	**1–4mg**	**24h**	May stick to plastic of syringe making titration difficult
Co-codamol Weak 8/500 (Not recommended for palliative care patients)	p.o.	1–2 Tabs.	4–6 h Max 8 in 24h	Codeine phosphate 8mg + paracetamol 500mg. Soluble preparations available. There is no evidence that 'weak co-codamol' is any more efficacious in pain control than paracetamol alone.[6]
Co-codamol **Strong** 30/500	p.o.	1–2 Tabs.	4–6 h Max 8 in 24h	Codeine phosphate 30mg + paracetamol 500mg e.g. Tylex, Solpadol. Soluble preparations available
Co-danthramer	p.o.	5–10ml 1–2 Caps.	nocte nocte	Stimulant (dantron) 25mg + softener (poloxamer) 200mg per Caps. or 5ml. Useful for drug induced constipation. 'Strong' capsules and Susp. also available. SE: May colour urine red. Do not use if incontinent as is associated with burning of perineal skin and excoriation Not licenced for patients with non-malignant disease as danthron is a potential carcinogen.
Co-danthrusate	p.o.	1–3 Caps. 5–15ml	nocte nocte	Stimulant (dantron) + softener (docusate) See co-danthramer
Co-dydramol	p.o.	1–2	4–6h max 8 in 24h	Dihydrocodeine 10mg + paracetamol 500mg. There are also combined preparations containing dihydrocodeine 20mg and 30mg

Drug	Route	Dose	Frequency	Indications/Side-effects/Remarks
Colestyramine	p.o.	4–8g	o.d.	Anion-exchange resin
				Pruritus associated with biliary obstruction, diarrhoea associated with ileal resection, radiation
				SE: Constipation and nausea
Cyproterone acetate	p.o.	300mg/24h	Divided doses	Anti-androgen
	p.o.	200–300mg/24h	Divided doses	Cover flare of initial gonadorelin therapy
				Long term palliative therapy where orchidectomy or gonadorelin analogues not indicated
Co-proxamol	p.o.	1–2 tabs	4–6 h	Paracetamol 325mg + Dextropropoxyphene 32.5mg. Some NMDA activity.
			max 12 in 24h	Relatively low dose of paracetamol. May increase risk of bleeding with warfarin.
Cyclizine	p.o.	25–50mg	t.d.s.	Antihistamine. Useful for vomiting of GI cause, or raised intracranial pressure. SC route may cause skin reaction. Supps. available by special order.
	SC	25–50mg	t.d.s.	
	PR	25–50mg	t.d.s.	
	CSCI	**100–150mg**	**24h**	
Dexamethasone	p.o.	Up to 16mg	in 24 h	2–4mg o.d. for appetite
	i/m	Up to 16mg	in 24 h	8–16mg daily for raised intracranial pressure, SVCO, spinal cord compression.
	i/v			
	CSCI	**Up to 16mg**	**24h**	2–6mg prevent chemotherapy emesis. Give a.m. to avoid excitation. Reduce dose ASAP. Watch glucose and proximal myopathy. Consider PPI prophylaxis in patients at risk of peptic ulceration. Prescribe PPI if taking NSAID. Separate syringe driver.

Diamorphine	**SC**	Titrated		Strong opioid analgesic. More soluble than morphine.
	CSCI	**Titrated**		SC diamorphine is three times as potent as oral morphine.
				Modify dose in elderly patients and in patients with renal failure.
				SE: see pain section
	Topical	20mg		Mix in lidocaine gel (topical)
Diazepam	p.o.	2–10mg	o.d.–t.d.s.	Anxiety; agitation; breathlessness; convulsions. Alternative
	PR	5–10mg	p.r.n.	is SC midazolam which is shorter acting.
			(Supps. or soln.)	
Diclofenac	p.o.	25–50mg	t.d.s.	Bone pain and other inflammatory conditions if paracetamol and weak
	p.o.	75mg (m/r)	b.d.	opioids found to be ineffective. May enhance the anticoagulant effect
	i/m	75mg	stat	of warfarin and caution required in patients with asthma.
	PR	100mg	o.d.	If ineffective, try another NSAID. Contra-indicated with active peptic ulcer,
	SC	**up to 150mg**	**24h**	GI bleeding or renal failure. Consider PPI prophylaxis in patients
				at risk of peptic ulceration.
				Use separate syringe driver. SE: Local irritation
Digoxin	p.o.	62.5–500 mcg	o.d.	Supraventricular tachycardia especially atrial fibrillation
		(maintenance)		Reduce dose in elderly, and if reduced renal function.
				Avoid if hypokalaemic
				SE: Anorexia, nausea, vomiting, diarrhoea.
				Abdominal pain, confusion.
				Do not give if ventricular rate is <60 beats per minute

Drug	Route	Dose	Frequency	Indications/Side-effects/Remarks
Dihydrocodeine	p.o. p.o. (m/r)	30–60mg 60–120mg	4–6h b.d.	Moderate pain. Similar efficacy to codeine orally—one tenth as potent as morphine. Increased risk of toxicity in renal failure requires dose reduction to 8h. Anticipate constipation.
Disodium pamidronate	i/v	30–90mg	In minimum 500ml sodium chloride 0.9% over 2–4h	Hypercalcaemia. Rehydrate first. max dose rate 1mg/min. Dose according to corrected plasma calcium concentration. Repeat after one week if poor initial response. Bone pain (especially breast cancer and multiple myeloma).Takes 7 days to produce maximal effect which lasts 2–3 weeks. Repeat every 3–4 weeks as long as benefit maintained.
Docusate sodium	p.o.	100–200mg	Daily	Softens stool. Weak stimulant. May help constipation in presence of partial bowel obstruction. Acts in 1–2 days.
Domperidone	p.o. PR	10–20mg 30–60mg	4–8h 4–8h	Antiemetic, bowel motility stimulant. Beware intestinal obstruction as may cause pain. Less extrapyramidal problems than with metoclopramide
Dosulepin	p.o.	50–150mg	nocte or b.d.	Tricyclic antidepressant Neuropathic pain. Lower doses start at 10mg nocte. Depression. Higher doses from 50mg SE: lowers convulsion threshold, dry mouth, urine retention, constipation, blurred vision

Epoetin	SC	150–300u/kg	Weekly	Recombinant human erythropoietin Anaemia associated with erythropoietin deficiency. Aim to elevate haemoglobin at a rate not exceeding 2g/100ml/month. If haemoglobin reaches 14 suspend until returns below 13g/100ml Contra-indicated in patients with chronic renal failure SE: Hypertension
Etamsylate	p.o.	500mg	q.d.s.	Useful for capillary bleeding
Fentanyl	transdermal	25, 50, 75, 100mg/h over 3 days	72 h	Strong opioid for severe pain. Due to slow onset of action, patients may need extra analgesia for up to 24 h after fentanyl patch is started. Laxatives may be reduced, as causes less constipation than other opioids. On removal of patch it may take 17 h or more for plasma levels to drop by 50%. Unsuitable for unstable pain due to slow onset of action. **Conversion:** Daily oral morphine mg Fentanyl patch delivery mcg/h 50–130 25 135–224 50 225–314 75 315–404 100 405–494 125 Caution: when changing from transdermal fentanyl to morphine; use lower morphine dose.
Fentanyl	OTFC Lozenge	200, 400, 600, 800, 1200 mcg	For breakthrough pain	Dose of breakthrough analgesia with OTFC is not related to background analgesic dose so start with 200 mcg. Mouth needs to be moist

Drug	Route	Dose	Frequency	Indications/Side-effects/Remarks
Fluconazole	p.o.	50 mg	o.d.	Candidiasis. Give 7–14 day course
Fludrocortisone	p.o.	50–300 mcg	o.d.	Mineralocorticoid Postural hypotension Adrenal replacement with hydrocortisone
Fluoxetine	p.o.	20mg	mane	Enervating antidepressant. Long half life (5 weeks) SE: anxiety. GI symptoms usually settle within a few days
Gabapentin	p.o.	Starting dose 100–300mg Doses above 1800mg/24h need specialist attention.	Initially nocte then t.d.s.	Neuropathic pain. Anticonvulsant. Higher benefit/side-effect ratio than most other agents used for neuropathic pain. Use lower dosing in elderly and if renal failure present. Standard dosing regime not established. BNF recommends 300mg day 1, 300mg b.d. day 2, 300mg t.d.s. day 3, then titrate according to response in 300mg steps to max. of 1.8mg/day Avoid abrupt withdrawal. (Withdraw over 1 week.) SE: drowsiness, fatigue, ataxia
Gliclazide i/r m/r	p.o. p.o.	40–80mg 30mg (equivalent to 80mg i/r)	o.d. o.d. max 120mg/24h	Sulphonylurea SE: Weight gain, hypoglycaemia, GI upset.
Glycopyrronium	p.o. **CSCI** SC	0.2–0.4mg **0.6–1.2mg** 0.2–0.4mg	4h **24h** t.d.s.	Dries secretions. Proven efficacy via continuous syringe driver route not from stat injections. Probably less central and/or cardiac side-effects than atropine or hyoscine.

(Zoladex, Zoladex LA)	(Long acting) Implant	3.6mg	12 weeks	early breast cancer. Implant in anterior abdominal wall with local anaesthetic. 'Flare' of androgen release when starting therapy can lead to increased activity of disease, and symptoms such as back pain need to be taken very seriously, if there are known spinal metastases, since spinal cord compression can be precipitated. (Flare can be covered with an anti-androgen, such as cyproterone acetate)
Granisetron	p.o.	1–2mg	Every 4 weeks	Serotonin antagonist. Nausea/vomiting especially post RT or C/T SE: Constipation
Haloperidol	p.o. SC **CSCI**	0.5–10mg 2.5–10mg **3–10mg**	o.d.–b.d. 4h p.r.n. **24h**	Antiemetic. Small doses (e.g. 1.5mg b.d.) for nausea, particularly drug or metabolic induced. Higher doses in psychosis and agitation. Beware extrapyramidal side-effects and avoid in Parkinson's disease
Hydromorphone i/r	p.o.	Titrated	4h	Alternative opioid. Caps. i/r 1.3, 2.6mg ×7.5 potency of morphine; i.e. 1.3mg hydromorphone = 10mg morphine
Hydromorphone m/r	p.o	Titrated	b.d.	Caps. m/r 2, 4, 8, 16, 24mg (12 h)

hydromorphone (mg) / morphine (mg):

hydromorphone (mg)	morphine (mg)
2	15
4	30
8	60
16	120
24	180

Hydromorphone inj	**CSCI** SC	Titrated	24 h 4 h	10mg/ml, 20mg/ml, 50mg/ml ×7.5 the potency of morphine Conversion factors from oral to SC hydromorphone range from equipotent to 3:1 Available as a 'special' from Martindale Pharmaceuticals

Drug	Route	Dose	Frequency	Indications/Side-effects/Remarks
Hyoscine butylbromide (*Buscopan*)	**CSCI**	**60–180mg (Intestinal obstruction)**	**24h**	Antimuscarinic, anticholinergic. Less sedating than hyoscine hydrobromide. Uses: intestinal colic, reduces bronchial secretions
		20–60mg (reduce bronchial secretions)		Very short half life
	SC	10–20mg	4h	
	p.o.	20mg	q.d.s.	Poor oral bioavailability
Hyoscine hydrobromide	SC	0.2–0.4mg	4–8h	Antimuscarinic, anticholinergic
	CSCI	**0.6–0.4mg**	**24h**	Antiemetic for refractory nausea
				Dries secretions second line to glycopyrronium
	SL	0.3mg	6h p.r.n.	SE: paradoxical agitation, sedation
	patch	1 patch	Change every 72h	
		1mg		
Ibuprofen	p.o.	200–600mg	t.d.s.	First line NSAID. Lower risks of side-effects than other NSAIDs. Topical preparations available. See diclofenac for contra-indications.
Ipratropium bromide	Neb.	0.25–0.5mg	6h	For breathlessness when there is bronchospasm, particularly if COPD present. Drying effect on secretions.

Ketamine	p.o.	25–100mg	t.d.s./q.d.s.	Under specialist supervision only. Neuropathic pain; build up dose slowly.
Ketamine	**CSCI**	**75–300mg** (Higher doses have been reported)	24h	May need prophylactic oral haloperidol 3mg nocte or a benzodiazepine to cover for psychomimetic side-effects. Oral solution available. May need to reduce opioids by 50%. Use separate syringe driver.
Ketorolac	p.o.	10mg	4–6 h (elderly 6–8 h)	Bone pain and other inflammatory conditions. Max 40mg p.o.
	SC	10–30mg	4–6 h	Max 90mg SC daily. See diclofenac warnings and cautions. Beware gastric bleeding.
Ketorolac	**CSCI**	**60–90mg**	**24h**	Use separate syringe driver With gastric protection (PPI)
Lactulose	p.o.	15–30ml	b.d.	Osmotic laxative. May cause abdominal bloating and wind. Requires a good fluid intake May take 48 h for full effect.
Lansoprazole	p.o.	30mg	o.d.	Proton pump inhibitor. Gastric and duodenal ulcer and oesophagitis Prophylaxis with NSAIDS and corticosteroids. Susp. available.

Drug	Route	Dose	Frequency	Indications/Side-effects/Remarks
Levomepromazine (methotrimeprazine)	p.o.	6.25–25mg (6.25mg = 1/4 Tab.)	o.d.–b.d.	Nausea and vomiting. Broad spectrum 'second line' antiemetic. SE: Sedation 6mg and 25mg Tabs.
Levomepromazine	**CSCI**	**6.25–50mg**	**24h**	SC route may cause skin reaction Dilute with sodium chloride 0.9% There is a 2:1 oral: SC conversion ratio
Levomepromazine	p.o.	6.25–200mg	o.d.–b.d.	Psychosis or severe agitation. Useful in terminal sedation. SE: May cause anticholinergic side-effects, hypotension and extrapyramidal symptoms
Levomepromazine	**CSCI**	**6.25–200mg**	**24h**	SC route may cause skin reaction. Dilute with sodium chloride 0.9%. Avoid in Parkinson's disease
Levomepromazine	SC	6.25–25mg	4–8 h	
Lidocaine (lignocaine)	Topical	5% ointment		Topical analgesia
Lithium (Carbonate/citrate)	p.o.	Dose adjusted to individual patient		Treatment and prophylaxis of mania, bipolar disorder, recurrent depression. Narrow therapeutic/toxic window. Target serum lithium concentration 0.4–1mmol/l, 12 h after a dose. Requires regular monitoring SE: GI upsets, tremor, renal impairment, oedema, blurred vision, drowsiness. Worse if sodium depleted, so beware if using diuretics. Drug interactions: Numerous—check each medicine.

Drug	Route	Dose	Frequency	Notes
Lofepramine	p.o.	140–210mg	Divided doses	Antidepressant. Lower incidence of antimuscarinic side-effects than amitriptyline
Loperamide	p.o.	2–4mg max. 32mg/24h	t.d.s. or with each loose stool	Useful for diarrhoea and the pain of bowel colic. No CNS effects.
Loratadine	p.o.	10mg	o.d.	Non-sedating antihistamine
Lorazepam	p.o./SL	0.5–2mg	b.d.	Anxiety/panic attacks. Shorter duration of action than diazepam. Useful sublingually in acute anxiety and breathlessness.
Macrogol (polyethylene glycol) (Movicol)	p.o.	Dissolve sachet in 125ml water	1–3 sachets/day up to 8 sachets/day for faecal impaction	Licenced for faecal impaction.
Medroxyprogesterone acetate	p.o.	400mg (double dose if poor response)	o.m.	Appetite stimulation in anorexia. Effect enhanced with concurrent NSAID. Takes 2–3 weeks to produce maximal effect. Hot flushes after surgical or chemical castration
	p.o.	5–20mg	b.d.–q.d.s.	
Megestrol acetate	p.o.	40–160mg	o.m.	Appetite stimulation in anorexia. Effect enhanced with concurrent NSAID. Take 2–3 weeks to produce maximal effect. Hot flushes after surgical or chemical castration

Drug	Route	Dose	Frequency	Indications/Side-effects/Remarks
Methadone	p.o	Titrated	b.d.–t.d.s	May be used for nociceptive and possibly neuropathic pain if no longer responsive to/tolerant of morphine.
	SC	Titrated	b.d.–t.d.s	Long half life.
	CSCI	**Titrated**	**24h**	Subcutaneously, use 50–70% oral dose. Can be used in renal failure.
				Prescribed differently from morphine, see pain chapter.
				SE: Long 1/2 life can lead to overdosing
Methotrimeprazine, see levomepromazine				
Methylphenidate	p.o.	5mg	o.d.–b.d.	Similar to dexamfetamine
				Uses: Opioid induced drowsiness.
				Mood while awaiting antidepressant to work
				SE: restlessness, confusion, sleep disturbance
Metoclopramide	p.o.	10–20mg	q.d.s.	Antiemetic, especially useful for drug related nausea, and also for cancer
	p.o.(m/r SC)	15mg	b.d.	related anorexia.
		10–20mg	q.d.s.	Increases gut motility and gastric emptying.
	CSCI	**30–90mg**	**24h**	Use cautiously in GI obstruction If makes GI cramps or diarrhoea worse stop.
				Extrapyramidal side-effects. (reversible with procylidine)
Metronidazole	p.o.	400mg	t.d.s.	Antibiotic for anaerobic infections.
	topical	1g	t.d.s.	Topically useful for fungating, odorous wounds
	PR		t.d.s.	SE: Nausea
Midazolam	SC	2.5–10mg	p.r.n.	Benzodiazepine. Shorter duration of action than diazepam
	Buccal			Single doses useful for quick, uncomfortable procedures, anxiety, agitation,
	intranasal			as replacement for anticonvulsants and sedation in the terminal phase.
	CSCI	**10–100mg**	**24h**	

Drug	Route	Dose	Frequency	Notes
Mirtazepine	p.o.	15–45mg titrate	Nocte	Some evidence of faster onset of action and promotion of appetite and sleep than other newer antidepressants. (Lower doses more sedating than higher, enervating, doses)
Morphine (i/r)	p.o.	Titrated	4 h	Pain/breathlessness 1/3 potent as subcutaneous diamorphine. Anticipate constipation. Oramorph 10mg/5ml, 100mg/5ml Single unit dose vials 10mg, 30mg, 100mg, all in 5ml. Sevredol Tabs.: 10mg, 20mg, 50mg.
	PR	Titrated	4 h	Supps. 10, 15, 20, 30mg
Morphine (m/r)	p.o.	Titrated	12 h	MST continuous 5, 10, 15, 30, 60, 200mg. MST Susp. 20, 30, 60, 100, 200mg (sachets). Zomorph 10, 30, 60, 100, 200mg. MXL 30, 60, 90, 120, 150, 200mg.
Morphine	p.o.	titrated	24 h	As for diamorphine, but high doses will require larger volumes.
	SC	Titrated	4 h	
	CSCI		24 h	Conversion: p.o. to SC 2:1.
Nabilone	p.o.	0.1–0.2mg	q.d.s.	Cannabinoid Breathlessness, nausea. SE: Sedation/dysphoria may occur with higher doses. Oral solution can be made up
Naloxone	i/v	0.1–0.2mg	every 2mins.	Reversal of opioid induced respiratory depression. Beware return of severe pain. Mix Amp. with 10ml of sterile water and give 1ml a minute titrating response. Beware that treating opioid induced respiratory depression may require repeated dosing and close monitoring for several hours.
	i/m/SC	0.1–0.2mg	every 2mins	

Drug	Route	Dose	Frequency	Indications/Side-effects/Remarks
Naproxen	p.o. PR	250–500mg 500mg	b.d. b.d.	Bone pain and other inflammatory conditions. If ineffective, try another NSAID. Beware with warfarin and in patients who are asthmatic. Contra-indicated with active peptic ulcer or GI bleeding See diclofenac for warnings and cautions
Nifedipine	p.o. SL	5mg 5mg	t.d.s. t.d.s.	Smooth muscle relaxant; useful for hiccups, oesophageal spasm and tenesmus. SE: Hypotension, peripheral oedema, headache
Nitrous oxide 50% +oxygen 50%				For incident pain. Produces analgesia without loss of consciousness. Exponents claim useful for changing painful dressings, etc. Patient must control administration
Nystatin	p.o.	1–5ml 100,000 u/ml	q.d.s.	Oral Candidiasis
Octreotide	SC **CSCI**	0.1–0.2mg **300–1000mcg**	t.d.s. **24h**	Somatostatin analogue. Very short duration of action. Carcinoid symptom control. Reduces GI secretions and motility. Useful in intestinal obstruction, enterocutaneous fistulae and intractable diarrhoea. Not sedative.
Sandostatin LAR	Depot injection	20mg/month × 3 months then review results		Expensive; use when other treatments have failed. Use with caution if patient has diabetes mellitus
Lanreotide	Depot injection	30mg/2 weeks × 3 months then review results		

Olanzepine	p.o.	5–10mg	o.d.	New generation antipsychotic
				Moderate to severe mania
				SE: less than with older antipsychotics but postural hypotension, extrapyramidal effects.
				Caution: Glaucoma, hyperglycaemia, elderly stroke patients with dementia.
Omeprazole	p.o.	10–20mg	o.d.	Proton pump inhibitor (PPI) Gastric and duodenal ulcer and reflux oesophagitis
Ondansetron	p.o.	8mg	b.d.–t.d.s.	Serotonin antagonist.
	i/v	8mg	b.d.–t.d.s.	Uses: Vomiting caused by RT or C/T, ovarian intestinal obstruction, hepatic
	PR	16mg	o.d.	cholestatic itch.
	CSCI	**8–24mg**	**24h**	Relatively more expensive than other antiemetics.
				Max. 8mg daily in severe hepatic failure.
				SE: Constipation
				Melt forms available
Oxybutynin	p.o.	2.5–5mg	b.d.–t.d.s.	Antimuscarinic
				Detrusor instability
				Urinary incontinence (urge)
				SE: Antimuscarinic effects
Oxycodone i/r	p.o.	Titrated	4–6h	Moderate to severe pain.
	PR	Titrated	8h	5mg, 10mg, 20mg Caps., Liquid 5mg/5ml, 10mg/ml
				20mg Oral morphine equivalent to 10mg oxycodone
				Oxycodone 30mg Supps. available. (Longer acting than morphine Supps.)
Oxycodone m/r	p.o.	Titrated	12h	Modified release Tabs. 10mg, 20mg, 40mg, 80mg 12 h.
				20mg oral morphine equivalent to 10mg oral oxycodone

Drug	Route	Dose	Frequency	Indications/Side-effects/Remarks
Oxycodone inj	SC	5–10mg	4h	10ml/ml
	CSCI	**Titrated**	**24h**	1ml and 2ml Amps. Twice as potent as oral oxycodone e.g. 20mg of oral oxycodone is equivalent to 10mg of injectable oxycodone.
Pamidronate (see Disodium pamidronate)				
Pancreatin (Creon 10,000)	p.o.	1–2 Caps. with meals		For fat malabsorption e.g. Creon 1–2 sachets with meals Preparations containing lipase 25000 and 40000 units available.
Paracetamol	p.o.	0.5–1g	4–6 h	Analgesic. Antipyretic. Available as Tabs, Caps., caplets, Susp., dispersible and 125 and 500mg Supps.
	PR	0.5–1g	4–6 h Max. 4g in 24h	
Parecoxib	i/m	40mg initially then 20–40mg	12 h	Cox-2 NSAID injection SE: as per other NSAID drugs
	i/v			
Paroxetine	p.o.	20mg	o.m.	SSRI antidepressant/ anxiolytic. Short half life. Used for itch and sweating. Withdraw slowly SE: extrapyramidal effects noted

Phenobarbital	p.o.	60–180mg	Nocte	Anticonvulsant. Useful as replacement oral anticonvulsant and in terminal sedation.
	i/m	50–200mg	b.d.	Use separate syringe driver.
	CSCI	**200–600mg**	**24h**	Max. 600mg daily
Pilocarpine	p.o.	5mg	t.d.s.	Cholinergic
		4% eye drops (orally)	t.d.s.	Sialagogue for dry mouth
Piroxicam	p.o.	20mg	b.d.	NSAID
	melt	20mg	b.d.	Inflammatory pain
				Melt useful when swallowing not possible.
				SE: as per diclofenac
Pregabalin	p.o.	75mg	b.d.	Neuropathic pain, epilepsy and anxiety. Similar mode of action to Gabapentin

Dose regime:

Normal Kidney Function				**Impaired Kidney Function**		
Time	Breakfast	Supper		Time	Breakfast	Supper
Step 1	75 mg	75 mg		Step 1	50 mg	50 mg
Step 2	150 mg	150 mg		Step 2	100 mg	100 mg
Step 3	300 mg	300 mg		Step 3	150 mg	150 mg

If necessary step 2 can be started after 3–4 days, and step 3 after a further 7 days
Common side-effects are sedation, dizziness, and headaches.
Potentiated by alcohol and oxycodone

Prochlorperazine	p.o.	5–10mg	t.d.s.	Neuroleptic.
	i/m	12.5mg	t.d.s. p.r.n.	Antiemetic. May be useful for metabolic/drug induced nausea.
	PR	25mg	t.d.s.	Too irritant to be given subcutaneously.
	buccal	3–6mg	b.d.	

Drug	Route	Dose	Frequency	Indications/Side-effects/Remarks
Procyclidine	p.o. i/m / i/v	2.5–5mg 5–10mg	t.d.s. p.r.n.	For management of extrapyramidal side-effects of neuroleptic drugs or dopamine antagonists. (max. 20mg daily)
Ranitidine	p.o.	300mg 150mg	nocte b.d.	Peptic ulceration. Steatorrhea due to bile duct obstruction. Less evidence of protection against NSAID induced gastric ulceration than PPIs.
Riluzole	p.o.	50mg	b.d.	Used to extend life (?) or the time to mechanical ventilation in patients with motor neurone disease. SE: Nausea, vomiting, abdominal pafin, circumoral paraesthesia, altered liver function tests
Risperidone	p.o.	0.5–2mg	b.d.	'Atypical antipsychotic' useful for psychoses in which both positive and negative symptoms are prominent. Extrapyramidal symptoms are less common than with traditional antipsychotics, but it is more expensive. In elderly start at 0.25 or 0.5mg nocte
Salbutamol	neb p.o. SC	2.5–5mg 8mg m/r 0.5mg	6–8h b.d. 4h	β agonist Bronchospasm Beware causes tachycardia and multiple doses can lead to agitation and anxiety.
Senna	p.o.	2–4Tabs.	nocte	Stimulant laxative. Acts in 8–12 h Avoid in bowel obstruction.
Sertraline	p.o.	50mg	o.d.	SSRI antidepressant. Caution in epilepsy as reduces fit threshold Reduce slowly SE: GI upset

Sodium valproate	p.o.	100–300mg	b.d.	Anticonvulsant Start at 100mg b.d. for neuropathic pain; 300mg b.d. for convulsions. Tabs., m/r Tabs., Supps. available by special order. SE: Nausea, blood dyscrasia, liver dysfunction
Spironolactone	p.o.	100–200mg Max. 400mg for ascites	o.d.	Potassium sparing diuretic. Sodium and fluid retention, malignant ascites. (Ascites dose regimes vary considerably). Trial with furosemide for few days. Avoid with ACE inhibitors, potassium supplements and potassium sparing diuretics as could cause hyperkalaemia. SE: Gynaecomastia
Sucralfate	p.o	2g	b.d.	Protects mucosa from acid-pepsin attack in gastric and duodenal ulcers and also protects oral mucosa. Paste/Susp.
Tinzaparin	SC	175u/kg	o.d.	Low molecular weight heparin (LMWH). Treatment dose for pulmonary embolus (PE) and deep venous thrombosis (DVT)
	SC	50u/kg	o.d.	Prophylaxis In cancer patients LMWH is now the treatment of choice if anticoagulation is required
Tizanidine	p.o.	2mg titrate 3 day intervals, 2mg steps Max. 36mg/day	o.d.	Muscle relaxant for spasticity associated with multiple sclerosis or spinal cord disease. Regular LFT monitoring for first four months

Drug	Route	Dose	Frequency	Indications/Side-effects/Remarks
Tramadol				May be useful for nociceptive and neuropathic pain.
i/r	p.o.	50–100mg	q.d.s.	Tramadol 50mg equivalent to morphine 10mg
m/r	p.o.	100–200mg (max 400mg/24h)	b.d.	Less constipating than codeine
Tranexamic acid	p.o.	1–1.5g	b.d.–q.d.s.	Useful for capillary bleeding e.g. surface bleeding from ulcerated tumours. Cautions if: 1. Haematuria, as may encourage clot formation and ureteric obstruction. 2. History of thromboembolism
Venlafaxine	p.o.	37.5–75mg	b.d.	SNRI antidepressant Used also for hot flushes and neuropathic pain
Warfarin	p.o.	As per INR	o.d.	Coumarin anticoagulant Takes 48–72 h to be fully effective Used to treat DVT and PE Used for prophylaxis with indwelling i/v lines and atrial fibrillation. Usual adult induction *10mg o.d. for 2 days then depending on INR target daily maintenance. * Lower dose if abnormal liver function, cardiac failure. Caution: Paracetamol, NSAIDs, Cranberry juice.
Zoledronic acid	i/v 15 minute 'push'	4–8mg	4–6 weeks	Bisphosphonate Bone pain and hypercalcaemia Monitor calcium levels in bone pain, as may require Vit D or calcium

6 Scottish Intercollegiate National Guidelines Network (2000) *Control of pain in patients with cancer: a national clinical guideline.* Edinburgh: SIGN (www.sign.ac.uk).

Syringe drivers

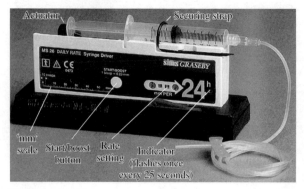

Fig. 4.2 A syringe driver

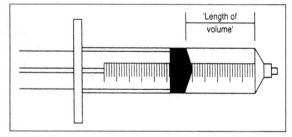

Fig. 4.3 A syringe

Syringe drivers are used to aid drug delivery when the oral route is no longer feasible.

Indications for use:
1 Intractable vomiting
2 Severe dysphagia
3 Patient too weak to swallow oral drugs
4 Decreased conscious level
5 Poor alimentary absorption (rare)
6 Poor patient compliance

Morphine conversion

Diamorphine can be administered subcutaneously in a smaller volume than morphine, and in countries where diamorphine is available is the preparation of first choice.

Oral morphine : Subcutaneous diamorphine

Ratio   3   :   1

When converting from opioids other than morphine, calculate the equivalent dose of oral morphine over 24 h and continue as above.

The following drugs may be mixed with diamorphine
- cyclizine
- haloperidol
- hyoscine hydrobromide
- metoclopramide
- octreotide
- granisetron
- glycopyrronium
- hyoscine butylbromide
- levomepromazine
- midazolam
- ondansetron

Drugs not suitable for subcutaneous usage:
- diazepam
- chlorpromazine
- prochlorperazine

Use separate syringe driver for:
- dexamethasone
- phenobarbital
- diclofenac
- ketamine
- ketorolac

Conversion of oral morphine (or oral morphine equivalent) to parenteral diamorphine

  morphine 3mg p.o. = diamorphine 1mg SC

Method add the total daily oral dose of morphine (or oral morphine equivalent) and divide by three.

  e.g.   morphine 10mg p.o. 4h
                 or
          MST 30mg b.d.   }= morphine 60mg p.o. 24h
                 or
          MXL 60mg o.d.
          morphine 60mg p.o. 24h = diamorphine 20mg SC 24h

General principles
- Care should be taken when mixing more than two drugs in a syringe and in ensuring that the diluent used is compatible with the drugs. The diluent of choice is water for injection except in the following where sodium chloride 0.9% for injection should be used:- diclofenac, granisetron, ketamine, ketorolac, octreotide and ondansetron
- If requiring more than three drugs in one syringe driver, re-assessment of treatment aims is required
- With combinations of two or three drugs in one syringe, a larger volume of diluent may be needed, e.g. 20ml or 30ml syringe

Preparation of syringe driver

The following is an example only, to illustrate the principle; local practices may differ. Training is essential.

Important—check type of portable Graseby syringe driver

Blue driver hourly rate	We strongly encourage the use of only the green Graseby MS 26, mm per 24 h syringe driver as having two different types can cause dangerous dose errors.
Green driver daily rate	

Draw up prescribed 24 h medication mixed with water for injection as diluent.(Use sodium chloride 0.9% as diluent with levomepromazine.)

Set the rate on the syringe driver.

(The rate of delivery is based on a length of fluid in mm per unit time).

For example:

MS 26—Green (mm per 24 h, a **daily** rate)

$$\text{rate} = \frac{\text{measured 'length of volume' in mm}}{\text{delivery time in days}}$$

e.g. 48mm = 48mm per day

Rate on dial is 48

MS 16 A—Blue (mm per h)

$$\text{rate} = \frac{\text{measured 'length of volume' in mm}}{\text{delivery time in h}}$$

e.g. $\dfrac{48 \text{ mm}}{24 \text{ h}} = 2\text{mm per h}$

Rate on dial is 02

Problems

Infusion running too fast:	Check the rate setting and recalculate.
Infusion running too slow:	Check start button, battery, syringe driver, cannula and make sure injection site is not inflamed.
Site reaction:	Cyclizine and levomepromazine cause site reactions most commonly. Firmness or swelling is not necessarily a problem but the needle site should be changed if there is pain or obvious inflammation. If there is no alternative to subcutaneous administration of drugs it may be helpful to add dexamethasone 1mg to the mixture.
	A plastic/teflon needle may reduce local irritation if there is a nickel allergy

Precipitation

Check compatibility of drugs.

Check solution regularly for precipitation and discolouration and discard if it occurs. Cyclizine may precipitate at high doses, particularly in combination with high doses of diamorphine. Other combinations may also cause cloudiness in the syringe. On rare occasions a patient may need two or three separate syringe drivers to separate the drugs.

Light flashing
This is normal. The light flashes:
Blue—Once per second   Green—Once per 25 seconds

Flashing will stop when the battery needs changing. The syringe driver will continue to operate for 24 h after the light has stopped flashing.

Alarm
This always sounds when the battery is inserted. It can be silenced by pressing Start/Test button.

Check for—empty syringe—kinked tube—blocked needle/tubing—jammed plunger.

Drug compatibilities—usually max. 3 drugs in one syringe

Table 4.1 Examples of commonly used syringe driver preparations

Diamorphine	+Haloperidol	+Cyciizine**
Diamorphirie	+Haloperidbl	+Hyoscine Hydrobromide
Diamorphine	+Haloperidol	+Hyoscine Butylbromide
Diarnorphine	+Haloperidol	+Levomepromazine***
Diamorphine	+Haloperidol	+Midazolam
Diarnorphine	+Cyclizine**	+Hyoscine Hydrobrornide
Diamorphine	+Cyclizine**	+Levomepromazine***
Diamorphine	+Cyclizine**	+Midazolam
Diamorphine	+Midazolam	+Hyoscine Hydrobromide
Diamorphine	+Midazolam	+Hyoscine Butylbromide
Diamorphine	+Midazolam	+Levomepromazine***
Diamorphine	+Midazolam	+Glycopyrronium
Diamorphine	+Levomepromazine***	+Hyoscine Hydrobromide
Diamorphine	+Levomepromazine***	+Hyoscine Butylbromide
Diamorphine	+Levornepromazine***	+Glycopyrronium

**Cyclizine is incompatible with normal saline.

If needing to use a dose of cyclizine greater than 75mg/24 h in conjunction with a dose of diamorphine greater than 160mg/24 h, a 20ml b.d. syringe should be used. This will enable dilution to 14ml so that the medication remains compatible in the syringe.

***Levomepromazine can be irritant.

If skin site soreness becomes a problem, it is recommended to dilute it with sodium chloride 0.9% rather than water for injections. However, please note if diamorphine is combined with levomepromazine, sodium chloride 0.9% can only be used when diamorphine concentration is less than 40mg/ml. If the diamorphine concentration exceeds 40mg/ml, water for injections should be used. If skin site soreness is a problem in this instance, increase the size of syringe used. If other drugs are in the syringe, check these are compatible with saline.

Table 4.2 Common drugs, doses and ranges for palliative care use with a 24 h syringe driver

The following is a guide to drugs that may be used in a 24 h subcutaneous syringe driver. They may be used alone or in combinations. Advice should be sought when combining drugs or in exceptional circumstances.

All drugs should be mixed with WATER unless otherwise indicated.

Drug class of drug/ (Amp. size)	Indications	Compatibility	Contra-indications	Possible side-effects	p.r.n. dose onset of action	24h infusion dose ranges
Cyclizine Antihistaminic, antimuscarinic antiemetic (50mg/1ml)	Nausea and vomiting associated with motion sickness. Anticipatory nausea. Pharyngeal stimulation. Mechanical bowel obstruction, Raised intracranial Pressure	Can precipitate with dexamethasone, diamorphine (in higher doses), metoclopramide, midazolam and saline	No absolute ones in patients with advanced cancer Do not give with metoclopramide Do not give with levomepromazine Do not give with buscopan	Drowsiness, dry mouth, blurred vision, hypotension Injection can be painful Can be sedating If syringe driver site is irritated try to dilute further.	50mg i/m / SC every 8 h Within 2 h	50-150mg usual dose
Dexamethasone Corticosteroid 4(mg/ml)	Antiemetic Pain relief Raised Intracranial pressure	Mixes with metoclopramide Precipitates with cyclizine,	Diabetes—may need supervision	Gastro-intestinal side effects, Impaired healing.	Discuss with oncology/palliative care team	4-16mg usual dose

	Spinal cord compression intestinal obstruction	midazolam, haloperidol, levomepromazine, Advisable to put in separate driver but can mix with diamorphine	weight gain, hirsutism, increased appetite	Not usually needed
Diamorphine Opioid analgesic (5mg, 10mg, 30mg, 100mg, 500mg)	Pain Dyspnoea Cough Diarrhoea	None if titrated carefully against a patients' symptoms Modify dose in renal failure	Nausea Drowsiness Dry mouth Constipation Confusion Twitching	With most drugs	One sixth of total 24h infusion dose Within 10–30mins	Variable depending on total oral intake of morphine Conversion of oral morphine to subcutaneous diamorphine is 3:1
Diclofenac NSAID Non-opioid analgesic (75mg/3ml)	Pain (particularly associated with tissue inflammation or bone pain/movement related pain)	Incompatible with most drugs. Give in a separate syringe driver Use sodium chloride 0.9% for dilution **Do Not Mix**	Active peptic ulceration Urticaria Rhinitis Asthma Angioedema	Skin ulceration especially with prolonged use (SC)	75mg SC every 12 h (do not give as well as the infusion) Within 20–30 mins	75–20mg usual dose

Drug class of drug/ (Amp. size)	Indications	Compatibility	Contra-indications	Possible side-effects	p.r.n. dose onset of action	24h infusion dose ranges
Glycopyrronium bromide Quaternary ammonium antimuscarinic (0.2mg/ml, 0.6mg/3ml)	Death rattle Colic in inoperable bowel obstruction. Reduction of secretion May be effective if no response to hyoscine Anti-secretory effect Does not cross the blood brain barrier so does not cause drowsiness	With most drugs	2–5 times more potent than hyoscine hydrobromide	Tachycardia Dry mouth	0.2mg SC every 6–8 h Within 20–40 mins	0.6–1.2mg usual dose
Haloperidol Butyrophenone Antipsychotic (5mg/ml)	Nausea and vomiting Psychotic symptoms Agitated delirium Intractable hiccup	With most drugs	Parkinson's disease Possible CNS Depression with anxiolytics & alcohol	Extra-pyramidal symptoms, dry mouth, sedation, drowsiness, difficulty in micturition, hypotension, blurred vision	1.5–3mg SC daily to every 8 h Within 10–15mins	2.5–5mg usual dose for nausea and vomiting
Hyoscine butylbromide Antimuscarinic antispasmodic antisecretory	Obstructive symptoms with colic and antisecretory effects, Death rattle	With most drugs, except cyclizine	Narrow angle glaucoma (unless moribund), Myasthenia gravis.	Does not cross blood brain barrier so does not cause drowsiness	10–20mg SC every 8 h Within 3–5 mins	Bowel obstruction with colic: 60–120mg usual dose

Drug	Indications/uses	Interactions	Cautions	Side effects	Dose	Dose range
Hyoscine hydrobromide 0.4mg/1ml or 0.6mg/ml	Death rattle Colic Reduce salivation Some antiemetic action			Sedation	0.4mg	1.2–2.4mg
Levomepromazine Antiemetic phenothiazine antipsychotic (25mg/1ml)	Nausea and vomiting Insomnia Terminal agitation Intractable pain. Useful as antiemetic and sedation Can be very sedating	Precipitates with dexamethasone Do not use with cyclizine	Parkinson's disease, Postural hypotension, Antihypertensive therapy, Epilepsy, Hypothyroidism Myasthenia gravis	Sedation, dose dependent postural hypotension	6.25–12.5mg i/m/SC every 4–6 h usual dose within 30 minutes	6.25–25mg usual dose for nausea & vomiting 25–150mg usual dose terminal agitation
Metoclopramide Prokinetic antiemetic (10mg/2ml)	Nausea and vomiting caused by gastric irritation Delayed gastric emptying Stimulation of the CTZ Obstructive bowel symptoms without colic Non-sedating	With most drugs	Concurrent administration with antimuscarinic drugs, Concurrent i/v administration of 5-HT$_3$ receptor antagonists Do not give in bowel obstruction if colic present	Dizziness Diarrhoea Depression Extra-pyramidal effects	10–30mg i/m/SC every 8 h	60–120mg

Drug class of drug/ (Amp. size)	Indications	Compatibility	Contra-indications	Possible side-effects	p.r.n. dose onset of action	24h infusion dose ranges
Midazolam Benzodiazepine (10mg/2ml) Anxiolytic	Sedation for terminal agitation, Multifocal myoclonus Epilepsy Intractable hiccup Muscle spasm	With most drugs	Drowsiness, Hypotension	Dizziness, drowsiness	2.5–10mg SC every 4 h Within 5–10 mins	10–60mg usual dose
Octreotide Somatostatin analogues FOR SPECIALIST USE ONLY 50mcg/ml 100mcg/ml 200mcg/ml 500mcg/ml	Intestinal obstruction associated with vomiting intractable diarrhoea Symptoms associated with hormone secreting tumours Bowel fistulae Injection can be painful (gently hand warm the vial)	Precipitates with dexamethasone	Caution in diabetes mellitus may potentiate hypoglycaemia	Dry mouth, nausea, vomiting anorexia abdominal pain, flatulence	50–100 mcg SC every 8 h Within 30 mins	Intestinal obstruction: 300–600 mcg usual dose

Further reading

Books

Dickman A. *et al*. (2005) The syringe driver: continuous subcutaneous infusions in palliative care. 2nd edn. Oxford: Oxford University Press.

Reviews

Scottish Intercollegiate Guidelines Network, (2000) *Control of Pain in Patients with cancer a National Clinical Guideline*. Edinburgh: SIGN.

Chapter 5

Oncology and palliative care

The best sentence in the English language is not 'I love you' but 'It's benign'.

Woody Allen, *Deconstructing Harry*, 1998

The commonest cancers are of the lung, breast, skin, gastrointestinal tract, and the prostate gland.

Introduction

Cancer is an important cause of morbidity and mortality, particularly in industrialized countries. Currently in the UK one person in three will be diagnosed with cancer during their lifetime and one in five will die of their disease.

As 60 per cent of all cancers are diagnosed in those aged over 65 years, our rapidly increasing older population suggests that cancer will become an even more common problem in the coming decades.

Cancers may develop in all body tissues. The cells that form cancers can be differentiated from cells in normal tissues in a number of ways, including:

1 Cell division that has escaped the control of normal homeostasis
2 Abnormalities of cell differentiation—in general terms cancer cells tend to be less well differentiated than their non-malignant counterparts
3 Resistance to programmed cell death
4 The potential for cancerous cells to invade local tissues and metastasize

The development of cancer is associated with the accumulation of defects or 'mutations' in a number of critical genes within the cell.

Many cancers, for example, are associated with mutations leading to overactivity of growth promoting genes known commonly as oncogenes. Conversely cancers may also be associated with mutations leading to underactivity of genes which act to suppress growth.

Although our understanding of the genetic abnormalities underlying cancer has grown exponentially over the last decade, the factors that cause these changes are not clear for most cancers.

There is evidence that exogenous carcinogens may be closely linked to some cancers. Smoking, for example, is a causative factor in lung, cervix and bladder cancer.

In other cancers there is an inherited susceptibility to particular types of malignancy. In the majority of common cancers, however, the cause remains elusive. It is likely that for many of these cancers both environmental and genetic factors are implicated.

Organization of cancer care

Optimal care of the patient with cancer requires input from a number of medical disciplines. Typically a provisional diagnosis of cancer is made by a surgeon or physician and confirmed by a pathologist following biopsy or fine needle aspiration. A surgeon or an oncologist may then undertake definitive treatment. Support of the patient through treatment may well involve input from a wide range of surgical, medical, allied medicine health professionals and laboratory disciplines.

Several factors facilitate this care:

1 Good organization of cancer services
2 Cancer site specialization for surgeons and oncologists
3 Multidisciplinary team working
4 Well-established links with laboratory and clinical cancer research

The disease journey

A close working relationship between oncology and palliative care professionals is important. In the past, this relationship was not optimal due to misunderstandings of their different rôles and treatment aims. Increasingly now the goals are shared and closer working relationships are being forged, at different points along the patient's disease journey.

At time of original diagnosis

Oncological services, specialist and generalist palliative care services, including the General Practitioner and community health team, need to share information quickly so, at this point, when patient and family feel particularly vulnerable, informed support can be maximized.[1]

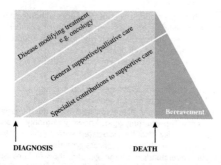

Disease modifying treatment e.g. oncology

General supportive/palliative care

Specialist contributions to supportive care

Bereavement

↑ **DIAGNOSIS**   ↑ **DEATH**

Traditionally palliative care services were only 'offered' to patients when 'there is nothing more that can be done'.

Increasingly palliative care is involved from the point of diagnosis with increasing input as the oncology needs decrease, maximizing at time of death and continuing on with bereavement support.

Through the period of staging and/or surgery

This can be a time of great uncertainty for patients, when communicating the often complex prognostic and treatment information is so important. Many find the issues very difficult to grasp, so vast are the associated life implications. An understanding of these issues and of the likely treatments by all those involved in the clinical and supportive care of patient and family can help to consolidate information transfer. It is often only a few days after a crucial oncology outpatient appointment that patients become receptive to important information.

If other healthcare professionals are hesitant or contradictory in their explanations of treatment options patient anxiety will be increased.

> 'When I was diagnosed with my bowel cancer I was simply devastated. You see, I had watched my father dying from lung cancer and I was sure I would go the same way. I could hardly get out of the hospital quickly enough to get my farm and affairs sorted out. The Doctor said something about treatment, but I knew from watching others with cancer that treatment was pointless, so I never went back for the cancer specialist appointment.
>
> It was only after my own Doctor came out and we had a good chat that I even thought that they could do anything for me. In the end I decided to go and see what they were offering, still never believing that they could do any good.
>
> I honestly believe if my own doctor hadn't taken the time to come and explain that there really was something they could do to help I would not been alive to enjoy these past six years.'

Through the period of treatment

While the majority of supportive care during this period tends to be linked through the oncology services, specialist and generalist palliative care teams need to be aware of the:
• Goals of treatment
• Side-effects of treatment
• Follow-up plans

The goals of oncology treatment

Before commencing any treatment it is important that both patient and carers are aware of the goals of treatment.

Frequently after what the consultant feels to have been a very full and frank discussion outlining these goals, a patient will ask a much more junior member of the team to clarify what has been said.

This may be because they do not wish to admit to not fully understanding what was being discussed; alternatively they may feel able to ask more questions from a member of the team whom they find more approachable.

It is also possible, particularly if the outlook is not good, that patients will ask different members of the team hoping to find a more optimistic prognosis. Clearly it is not in the patient's interest to hear conflicting opinions about their prognosis and this should be avoided.

1 National Council for Hospice and Specialist Palliative Care Services (2002) *Definitions of Supportive and Palliative Care*. London: NCHSPCS (Briefing Bulletin 11).

Openness regarding realistic treatment outcomes is also important in maintaining staff morale. While the death of a patient is often difficult, particularly for the nurses who are most closely involved in care, this is especially so if unrealistic expectations of treatment are fostered.

Radical oncological treatment

Radical oncological interventions are curative in intent. They may involve surgery, radiotherapy or chemotherapy (or a combination of these modalities).

Because the potential benefits of treatment are great, a relatively high incidence of drug toxicity side-effects is more acceptable.

Providing patients with good symptom control and emotional support through radical treatment is important. They need to be encouraged to complete what is often a very demanding treatment course in order to benefit maximally.

Without such encouragement patients may miss the only opportunity they have of cure.

Increasingly there is an appreciation that such treatments may be associated with long term toxicities/side-effects (which may be especially relevant for children). Clearly in this potentially curative group care must be taken to minimize the potential for cumulative dose toxicities such as cardiotoxity caused by anthracyclines.

Adjuvant oncological treatment

Many patients suffer tumour relapse following apparently curative surgery for their primary tumour. This is believed to be due to the presence of micrometastatic disease that is not clinically apparent at the time of the primary treatment.

Anticancer treatment (usually chemotherapy) given at this stage has been shown to improve long-term survival for some tumours.

This approach has proven successful even for tumours where chemotherapy is not curative in the metastatic setting, and is presumably related to the increased chemosensitivity associated with microscopic volumes of disease.

The absolute gains in survival from adjuvant chemotherapy are generally small but real. (Adjuvant chemotherapy in premenopausal women with breast cancer, for example, is associated with an approximately 30 per cent relative improvement in 10 year survival). At present there are few predictive factors to identify patients most likely to benefit from adjuvant therapy. The decision to proceed is often based on the statistical likelihood of relapse, with those at highest risk benefitting most.

The fact remains that the majority of patients will not benefit from adjuvant therapies. Such treatments should therefore have manageable acute toxicities and a low incidence of long-term toxicities.

Palliative oncological treatment

Palliative treatment is indicated when curative treatment is not possible but where treatments may have sufficient anticancer activity to improve cancer-related symptoms. In many cases improvement of symptoms is accompanied by tumour shrinkage detectable clinically or by radiological methods such as

CT scan or MRI. Increasingly, however, it is recognized that there may be a palliative benefit even in the absence of tumour shrinkage.

As the primary object of therapy is to improve quality of life, such treatments should be well tolerated with a low incidence of acute side-effects. Long-term toxicities are generally not relevant.

In some cases the distinction between radical and palliative treatment may not be absolutely clear cut. Indeed the aims of treatment may change as the disease progresses.

Patients presenting with advanced ovarian cancer, for example, have largely incurable disease. However, the tumour is often chemosensitive and lengthy remissions are often seen following primary chemotherapy. In such patients a relatively high incidence of acute toxicity may be acceptable, with efforts being focused on managing chemotherapy-related symptoms. Conversely, a patient presenting with relapsed ovarian cancer following first line chemotherapy has a low expectation of benefit from further chemotherapy. Consequently only a low incidence of acute toxicity is acceptable with second line chemotherapy, from which expectation of benefit is very limited.

For patients and carers who have been through radical or adjuvant therapy the switch to palliative treatment can be difficult to understand. Perhaps much of the 'bad press' that oncological care has received has been due to patients and relatives feeling that they were being given so called 'curative' treatments beyond the point when any cure was possible.

In particular patients and carers can be bemused that unlike when they were receiving radical or adjuvant therapy there is little emphasis placed on assessment scans and X rays as the key question now relates purely to how the patient is doing symptomatically.

Managing patients receiving oncology treatments

Chemotherapy and radiotherapy is now given largely on an outpatient basis. Surgical patients also spend less time in hospital than in the past. This allows patients to spend more time at home, but inevitably places an increased burden of care on those providing support in the community, particularly where the cancer centre is a long distance from home. Thus a general understanding of the particular side-effects, and the appropriate treatment for such complications, is needed increasingly by healthcare professionals in the community and those providing on-call services.

It should not be assumed automatically that a new symptom developing in a patient undergoing treatment for cancer is related to the side-effects of treatment or to the cancer itself, although the high possibility of this must be considered. (*Chemotherapy does not prevent patients developing appendicitis!*) Thus the health professional needs to assess each new symptom independently, and be aware of the side-effects of commonly used oncological treatment regimes. (📖 See the sections on chemotherapy and radiotherapy.)

Supportive teams need to know the significance and *appropriate responses for individual patients* to such side-effects as:

Clinical anaemia

Nausea and Vomiting

Pain

Pyrexia and possible infection
  What are the risks of neutropaenia for this patient?

Increased drowsiness

Confusion
  Could this patient be opioid toxic, hypercalcaemic, or developing renal failure?

Hair loss

Altered sensation, back pain, incontinence
  Could this patient be developing spinal cord compression?

The appropriate response and management will differ according to what the patient and their family want, the disease process, and where the patient is on their disease journey.

Treatment planning

It is important that treatment plans are communicated adequately to patients, families, and professional carers to ensure that appropriate support is given.

A basic management plan should include:

- Details of proposed diagnostic and staging investigations
- Proposed treatment plan for surgery, chemotherapy and radiotherapy where appropriate. The plan should include details regarding the duration of treatment and timing of interval investigations to assess response to therapy. (Patients can be understandably anxious in the days preceding a scan aimed at assessing response to treatment.)
- Changes to treatment dosages or frequency including reasons for change
- Particular side-effects of treatment to watch out for, and specific advice on what to do if these signs or symptoms develop
- Clear instructions about how long treatments such as antibiotics or steroids should be administered or tailed off
- Treatment goals
- Details of significant conversations with patients and their carers relating to their understanding of their disease and their wishes for further treatment
- Clear details of who to contact in case of treatment complications

No single set of healthcare professionals can manage the many needs that patients have on their disease journey. Holistic, patient-centred, care requires a multi-professional and multi-disciplinary approach that places the patient and their family at the centre.

To facilitate improvements in communication many centres are now using patient-held records on which the different professionals record their findings and management plans, thus improving the continuity of care. With the increasing demand for transparency in care from patient groups, and the importance of ongoing care, such systems may well become normative in the UK.

Clinical trials

Clinical research is necessary in order to improve outcomes for patients with cancer. The link between the laboratory and the clinic is developing and increasingly patients are being recruited into trials.

There are three main types of clinical trial:

Phase I

Aim:
- To establish the human toxicity of a new drug through delivering carefully selected increasing doses to patients
- To establish the safe dose at which to start further trials with the drug
- To evaluate the body's handling of the drug by pharmacokinetic studies

Eligible patients
- Patients who have progressive disease despite standard oncological therapy or those for whom no standard therapy exists
- Patients must be aware that the primary objective of the studies is to assess toxicity. There is little expectation of benefit for themselves, with a response rate of approximately 5 per cent
- Patients recruited to Phase I trials usually have a high performance status and are highly motivated individuals, since involvement often requires intensive lengthy monitoring as an inpatient

Phase II

Aim:
- To establish the antitumour activity of the drug for a particular tumour type

Eligible patients
- Patients who have progressive disease despite standard chemotherapy or for whom no standard therapy exists
- Patients usually have a high performance status and are highly motivated
- Patients are closely monitored with toxicity and response assessments but not as intensively as those in Phase I studies

Phase III

Aim:
- To compare the new drug or drug combination with conventional therapy.

Eligible patients
- Patients for whom a standard therapy exists. (New drugs may also be compared with 'best supportive care' where no standard therapy exists.)

Important and common end points include disease free survival (in adjuvant studies), and overall survival (in palliative studies). Increasingly more clinically relevant end points such as improvements in pain, performance status and weight gain and quality of life are being used in Phase III trials of palliative agents.

Typically Phase III trials are much larger than Phase I/II trials and patients require less frequent monitoring.

Oncological surgery[2]

Surgery remains the modality of treatment most likely to cure patients diagnosed with solid tumours. It has most potential when the cancer is localized, though results are improving for patients with certain types of metastatic tumours.

Surgery has three main rôles in cancer management.

1 Diagnosis and staging
2 Curative treatment
3 Palliative treatment

Diagnosis and staging

In the past, many patients suspected of having cancer required surgery to confirm the diagnosis. The development of cross-sectional radiology and the ability to perform diagnostic biopsies using radiological guidance or endoscopy now often allows accurate diagnosis.

Patient morbidity has significantly reduced now that major diagnostic surgical procedures are no longer needed. The number of 'open and close' laparotomies for unresectable cancer, for example, has reduced to <5 per cent in recent years, largely due to these advances.

However surgical staging remains important in a number of common tumours:

- Axillary lymph node dissection for patients with breast cancer, for example, allows assessment of these nodes for involvement by tumour. Such information is important in determining prognosis and guiding decisions regarding adjuvant treatments
- Ovarian cancer spreads mainly via the transperitoneal route leading to tumour deposits in peritoneal surfaces and the omentum—sites poorly visualized on conventional imaging. A laparotomy for patients with ovarian cancer therefore allows a more accurate staging of disease than is currently possible with non-invasive means. Again such information is vital in determining prognosis and guiding further treatment

Curative surgery

Non-metastatic disease

Surgery is most commonly curative in intent for localized cancers and is generally dependent on complete resection of the tumour with a margin of normal tissue.

In some tumours with a propensity to spread to lymph nodes, resection of the draining lymph nodes may improve local control (e.g. vulval tumours). In other tumours the value of lymphadenectomy is uncertain and is the subject of ongoing clinical trials (e.g. endometrial cancer).

Unfortunately surgery still fails to cure many patients. There are a number of reasons for this:

1 Development of metastatic disease—this is due to the presence of micro-metastatic disease unidentifiable at the time of surgery. This is a common reason for failure of surgery to cure breast and bowel tumours
2 Development of local relapse—outcomes from surgery are often closely linked to the margin of normal tissue excised in continuity with

the tumour. The amount of tissue that can be resected may be limited by patient-related factors (e.g. only a partial lobectomy may be possible in patients with lung cancer due to the patients' underlying poor respiratory function) or by tumour related factors. (e.g. invasion by tumour of a vital structure such as the aorta.)

Metastatic disease

Although much less common, surgery may be curative in a limited number of tumours in the metastatic setting. The rôle for potentially curative surgery is best established in a small number of instances. These include:

- Pulmonary metastases from osteosarcoma
- Pulmonary metastases from soft tissue sarcoma
- Liver metastases from colorectal cancer
- Residual masses following chemothearpy for metastatic teratomas.

In each of these cases best results are seen with careful patient selection according to well defined criteria. In general terms the best long-term results are seen in patients who relapse after a long period from initial tumour diagnosis and who have low volume disease and a good performance status.

Palliative surgery

Surgery may provide very effective palliation in a number of situations. Given the specific problems of oncology patients in the palliative situation (limited life expectancy, poor performance status, rapid tumour progression), the decision to proceed with surgery must involve a careful weighing up of the benefit/harm of such procedures. These decisions are best made with a multidisciplinary approach by surgeons specialized in oncology and experienced in palliative management.

Bowel obstruction

Patients with colonic or ovarian cancer form the majority of patients with bowel obstruction referred for surgery. Surgery to relieve the obstruction is warranted even if disease is incurable (due to liver metastases or locally advanced disease for example) as such patients may live for many months. Where possible these patients should have the primary tumour excised and a primary anastomosis performed.

Patients with ovarian cancer commonly present with obstructive bowel symptoms. At initial presentation debulking surgery provides excellent palliation. Patients presenting with relapsed disease and obstructive symptoms often have multiple sites of obstruction due to widespread intraperitoneal dissemination of their disease. In this instance surgery is much less likely to be useful.

Fistulae

Fistulae may arise as a result of pelvic tumours or as a complication of radiotherapy. They are often associated with unpleasant symptoms. Optimum preoperative assessment requires imaging to delineate exactly the site of fistula formation and to guide surgical decisions. Surgery may provide excellent palliation but may not be useful in those with multiple

2 Cassidy J., Bissett D. et al. (2002) Oxford Handbook of Oncology. Oxford: Oxford University Press.

sites of fistulae or rapidly advancing intra-abdominal disease where life expectancy is limited.

Jaundice

Obstructive jaundice due to extrinsic pressure by lymph nodes on the biliary system, or due to intrinsic lesions such as cholangiocarcinoma, are commonly well palliated by radiological and endoscopic placement of stents.

The complications of stents include infection and blockage with consequent need for replacement.

Surgical relief of obstructive jaundice (e.g. by choledochoenterostomy) avoids problems associated with stents and may be indicated in a small minority of patients with an excellent performance status and slow-growing disease.

Pain

Surgical debulking of large slow-growing tumours can reduce pain and is justified in patients where the expected morbidity of the procedure is low. Neurosurgical approaches such as cordotomy are only infrequently considered.

Gastrointestinal bleeding

A wide range of endoscopic techniques have been developed to stop bleeding from benign and malignant causes. This may avoid the need for more major surgery in patients who have a limited life expectancy.

These include:

- Sclerotherapy
- Laser coagulation
- Radiological embolization

Bone metastases

Metastases to bones can cause major palliative problems. Specific problems include pain and pathological fracture. Factors that identify patients most at risk of pathological fracture include:

- Site—lesions in weight-bearing bones
- Extent of destruction—destruction of >50 per cent of cortex
- Symptoms—patients complaining of pain, particularly on weight bearing
- Type of lesion—lytic lesions > blastic lesions

Such patients may benefit (both in terms of reduced pain and reduced risk of fracture) from prophylactic fixation of a long bone. The type of internal fixation used depends on the site of fracture and the patient's performance status. In all cases internal fixation of the bone should be followed by radiotherapy to control tumour growth and promote healing.

Techniques such as vertebroplasty are available to manage pain in vertebrae.

Chemotherapy

I am dying from the treatment of too many physicians

Alexander the Great

Identification of agents

Chemotherapy generally refers to a group of agents used in the systemic management of cancer. A disparate group, they are linked by having demonstrated evidence of anticancer activity and a common range of side-effects.

The anticancer activity of these agents has been identified in a number of ways. For some the discovery of antineoplastic activity was serendipitous. Cisplatin was discovered because of using platinum electrodes in an antibiotic experiment.

For others this activity was identified during screening of a wide range of natural products (e.g. paclitaxel). Some of these agents have been biochemically modified to reduce their toxicity while retaining their anti-neoplastic activity (e.g. carboplatin).

Mechanism of action

Chemotherapy exerts its anticancer action by a wide variety of mechanisms which are, as yet, incompletely understood (see Table 5.1).

For many, DNA is believed to be the most important cellular target—irinotecan for example inhibits the topoisomerase I enzyme thereby causing double strand breaks in DNA. For other agents, microtubules, particularly those involved in formation of the mitotic spindle, appear to be the vital target—paclitaxel for example promotes tubulin polymerization and so arrests cells in metaphase.

A number of factors determine the likelihood of achieving a useful response to chemotherapy. Some tumours are inherently more sensitive to chemotherapy than others. In general terms chemotherapy tends to be most effective in tumours with fast cell turnover such as acute leukaemias and high grade lymphomas. Seminomas, however, a tumour with a long natural history, are also very chemosensitive. Clearly there are other factors, as yet poorly understood, that determine a tumour's chemosensitivity.

Patient-related factors are also important in determining likelihood of response. Patients with poor performance status, for example, respond less well than those with good performance status. The reasons for this are poorly understood but are probably due at least in part to a reduced tolerance to the acute toxicity of chemotherapy.

While chemotherapy may induce a partial or even complete response, the tumour may regrow with disease that has become chemoresistant. There is evidence in some cases that the tumour may have become more efficient at 'effluxing' the drug from the cell. Increasingly it is recognized that the ability of cells either to repair or tolerate the damage inflicted by chemotherapy may lead to chemoresistance. The causes of chemoresistance and the development of agents to overcome such mechanisms are active areas of research at present.

Tumours which divide rapidly with short doubling times respond best to chemotherapy.

Adverse effects of chemotherapy

Although the specific side-effect profile varies between agents, there are a number of side-effects common to most agents.

- *Alopecia* is a common and often distressing side-effect associated with many agents. Patients can be reassured that hair almost always regrows following chemotherapy although they may notice some changes. The hair may change colour and there can be a change in curliness

- *Nausea and vomiting* are common with many agents, although the degree to which this is a problem varies both between agents and between patients. The development of 5-HT$_3$ antagonists (e.g. tropisetron, granisetron) has greatly aided the management of this troublesome side-effect. The efficacy of 5-HT$_3$ antagonists can be improved by the addition of steroids

- *Myelosuppression* is another troublesome effect associated with chemotherapy. The white cells (in particular the neutrophils) are most commonly affected between 1 to 2 weeks following chemotherapy. Patients should be warned of the possibility of developing infection during this time and the urgency with which they should seek help, as they will require immediate treatment with broad spectrum antibiotics. The development of granulocyte colony stimulating growth factors has reduced this toxicity by shortening the duration of neutropaenia. This has allowed higher doses of chemotherapy to be given more safely in certain situations

- *Anxiety* The prospect of chemotherapy is a frightening concept for many patients—not least due to the (often mistaken) view of the difficult side-effects. It is important that the patient and their carers are fully educated about the type of side-effects they are likely to encounter during treatment and how best to deal with them. Most patients are extremely anxious during this difficult time and information may have to be repeated a number of times. It is very useful to have written information to supplement what has been said in consultations. It also useful if a relative or friend attends with the patient—they will often be able to help the patient review the information at a later date

Chemotherapy regimens

A wide and somewhat bewildering number of chemotherapy regimens are used in the treatment of patients with cancer. In general terms the tendency has been to combine drugs that demonstrate activity as single agents but which do not share the same side-effects.

More sophisticated techniques to examine synergy and pharmacokinetic interactions in a pre-clinical setting are now developing, and this will guide a logical approach to optimal combinations of agents.

Chemotherapy may be given in the following situations:

- Curative
- Adjuvant
- Neo-adjuvant
- Palliative

Curative

A small number of solid malignancies are curable by chemotherapy alone. Such tumours include germ cell tumours, lymphomas and certain childhood tumours.

In general terms chemotherapy regimens used in the treatment of these diseases are intensive and associated with a high incidence of acute toxicity. It is important that patients receive chemotherapy on schedule, with no delays, as there is evidence that dose reductions and prolonging treatment times may adversely affect outcome. Consequently treatment can exact a high physical and psychological toll on patients and their relatives.

Given that the long term aim of treatment is cure, patients and their carers need encouragement to persevere, which will be easier if physical symptoms are optimally managed. The palliative care team may well provide expert assistance at this stage of the patient's management.

Increasingly it is becoming clear that patients who are cured following chemotherapy are at risk of long-term toxicity from their treatment. Such problems include secondary leukaemias and solid tumours, fatigue, infertility and cardiomyopathy. These problems have only become appreciated in recent times. Undoubtedly as more people become long-term survivors of cancer, more problems will emerge. For this reason it is important that long-term survivors of cancer remain on long term follow-up.

Adjuvant

Many patients presenting with apparently localized cancer are known to be at high risk of developing metastatic disease. This is presumed to be due to the presence of micrometastases not apparent by current imaging modalities. Chemotherapy given following successful primary treatment for apparently localized cancer may reduce the risk of developing clinical metastatic disease.

Cancers where adjuvant chemotherapy is commonly used include breast and colorectal cancer where large multi-centre randomized controlled trials and subsequent meta-analysis have confirmed the survival gain.

At an individual level these gains are small, with absolute improvements in overall survival of 5–15 per cent after five years. At a population level, however, this represents a large number of lives saved in diseases as common as breast and bowel cancer.

Presently surrogate markers such as tumour size, grade and lymph node involvement are commonly used to assess risk of disease relapse and thereby identify those most likely to benefit from adjuvant therapy. Much current research is directed at developing predictive markers to identify more precisely those most likely to benefit.

Given that the majority of patients treated will not benefit from treatment as their disease will relapse anyway or because primary treatment has been curative, adjuvant regimens must therefore be well tolerated with a low incidence of serious acute side-effects and long-term side-effects.

Again, as with treatment in the curative setting, positive outcomes from treatment are closely linked to maintaining dose intensity and avoiding delays in chemotherapy. Where acute toxicities are a problem, involvement of the palliative care team may improve symptom management and facilitate delivery of treatment on schedule.

Neo-adjuvant

Chemotherapy may be used 'up front' in non-metastatic tumours prior to definitive treatment (usually surgery) for the tumour. This may be done in the case of a large inoperable primary tumour to shrink the cancer and facilitate surgery. Such an approach is standard practice for example in very large primary breast tumours or those with skin involvement.

Increasingly neo-adjuvant therapy is being utilized for tumours that are operable. Potential advantages of this approach include less extensive surgery in a tumour that has shrunk. From a research point of view a neo-adjuvant approach with biopsies before and after therapy may allow molecular markers that predict chemosensitivity to be identified.

Conversely there are a number of potential problems with neo-adjuvant chemotherapy. First, in a responding tumour there may be a loss of potentially useful prognostic information from the subsequently resected tumour specimen. There is also the risk that such an approach may allow interim tumour progression in a lesion that does not respond to chemotherapy. Finally performing less radical surgery in a tumour that has responded to chemotherapy may compromise local control.

This approach is being examined with particular interest in a number of tumours including oesophageal, gastric and breast tumours.

> Growth for the sake of growth is the ideology of the cancer cell.
> Edward Abbey 1927–1989

Palliative

The majority of solid cancers are not curable in the metastatic setting. Chemotherapy, however, may have a valuable rôle to play in the palliative treatment of such patients. Research now includes end points such as quality of life and toxicity, which is more clinically relevant in this setting than assessing overall survival as a sole entity.

Given that improvement or maintenance of quality of life is the most important aim of palliative chemotherapy, acute toxicities must be infrequent and easily managed.

Optimally a patient is best managed when chemotherapy is administered *in conjunction with* input from the palliative care team. Such input also facilitates the gradual handing over of care to the palliative care team as the patient's disease progresses. Such a team-based approach reduces problems of patients feeling neglected by their oncologist when chemotherapy is no longer useful.

Indications for palliative chemotherapy

> 'Treatment decisions are based on a consideration of the balance between the benefits expected and the toxicity and risks of chemotherapy which are different for each patient'.[3]

1 Maintaining or improving quality of life: This is the single most important aim of palliative chemotherapy. Chemotherapy may alleviate specific symptoms such as dyspnoea or chest pain in a patient with lung cancer. It may also improve or maintain general well-being with improvements in such factors as appetite and energy. The development of quality of life assessment tools, especially those with disease-specific elements, has greatly facilitated the assessment of the effect of chemotherapy on quality of life

---

3 McIllmurray M. (2004) Palliative medicine and the treatment of cancer. In D. Doyle, G. Hanks, and N. Cherney (eds). *Oxford Textbook of Palliative Medicine*, p 232. Oxford: Oxford University Press.

2 **Improving survival:** While this is a secondary objective in most cases, it is quite clear that chemotherapy given with palliative intent frequently prolongs survival. The extent to which it is expected that survival may be prolonged varies between diseases. Chemotherapy in pancreatic cancer is associated with an improvement in survival of only a few weeks, whereas patients receiving chemotherapy for ovarian cancer may have improved survival of many months or even years

3 **In emergency situations:** Potentially life-threatening tumour-related emergencies such as spinal cord compression or superior vena cava compression may be treated with chemotherapy where the primary tumour is very chemosensitive. Such tumours include lymphoma and small cell lung cancer

Chemotherapy within the palliative setting is increasingly common because of:

Earlier referral for palliative care services
Chemotherapeutic services and palliative care services will only be enhanced by a close working relationship with good lines of communication, early referral, and a seamless highway of care along which a patient can receive the specific form of care they need for the particular part of their journey. The journey from diagnosis to death is not linear but dynamic with different interventions governed not by the passage of time but by a patient's particular needs. With an integrated service and earlier referral patterns there will be an ever increasing number of patients in the palliative care setting who have just had, are having, or are just about to have, chemotherapy. In many cancer centres patients will be introduced to the palliative care team as part of their initial contact with 'the cancer service'.

Increasing indications for chemotherapy
Over the last decade there has been a huge increase in the number of drugs available to treat cancer patients and clinical trials have identified that these agents may provide palliative benefit in those for whom no treatment would have been available 20 years ago.

Patients undergoing clinical trials
Patients who have relapsed from their initial chemotherapy may well be involved in clinical trials of other agents if their overall fitness and clinical condition permits. As trials often involve treatments where conventional regimes have failed, such patients are often quite advanced in their disease, and in need of increasing palliative care input.

When is chemotherapy offered in the palliative care setting?
The decision to use chemotherapy with palliative intent is often a complex matter, and a number of factors must be taken into consideration:
• **Patient fitness**—Generally patients with ECOG performance status (see the box on p.xxxi) >2 tolerate chemotherapy very poorly—chemotherapy is contra-indicated in such patients. Possible exceptions include patients with very chemosensitive tumours that may be expected to respond quickly such as small cell lung cancer and lymphoma

- **Patient symptoms**—Chemotherapy in the palliative setting is generally delayed until the patient develops symptoms. The potential danger with this approach is that the patient may rapidly develop symptoms which render them unfit for chemotherapy. In some cases, therefore, oncologists may choose to monitor disease and institute treatment when there is evidence that disease, although asymptomatic, is progressing
- **Disease sites** —Generally large volume disease at life-threatening sites such as the liver requires urgent chemotherapy even in the absence of disease-related symptoms, unless the patient is imminently dying, as patients are likely to become symptomatic very quickly. Close relationships may build up between doctors and patients over many years. It may be difficult for doctors to withdraw toxic oncological treatment from a patient who continues to demand it, even if it has now become clearly inappropriate. Clear and open discussion with patients and their family about the potential benefits and risks of chemotherapy, the aims of treatment and, in particular, agreements for stopping treatment is important. The palliative care team may be helpful in supporting the oncology team with these discussions

How will chemotherapy affect the patient and family?'

Each individual patient and family will have their own particular response to chemotherapy in the palliative care setting. Certain themes may be common to many such individuals. The following are some of the scenarios encountered in GP surgeries, oncology services and palliative care units.

1 **'We've got to keep on trying.'** Having endured the rigours of their disease and its management, some patients reach the palliative setting protesting their capacity as 'fighters'. (There is now evidence that psychological disposition has no bearing on disease outcome.) They have coped with their disease by trusting in the system and in being 'active' in fighting their cancer. It is very hard to wean such patients off chemotherapy or to stop active treatment as to do so seems, in their eyes, to admit defeat. Such patients will ask to be put into trials and see their rôle as patients as being fulfilled only so long as they are participating in active treatment

2 **'It was not half as bad as I thought it was going to be.'** Increasingly due to improved symptom control measures and a more holistic approach, patients may be pleasantly surprised by their tolerance of chemotherapy. Most people have had a previous contact with someone going through chemotherapy and their expectations are often adversely affected by this

3 **'He has suffered enough.'** Other families come through their disease journey with very ambivalent attitudes towards the system and to chemotherapy. They arrive in the palliative care setting determined that further suffering should be kept to a minimum. They can be reluctant to consider any intervention at all, other than the administration of pain controlling medications. For such a family the prospect of chemotherapy entering into the palliative setting is anathema, and time may need to be taken to explain the benefits in certain situations, if appropriate

4 **'Her hair fell out, then she died.'** Many patients and families come with memories and histories of relatives who have received chemotherapy in the past. Memories seldom show clearly the distinction between problems caused by the illness itself and problems caused by side-effects. The two merge into a mess of suffering leaving the patient and the family convinced that there is only one thing worse than dying with cancer—and that is dying from cancer with the side-effects of chemotherapy. Doctors and nurses are not inured from such emotional responses

5 **'Whatever you say Doctor.'** Another group of patients cope with their disease by investing their trust in 'the doctor' looking after them. Such an approach runs contrary to non-patronizing modern trends but is still present particularly among older patients. To present such patients with a meta-analysis of the benefits of one form of chemotherapy or another and to ask the patient which one he wants to choose would be inappropriate

6 **'What about Mexican dog weed.'** Some patients and relatives may come into the palliative care setting clutching reams of printouts from the Internet about treatments from clinics around the world. They will often be very articulate and questioning of every intervention. Some will have an alternative medicine approach and be very sceptical of western medicine. Honest communication needs to include how health professionals interpret the clinical research literature and what they would be prepared to do in terms of agreeing to provide a treatment that is controversial, unproven and unlicenced. Boundaries need to be set and unrealistic expectations dispelled alongside not removing hope that a reasonable quality of life can still be achieved

7 **'I've had a good life.'** A section of patients come into the palliative setting without illness at the centre of their lives. Instead they are focused on their living and their dying, with its important stages and goodbyes. Such patients have accepted the inevitability of their death and have moved on to preparing for it. They have things that they want to do. When it comes to the possibility of chemotherapy for such people their main concern is, 'Will it interfere with what I still have to do?' They are strangely neutral about chemotherapy and it is almost as if they are humouring the professionals by agreeing to it, while they get on with the real business of living

8 **'I just can't face it.'** Some patients have been so worn down by their disease and treatment that the prospect of any more chemotherapy fills them with fear and dread. Sometimes the fears are justified and sometimes they are not. Sometimes their expression of fear about chemotherapy is a way of verbalizing fears about other matters which should be explored. They face the dilemma of risks and fears whether or not they accept chemotherapy and will need a lot of support in reaching a treatment decision

Cytotoxic drugs

Alkylating agents
Damage DNA by addition of an alkyl group eg. cyclophosphamide, ifosfamide, melphalan, busulphan.

Platinum agents
Damage DNA by addition of platinum adducts e.g. cisplatin, carboplatin, oxaliplatin.

Antimetabolites
Inhibit production of pyrimidine and purine metabolites e.g. fluorouracil, methotrexate, capecitabine, mercaptopurine, gemcitabine.

Antitumour antibiotics
Variable mechanism e.g. doxorubicin, epirubicin, mitoxantrone, bleomycin.

Vinca alkaloids
Bind to the tubulin blocking microtubule and therefore interfere with spindle formation at metaphase e.g. vincristine, vinorelbine, vinblastine.

Taxanes
Promote tubulin polymerization and arrest cells at metaphase e.g. paclitaxel, docetaxel.

Topoisomerase I inhibitors
Inhibit topoisomerase I leading to DNA damage e.g. irinotecan, topotecan.

Hormonal agents
Selective Oestrogen Receptor Modulators (SERMs)
Partial antagonists of the oestrogen receptor e.g. tamoxifen.

Aromatase inhibitors
Inhibit extragonadal oestrogen production e.g. anastrozole, letrozole.

Gonadorelin analogues
Inhibit gonadal production of oestrogen and testosterone e.g. leuprorelin, goserelin.

Anti-androgens
- Testosterone receptor antagonists
- Cyproterone acetate

Immunomodulatory
- e.g. Interferon

Novel agents
Many anticancer agents currently in development have been rationally developed to antagonize elements of the neoplastic process at a cellular level. While most of these agents are still in preclinical or early clinical testing, a number have already entered routine clinical practice. As a rule these agents are much better tolerated than conventional cytotoxic drugs with less myelosuppression, alopecia and emesis. Preclinical testing

suggests that many may act as cytostatics rather than cytotoxics and that there may be syergistic interactions with other drugs. The challenge in the future will be the rational design of clinical trials to investigate how these agents are best used.

Antibodies

- **Herceptin**—a monoclonal antibody to HER-2—a member of the epidermal growth factor receptors over-expressed in approximately 25 per cent of all breast cancers and associated with poor prognosis. Herceptin has demonstrated activity in HER-2 over-expressing tumours both alone and in combination with chemotherapy
- **Rituximab**—a monoclonal antibody to CD-20, a protein expressed in some lymphomas. Again rituximab is active both alone and in combination with chemotherapy

Tyrosine kinase inhibitors

Many of the signalling pathways within a cell involved in the cancer phenotype rely on enzymes called tyrosine kinases. Interruption of this activity may interrupt signalling pathways involved in cancer.

- **Iressa**—inhibits the tyrosine kinase activity of the epidermal growth factor receptor activity demonstrated as a second line agent in non-small cell lung cancer. Common side-effects include diarrhoea and skin rashes
- **Imatinib**—inhibits the tyrosine kinase activity of the S-kit proteins found in gastrointestinal stromal tumours and also of the BCR/ABL fusion protein found in chronic myeloid leukaemia

Table 5.1 Classification of anticancer agents

Class of agent		Mode of action	Examples in common usage
Cytotoxics	Alkylating agents	Damage DNA by addition of an alkyl group	Cyclophosphamide, ifosfamide, melphalan, busulphan
	Platinum agents	Damage DNA by addition of platinum adducts	Cisplatin, carboplatin, oxaliplatin
	Antimetabolites	Inhibit production of pyrimidine and purine metabolites	fluorouracil, metotrexate, capecitabine, mercaptopurine, gemcitabine
	Antitumour antibiotics	Variable	Doxorubicin, epirubicin, mitoxantrone, bleomycin
	Vinca alkaoids	Bind to tubulin blocking microtubule and therefore spindle formation at metaphase	Vincristine, vinorelbine, vinblastine
	Taxanes	Promote tubulin polymerization and arrest cells at metaphase	Paclitaxel, docetaxel
	Topoisomerase I inhibitors	Inhibit topoisomerase I leading to DNA damage	Irinotecan, topotecan
Hormonal agents	Selective oestrogen receptor modulators (SERMs)	Partial antagonists of the oestrogen receptor	Tamoxifen
	Aromatase inhibitors	Inhibit extragonadal oestrogen production	Anastrozole, letrozole
	Gonadorelin analogues	Inhibit gonadal production of oestrogen and testosterone	Leuprorelin
	Antiandrogens	Testosterone receptor antagonists	Cyproterone acetate
Immuno- modulatory	Interferon		
'Novel' agents	Antibodies	Opsonization, interrupt growth stimulatory pathways	Rituximab, trastuzumab
	Signal transduction inhibitors	Interrupt growth stimulatory pathways	Imatinib, iressa
	Vascular targeting agents	Target 'new' vessels associated with tumours, not in use outwith a clinical trial	Bevacizumab

Table 5.2 Commonly used anticancer drugs (new drugs are regularly being introduced)

Drug	Administration	Excretion	Side-effects	Indications
Bleomycin *Cytotoxic antibiotic*	i/v	Excretion: Urine	'Flu symptoms; Hyperpigmentation; Allergic reactions; Pulmonary fibrosis— common with doses >300 mg	Germ cell tumours Lymphoma
Busulphan *Alkylating agent*	p.o	Excreted in urine	Myelosuppression; Hyperpigmentation Pulmonary interstitial fibrosis; Hepato-venous occlusion	Leukaemia
Caelyx see doxorubicin				
Carboplatin	i/v	Renal	Myelosuppression especially thrombocytopaenia; Emesis	Ovarian cancer
Capecitabine *Antimetabolite*	p.o	Renal	'Hand foot' syndrome; Diarrhoea Stomatitis	Colorectal cancer Breast cancer
Cisplatin	i/v	Renal	Emesis; Renal Failure; Peripheral neuropathy; Ototoxicity; Allergic reactions	Germ cell tumours Lung cancer
Cyclophosphamide *Alkylating agent*	p.o	Hepatic and renal	Myelosuppression; Alopecia; Emesis Haemorrhagic cystitis (reduced by mesna)	Breast cancer Lymphoma
Cytarabine *Antimetabolite*	i/v, i/t, SC	Hepatic and renal	Myelosuppression; Diarrhoea; Stomatitis	Leukaemia
Dactinomycin *Cytotoxic antibiotic*	i/v	Hepatic and renal	Myelosuppression; Mucositis; Diarrhoea Alopecia	Choriocarcinoma Ewing's sarcoma

Drug	Administration	Excretion	Side-effects	Indications
Docetaxel *Taxane*	i/v	Hepatic	Myelosuppression; Fluid retention Alopecia; Peripheral neuropathy	Breast cancer
Doxorubicin (Adriamycin) *Cytotoxic antibiotic*	i/v and intravesical	Hepatic	Emesis; Myelosuppression; Mucositis Alopecia; Cardiomyopathy—risk related to total cumulative dose.	Breast cancer Sarcoma
Doxorubicin Liposomal (Caelyx) *Cytotoxic antibiotic*	i/v	Hepatic	Palmar-plantar erythrodysaesthesia; Stomatitis	Ovarian cancer Breast cancer Kaposi's sarcoma
Etoposide	i/v	Renal	Myelosuppression; Emesis; Alopecia Secondary leukaemia	Lung cancer Germ cell tumour
Epirubicin *Cytotoxic antibiotic*	i/v	Hepatic	Similar to Doxorubicin but less cardiotoxic	Breast cancer
Fluorouracil *Antimetabolite*	i/v, topical cream	Liver and renal	Mucositis; Diarrhoea; Hand-foot syndrome; Myelosuppression; Gastrointestinal upsets; Cerebellar ataxia (rare); Gritty eyes and blurred vision	Colorectal cancer Breast cancer
Gemcitabine *Antimetabolite*	i/v	Renal	Myelosuppression; 'Flu like symptoms; Fatigue; Pneumonitis	Pancreatic cancer Bladder cancer Lung cancer

Drug	Route	Elimination	Side effects	Indications
Ifosfamide *Alkylating agent*	i/v	Hepatic and renal	Alopecia; Emesis; Haemorrhagic cystitis; Encephalopathy	Sarcomas
Irinotecan *Topoisomerase inhibitor*	i/v	Hepatic and renal	Cholinergic syndrome—associated with infusion; Delayed diarrhoea; Nausea and vomiting; Myelosuppression; Alopecia	Colorectal cancer
Mercaptopurine *Antimetabolite*	p.o	Peripheral tissues	Myelosuppression; Hepatic dysfunction; Stomatitis	Leukaemia
Methotrexate (+ folinic acid) *Antimetabolite*	p.o, i/v, i/m, i/t p.o.	Renal	Myelosuppression; Mucositis; Skin pigmentation; Nephrotoxicity	Osteosarcoma Breast cancer Leukaemia and lymphoma
Mitomycin *Cytotoxic antibiotic*	i/v or intravesical	Hepatic metabolism	Myelosuppression; Lung fibrosis; Nephrotoxicity Stomatitis; Diarrhoea; Haemolytic uraemic syndrome	Anal Bladder

Drug	Administration	Excretion	Side-effects	Indications
Mitoxantrone *Cytotoxic antibiotic*	i/v	Excretion: Bile > urine	Myelosuppression; Emesis; Alopecia; Mucositis; Cardiotoxicity	Lymphoma Leukaemia
Oxaliplatin	i/v	Renal	Peripheral neuropathy; Myelosuppression; Nausea and vomiting; Laryngeal spasm	Colorectal cancer
Paclitaxel *(Taxane)*	i/v	Hepatic	Myelosuppression; Alopecia; Hypersensitivity reactions; Peripheral neuropathy	Ovarian cancer Lung cancer Breast cancer
Temozolomide *Alkylating agent*	p.o.		Emesis; Myelosuppression	Astrocytomas Melanoma
Tioguanine *Antimetabolite*	p.o. (40 mg)	Renal	Myelosuppression; Mucositis; Diarrhoea; Hepatic dysfunction	Leukaemia
Thiotepa *Alkylating agent*	i/v	Excreted more in urine than bile	Myelosuppression	Leukaemia

Topotecan *Topoisomerase inhibitor*	i/v	Liver metabolism Urine excretion	Myelosuppression; Emesis; Alopecia; Diarrhoea	Ovarian cancer
Vinblastine *Mitotic spindle inhibitor*	i/v	Hepatic	Myelosuppression constipation and stomatitis Rare: hair loss or peripheral neurotoxicity	Lymphoma Germ cell tumours
Vincristine *Mitotic spindle inhibitor*	i/v	Hepatic	Peripheral neuropathy; Autonomic neuropathy	Lymphomas Leukaemia
Vindesine *Mitotic spindle inhibitor*	i/v	Hepatic	Myelosuppression: Mild neurotoxicity; Autonomic neuropathy	Leukaemia
Vinorelbine *Mitotic spindle inhibitor*	i/v	Hepatic	Myelosuppression: Phlebitis; Peripheral neuropathy	Breast cancer Non-small cell lung cancer

Table 5.3 Hormone and anti hormone drugs

Drug	Administration	Side-effects	Comments
SERMs			
Tamoxifen	p.o.	Menopausal symptoms Thromboembolic event Endometrial hyperplasia and cancer	Used first line in adjuvant treatment of ER/PR +ve breast Cancer
Anti-androgens			
Bicalutamide	p.o.	Hepatotoxicity	Used in prostatic cancer sometimes
Cyproterone acetate		Gynaecomastia	in combination with gonadorelin
Flutamide			analogues
Aromatase inhibitors			
Anastrozole	p.o.	Menopausal symptoms?	Used in post-menopausal breast cancer
Formestane	i/m	Increased fractures	
Letrozole	p.o.		
Gonadorelin analogues*			
Buserelin	SC and intranasal	Gynaecomastia, impotence,	Prostate cancer
Goserelin	implant	nausea, fluid retention	Breast cancer
Leuprorelin	i/m	Menopausal symptoms	
Triptorelin	i/m		

*Beware initial flare of symptoms when start use in men with prostate cancer. This should be 'covered' with the concomitant use of antiandrogens for the first few weeks of therapy.

Table 5.4 Emetic risk of common chemotherapy drugs

Cytotoxic agents	Risk
Cisplatin*	High
Cyclophosphamide >1000 mg/m²*	
Ifosfamide*	
Melphalan*	
Actinomycin	Moderate
Amsacrine	
Busulphan	
Carboplatin*	
Chlorambucil	
Cladribine	
Cyclophosphamide <1000 mg/m²	
Cytarabine >150 mg/m²	
Dacarbazine	
Daunorubicin	
Daunorubicin liposomal	
Doxorubicin	
Epirubicin	
Lomustine	
Methotrexate >1G/m²	
Mitoxantrone	
Procarbazine	
Bleomycin	Low
Cyclophosphamide <300 mg/m²	
Cytarabine <150 mg/m²	
Etoposide	
Fludarabine	
Mercaptopurine	
Methotrexate <IG/m²	
Tioguanine	
Thiotepa	
Vinblastine	
Vincristine	

*Delayed emesis risk.

Radiotherapy

Radiotherapy is the most important type of non-surgical treatment for patients with common cancers. The proportion of these treated by radiotherapy at some time during their illness has risen steadily and is now well over 50%.

Tobias, UCH London

Introduction

Radiotherapy as a therapeutic modality developed shortly after the discovery of x-rays at the end of the nineteenth century. Clinical and technological advances subsequently have made it one of the most successful modalities in the treatment of patients with cancer, both in the curative and palliative settings.

Mechanism of action

Radiotherapy is the therapeutic use of ionising radiation to destroy cancerous cells. The critical cellular target is, in common with chemotherapy, the nuclear DNA. Double-stranded breaks in the DNA molecule appear to be the lesion responsible for cell death. Cell death takes place during subsequent mitotic cell division, hence the term mitotic cell death. Much less commonly, certain tissue types, such as lymphocytes and parotid acinar cells, undergo cell death without attempting mitosis, a process known as interphase cell death. Not all double-stranded DNA breaks, however, result in cell death, indeed most are repaired by the cell's DNA repair enzyme apparatus. The success or otherwise of the repair process determines the fate of the cell.

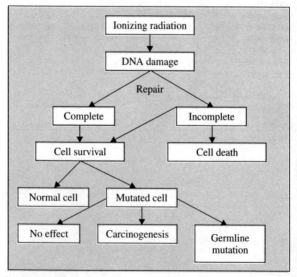

Fig. 5.1 The cell repair process after radiotherapy

Response of normal tissues to radiation

Different types of normal tissue respond differently to radiation. Homeostatic mechanisms control cell populations by balancing cell death with new cell growth through the proliferation of stem cells. If a proportion of these stem cells are destroyed by radiation, the rate of renewal of normal cells will be reduced. The time of appearance of this tissue damage is determined by the lifespan of the mature cells within that tissue. For certain tissues such as skin and mucosa, this lifespan is short as cells are quickly lost by desquamation, and hence tissue damage is manifest during the radiation course. For other tissues, cell turnover is much slower and radiation damage will only become apparent many months or years after radiation exposure. This gives rise to the distinction between the acute and late effects of irradiation.

Acute effects of radiation

This refers to the normal tissue reactions during a course of radiotherapy. The mucosa and haemopoetic system, i.e. tissues with a fast normal cellular turnover, display effects of irradiation earliest. For example, patients receiving radiotherapy to the head and neck area may develop severe oral mucositis, and those receiving radiotherapy to significant volumes of bone marrow, may develop bone marrow suppression.

Acute reactions are usually observed during the course of conventionally fractionated radiotherapy (1.8–2 Gy per fraction five times a week).

Late effects of radiation

These occur predominantly in slowly proliferating tissues (lung, kidney, heart, liver and CNS). By definition, late reactions occur more than 90 days after commencing a course of radiation.

In addition some of the tissues which develop their effects early, can also demonstrate late effects such as fibrosis or telangiectasia in the skin. This reflects the differing populations of cells (fibroblasts, endothelium etc.) which exist within a single organ.

Normal tissue tolerance

Not only do different tissues respond at different rates to irradiation, they also vary in their sensitivity. Certain tissues e.g. the lens, exhibit damage at very low doses while other tissues demonstrate marked resistance to the effects of radiation, e.g. uterine cervix. The situation is analogous among cancers. Lymphomas and seminomas show sensitivity to radiation while renal cell carcinomas and melanomas are radioresistant.

A number of treatment and patient factors influence tissue tolerance to radiation. These include:
- Total radiation dose given: higher doses are more toxic
- Fraction size: late responding tissues more sensitive to large fractions
- Overall longer treatment time: better tolerated by normal tissues
- Treatment volume: larger volumes are generally more toxic
- Quality of the radiation: neutrons are more damaging than photons or electrons
- Concomitant therapy: oncurrent chemotherapy reduces tolerance

Patient factors adversely influencing tissue tolerance:
- Older age
- Haemoglobin level
- Smoking
- Diabetes mellitus
- Connective tissue disorders
- Genetic syndromes (e.g. ataxia telangiectasia)

Tolerance doses for specific tissues

The following tissues suffer a 5 per cent incidence of toxicity at five years when conventional radiotherapy is given in fraction dose sizes of 1.8–2 Gy per fraction at the doses stated for each tissue type.

Table 5.5 Normal tissue tolerance

Tissue	Injury	Tolerance
Brain	Necrosis	60 Gy
Spinal cord	Myelopathy	45 Gy (<1% incidence)
Lens*	Cataract	10 Gy
Small intestine	Ulceration/perforation	45–50 Gy
Kidney*	Clinical nephritis	23 Gy
Lung*	Pneumonitis	18–20 Gy
Heart*	Pericarditis	40 Gy

*Whole organ.

Retreatment

Traditional teaching precluded retreating areas that had already received a maximal radiation dose. Recent studies have shown some tissues and organs have a greater capacity to recover from subclinical radiation injury than was previously thought. For example the large capacity of long-term regeneration of the CNS allows new possibilities for retreating recurrent neurological tumours with irradiation.

Table 5.5 Radiation effects within specific tissues (following standard radical doses)

Skin	Acute reaction—erythema begins week 3–4 Dry or moist desquamation later	Reaction settles within 2–4 weeks of completion of therapy
	Late reaction—fibrosis, atrophy, telangiectasia	
Oral mucosa	Acute reaction—erythema/oedema from wk 2–4 Patchy followed by confluent mucositis later	Reaction settles within 2–4 weeks of completion of therapy
Gastrointestinal tract	Acute reaction—mucositis causes nausea, anorexia, cramps, and diarrhoea	Reaction settles within 2–4 weeks of completion of therapy Treat symptomatically
	Late reaction—ulceration and fibrosis leading to strictures, fistulae, and malabsorption	Usually >6 months post RT
Brain	Acute reaction—lethargy common Occasionally cerebral oedema	
	Late reaction—somnolence syndrome at 1–3 months post RT Brain necrosis at 6 months to 3 years	Resolves spontaneously with/without help of steroids Indistinguishable clinically from recurrent tumour
Spinal cord	Late reaction—Lhermitte's syndrome 2–18 months after RT Radiation myelopathy at 6–12 months	Resolves spontaneously. Does not progress to myelopathy. Irreversible
Lung	Early/intermediate reaction—pneumonitis at 1–3 months Results in pulmonary fibrosis	Classical straight-edged appearance on chest x-ray
Kidney	Late reaction—proteinuria, hypertension, renal failure	May take up to 10 years to develop
Heart	Late reaction—pericarditis/effusion Most within 6 months of RT Cardiomyopathy Coronary artery disease	Most resolve spontaneously; may develop into a constrictive process 10–20 years post RT 10–15 years post RT

NB Patients undergoing radiotherapy usually experience lethargy as a general side-effect.

Types of radiation therapy

There are three main types of radiation therapy:

1 External beam radiotherapy, delivered by radiotherapy machines
2 Brachytherapy, solid radiation sources delivered directly into tumours
3 Unsealed source or radioisotope therapy, given by mouth, intravenously or into tissue spaces

External beam radiotherapy

External beam radiation consists of different energies, as shown in Table 5.7.

Table 5.7

Type of radiation	Energy	Use
Superficial X-rays	80–150 kV	Skin tumours
Orthovoltage X-rays (DXT)	200–400 kV	Thick skin tumours Superficial tumours e.g. ribs
Megavoltage radiation		
γ rays—cobalt 60	1.25 MV (mean)	Deep tumours
X rays—linear accelerator	4–25 MV	Deep tumours
Electrons	4–20 MeV	Skin tumours Superficial tumours

Superficial X-rays use relatively low energy x-ray photons in the range 80–400 kV. These x-rays are relatively non-penetrating, depositing the majority of their energy in the most superficial few millimetres of skin. They therefore deliver a high dose to the skin with rapid fall-off with increasing depth and are thus appropriate for the treatment of superficial skin lesions such as basal cell cancers.

Orthovoltage energy X-rays are slightly more penetrating and deliver sufficient dose at depth to treat adequately thicker skin or subcutaneous lesions such as rib metastases. (Both superficial and orthovoltage x-rays suffer the disadvantage of delivering a higher absorbed dose to bone compared to soft tissue, thus increasing the risk of osteoradionecrosis if a lesion is positioned too close to underlying bony tissue.)

Megavoltage X-ray photons possess energies 50–200 times those of superficial x-rays. (1–20MV) In contrast to superficial/orthovoltage x-rays, megavoltage photons are produced by the acceleration of electrons along a linear tube (wave guide) before striking a target. This is done within a machine called a linear accelerator. The interaction of these high energy electrons with the target material generates high energy x-rays.

High energy x-rays are very penetrating and give a much higher dose at a given depth within a tissue than superficial x-rays.

Megavoltage x-rays possess the advantage of relative sparing of the superficial skin tissues as the maximum absorbed dose occurs up to several centimetres below the skin surface. There is also no increased absorption of dose in tissues containing elements of high atomic mass such as bone.

Electron therapy

Electrons may be generated using a linear accelerator. In this situation the accelerated electron beam exits the linear accelerator without striking the target. Electron therapy is used to treat superficial tumours, most often of the skin. It is their characteristic deposition of dose with depth which makes electrons ideal for this purpose: >90 per cent of the dose is deposited in the first few centimetres of tissue with very rapid dose fall-off thereafter, thus sparing underlying structures.

Treatment planning

This is the essential prerequisite step before treatment delivery. During the process of treatment planning questions such as 'where to treat?', 'what to treat?', 'what not to treat?', 'how to treat and how much to treat?' are addressed. It is essentially an iterative process with changes being made at various stages to facilitate the design of an optimal treatment schedule. There are several rungs in the planning ladder (Fig. 5.2).

The complexity of treatment planning depends upon the tumour and the intent of therapy. Radical plans are generally more complicated and time-consuming than those with palliative intent.

Immobilization is relatively more important for those tumours positioned close to sensitive normal tissue structures and for radical, high-dose, treatments.

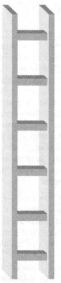

Patient positioning	Appropirate, comfortable and reproducible position makes therapy more tolerable and enables more reliable delivery
Immobilization	Immobilizaton will vary with the intent of treatment and the tumour site e.g. Perspex shells for head and neck cancers
Localization of the tumour	This may be clinical or using various imaging modalities e.g. fluroscopy, CT scanning
Target definition	The demonstrable tumour is outlined with additional margins allowed for microscopic extension and patient/organ movement
Generation of optimal dose distribution	Simple arrangement of x-ray beams used for palliative situations. Radical plans require more complex multiple beam configurations
Verification	Essential prior to treatment delivery to ensure target covered and critical normal organs protected

Fig. 5.2 The treatment ladder

The tumour is **localized** either by clinical examination e.g. skin tumours, or by imaging, most commonly fluoroscopy or CT scanning. Newer technology permits the fusing of various imaging modalities e.g. CT/MRI images, PET/CT images.

Once the tumour is localized the **target volume is defined**. This encompasses the tumour with a safety margin. This margin is added to allow for microscopic tumour extension, the so-called clinical target volume. Additionally, the margin will also accommodate movements in the organ containing the tumour, and uncertainties inherent in the treatment delivery system.

After the target has been delineated differing beam arrangements are generated. The arrangement is chosen which best covers the target volume and most successfully spares the normal tissue structures.

The final step in treatment planning is **verification**. This is an essential step to ensure that a plan generated on a planning computer actually fits the patient i.e. the tumour is accurately targeted and critical structures such as spinal cord are adequately spared. The verification process continues through treatment with dose measurements confirming appropriate dose delivery.

Radiotherapy dose prescription

Once the final treatment plan is decided upon, the radiation dose must be prescribed. There are several constituents that together make up the prescription:

- Total dose
- Number of fractions (fraction size)
- Overall treatment time

Total dose/number of fractions

Rather than deliver the entire dose of radiation in a single treatment, the dose is divided up into smaller quanta. This is the process of fractionation, each treatment dose being known as a fraction. Fractionation is performed to permit repair of normal tissue radiation damage. Fractionation will also permit repair to occur within tumour tissue, although this is relatively less efficient. In consequence, when a treatment course is fractionated, the total dose of radiation must be increased. Early studies showed that changing from a single dose to a six-week fractionated course of therapy required an increase in the total dose by a factor of three in order to achieve the same biological effect.

- The relationship between total dose and number of fractions is, however, complex and mathematical models are used to help predict the biological effects

Small numbers of fractions are convenient for the patient as travelling is kept to a minimum, however, the fraction size is in consequence larger; this increases the biological effectiveness of each fraction resulting in more severe damage to late-responding tissues. The total dose in such hypofractionated courses must be reduced to maintain an acceptable level of late tissue damage.

Hypofractionated treatment courses are often employed in the palliative setting on account of their convenience for patients and the relative unimportance of adverse long-term effects of radiation in patients with limited life expectancy.

Overall treatment time

Standard radical fractionation schedules involve treating once per day, Monday to Friday, for four to seven weeks. As treatment usually extends beyond four weeks, tumour cell repopulation becomes a problem.

As the number of tumour stem cells and mature functional tumour cells are depleted as a result of radiotherapy, the remaining stem cells sense this loss and begin to replicate actively to counteract this deficit. This is known as *tumour repopulation*. It appears that there is a lag period of approximately 3–4 weeks before this phenomenon occurs. Each fraction of radiotherapy delivered after the onset of repopulation is therefore relatively less effective, since part of the fraction must counteract this increase in the number of tumour cells resulting from repopulation.

A means of circumventing this effect of tumour repopulation is to *accelerate* the radiotherapy course so that the dose is delivered over a shorter time period, preferably less than the 3–4 weeks required for the onset of repopulation. A large randomized controlled clinical trial[4] of accelerated radiotherapy in non-small cell lung cancer has demonstrated that such an approach can be effective, with an increased rate of local tumour control and overall survival.

Brachytherapy

Here the radiation source is closely applied to the tumour. (Literally: therapy at a short distance, from the Greek βραχυς, brachys, short).

The underlying principle is the inverse square law, which states that the intensity of radiation, R, at a given distance, D, from a radioactive source, and therefore the absorbed dose, is inversely proportional to the square of that distance. Put simply, doubling the distance between the radiation source and the tissue reduces the dose absorbed by the tissue by a factor of four (rather than a factor of two as might be expected if the relationship was linear).

$$R \propto \frac{1}{D^2}$$

The beauty of brachytherapy lies in the ability to administer high doses of radiation to the tumour with relative sparing of neighbouring normal tissue because of rapid fall-off of absorbed dose with distance.

Brachytherapy is also known as **sealed source therapy** because the radioactive substance (often a metal) e.g. Iridium[192], is usually encased or sealed within a metal casing such that the radioactive substance does not actually physically touch the tissue even when inserted directly into the tumour (see below).

Brachytherapy takes three main forms:

- **Interstitial:** The radiation source is inserted directly into the tumour tissue
- **Intracavitary:** The radioactive source is inserted into a body cavity such as the uterus or the vagina when treating endometrial or cervical cancer
- **Intraluminal:** The radioactive source is positioned in the lumen of a hollow viscus e.g. bronchus, oesophagus

Brachytherapy, because it involves the placing of radioactive sources in close proximity to the patient, must of necessity make staff vulnerable to the risk of radiation exposure.

Decreasing the time during which exposure might occur, maximizing the shielding between source and staff, and most importantly increasing the distance from source to personnel all help to diminish risk.

In practice the brachytherapist places hollow tubes into the tumour, cavity or lumen, through which the source may subsequently be driven mechanically. Thus the radioactive source is brought into very close proximity to the tumour but staff experience no significant exposure.

Unsealed source therapy

This involves administering radioactive substances directly into the patient either in the form of liquids for ingestion or solutions for intravenous administration.

Unsealed source therapy is most often used as a palliative manoeuvre, although radioactive iodine[131] is employed as an adjuvant to curative surgery for well-differentiated thyroid cancer and indeed is often used to treat thyrotoxicosis, a non-malignant condition.

Radiation protection issues are to the fore as patients emit radiation for a variable period after administration of the radioisotope depending on the half-life of the isotope. They are carefully instructed regarding the precautions necessary to prevent excess exposure to others, most notably family members. Such precautions include double flushing of the toilet after micturition, and refraining from close contact with children and avoiding places of entertainment or work for a specified period of time post-treatment.

A number of radioisotopes are commonly used:

- **Strontium[89](Sr^{89}):** Often used for the relief of bone pain due to metastatic bone disease. A disadvantage is the relatively long half-life which poses radiation protection problems, especially if the patient dies within a short period after treatment. Some patients experience a flare up in their bone pain within a few days of treatment. This usually settles with appropriate analgesia. As strontium is absorbed into bone tissue, bone marrow toxicity may occasionally occur, and regular blood count monitoring after treatment is advised

- **Samarium[153](Sm^{153}):** Used less commonly than Sr^{89} but indicated likewise for the relief of pain from bony metastatic disease. It has the advantages of a shorter half-life and the production of photons as part of its decay pathway. These photons permit scintigraphy and thus bone scan images may be obtained. The propensity to pain flare and marrow toxicity pertain as for Sr^{89}

- **Iodine[131]:** Both normal thyroid and well-differentiated thyroid cancer (papillary and follicular variants) selectively take up and concentrate iodine. This can be exploited therapeutically using I^{131}. Due to this concentrating effect within thyroid tissue, high doses can be selectively delivered to the normal or malignant thyroid tissue leading to its destruction. In the case of normal thyroid tissue, hyperthyroid patients may be rendered euthyoid with a relatively low dose of I^{131}; in the case of malignancy, I^{131} is used as an adjuvant treatment following surgery to ablate the remaining normal thyroid tissue and any potential microscopic residual tumour

- **Phosphorus^{32}:** P^{32} has proved useful in the treatment of polycythaemia rubra vera although, because it may increase the risk of subsequent development of leukaemia, it is generally reserved for patients over 70 years of age

4 Saunders M., Dische S. *et al.* (1999) Continuous, hyperfractionated, accelerated radiotherapy (CHART) versus conventional radiotherapy in non-small cell lung cancer: mature data from the randomised multicentre trial. *Radiotherapy and Oncology*, **52**: 137–48.

Radiation therapy

Radiotherapy is used for about half of the 200,000 patients who develop cancer in the UK each year. It has a curative rôle in two-thirds, and a palliative rôle in the remainder.

Horwich, Royal Marsden

Radiotherapy may be administered in differing clinical situations and with varying intents.

Treatment can be:
- **Radical**—Curative intent
- **Adjuvant**—Postoperative
- **Palliative**—Symptom control

Radical radiotherapy

Radiotherapy may be administered with the intent of cure either as the preferred primary therapy (e.g. early stage Hodgkin's disease), or as an alternative to surgery.

In the latter situation it has the advantage of preserving normal anatomy e.g. anal canal cancer, bladder cancer. Additionally, acute morbidity is often less severe. However, as no surgical specimen is obtained, there can be no pathological data to permit accurate staging. Stage must therefore be assessed by clinical or radiological methods. Late effects of radiation, such as fibrosis, may also make subsequent assessment of the tumour site for local recurrence difficult.

Radical radiation is reserved for tumours which can be encompassed within a reasonable radiation treatment volume, i.e. localized, as opposed to widely metastatic disease; this presupposes accurate staging investigations.

Treatment is often complex, with effort given to rigid immobilization and the use of complicated beam arrangements to obtain a uniform dose distribution confined to the tumour with preservation of normal surrounding structures. A high dose of radiation is necessary for all but the most radiosensitive of tumours, and treatment is delivered in conventional (small) fraction sizes in order to reduce the late adverse effects of radiation.

Examples of radical radiotherapy include:
- **Head and neck tumours:** Many squamous cell tumours of the head and neck region can be cured by radical radiotherapy (often combined with synchronous chemotherapy) e.g. early stage cancers of the larynx are frequently cured with preservation of good quality phonation
- **Anal canal cancer:** A radical approach using concurrent chemo-radiotherapy has been shown to be effective management for epidermoid anal canal cancer. Additionally between 60–70 per cent of patients retain a functioning anal sphincter after treatment. A common alternative to such an approach is primary abdominoperineal excision of the rectum and anal canal, which results in a permanent colostomy

- **Lung cancer:** Radical radiotherapy is not infrequently employed as a second-best option in the management of lung cancer. The patients considered for such treatment are not deemed sufficiently fit to undergo radical surgery but may be fit for radiation treatment

Adjuvant radiotherapy

Adjuvant radiotherapy is administered as an adjunct to potentially curative surgery. The principle underpinning such treatment is the possibility of microscopic residual disease, either within the tumour bed, lymphatic channels or regional lymph node drainage. The aim of adjuvant radiotherapy is the eradication of this microscopic disease and thereby to reduce the rate of local relapse and improve overall survival.

Examples of adjuvant radiotherapy:

- **Breast cancer:** This is perhaps the best example and is certainly the most common exemplifier of adjuvant radiation. Up to 50 per cent of the workload of many UK radiotherapy centres is devoted to adjuvant breast irradiation. Local relapse rates following partial mastectomy may reach 30 per cent. Postoperative breast irradiation can reduce this figure by three to fourfold. Local control rates then conform to those achieved after mastectomy but with a superior cosmetic outcome

- **Head and neck cancer:** Surgery for squamous tumours of the head and neck is complex. Due to the close proximity of tumours to important structures, surgical margins may often be inadequate because compromise must be made to retain acceptable functional and cosmetic outcomes. Adjuvant irradiation is employed if margins are unsatisfactory or following radical neck surgery which demonstrates multiple involved lymph nodes. Classically adjuvant radiotherapy is administered after surgery has been performed

However, in some situations, although surgery remains the mainstay of treatment, radiotherapy may be delivered as a prelude to a surgical procedure.

True **neo-adjuvant radiation** is administered in order to shrink or downstage the tumour, thus facilitating subsequent surgery. In this case time must elapse between irradiation and surgery to allow tumour reduction. An illustration of this technique is preoperative rectal radiotherapy for tethered or fixed rectal adenocarcinoma. Treatment is delivered over 4–5 weeks after which there is a gap of about six weeks during which tumour shrinkage occurs. Surgery is then often made possible, when pre-radiotherapy it would not have been.

Short fractionation preoperative rectal radiotherapy, by contrast, is delivered over the week immediately prior to surgery. No time is permitted for tumour shrinkage. Trials have, however, confirmed a significant improvement in local control and overall survival with this approach.

Adjuvant radiation treatment courses typically extend over 4–6 weeks. The general principles applied to radical radiotherapy also hold for the adjuvant setting as treatment intent is curative i.e. immobilization, careful avoidance of critical organs at risk, and low dose per fraction. Total doses tend to be slightly lower since the target is microscopic residual disease. It must, however, be remembered that following surgery the vascular supply to tissues is disrupted resulting in areas of tissue hypoxia. **Radiation is relatively less effective in an environment that is poorly oxygenated**.

Palliative radiotherapy

When radiotherapy is administered in the palliative setting, the focus of interest is the control of distressing symptoms. The disease is, by definition, incurable. These factors impact upon treatment in a variety of ways:

- Only symptomatic sites of disease are targeted
- Sites at high risk of producing symptoms may receive prophylactic treatment
- Fractionation regimens are kept short
- Moderate doses of radiation are employed
- Palliative benefit must outweigh treatment-related toxicity

Palliative radiotherapy may produce prolongation of survival but this is not its primary aim, rather it is the quality of that survival which is the goal. Palliative radiotherapy often produces significant symptomatic gain.

There are several clinical scenarios in which palliative radiotherapy commonly proves useful.

Pain

Bone metastases, pain due to nerve compression or soft tissue infiltration will usually respond to radiation treatment and will respond to large single fractions of radiotherapy as effectively as more prolonged treatment schedules.

The former are more patient-friendly and may be repeated if necessary. If pain is diffuse, affecting many disparate sites within the skeleton, wide field—hemibody—irradiation often produces relief. An alternative is radioisotope therapy with Sr^{89} or Sm^{153}.

Osteolytic tumour deposits in weight-bearing bones are at risk of fracture and are best fixed prophylactically by orthopaedic intervention. This is often followed by postoperative irradiation, although good evidence of benefit is lacking. Rarely radiation is given without prophylactic surgical intervention.

Haemorrhage

Haemoptysis, haematuria, haematemesis, and rectal bleeding all respond to radiation. A hypofractionated treatment course often produces prompt sustained benefit (at least 70 per cent in carcinoma of the bronchus).

Obstruction

Any hollow viscus may undergo obstruction caused by a malignant process. Several organs may commonly be obstructed by cancer:

- Superior vena cava (SVC)
- Upper airways i.e. trachea, bronchus
- Oesophagus

Prompt, if not immediate, relief is frequently afforded by stent insertion under the care of the interventional radiologists for SVC or oesophageal obstruction. There is a rôle for palliative radiotherapy in some patients who are unsuitable for such procedures, or in the case of stent overgrowth by tumour.

Radiotherapy is most often used for bronchial obstruction due to lung cancer; laser resection or stent insertion are less commonly employed alternatives.

Radiotherapy probably remains the treatment modality of choice for SVC obstruction caused by radiosensitive tumours, for example, small cell lung cancer.

Neurological symptoms
- Spinal cord compression
- Brain metastases
- Cranial or peripheral nerve compression
- Malignant meningitis
- Choroidal or orbital metastases

Radiotherapy is the most common means of treating spinal cord compression. There are a number of important indications for surgical as opposed to radiotherapeutic intervention (e.g. uncertain pathology, unstable spine).

Radiotherapy often improves pain associated with the compression, but neurological recovery is less predictable and mainly depends on the degree of weakness prior to therapy and the particular histological tumour type.

Brain metastases are increasing in incidence as oncological management improves and patients survive long enough to develop relapse within the brain. Steroids can produce significant benefit if the effects are due to oedema or compression rather than tissue destruction. However, their beneficial effects tend to be short-lived. Prolongation of symptom control and a small gain in survival (1–2 months) can additionally be obtained with cranial irradiation, usually at the cost of alopecia and lethargy. Those with good pre-treatment neurological function and sensitive tumours stand to gain most.

Cranial or peripheral nerve compression most often occurs with breast or prostate neoplasms. Pain is often improved but nerve palsies seldom show significant recovery.

Fungating tumours
Locally advanced breast tumours, skin tumours, metastatic skin or lymph node deposits, can all lead to fungation. If surgical intervention is not possible or felt to be inappropriate, radiotherapy can reduce the tumour mass, serous ooze or haemorrhage, and promote healing.

Managing side-effects of radiotherapy

Skin

General advice
- Skin reactions tend to be worse in the skin folds i.e. inframammary fold, axilla, groin and perineum
- Deodorants should be avoided within the treatment area
- Avoid aftershave lotions or astringent cosmetics
- Mild soaps are permitted, and washing should be gentle (no vigorous rubbing) and the area patted dry
- Care must be taken not to remove skin markings delineating the treatment fields

Mild reactions
- Skin pink or slightly red
- Apply aqueous cream frequently

Moderate reactions
- Skin red, dry and scaly; some pruritus/tingling
- Apply aqueous cream frequently
- If itch is problematic, 1% Hydrocortisone cream q.d.s. useful

Severe reactions
- Skin inflamed patchy areas of moist desquamation
- Epidermis may blister and slough exposing the dermis leading to pain and serous ooze with increased risk of infection
- Hydrogel or alginate dressing to moist areas; Diprobase® cream to intact epidermis
- Swab if evidence of infection

Mouth and throat care
This is particularly important for patients receiving radiotherapy for head and neck lesions

General advice
- The patient needs a dental assessment and any dental treatment should be carried out before radiotherapy begins
- A good fluid and nutritional intake is very important and nutritional support by NG feeding is indicated if >10 per cent weight loss occurs.
- Cessation of smoking should be strongly encouraged
- Avoid alcohol and spicy foods
- The voice should be rested as the radiotherapy reaction becomes established

Treatment of mucositis
- Normal saline or bicarbonate mouth washes often help
- Antiseptic mouth washes, e.g. chlorhexidine, keep the mouth clean but can cause pain due to their alcohol content
- Oropharyngeal candida infection should be actively sought and treated

- Local analgesics include:
  - aspirin (which may be gargled)
  - paracetamol (which may be gargled)
  - benzydamine (Difflam®)
  - local anaesthetics (Xylocaine®)
  - topical steroids (Adcortyl in orobase®, Corlan pellets®)
  - coating agents (Sucralfate®, Gelclair®)

Dysphagia
Thoracic radiotherapy can lead to oesophagitis which needs explanation and symptomatic treatment. Smoking should be strongly discouraged; spirits and spicy food should be avoided.

An antacid e.g. Gaviscon®, soluble paracetamol or aspirin may all help. A non-steroidal anti-inflammatory drug either orally or by suppository may be used. The oesophagus can be coated with some effect by Sucralfate®.

Nausea and vomiting
Radiotherapy to the abdomen often causes nausea due to serotonin release. All patients should thus be considered for prophylactic antiemetic therapy, e.g. ondansetron.

Diarrhoea
This side-effect frequently accompanies radiotherapy to the abdomen or pelvis. Dietary modification i.e. reduction in dietary roughage, may sometimes relieve the diarrhoea. Anti-diarrhoeal drugs (e.g. loperamide) should be provided to all patients with clear instructions of when and how they should be taken. Proctitis often accompanies rectal or prostatic irradiation and should be treated with rectal steroids either by suppository or enema.

Pneumonitis
Acute radiotherapy-induced pneumonitis can develop one to three months after treatment and is associated with a fever, dry cough and breathlessness. The main differential diagnosis is pneumonia and this should be excluded where possible. The diagnosis can be confirmed by a chest x-ray, which shows lung infiltration confined within the treatment volume. Treatment is with a reducing course of steroids i.e. a starting dose of prednisolone 40 mg.

Cerebral oedema
This can occur during or after cranial irradiation, particularly if no surgical decompression of the brain tumour or metastasis has been undertaken. Oedema usually responds to an increase in the dose of oral steroids.

Somnolence syndrome
This occurs within a few weeks of completion of brain irradiation and may manifest itself with nausea, vomiting, anorexia, dysarthria, ataxia and profound lethargy. Recovery occurs spontaneously but can be accelerated with steroids.

New developments

Radiotherapy has advanced markedly since the early days of the nineteenth century. Progress is still being made to improve the quality and effectiveness of treatment for patients.

There are a number of areas of development:

Defining tumour volume

Improvements in imaging have enabled tumours to be targeted more accurately. This reduces the risk of missing the tumour, and also allows the treatment volume to encompass the tumour more closely. The dose of radiation can therefore be higher (giving improved tumour control) without risking additional toxicity to normal tissues.

Imaging

Refinements in CT scanning technology have led to the advent of the multi-slice CT scanner that provides multiple high quality images rapidly, from which tumour volumes may be defined not only in two but also in three dimensions.

Images can now be fused from different imaging modalities, e.g. MRI/CT image fusion. The new development of co-registered CT/PET scanning combines functional data (through PET scanning) and high quality spatial information (through CT scanning) providing opportunity for optimal target volume definition.

Conformal therapy

Imaging improvements provide the ability to identify the tumour target more accurately. This reduces the risk of missing the tumour, but it also provides the opportunity of conforming the treatment more closely to the tumour volume and thereby lessening damage to surrounding normal tissues. Taken further, conformal therapy may permit dose escalation with resulting improved tumour control rates, but without increased toxicity. Multileaf collimators within the treatment unit can automatically shape the treatment field, conforming it to the desired target shape.

Intensity Modulated Radiotherapy (IMRT) takes this a step further. With IMRT the intensity of the treatment beams are modified in such a way that almost any three-dimensional volume may be generated. Even concave volumes may be created and so targets which envelop the spinal cord, e.g. thyroid, can be treated much more satisfactorily than with conventional techniques.

Fractionation/combined modality treatment

Advances in the understanding of the principles of fractionation have led to improved treatment outcomes for patients, e.g. CHART in non-small cell lung cancer. Further research with hypo/hyperfractionation and acceleration is ongoing in other tumour types.

The integration of chemotherapy with radiation treatment has provided benefit in a number of tumour sites, e.g. cervical cancer. Research seeks to refine this further and also to incorporate the newer molecular agents into radiation therapy.

Individualization of therapy

Two patients with ostensibly similar tumours receiving identical treatments may respond differently, one being cured and the other dying from cancer in a short time. There are clearly factors inherent within tumours which predict for response to radiotherapy. If such variables could be identified before a treatment course commences, the chance of response would be defined which would help clinicians in deciding whether or not radiotherapy would be a good treatment option. Furthermore, it might be possible, knowing the particular tumour characteristics, to adapt the treatment course accordingly perhaps by modifying the dose prescribed, altering the fractionation schedule such that the prospect of cure could be enhanced. Predictive assays are being developed to realize this possibility. New microchip technology may help elucidate the genes behind the differing responses to therapy, and more importantly, offer patients the possibility of treatment tailored to their individual needs.

Common cancers

Incidence

There are huge variations in cancer incidences across the globe, reflecting the impact of environmental and genetic factors on the causes of cancer.[5]

Table 5.8 The eight commonest cancer types affecting men and women worldwide

Cancer type	Ratio, high:low rate	High incidence	Low incidence
Oesophagus	200:1	Kazakhastan	Holland
Skin	200:1	Australia	India
Liver	100:1	Mozambique	UK
Nasopharynx	100:1	China	Uganda
Lung	40:1	UK	Nigeria
Stomach	30:1	Japan	UK
Cervix	20:1	Hawaii	Israel
Rectum	20:1	Denmark	Nigeria

Table 5.9 The eight commonest cancer types effecting men and women in the UK[5]

Men	Women
Lung	Breast
Colorectal	Lung
Skin	Colorectal
Prostate	Skin
Stomach	Stomach
Pancreas	Ovary
Oesophagus	Cervix
Leukaemia	Pancreas

In this Handbook it is not possible to outline oncological management of all cancer types. The following cancers are the commonest, and those for which the palliative care team has a particular rôle to play.

Table 5.10 Common cancers

Cancer Type	Page	Cancer Type	Page
Lung	132	Upper GI	154
Colorectal	138	Bladder and ureter	158
Breast	142	Brain	160
Prostate	146	Haematological	164
Gynaecological	150	Unknown primary	166

5 Souhami R. L., Tobias J. D. (2003) *Cancer and its Management.* 4th edition. Oxford: Blackwell Science.

Patients with lung cancer

Background
- Most common cancer in men and women in the UK and the US
- Eighty per cent due to smoking
- Eighty per cent are non-small cell subtype (squamous, adenocarcinoma or large cell)
- Twenty per cent are small cell subtype

Symptoms at presentation
- Cough
- Haemoptysis
- Chest pain
- Recurrent chest infection
- Hoarseness

Diagnosis and staging
Diagnosis
- CXR
- Sputum cytology
- Bronchoscopy with biopsy
- Bronchial brushings and washings
- CT guided biopsy

Staging
- Bronchoscopy
- CT scan of chest, liver and adrenals
- Mediastinoscopy
- Pleural aspiration, pleural biopsy
- Bone and brain scan if symptomatic

Small cell lung carcinoma (SCLC)
This is generally believed to be a systemic disease at the time of diagnosis; thus surgery generally plays no part in the management of this disease

Staging
- Limited stage disease—disease confined to one hemithorax
- Extensive stage disease—disease present beyond one hemithorax

Management
- Because of chemoresponsiveness and frequent dissemination at diagnosis combined chemotherapy is the treatment of choice.
- Many chemotherapeutic agents have demonstrated activity in this disease. Commonly used regimes include cisplatin/etoposide and cyclophosphamide/doxorubicin/vincristine
- For patients with limited stage disease, thoracic irradiation in addition to chemotherapy improves local disease control and prolongs survival when compared with chemotherapy alone. Prophylactic cranial irradiation reduces the incidence of brain metastases but has not been shown to prolong survival
- Further radiotherapy may be a useful palliative treatment for patients relapsing after or resistant to chemotherapy

Prognosis

Approximately 80 per cent of patients respond to chemotherapy but the majority relapse and only approximately 10 per cent of patients are alive two years following diagnosis.

Non-small cell lung carcinoma (NSCLC)

Non-small cell lung cancer metastasizes later in its course than small cell lung cancer and consequently surgery offers the best chance of cure. All patients being considered for surgical treatment must be carefully staged to determine tumour operability. The patient must also be carefully assessed preoperatively to assess fitness for surgery.

Postoperative mortality rate should be less than 5 per cent.

Table 5.11 TNM staging of lung cancer

T_1	Tumour <3 cm diameter; distal to main bronchus
T_2	Tumour >3 cm diameter; or involve main bronchus 2 cm distal to carina; or invading visceral pleura; or atelectasis extending to hilum
T_3	Tumour invading chest wall, diaphragm, mediastinal pleura or pericardium; or tumour in main bronchus <2 cm distal to carina or atelectasis of whole lung
T_4	Tumour invading mediastinum, heart, major vessels, trachea, oesophagus, vertebra or carina; or malignant pleural effusion
N_0	No regional node metastases
N_1	Ipsilateral peribronchial or peribronchial or hilar nodes
N_2	Ipsilateral mediastinal or subcarinal nodes
N_3	Contralateral mediastinal nodes; scalene or supraclavicular nodes

Table 5.12 Stage grouping

I	$T_{1-2} N_0$
II	$T_{1-2} N_1$ or $T_3 N_0$
IIIA	$T_{1-2} N_2$ or $T_3 N_{1-2}$
IIIB	T_4 any N M_0; or any $N_3 M_0$
IV	Any M_1

Management

Surgery

Surgical resection offers the best chance of cure in this disease. The aim of surgery is to resect the primary tumour with clear lateral and bronchial margins with draining peribronchial and hilar lymph nodes. Lobectomy is the most commonly performed operation but a bilobectomy or pneumonectomy may be performed for more extensive tumours.

Conversely in less fit patients with limited respiratory reserve only a partial lobectomy may be tolerated, although the results from this surgery in terms of the risk of tumour recurrence may be inferior.

NSCLC radiation therapy

Radical radiotherapy

Selected patients with stage I–III disease who are unfit for surgery may be suitable for radical radiotherapy. Five year survivals of 15–20 per cent have been reported in this highly selected patient group.

The benefit of adjuvant radiotherapy following surgery for high risk disease is uncertain but may reduce the risk of local disease relapse.

Palliative radiotherapy

Radiotherapy is a key component of symptomatic treatment for
- Haemoptysis
- Chest pain
- Dyspnoea
- Cough.

NSCLC chemotherapy

NSCLC is much less chemosensitive than SCLC. Cisplatin-based therapy, however, has recently been demonstrated to improve quality of life with some improvement in survival in the palliative setting. Commonly used regimens include cisplatin/paclitaxel and cisplatin/vinorelbine.

Chemotherapy may also be used in the neo-adjuvant setting to down stage a tumour prior to consideration of surgery. Adjuvant chemotherapy following surgery may also confer a small survival benefit.

Table 5.13 Prognosis

Stage	Five year survival(%)
I	60–80
II	25–40
IIIA	10–30
IIIB and i/v	< 5

General issues

Lung cancer, because of its link with smoking, both active and passive, may be associated with emotional distress in the patient and their carers. Lung cancers often occur on top of a background of pre-existing lung disease which may alter the patient's perception of breathlessness and cough.

Specific pain issues
- **Pleuritic pain** may be associated with the tumour itself, metastases in ribs or local inflammation. This type of pain responds well to non-steroidal anti-inflammatory drugs (NSAIDs). It may also be helped by local nerve blockade
- **Pancoast tumour** can produce severe neuropathic pain which may only be partially opioid-responsive and will need adjuvant analgesics. Early referral for specialist help should be considered
- **Bone metastases** may occur, putting the patient at risk of pathological fractures and spinal cord compression. Management of subsequent pain may be difficult and specialist advice should be sought

Other complications

- **Breathlessness** is common and can be very distressing for carers (📖 see respiratory section). Treat reversible causes such as anaemia and pleural effusion, where appropriate. Give clear explanations of what is happening. Ensure that practical measures such as sitting upright, opening windows and using fans have been discussed with the family. Regular doses of short-acting oral morphine every 2–4 h may decrease the sensation of breathlessness. Other more specialist interventions such as palliative radiotherapy, endobronchial laser therapy and stenting may help some patients. Panic and anxiety are frequently associated with breathlessness and may be helped by simple relaxation techniques. A low dose of an anxiolytic such as diazepam may be helpful

- **Haemoptysis** is a frightening symptom. Palliative radiotherapy may be effective if the patient is fit enough. Oral anti-fibrinolytics such as tranexamic acid may help. Occasionally frequent small episodes herald a catastrophic haemoptysis. This is rare, but is a difficult situation to manage and early involvement of specialists should be considered. The risks of frightening a family with information about a possible risk of catastrophic haemoptysis need to be balanced against the potential distress that could be caused by leaving a patient and family unprepared

- **Cough** can exacerbate breathlessness and pain, and affect sleep and a patient's ability to eat. Its management will depend on the cause, but it is often appropriate to try and suppress the cough pharmacologically using codeine linctus or morphine. If not responding to simple measures refer for specialist assessment

- **Hypercalcaemia** may occur. It should be considered in any patient with persistent nausea, thirst, altered mood or confusion (even if intermittent), worsening pain and/or constipation. It should be treated with i/v hydration and bisphosphonates unless the patient is clearly dying, in which case treatment is not appropriate

- **Cerebral metastases** are common. Decisions about investigation and management may be complex and need to be made on an individual basis. Altered behaviour and personality, as well as problems of comprehension and communication, can be very distressing for relatives. Persistent headache, worse in the mornings and unexplained vomiting may be early signs of this diagnosis. There is a risk of epileptic fits and prophylactic anticonvulsant medication may be appropriate

- **Hyponatraemia** and other biochemical imbalances are particularly common in small cell lung cancer. Management can be complex and needs specialist input

- **Altered taste and anorexia** are common. Good oral hygiene, and effective treatment of oral candidiasis may help. Carers may find it helpful to talk through different ways of encouraging the patient to eat, such as freezing supplement drinks and making small meals frequently etc.

- **Superior vena cava obstruction (SVCO)** can occur, particularly in patients with right-sided lung cancers. Management includes consideration of vascular stenting, radiotherapy and high dose oral steroids in a single daily dose

Mesothelioma

General comments

This usually affects the pleura but can affect other mesothelial linings, most commonly the peritoneum. It is associated with exposure to asbestos, although unlike patients with asbestosis the history may be difficult to elicit, as the risk of mesothelioma appears unrelated to the length of exposure to asbestos and may occur many years after such exposure. It is a relentlessly progressive tumour.

It is important that the patient is aware that they may be entitled to *compensation* and should consult a specialist lawyer about this.

> All deaths due to mesothelioma should be discussed with the coroner who will most probably carry out a post-mortem, unless the disease was clearly non-industrially related. The patient and family should be made aware that the coroner will be contacted (regardless of any compensation claims or litigation), to try and minimize distress at the time of death.

Diagnosis

- CXR
- CT scan of chest
- Pleural biopsy
- Thoracoscopic biopsy

There is a high incidence of false negative biopsies—in some cases these may need to be repeated a number of times to make a diagnosis.

Treatment

Surgery

Radical surgery is of uncertain value, with a high mortality and few long term survivors reported. Palliative surgery with parietal pleurectomy and decortication of the lung may offer excellent palliation with minimal morbidity.

Radiotherapy

The tumour may grow along the track of a biopsy or drainage needle to produce a cutaneous lesion. These areas can become painful, ulcerated and can be difficult to manage. Palliative radiotherapy is given prophylactically following the biopsy. It may also be used locally for established cutaneous spread.

Chemotherapy

The value of chemotherapy in this disease is uncertain. Recent reports however suggest that selected patients may respond to platinum-based regimes with some palliative benefit.

Specific problems in the management of mesothelioma

- **Pleural effusions** are common, frequently blood stained and become increasingly difficult to aspirate as the disease progresses. Surgical intervention to prevent re-accumulation of fluid may be helpful if carried out early enough
- **Breathlessness** can be severe due to pleural disease limiting the capacity of the lung as well as the occurrence of pleural effusions.

Give clear explanations of what is happening. Ensure that practical measures such as sitting the patient up, opening windows and using fans have been discussed with the family. Regular doses of short acting oral morphine every 4 h may decrease the sensation of breathlessness. Panic and anxiety are frequently associated with breathlessness and may be helped by simple relaxation techniques. A low dose of an *anxiolytic* such as diazepam may be helpful. Other treatment options are limited

● **Ascites** occurs with peritoneal mesothelioma. The ascitic fluid is frequently blood stained and becomes increasingly difficult to aspirate as the disease progresses.

Specific pain complexes

Mesotheliomas can produce severe neuropathic pain which may only be partially opioid responsive and may need adjuvant analgesics. Early referral for specialist help should be considered. Local nerve blockades can help in some cases.

Colorectal cancer

Background

- Fourth commonest cancer worldwide
- Approximately 50 per cent of tumours occur in the rectum or sigmoid colon
- Dietary factors are thought to be important
- 6–8 per cent of cases are familial
- Associated syndromes include Familial Adenomatous Polyposis Coli and Hereditary Non-polyposis Coli

Common presentations

- Iron deficiency anaemia
- Abdominal pain
- Altered bowel habit
- PR bleeding

Staging and diagnosis

- Barium enema
- Colonoscopy—all patients must have full evaluation of the colon prior to surgery
- Sigmoidoscopy
- CT/Ultrasound scan of abdomen
- MRI/endorectal ultrasound may be useful to assess local extent of tumour in the rectum

Table 5.14 TNM staging for colorectal cancer

T_1 Invades submucosa	Stage I—T_1/T_2, N_0 M_0
T_2 Invades muscularis propria	Stage II—$T_{3/4}$, N_0 M_0
T_3 Invades subserosa	Stage III—T_{1-4}, N_1/N_2 M_0
T_4 Invades through serosa	Stage i/v—T_{1-4} N_{1-2} M_1
N_0 N_0 lymph node involvement	
N_1 1–3 nodes involved	
N_2 4 or more nodes involved	
N_3 Central nodes involved	
M_0 No distant metastases	
M_1 Distant metastases	

Management

Surgery of primary disease

Surgery is the mainstay of therapy for colorectal cancer.

For colonic tumours a segment of colon with its blood supply and draining nodes is excised. Depending on the site of the tumour this may involve a right or left hemicolectomy or a sigmoid colectomy.

Traditionally surgery for rectal tumours has involved an abdomino-perineal approach. In the absence of radiotherapy local relapse rates of 25–30 per cent have been reported. Traditionally radiotherapy has been used postoperatively but increasingly a short course of radiotherapy is being used to 'sterilize' the area prior to surgery. Some surgeons now advocate more extensive local surgery in the form of a total mesorectal excision, where the rectum is excised en bloc with the adjacent perirectal tissue. This has reduced local relapse rates to less than 10 per cent.

Surgery for hepatic metastases

The majority of patients develop liver metastases as the first site of disease progression following definitive first line treatment.

A proportion of these patients may be suitable for metastatectomy. Up to 40 per cent five-year survival has been reported for carefully selected patients.

Chemotherapy

Adjuvant chemotherapy of colorectal cancer

Several large randomised controlled trials have demonstrated a small but definite survival advantage to fluorouracil-based therapy for patients with Stage III disease.

The value of adjuvant chemotherapy for patients with Stage I/II disease is uncertain and is being addressed in a number of ongoing trials.

Advanced colorectal cancer

Fluorouracil-based chemotherapy has also been demonstrated to confer a palliative benefit in patients with metastatic disease. There also appears to be a survival advantage to chemotherapy of at least six months. Combination regimes with fluorouracil and oxaliplatin or irinotecan may be superior to single agent fluorouracil.

Capecitabine, a recently developed orally available fluorouracil analogue has also been demonstrated to have activity in this disease.

Radiotherapy

Adjuvant treatment

Pelvic radiotherapy with concurrent chemotherapy reduces risk of pelvic relapse for patients with Stage II and III rectal cancer.

Pelvic chemoradiotherapy may also be useful for patients with large fixed rectal tumours to reduce tumour volume prior to consideration of surgical resection.

General comments

- **Liver metastases** often occur and may cause capsular pain. This usually responds well to non-steroidal anti-inflammatory drugs (NSAIDS) or steroids. Liver metastases may also lead to hepatomegaly, causing squashed stomach syndrome with delayed gastric emptying and a feeling of fullness. This may respond to a prokinetic agent such as metoclopramide
- **Perineal and pelvic pain** may be caused by advancing disease or be iatrogenic. There is nearly always a neuropathic element to the pain which will only be partially opioid sensitive. Tenesmus is a unique type of neuropathic pain which requires specialist assessment. It may respond to drugs that have an effect on muscle tone such as nifedipine, baclofen, or nitrates

- **Bone metastases** are rare but can occur with colonic cancer
- **Bowel obstruction**, unless it can be palliated surgically, should be managed medically using a syringe driver containing a mixture of analgesics, antiemetics and anti-spasmodics. Multiple levels of obstruction of the bowel, which is not infrequent, may make surgery inappropriate. Differentiating between a high blockage (where vomiting is a feature) and blockage lower in the bowel can be useful in targeting treatment strategies. Imaging techniques may also be helpful to delineate the level of obstruction
- **Fistulae** between the bowel and the skin or bladder may occur. These can be very difficult to manage and require a multidisciplinary approach with specialist input
- **Poor appetite** is not uncommon and can be helped with the use of steroids
- **Rectal discharge and bleeding** are unpleasant and difficult symptoms to manage. Referral to a clinical oncologist is appropriate as radiotherapy may be of benefit
- **Hypoproteinaemia** is common due to poor oral intake and poor absorption from the bowel and may lead to lower limb oedema
- **Cerebral metastases** are not common with colonic cancers

Breast cancer

Background
- Accounts for 20 per cent of all cancers
- Life time risk 1/12
- Factors which increase the risk of breast cancer include increasing age, a family history of breast cancer, nulliparity and use of HRT
- Incidence of breast cancer is increasing although overall mortality is decreasing
- Male breast cancer is rare—accounting for only 0.7 per cent of all breast cancers

Genetics of breast cancer

Five to ten per cent of breast cancers are believed to be hereditary. Many of these cancers are due to germline mutations in the tumour suppresser genes BRCA1 or BRCA2. For patients with proven mutations in the BRCA1 or BRCA2 gene prophylactic subcutaneous mastectomy reduces the incidence of breast cancer.

At present treatment for a breast tumour arising in a mutation carrier is the same as for non-mutation carriers.

Presentation
- Breast lump
- Nipple inversion or discharge
- Mammographically detected lesion—increasingly common mode of presentation

Diagnosis
- Mammogram
- Ultrasound
- Fine needle aspiration cytology
- Core biopsy

Pathology

Table 5.15 Pathology

Preinvasive lesions
Lobular carcinoma in situ (LCIS)—significance uncertain
Ductal carcinoma in situ (DCIS)—usually detected mammographically may progress to invasive disease
Invasive lesions
Ductal carcinoma—not otherwise specified—accounts for approximately 80% of all tumours
Lobular carcinoma
Tubular carcinoma
Medullary carcinoma

Presentation and staging

Breast cancer is diagnosed by a 'triple assessment'.

1 Clinical examination
2 Bilateral mammography
3 Fine needle aspiration cytology or core biopsy

This approach has >90 per cent sensitivity and specificity.

All patients with proven invasive disease should have axillary node dissection as a staging procedure to assess axillary node involvement. Staging investigations are more likely to reveal metastases in patients presenting with node-positive disease than in those with disease localized to the breast.

Prognostic factors

Include:

- Axillary node involvement—most important prognostic criterion
- Five years survival node +ve patients 20–30 per cent, node –ve patients 70–80 per cent
- Tumour size
- Tumour grade
- Oestrogen receptor (ER)/Progesterone receptor (PR) status. More favourable prognosis if ER/PR positive
- Patient age—<35yrs is an adverse independent prognostic factor, see Table 5.16 overleaf

Common problems

Bone pain due to bone metastases

- **Pathological fractures** may occur without obvious trauma
- **Spinal cord compression** requires prompt diagnosis, high dose oral steroids and urgent referral to the oncologist. The steroids should be continued at a high dose until a definitive plan has been made
- **Neuropathic pain** can be a particular problem especially if there has been spread into the brachial plexus
- **Liver metastases** are common and may require steroids or NSAIDs to reduce the pain of liver capsule stretch. Surgery may be appropriate
- **Hypercalcaemia** may occur. In many cases treatment should be considered with i/v hydration and i/v bisphosphonates on a monthly basis
- **Lymphoedema** can develop, at any point in the course of the disease, affecting the arm following surgery and/or radiotherapy. Early referral to a lymphoedema specialist provides the best chance of minimising the morbidity and distress caused. Management includes good skin care, avoiding additional trauma to the affected arm (including taking of blood tests and BP measurement) and appropriately fitting compression garments
- **Lung and pleural spread** are common causes of breathlessness and cough. These symptoms need to be investigated thoroughly. Drainage of a pleural effusion may be a useful symptomatic procedure and pleurodesis should be considered
- **Psychosocial problems.** A section of these patients will be mothers with young children for whom the trauma of disease is worsened by fears for their children. A multidisciplinary supportive approach at a pace dictated by the patient can help to reduce some of the distress for the patient and her family

Management

Table 5.16 Management

Non-invasive breast cancer DCIS and LCIS	Simple mastectomy OR Partial mastectomy and postoperative radiotherapy. Axillary dissection not indicated.
Early breast cancer T$_{1-3}$, N$_{0-1}$	**Surgery:** either simple mastectomy or partial mastectomy (lumpectomy) and axillary node dissection.
	Loco-regional radiotherapy: indicated for all patients with partial mastectomy and for mastectomy patients at high risk of local relapse (e.g. patients with >4 nodes positive).
	Adjuvant endocrine therapy: Tamoxifen indicated for all ER- or PR-positive tumours. Approximately 30% relative reduction in mortality. Value of aromatase inhibitors is being examined in randomized controlled trials.
	Adjuvant chemotherapy: Combination chemotherapy reduces recurrence and improves overall survival. Anthracycline based regimens are probably slightly more effective than non-anthracycline based regimens but with a higher incidence of cardiotoxicity. Absolute 10 year survival benefit: 7–11% <50 years; 2–3% > 50 years. Commonly used regimens include Adriamycin/cyclophosphamide (AC), fluorouracil/epirubicin/cyclophosphamide (FEC), cyclophosphamide/methotrexate/fluorouracil (CMF). The benefit risk ratio for chemotherapy must be assessed on an individual patient basis.
	Neo-adjuvant therapy: Not yet fully evaluated. May have some advantage in allowing more patients to have breast conserving surgery. Trials to assess the value of a neo-adjuvant approach are ongoing.
Locally advanced breast cancer *(Presence of infiltration of the skin, chest wall or fixed axillary nodes)*	The presence of infiltration of the skin, chest wall or fixed axillary nodes requires a *neo-adjuvant* approach. Younger patients and those with ER/PR negative disease may need chemotherapy. Elderly patients with ER or PR positive disease may be treated with hormonal therapy alone. In this situation aromatase inhibitors increasingly appear to be superior to tamoxifen.

Metastatic breast cancer
The aim is palliation. Usual sites of metastases: lung, liver, bone, brain

Bone metastases often respond to hormone manipulation with e.g tamoxifen

Such patients may survive for many years

Endocrine therapy: indicated in those patients with ER- or PR-positive disease and slowly progressive disease. Responses tend to be slower in onset (3–6 months) than with chemotherapy but also tend to be more durable. Expected response rates of 40–60% to first line hormonal therapy in those with ER- and/or PR-positive tumours. Disease that responds to endocrine therapy and then progresses has a 25% response with second line treatment. Response to a third hormonal agent is 10–15%.

Chemotherapy: indicated in situations where a high response rate and rapid time to response are required. Anthracycline based regimens are used first line. Combinations such as FAC produce response rates of 40–60% with a median time to progression of 8 months. Taxanes are used in patients who have had prior exposure to anthracyclines—response rates 40–60%. In patients with HER-2 over expression addition of Herceptin (trastuzumab) to Taxotere (docetaxel) increases response rate and prolongs survival. In patients unfit for a taxane Herceptin may be used as a single agent. Other agents which may be used include capecitabine, vinorelbine and Caelyx (liposomal doxorubicin).

Radiotherapy: useful for palliation of painful bone metastases or of soft tissue metastases causing pressure effects.

Bisphosphonates: useful in the treatment of malignancy related hypercalcaemia. As a maintenance treatment in patients with bone disease, they have been demonstrated to reduce bone pain, skeletal events related to malignancy, and the incidence of hypercalcaemia.

Prostate cancer

Background
- Accounts for approximately 30 per cent of all cancers in men
- Second to lung cancer as a cause of cancer deaths in men
- Increasing age is major risk factor—70 per cent of men >80yrs have some evidence of prostatic cancer
- Appears to be linked to androgen exposure—rare in men castrated before 40yrs
- Incidence of prostate cancer is rising—in part this is due to increased detection of early disease by PSA screening
- Many PSA-detected cancers are clinically unimportant—more work needs to be done to distinguish patients with raised PSA levels who are at risk of developing metastatic disease

Presentation
- Urinary outflow symptoms
- Haematuria
- Back pain

Diagnosis and staging
- PSA assessment: PSA >4 ng/ml: clinical suspicion, requires transurethral ultrasound and needle biopsy
- PSA >50 ng/ml: often distant metastases
- Transurethral ultrasound and biopsy
- CT/MRI—may help to assess lymph node involvement
- Isotope bone scan

Table 5.17 TNM staging of prostate cancer

T_1—Clinically inapparent
T_2—Palpable tumour confined to prostate
T_3—Tumour extends through capsule
T_4—Tumour is fixed or invades structures other than seminal vesicles
N_0—N_0 regional nodes
N_1—Regional lymph node metastases
M_0—N_0 metastases
M_1—Metastases present

Management
Many prostate tumours are clinically insignificant and will not cause symptoms in the patient's lifetime. It is important, however, to recognize those patients whose tumours are likely to become clinically apparent.

Prognostic factors in patients with cancer confined to the prostate:
- Tumour grade—assessed by Gleason Score
- Tumour stage
- Patient age—younger patients are more likely to develop problems than older patients

Cancer confined to prostate gland

If aged <70 and fit, consider radical local therapy:

• Prostatectomy
• Radiotherapy

There are currently no trials directly comparing these approaches. In general terms fitter patients tend to be treated with surgery rather than radiotherapy.

Complications:

• Prostatectomy: 50 per cent impotence; 8–15 per cent long term incontinence
• Radiotherapy: 40 per cent impotence; rectal stricture/bladder irritation but no incontinence

If over 70 years:

• 'Wait and see' policy

Locally extensive disease (T_3/T_4) or Node N_1 disease

• Neo-adjuvant anti-androgen therapy
• Radical radiotherapy

Metastatic disease

The natural history is very variable, with a number of patients with metastatic bone disease living for >5years following diagnosis.

The majority of tumours are sensitive to androgens. Hormonal manipulation aimed at reducing the effect of androgens (mainly testosterone) at a cellular level will produce responses in around 70 per cent of men with bone metastases with a median response duration of 12–18 months.

Commonly used hormonal treatments include:

• Medical castration with gonadorelin analogues. (These can induce a flare of hormone induced activity on initiating therapy which needs to be suppressed with anti-androgens for the initial two weeks.)
• Anti-androgens (cyproterone acetate, flutamide, bicalutamide). These may be used alone or in combination with gonadorelin analogues. The value of the combination is, however, uncertain
• Oestrogens are only used by oncologists as third line therapy because of the high incidence of thromboembolic side-effects
• Bilateral orchidectomy—less popular due to availability of medical methods of castration

The side-effects of these hormone treatments include:

• Loss of libido and potency
• Hot flushes
• Change in fat deposition
• Osteoporosis
• Poor concentration
• Decreased energy and drive

Local radiotherapy may be useful as an additional palliative measure particularly for bone pain. Strontium[89] (i/v), a bone-seeking radio isotope, has proved an effective, though expensive, treatment for reducing bone pain.

Hormone refractory prostate cancer

The prognosis for patients whose disease has progressed through anti-androgen therapy is poor.

Therapeutic options at this stage include:

- Anti-androgen withdrawal—this results in a response in a small number of patients
- Chemotherapy—prostate cancer is relatively chemoresistant and no standard regimen has been established. Mitoxantrone however has been used in this disease with some evidence of useful clinical activity

Common palliation issues

- **Pathological fracture** may occur without obvious trauma. These may need orthopaedic intervention (pinning or joint replacement) and radiotherapy. Prophylactic orthopaedic intervention may also be required for bone lesions at high risk of fracture
- **Spinal cord compression** requires prompt diagnosis and treatment with high dose steroids and radiotherapy. A minority of cases may be suitable for surgical intervention. Such patients include those with a single site of disease and those in whom there is uncertainty regarding the diagnosis. These patients should be discussed with a neurosurgeon
- **Neuropathic pain** Local recurrence of tumour, pelvic spread or a collapsed vertebra may cause neuropathic pain. Such pain is partially opioid sensitive but adjuvant analgesics are usually required to supplement the effect of the opioid
- **Bone pain** Specialist advice should be sought about the appropriate use of radiotherapy and radioactive strontium as well as nerve blockade. Bisphosphonates such as pamidronate and zoledronate help to reduce bone pain and also reduce the number of cancer-associated skeletal events and incidence of hypercalcaemia
- **Bone marrow failure** may occur in patients with advanced disease. Typically the patient has symptomatic anaemia and thrombocytopenia. Support with palliative blood transfusions may be appropriate initially, but their appropriateness should be discussed with the patient and their family when there is no longer symptomatic benefit gained from transfusion
- **Retention of urine** Problems with micturition including haematuria may lead to retention of urine. This may be acute and painful or chronic and painless. If the patient is unfit for transurethral resection of the prostate (TURP) then consider a permanent indwelling urinary catheter. Chronic urinary retention can lead to renal failure
- **Lymphoedema** of the lower limbs and occasionally the genital area is usually due to advanced pelvic disease. It needs to be actively managed if complications are to be avoided
- **Altered body image** and sexual dysfunction can result from any of the treatment modalities, hormone manipulation, radiotherapy, or surgery. This may be exacerbated by apathy and clinical depression. Specialist mental and psychological health strategies may be required

Gynaecological cancer

Ovarian carcinoma

Background

- Fifth commonest cancer in women
- Median age at diagnosis 66yrs
- Approximately 5 per cent are familial
- 95 per cent of tumours are epithelial in origin
- Risk is reduced by factors that reduce the number of ovulatory cycles e.g. pregnancy, use of oral contraceptive pill

Presentation

Ovarian cancer spreads mainly intraperitoneally and may remain silent until late: 80 per cent of patients therefore, present with disease which has spread beyond the pelvis.

Commonly presenting symptoms include:

- abdominal distension
- abdominal pain
- altered bowel habit
- weight loss

Diagnosis and staging

Table 5.18 Diagnosis and staging

Stage	Description	Five year survival (%)
Stage I	Confined to ovaries but without pelvic extension	75
Stage II	Tumour with pelvic extension	45
Stage III	Tumour with peritoneal spread outside the pelvis, or involves small bowel; retroperitoneal or inguinal nodes	20
Stage IV	Distant metastases	<5

Preoperatively a diagnosis of ovarian cancer may be suspected if the marker CA 125 is raised (elevated in approximately 85 per cent of patients with stage III/i/v disease) and the presence of a pelvic mass or ascites on CT scan.

Confirmation of the diagnosis requires histology. Adequate staging and initial disease management requires total abdominal hysterectomy, bilateral salpingo-oophorectomy, omentectomy, lymph node sampling, and multiple peritoneal biopsies.

Management

Radical surgery has an important rôle in treatment and retrospective studies demonstrate significantly improved survival in patients whose disease has been optimally debulked (i.e. no tumour remaining measuring >1 cm in diameter). Where optimal debulking is not possible initially there may be a survival benefit to performing debulking surgery after three cycles of chemotherapy—so called interval debulking.

First line chemotherapy

A platinum/taxane combination is considered by most oncologist to be the optimum treatment for ovarian cancer, the most commonly used combination being carboplatin and paclitaxel (Taxol). Response rates are approximately 70–80 per cent, and median survival is 2–3 years with such treatment.

Although the introduction of paclitaxel has improved the median survival in this disease, the majority of patients develop progressive disease and 5 year survival is still less than 20 per cent.

Treatment at relapse

The vast majority of patients who relapse after first line therapy are incurable. Secondary surgical debulking may be useful in selected patients, but its value is uncertain. The choice of further chemotherapy depends on the interval between completion of previous chemotherapy and relapse.

Patients relapsing more than six months after completion of platinum-based therapy may respond to further chemotherapy and should generally be rechallenged with a platinum agent. The response rate depends on the 'time out' from treatment ranging from very low <6 months to 60 per cent >2 years.

Patients relapsing less than six months after completion of platinum-based chemotherapy are unlikely to respond to further platinum based therapy. Fit patients should be considered for Caelyx or topotecan.

Eventually all patients who relapse following primary chemotherapy will develop chemotherapy-resistant disease. The majority of these patients will have symptoms related to intra-abdominal disease, including abdominal pain and bowel obstruction. Management of these symptoms can be very challenging and requires a multidisciplinary approach with involvement of palliative physicians, surgeons and oncologists.

Carcinoma of the cervix

Background

- Strongly associated with Human Papilloma Virus (HPV) 16 (and also, but less strongly, with HPV 18 and 31)
- 30–40 per cent of patients with untreated cervical intraepithelial neoplasia progress to invasive squamous cell carcinoma with a latent period of 10–20yrs
- Commonest female cancer in South East Asia, Africa and South America
- In the UK incidence and mortality have fallen by approximately 40 per cent since the 1970s

Presentation

- Generally asymptomatic until late
- Post coital bleeding
- Intermenstrual bleeding

Staging

Table 5.19 Staging

	FIGO staging system
Ia	Micro-invasive disease (max. depth 5 mm, max. width 7 mm)
Ib	Clinical disease confined to the cervix
IIa	Disease involves upper 2/3 of vagina but not parametrium
IIb	Disease involves parametrium but not pelvic wall
IIIa	Disease involves lower 1/3 of vagina
IIIb	Disease extend to pelvic side wall
IVa	Spread of tumour to adjacent pelvic organs
IV	Spread of tumour to distant organs

MRI plays an increasingly important rôle in the preoperative staging of these tumours.

Management

Management depends largely on disease stage. Patients with stage Ia may be treated with simple hysterectomy or a conisation procedure in those patients wishing to preserve their fertility.

For Stage Ib or IIa disease, radical hysterectomy appears equivalent to radical pelvic radiotherapy. For patients with Stage IIb to IVa disease, recent evidence suggests that combined radical pelvic radiotherapy with platinum-based chemotherapy gives best results. Chemoradiotherapy may also be indicated for patients with Stage Ib and IIa disease with adverse prognostic factors, such as those with bulky tumours.

For patients with Stage IVb disease pelvic radiotherapy may be useful in palliating troublesome pelvic symptoms. Cervical cancer is only moderately chemosensitive with responses to single agents of around 20–30 per cent. Agents with some activity in this disease include cisplatin, ifosfamide and paclitaxel.

Palliative issues in gynaecological cancers

- Primary treatment often affects sexual function, fertility and body image, which may impact on coping strategies and need specialist counselling. Ovarian and vulval cancers often present late and specialist palliative care input from the point of diagnosis may be appropriate. Genetic counselling should be considered for close female relatives of patients with ovarian cancer, particularly if there is also a strong family history of breast cancer
- **Perineal and pelvic pain** is common in all three of the common gynaecological malignancies; cervical, ovarian and vulval carcinomas. There is nearly always a neuropathic element to the pain which may be only partially opioid-sensitive
- **Lymphoedema affecting one or both limbs** develops with uncontrolled pelvic disease. It can develop at any time in a patient's cancer journey and frequently affects both lower limbs. It needs to be actively managed if complications are to be avoided. Management includes good skin care, avoiding additional trauma to the affected leg(s), and appropriately fitting compression garments
- **Ascites** is particularly common with ovarian cancer and can be difficult to manage. Oral diuretics, particularly spironolactone in combination with a loop diuretic such as furosemide, may help a little. Repeated paracentesis may be needed. Consideration of a peritoneovenous shunt may be appropriate in some cases where prognosis is thought to be longer than three months
- **Complete or subacute bowel obstruction** is often not amenable to surgical intervention and should be managed medically using subcutaneous medication via a syringe drive. Nasogastric tubes are rarely needed, and hydration can often be maintained orally if the nausea and vomiting are adequately controlled
- **Renal impairment** can develop in any patient with advanced pelvic disease. It may be a pre-terminal event. Ureteric stenting may be appropriate depending on the patient's perceived prognosis, the patient's wishes and future treatment options. Renal impairment increases the risk of a patient developing opioid toxicity as renal excretion of opioid metabolites may be reduced
- **Vaginal or vulval bleeding** may respond to antifibrinolytic agents such as tranexamic acid, radiotherapy and/or surgery
- **Offensive vaginal or vulval discharge** can cause considerable distress to both patient and carers. Topical or systemic metronidazole may help as can barrier creams. Deodorizing machines may also help if the patient is confined to one room
- **Vesico-colic and recto-vaginal fistulae** need surgical assessment. These can be very difficult to manage and require a multidisciplinary approach with specialist input

Upper gastrointestinal tract cancer

Stomach cancer

Background

- Second most common cancer worldwide
- Sixth most common cancer in the UK
- More common in males than females (2:1)
- 90–95 per cent of gastric tumours are adenocarcinomas
- In the UK incidence of cancer of the distal stomach is falling but incidence of tumours of the cardia or gastro-oesophageal junction is rising

Presentation

- Anaemia
- Weight loss
- Dyspepsia

Diagnosis and staging

- Endoscopy and biopsy
- Endoluminal ultrasound to assess depth of invasion and lymph node involvement
- CT scan to assess lymph node involvement and distant metastases
- Laparoscopy—may be indicated to assess peritoneal disease if surgery is being considered

Treatment

Resectable disease

Surgery remains the only potentially curative modality of treatment. Partial or total gastrectomy (depending on tumour site and mode of spread) and regional lymphadenectomy is the most commonly performed operation. Factors determining outcome include:

- Tumour location—patients with distal tumours do better than those with more proximally located tumours
- Tumour extent—patients with tumours beyond the gastric wall have a worse prognosis
- Extent of lymph node involvement

Following surgery many patients remain at high risk of local and distant disease relapse. Recent trials have suggested that such patients may benefit from adjuvant chemoradiation.

Neo-adjuvant approaches are also being investigated.

Locally advanced/metastatic disease

Palliative operations can be performed to control pain or bleeding or to relieve obstruction for patients with advanced disease. The type of operation performed depends to a large extent on the status of the patient and anticipated disease course.

Chemotherapy has also been demonstrated to have a palliative benefit for patients with locally advanced or metastatic gastric cancer and may also improve survival by some months. Endoscopic procedures such as stenting or laser coagulation may also provide useful palliative benefits.

Radiotherapy may provide useful palliation for e.g. bleeding from locally advanced tumours. It may also be useful in palliating pain caused by metastatic disease, e.g. bone metastases.

Oesophageal carcinoma

Background

- Eighth most commonly occurring cancer in the UK
- More common in males than females (2:1)
- Tumours in the upper two-thirds of the oesophagus are usually squamous cell cancers
- Tumours in the lower third are usually adenocarcinomas
- Adenocarcinoma often arises in a Barrett's oesophagus—endoscopic screening may reduce the incidence

Symptoms

- Dysphagia
- Chest pain
- Dyspepsia

Diagnosis and staging

- Endoscopy and biopsy
- Barium swallow—demonstrate tumour length
- Endoluminal ultrasound—demonstrates extent of local invasion and lymph node involvement
- CT scan—assesses nodal involvement and distant metastases.

   Staging investigations include:

- Laparoscopy
- Mediastinoscopy
- PET scanning

Treatment

Resectable disease

Surgery remains the only potentially curative modality for tumours in the lower two-thirds of the oesophagus. Unfortunately, however, due to the tendency of the tumour to spread longitudinally via the submucosa, circumferentially to other mediastinal structures and to lymph nodes early in its course, the results are poor with five year survival of <30 per cent. Neo-adjuvant approaches examining preoperative chemotherapy or chemoradiotherapy are currently under investigation.

   Tumours in the upper third of the oesophagus are inoperable but may be suitable for radical radiotherapy treatment.

   Radiotherapy may also be used with radical intent in tumours in the lower two-thirds of the oesophagus in patients who are unfit for surgery.

Unresectable disease

Endoscopic placement of stents or radiotherapy may provide excellent palliation. Platinum-based chemotheraphy may also be useful in palliating symptoms in patients who are fit.

Pancreatic carcinoma

Background

- Seventh most common cause of cancer death in the UK
- Seventy-five per cent arise from the head of pancreas, 15 per cent from the body, 10 per cent from the tail
- Risk factors include:
  - smoking
  - chronic pancreatitis
  - diabetes mellitus
- 90 per cent are adenocarcinomas

Presentation

- Insidious onset of symptoms
- Jaundice
- Weight loss
- Backache

Investigations

- CA19–9—elevated in majority of cancers but low sensitivity
- ERCP with brushings or biopsy
- Ultrasound scan or CT with FNA or biopsy of pancreatic mass
- CT chest abdomen and pelvis
- Laparoscopy—may be required to assess peritoneal involvement prior to surgery

Management

Surgery is the only potentially curative modality of treatment. Unfortunately less than 20 per cent of patients present with surgically resectable disease. A pancreaticoduodenectomy is the operation of choice. However even in those patients who are suitable candidates for this surgery five year survival is less than 30 per cent.

The majority of patients will present with advanced unresectable disease, although surgical bypass procedures may be possible. Primary treatment is aimed at relief of jaundice, which is generally achieved by endoscopic or percutaneous transhepatic placement of a stent.

Chemotherapy (e.g. gemcitabine) can provide a small survival benefit and should be considered in patients with unresectable disease and a ECOG performance status of less than three.

Palliative issues for patients with upper gastrointestinal tract cancer

Mild and non-specific symptoms often precede the onset of dysphagia for many months in oesophageal carcinoma. Stomach cancer often presents late and is frequently metatstatic at presentation.

- **Liver capsular pain** due to liver metastases is common. This is only partially opioid responsive but responds well to NSAIDs or oral steroids
- **Oesophageal spasm** may occur and can be difficult to manage. Specialist advice should be sought. It may be aggravated by oesophageal candidiasis, which needs systemic treatment with oral systemic. antifugals. Smooth muscle relaxants such as nifedipine may also help
- **Involvement of the coeliac plexus** causes a difficult pain syndrome with non-specific abdominal pain and mid back pain. Blockade of the plexus using anaesthetic techniques can be useful
- **Dysphagia** can occur in both oesophageal and stomach cancer. It may be helped by stenting. Oncological treatment of the tumour may provide temporary relief. Advice about appropriate diet and consistency of the food may also help. Feeding gastrostomies are sometimes used prior to aggressive treatment to improve functional status and the ability to tolerate such intervention. Gastrostomies can also improve nutrition and quality of life but should only be inserted after careful multidisciplinary discussion involving the patient and their family. Ethical dilemmas can arise towards the end-of-life when issues of avoiding the prolongation of an uncomfortable dying period (by reducing or stopping artificial feeding) may need to be discussed. There is no evidence that the insertion of feeding tubes in the dying either extends life or improves symptoms
- **Anorexia** is frequent and often profound. There may be a fear of eating because of pain. This may bring the patient and their carer into conflict about food and the 'need to eat'. Open and honest explanation can help to relieve anxiety and provide practical approaches to dealing with the situation
- **Weight loss and altered body image** can be profound with these cancers and can cause distressing problems for the patient and their family
- **Nausea and vomiting** can be persistent and difficult to control. Specialist advice is often needed and drugs may need to be given by routes other than oral. Small frequent meals may improve the frequency of vomiting
- **Haematemesis** may be one of the presenting symptoms but can also occur as the tumour progresses. Where possible local treatment may help and brachytherapy and laser therapy, where available, can reduce the incidence. There is risk of a major bleed. This is a difficult situation to manage and early involvement of specialists should be considered

Cancer of the bladder and ureter

Background
- Account for 1 per cent of all cancers
- 90 per cent are transitional cell carcinomas (TCC)
- Risk factors for TCC include:
  - smoking
  - occupational exposure to aromatic amines and azo dyes
- Squamous cell carcinoma of the bladder is less common and associated with schistosomiasis and bladder calculi

Presentation
- Haematuria
- Frequency
- Urgency

Diagnosis and staging
- Cystoscopy and biopsy
- CT/MRI

Treatment
- 70–80 per cent of all bladder cancers are 'superficial'—that is, they do not invade the muscularis mucosa

'Superficial' tumours
- Treated with transurethral resection of tumour
- Many will recur and follow-up with regular cytoscopy is required
- Factors which identify patients likely to develop invasive disease include:
  - high grade tumours
  - tumours have breached the basement membrane
  - multiple tumours

Such patients may benefit from intravesical chemotherapy or immunotherapy.

'Invasive' tumours
Disease which invades the muscularis mucosa of the bladder may be treated with radical cystectomy or radiotherapy. These modalities have not been directly compared and decisions regarding the choice of therapy tend to be based on performance status, with surgery reserved for the younger and fitter patients.

Bladder cancer is moderately chemosensitive—patients with locally advanced or metastatic disease may benefit from palliative chemotherapy. Active agents include cisplatin, gemcitabine and paclitaxel. No regimen is considered standard and these patients should be considered for entry into clinical trials.

Common problems
- **Bladder spasm** can be frequent and troublesome leading to urinary frequency as well as pain
- **Pelvic pain** is common in advanced disease due to tumour progression. This pain can be extremely difficult to control as it is often complex and includes neuropathic elements. Anaesthetic interventions, including intrathecal and epidural procedures, may be needed to gain pain control

- **Recurrent haematuria** is common and may be sufficient to cause anaemia, and urinary retention due to clot retention. Catheter blockage may be a problem
- **Urinary incontinence** may occur
- **Urinary tract infections** due to long term indwelling catheters are common but not necessary to treat unless symptomatic
- **Lymphoedema** of the lower limbs and genital area may occur and requires specialist management to prevent complications
- **Fistulae** may occur which are often suitable for surgery. If surgery is not possible the risks of skin breakdown are high
- **Renal failure** may occur. Stenting the renal tract may be possible but, may not be appropriate and needs full discussion
- **Altered body image** and problems with sexual function are understandably common
- **Depression** is common because of the long course of the disease, sleep disturbance, and damage to self-esteem

Tumours of the central nervous system

To expect a personality to survive the disintegration of the brain is like expecting a cricket club to survive when all of its members are dead.

Bertrand Russell

Background
- About a third of all brain tumours are metastatic from primary sites outside the CNS
- Primary brain tumours account for approximately 2 per cent of all cancers
- Primary brain tumours tend to remain localized to the CNS
- Primary brain tumours include:
  - astrocytomas—account for 80 per cent of gliomas most commonly occurring primary brain tumour grade is important in determining prognosis oligodendroglioma—account for 5 per cent of gliomas commonly occur in the frontal lobes longer prognosis
  - ependymoma—tend to occur in children and young adults may metastasise within the CNS
  - medulloblastoma—accounts for 25 per cent of all childhood tumours
  - cerebral lymphoma—increasing in incidence partly due to HIV-associated malignancy

Symptoms
- Headache
- Epilepsy
- Neurological symptoms

Investigations
- Contrast-enhanced CT scan
- Gadolinium-enhanced MRI scan
- If CSF spread is anticipated (e.g. for high grade ependymoma) a neuroaxis MRI +/– CSF cytology is required
- Biopsy is usually required to confirm diagnosis

Primary brain tumours
Surgery

Where possible surgical resection for some low grade tumours may be curative. For higher grade lesions decompression of the tumour may provide palliation and facilitate postoperative radiotherapy.

Radiotherapy

For high grade gliomas postoperative radiotherapy prolongs the effectiveness of surgery and increases median survival. For tumours with a propensity for leptomeningeal spread, such as high grade ependymoma or medulloblastoma, cranio-spinal irradiation improves prognosis.

Chemotherapy

Chemotherapy has a limited rôle to play in the treatment of most brain tumours and its use remains to be clearly defined.

As a general rule in patients with brain tumours poorer prognosis is related to:
- High tumour grade
- Neurological deficit at presentation
- Older age at presentation

Secondary brain tumours

Brain metastases

Cerebral metastases account for approximately a third of all brain tumours. The commonest primary cancer sites include lung, melanoma and breast. Autopsy reveals that metastases are commoner than revealed clinically (60 per cent in small cell lung carcinoma and 75 per cent in melanoma). Carcinoma of the prostate, bladder and ovary rarely metastasise to the brain. Only 5–10 per cent of all patients with cerebral metastases will develop clinical problems.

Assessment—clinical history

Neurological examination of higher cortical function, cranial nerves, musculoskeletal system, sensation, cerebellar function and gait.

Clinical features

Symptoms and signs can evolve over days to weeks. Multiple deposits are present in over two-thirds of patients and clinical signs depend on the anatomical site.
- Focal neurological disturbance consists of motor weakness including hemiparesis (30 per cent), dysphasia and cranial nerve palsies
- Epileptic seizures (15–20 per cent)
- Raised intracranial pressure e.g. headache (50 per cent), nausea, vomiting and lethargy
- Change in mood, cognitive function or behaviour

Investigations

CT scan or MRI scan (better for tumours situated in the posterior fossa or brain stem) show the location of metastases, surrounding oedema and mass effect.

Management

Surgery may be suitable for a very small percentage of patients who are young, fit, with no disease elsewhere, a long treatment-free interval and with a solitary metastasis that will not respond well to radiotherapy, such as adenocarcinoma of the colon or renal carcinoma.

Patients who might benefit from radical treatment should be identified, including those with chemosensitive tumours such as the haematological malignancies, small cell lung cancer and possibly breast cancer.

Palliative radiotherapy with corticosteroids is the most usually appropriate treatment and may improve neurological symptoms and function in over 70 per cent (with a median survival 5–6 months), enabling a gentle reduction and sometimes withdrawal of steroids 4–6 weeks following treatment. Benefit may not be gained in those patients with poor prognostic factors which include poor performance status, over 60 years of age, non-breast primary site, multiple lobe involvement, short disease-free interval and overt uncontrolled metastases elsewhere. Decisions regarding treatment should be, as ever, tailored to the problems of the individual patient.

Cranial irradiation may cause some degree of scalp and upper pinna erythema and irritation. Temporary alopecia is universal in a population whose prognosis is unlikely to allow regrowth of hair within the remaining lifespan. The start of treatment may induce an increase in cerebral oedema which may require steroid dose readjustment. Other effects include transient somnolence, occurring within a few weeks, and longer term impairment of memory and cognition. These are significant problems in very few people and most patients do not survive long enough for late radiation changes in the CNS to develop.

Corticosteroids

High dose corticosteroids (dexamethasone 16 mg/day initially) reduce cerebral oedema and associated symptoms of headache and vomiting may be helped rapidly. In certain situations, particularly if metastases are in the posterior fossa, hydrocephalus may be present, in which case a ventricular shunt may be required for symptom control.

The short prognosis for most patients means that the issue of long term side-effects of steroids may not be a problem. It is best practice, however, gradually to reduce the dose to the lowest possible over a few weeks to minimize potential side-effects since difficulties may build up insidiously.

A stage may be reached when the dose necessary to control the cerebral oedema causes significant side-effects. Disabling problems such as obesity (and associated problems with immobility management), body image problems, proximal myopathy, mood swings, fragile skin and diabetes may then develop. There should be open dialogue (particularly while the patient is *compos mentis* and can join in discussions) about the ongoing use of steroids in the event that quality of life becomes adversely affected. Patients and families may view the steroids as agents to control the disease and resist attempts to reduce the dose, fearing the return of symptoms of raised intracranial pressure.

On the other hand, patients may have recognized that their quality of life is deteriorating despite continuing steroids and may then be happy for (or request that) steroids should be withdrawn. This should generally be done slowly while controlling the symptoms of raised intracranial pressure by other means.

When patients become moribund and can no longer swallow, steroids can generally be stopped but this may depend on the particular clinical circumstances and may need negotiation with the patient/family. There should be adequate medication provision (subcutaneous) for analgesia, antiemetics, anticonvulsants and sedatives as necessary.

Multiple complex physical and psychological problems including poor mobility, heavy care needs, swings in mood, and confusion can completely exhaust even the most caring family who need the expert support of an experienced multi-disciplinary team (MDT).

Prognosis

Although some patients, particularly with metastases from breast cancer, may survive relatively longer, most patients with brain metastases from solid tumours have a survival in the order of a few weeks or months at best.

Metastatic disease of the leptomeninges (meningeal carcinomatosis)

Five per cent of patients with tumours may develop clinical signs and symptoms of leptomeningeal disease, although the autopsy rate is higher (10 per cent). It is most commonly seen in lymphoma and leukaemia although it may occur in breast cancer, small cell lung cancer and melanoma.

Clinical features

The presenting features may be varied and fluctuating and the diagnosis should be considered in any unexplained neurological disturbance in a patient with cancer. The most frequently encountered are cranial nerve problems (75 per cent), headache (50 per cent), radicular or back pain (40–45 per cent) and weakness in one or more limbs (40 per cent). Other presentations include meningism, altered consciousness, confusion, sphincter disturbance and seizures. Abnormal physical signs are more prominent than symptoms, with lower motor neurone lesions predominating.

Investigations

- Lumbar puncture if there is no evidence of raised intracranial pressure (90 per cent will have positive cytology and increased protein on CNS analysis)
- MRI scan

Management

This may include intrathecal chemotherapy, depending on the tumour type and radiotherapy. The aim is to halt progression of disease and relieve symptoms but is essentially palliative except for a curable sub-group of leukaemia or lymphoma. Steroids and NSAIDs may help symptoms.

Prognosis

Without treatment patients may survive for several months, depending on the tumour type, with relentless progression of neurological symptoms. Even with treatment, prognosis is usually less than six months and is worst in small cell lung cancer, widespread disease, poor performance status and where there are widespread neurological signs.

Chronic leukaemia and myeloma

General comments

The clinical course tends to be very variable, but is characterized by a *protracted cycle of relapses and remissions*. This can cause considerable distress as the patients and their carers have to live with uncertainty about the future. Both patient and professionals involved with their care may find it hard to accept that a patient is entering the terminal phase.

Infection is a frequent and unpredictable complication of both the disease process and its treatment. It can be fatal and this makes the prognosis even more uncertain.

Chemotherapy may continue in advanced illness because of the possibility of a further remission and/or useful palliation.

Specific pain complexes

- **Bone pain** is very common. The pain is often worse on movement or weight-bearing, which makes titration of analgesics very difficult. The pain often *responds well to radiotherapy and/or oral steroids*. NSAIDs may help but must be used with caution because they may interfere with platelet and renal function
- **Pathological fractures** are particularly common in myeloma due to the lytic bone lesions. These often require *orthopaedic intervention* and subsequent *radiotherapy*. Prophylactic pinning of long bones and/or radiotherapy should be considered to prevent fracture and reduce the likelihood of complex pain syndromes developing
- **Spinal cord compression** requires prompt diagnosis, high dose oral steroids in a single daily dose and urgent discussion with an oncologist. The steroids should be continued at a high dose until a definitive plan has been made. They may then be titrated down in accordance with the patient's condition and symptoms
- **Wedge and crush fractures of the spinal column** can lead to severe back pain which is often associated with nerve compression and neuropathic pain. Such pain is partially opioid sensitive but adjuvant analgesics in the form of antidepressants and/or anticonvulsant medication are usually required to supplement the effect of the opioid. Specialist advice is frequently needed to maintain symptom control

Other complications

Bone marrow failure is usual. Recurrent infections and bleeding episodes can leave the patients and carers exhausted. Patients often feel dependent on the administration of blood and platelet transfusions, unable to consider reducing the frequency of life-sustaining treatment. Difficult decisions about reducing regular transfusions or stopping them if they are providing no further benefit may need to be faced with patients and families.

Night sweats and fever are common, imposing a heavy demand on carers, particularly as several changes of night and bed clothes may be needed. Specialist advice may help in relieving the symptoms, as there are a number of drugs that appear to be effective. (📖 See Chapter 6d, p. 289.)

Hypercalcaemia may occur, especially in myeloma. It should be considered in any patient with persistent nausea, altered mood or confusion (even if this is intermittent), worsening pain and/or constipation. Treatment with i/v hydration and i/v bisphosphonates should be considered. Resistant hypercalcaemia may be a pre-terminal event when aggressive management would be inappropriate

Palliative care of patients with carcinomatosis of unknown primary

Background

Approximately 3 per cent of patients present with metastases from an unknown primary site. As a group the prognosis for these patient is poor, with median survival of 3–4 months.

Investigations

- Serological tumour markers including CA19–9, CEA, CA125, αFP, βHCG, PSA, and paraproteins
- Biopsy—thorough pathological assessment with immunohistochemistry may provide clues to the primary site
- CT scan of chest, abdomen and pelvis

In some instances the site of metastatic disease may suggest a probable primary site, e.g. adenocarcinoma in axillary nodes suggest a breast primary.

Particularly in young patients it is important to rule out the possibility of a potentially curable germ cell tumour. This may be suggested by elevated αFP or βHCG.

In a substantial number of patients a primary site is not identified. In this instance exhaustive investigations are not appropriate.

Treatment

In some patients where the clinical presentation suggests a primary, even if a tumour cannot be detected in that organ, it may be appropriate to treat the patient in the usual manner. For example, a patient presenting with ER-positive adenocarcinoma in an axillary node could reasonably be treated as if breast cancer was the primary.

For patients in which there is little evidence of a primary site (e.g. those presenting with liver metastases) the choice is much more difficult. As the primary is unknown it is impossible to give patients an idea of the like-lihood of a treatment response or of how durable such a response is likely to be. Any potential benefit of treatment must be carefully balanced against possible toxicity and a decision to proceed with chemotherapy should only be undertaken following a very full discussion with the patient and carers, outlining the uncertainties and limitations of treatment and overall limited prognosis.

Anxiety is common in this group of patients. Not knowing the site of the primary tumour causes considerable distress. Extensive investigations may raise false expectations and may exhaust the patient. Equally patients and carers may feel cheated of the chance to have effective treatment if the primary is not looked for.

Carers may find coming to terms with the patient's death due to an 'unknown primary' difficult, and are perhaps at greater risk of an adverse bereavement reaction.

Key points

- Anxiety
- Anger
- Risk of over investigation
- Adverse bereavement reaction

Further reading

Cassidy J., Bissett D. et al. (2002) *Oxford handbook of oncology.* Oxford: Oxford University Press.

Kirkham S. (1988) The palliation of cerebral tumours with high dose dexamethasone: review. *Palliative Medicine,* 2: 27–33.

Souhami R. L., Tobias J. D. (2003) *Cancer and its management.* 4th edition. Oxford: Blackwell Science.

Thomas K. (2003) *Caring for the dying at home: companions on the journey.* Oxford: Radcliffe Press.

The management of pain

> To Each his sufferings, all are men,
> Condemned alike to groan;
> The tender for another's pain,
> Th'unfeeling for his own.

Thomas Gray, *Ode on a Distant Prospect of Eton College* (1747).
London: R. Dodsley.

The intricacy of the human condition and the constantly changing interface between the external and the internal allows pain to be experienced in myriad different modalities. This ever-fluxing dynamic interaction between external stimuli and the individual's capacity to deal with those stimuli can greatly increase the complexity of pain management. What may be experienced as terrible pain by one individual may be brushed aside by another. Further, even individuals presented with the same painful stimuli at different times in their lives may be affected in a completely different manner. Stories abound of soldiers wounded in battle being able to ignore pain which, had it resulted from an accident at home, would have completely incapacitated them.

Pain is experienced by people and families not by nerve endings.

Experts in torture have used the huge and varied capacity to experience pain in plying their evil arts. Conversely, as the capacity to experience pain is so varied, so the methods used to alleviate pain need to be multidimensional.

A mother kissing away the pain of her child who has just had a fall, and an anaesthetist inserting a spinal catheter are both involved in the process of pain alleviation. Ensuring that the intervention used is appropriate for individuals and their families is crucial, but so also is ensuring that other causes, contributory factors and healing potentials are not ignored.

In the centre of Kathmandu there is a tree shrine to the God of toothache, to which sufferers go to hammer in a coin to help alleviate their pain. The tree is covered with thousands of coins. In a city which until very recently had only a handful of dentists, such an approach to pain control may not be as simplistic as it might first appear to western eyes which have had the benefits of modern anaesthetics and dentistry for a few generations.

The arrogance of healers who believe that their approach to pain alleviation is the only effective method does not stand up to the experience of life, and the reality that there are many ways in which pain is experienced and dealt with.

For health workers involved in dealing regularly with patients' pain there is a tension between two extremes of care.

The scientific clinician can be so specialized in synapse research that his model of pain control can sound mechanistic, simplistic and unbelievable.

The holistic clinician on the other hand can view patients' pain with such a wide angle lens that appropriate analgesic intervention with enough focused attention to relieve the symptoms is not achieved.

Of necessity this section will look at aspects of pain control in isolation, but quality pain management always involves both a holistic approach to patient care and a scientific approach with meticulous attention to diagnostic and management detail.

He was around 25 and obviously embarrassed to be at the surgery.

'It's these pains in my gut doctor, they are really bad'. A pause, a whiff of a hidden agenda hung in the air.

'How long have you had this problem?'

'Only these last two weeks, it's really bad in the morning, and if I don't eat.'

A shifty look is followed by a blank stare at the floor.

'Have you any idea what might have brought the pain on?'

No answer, just an uncomfortable silence.

'Have you been worried about anything recently?'

A look combining fear and hope crosses his face, 'It's hard to talk about.'

'Often problems like this come from stress and worry, so what you're experiencing is not all that unusual. Anything that we discuss will, of course, be totally confidential'.

The story unfolds of sudden onset impotence following a relationship with a new partner while still harbouring strong feelings for his previous girl friend. Explanation and reassurance transform the man's demeanour, and he bounces out of the surgery relieved and unburdened.

I patted myself on the back for my ability to see beyond the offered reason for consulting to the deeper hidden meaning ignoring the fact that the doctor who treats 'just' the covert cause of pain is at similar risk as his colleague who focuses on 'just' the overt cause. Both lull themselves into the false sense of security that they have met the patient's real need.

Two weeks later the patient makes telephone contact.

'How are things?'

'Couldn't be better. I'm right back on form. It really made a difference talking with you, but, …'

'Yes?'

'But this pain in my stomach is still really bad. The only thing that seems to help is taking some of my mum's Zantac. Could you give me a script Doctor?'

Table 6a.1 Definition of pain terms[1]

Allodynia	Pain caused by a stimulus which does not normally provoke pain
Analgesia	Absence of pain in response to stimulation which would normally be painful
Causalgia	A syndrome of sustained burning pain, allodynia and hyperpathia after a traumatic nerve lesion, often combined with vasomotor dysfunction and later trophic changes
Central pain	Pain associated with a lesion in the central nervous system (brain and spinal cord)
Dysaesthesia	An unpleasant abnormal sensation which can be either spontaneous or provoked
Hyperaesthesia	An increased sensitivity to stimulation
Hyperalgesia	An increased response to a stimulus that is normally painful
Hyperpathia	A painful syndrome characterized by increased reaction to a stimulus, especially a repetitive stimulus, as well as an increased threshold
Neuralgia	Pain in the distribution of a nerve
Neuropathy	A disturbance of function or pathological change in a nerve
Neuropathic pain	Pain which is transmitted by a damaged nervous system, and which is usually only partially opioid sensitive
Nociceptor	A receptor preferentially sensitive to a noxious stimulus or to a stimulus which would become noxious if prolonged
Nociceptive pain	Pain which is transmitted by an undamaged nervous system and is usually opioid responsive
Pain	An unpleasant sensory and emotional experience associated with actual or potential tissue damage or described in terms of such damage
Pain threshold	The least experience of pain which a subject can recognize
Pain tolerance level	The greatest level of pain which a subject is prepared to tolerate

Mersky H., Bogduk N. (1994) *Classification of Chronic Pain.* 2nd edn. Seattle: IASP Press.

Pain is a common symptom

> For frequent tears have run
> The colours from my life.
>
> Elizabeth Barrett Browning 1806–61: *Sonnets from the Portuguese* (1850

- 'Pain is an unpleasant sensory and emotional experience associated with actual or potential tissue damage or described in terms of such damage. In other words, pain is a somatopsychic phenomenon.' (Robert Twycross)
- Pain is a complex physiological and emotional experience and not a simple sensation

Pain involves
- Unpleasant sensory experience
- Unpleasant emotional experience
- Social and spiritual components

Incidence of pain in cancer
- One quarter of patients *do not experience pain*
- One third of those with pain have a single pain
- One third have two pains
- One third have three or more pains

Causes of pain in patients with cancer
- Caused by cancer itself (85%)
- Caused by treatment
- Related to cancer and debility
- Unrelated to cancer

Perception of pain is modulated by
- The patient's mood
- The patient's morale
- The meaning of the pain for the patient

Patients with palliative care needs most commonly have *chronic malignan pain*. However, patients with *acute pain* or *chronic non-malignant pai* sometimes require the help of palliative care services. For these reasons i is important to assess each specific pain and to identify the likely cause.

Common causes of pain in patients with cancer
Cancer-related
- Bone
- Nerve compression/infiltration
- Soft tissue infiltration
- Visceral
- Muscle spasm
- Lymphoedema
- Raised intracranial pressure

reatment-related
  Surgery: postoperative scars/adhesions
  Radiotherapy: fibrosis
  Chemotherapy: neuropathy

Associated factors–cancer and debility
  Constipation
  Pressure sores
  Bladder spasm
  Stiff joints
  Post-herpetic neuralgia

Unrelated to cancer
  Low back pain
  Arthritis
  Angina
  Trauma

The experience of pain can

- Induce depression
- Exacerbate anxiety
- Interfere with social performance
- Negatively impact on physical capability
- Prevent work
- Decrease income
- Encourage isolation
- Impair the quality of relationships
- Create family disharmony and stress
- Challenge existential beliefs

These secondary effects are constantly affecting the patient's experience of pain.

Assessment of pain

When sorrows come, they come not single spies,
But in battalions.

William Shakespeare1564–1616: *Hamlet* (1601)

Assessment of a patient's pain is a crucial skill, which requires a structured approach, a closely listening ear and a sharp eye. Accurate assessment is also helped by experience, and is not a 'one-off' event—but needs to be constantly re-evaluated by the healthcare team as more information is gathered.

Assessment questions

There are many approaches to assessing pain, and each professional will develop his/her own approach to taking a *pain history*. The specifics of pain history questions are not crucial. What is important is that there is a logical outline scheme which works. Having good assessment technique is the basis for effective palliative care, and for prompt appropriate management of a patient's pain.

Pain History Principles

1 Seek to establish a relationship with the patient
2 Encourage the patient to do most of the talking
3 Begin with a wide angle open question before clarifying and focusing with more specific ones
4 Watch the patient for clues regarding pain
5 Avoid jumping to conclusions.

Remember, as you are assessing patients, they are assessing you.

- Eye to eye level contact
- Clear introduction
- Avoid over familiarity
- Explain what you plan to do
- Summarise back to the patient 'Have I heard things correctly'
- Avoid patronizing
- Use language and terms appropriate to patient

The most extreme agony is to feel that one has been utterly forsaken.

Bettelheim, Bruno (1979). *Surviving and Other Essays*. New York: Knopf.

Table 6a.2 One scheme of pain assessment questions

Is the patient currently in distress due to pain?	Before embarking on a full assessment it is important to achieve sufficient comfort for the patient to go through the assessment.
Is the pain related to movement?	Fractures/inflammation/peritonitis/pleurisy?
Is the pain periodic?	Colic: due to gastrointestinal or renal tract problems?
Is the pain worse on eating?	Mouth, oesophagus or stomach problems?
Is the pain associated with passing urine or stool?	Constipation, haemorrhoids, tenesmus, infection?
Is the pain associated with skin changes of colour, temperature or swelling?	Pressure sore/infection/ischaemic limb/DVT/skin tumour?
Is the pain associated with altered sensation?	This implies nerve damage: *neuropathic pain* which may occur in a dermatome (an area supplied by a peripheral nerve) *sympathetic pain* which occurs in the same distribution as the arterial blood supply.
Is the pain persisting?	Fear or depression, poor compliance with medication, inappropriate treatment or a new pain?
What relieves the pain?	What has already been tried which worked? e.g. change in position, distraction, medication?

Adapted from Thompson and Regnard.[2]

2 Thomson J. W., Regnard C. (1995) Pain. In C. Regnard, J. Hockley (eds) *Flow Diagrams in Advanced Cancer and Other Diseases*, pp. 5–10. London: Arnold.

Pain assessment tools

Symptom monitoring by patients can be used to enhance understanding of the symptoms and improve assessment of the effectiveness of management strategies. As an example of symptom monitoring, pain assessment charts and scales have been used extensively.

Used appropriately such evaluation tools provide a very useful quantifiable measure which both patient and healthcare professional can use to chart the effectiveness of pain reducing interventions.

However, for those patients who may ruminate about their 'pain scores', the use of such a method of assessment exacerbates pain, and pain awareness. Other patients who are in the advanced stages of illness will find the completion of pain charts an unnecessary burden.

From the health professional viewpoint, the collection of such data can be very useful, depending on the quality of the data collection, and can enhance understanding of how the patient perceives pain. However filling forms may draw the professional's attention away from the patient.

Pain is a multidimensional experience and as such requires a multidimensional assessment tool. The European Pain Group recommends two, the Brief Pain Inventory (BPI) and the McGill Pain Questionnaire (MPQ), as both have been well validated in a number of different languages.[3]

While such assessment tools cannot provide objective evidence of pain management, if applied appropriately they can provide clear evidence of trends experienced by individual patients.

A number of self report tools have been tested for use in palliative care to measure pain intensity in a reliable and valid way.

These include:

Visual analogue scales (VAS)
The VAS is an unmarked line with extremes marked as no pain and worst pain. Patients are asked to mark the point in the line that describes their pain.

No pain_____Worst pain

Categorical verbal rating scales (VRS)
A VRS involves a sequence of words describing different intensity levels of pain such as:

None   Mild   Moderate   Severe

Categorical numerical rating scales (NRS)
The NRS is similar to the VAS but uses numbers or gradations that indicate the severity of the pain experience

0____1____2____3____4____5____6____7____8____9____10
no pain   worst pain

3 Caraceni A., Cherny N., Fainsinger R., Kaasa S., Poulain P., Radbruch L., *et al.* (2000) Pain measurement tools and methods in clinical research in palliative care: recommendations of an expert working group of the European Association of Palliative Care. *Journal of Pain and Symptom Management.*

Brief Pain Inventory

Date: ___/___/___

Name: _____

Last   First   Middle Initial

Phone: (___) _____   Sex: ☐ Female   ☐ Male

Date of Birth: ___/___/___

1) Marital Status (at present)
     1. ☐ Single   3. ☐ Widowed
     2. ☐ Married   4. ☐ Separated/Divorced

2) Education (Circle only the highest grade or degree completed)
Grade   0   1   2   3   4   5   6   7   8   9
       10   11   12   13   14   15   16   M.A./M.S.
          Professional degree (please specify) _____

3) Current occupation_____
    (specify titles; if you are not working, tell us your previous occupation)

4) Spouse's Occupation_____

5) Which of the following best describes your current job status?
   ☐ 1. Employed outside the home, full-time
   ☐ 2. Employed outside the home, part-time
   ☐ 3. Homemaker
   ☐ 4. Retired
   ☐ 5. Unemployed
   ☐ 6. Other

6) How long has it been since you first learned your diagnosis? _____ months

7) Have you ever had pain due to your present disease?
   1. ☐ Yes   2. ☐ No   3. ☐ Uncertain

8) When you first received your diagnosis, was pain one of your symptoms?
   1. ☐ Yes   2. ☐ No   3. ☐ Uncertain

9) Have you had surgery in the past month? 1. ☐ Yes   2. ☐ No

10) Throughout our lives, most of us have had pain from time to time (such as minor headaches, sprains, and toothaches). Have you had pain other than these everyday kinds of pain during the last week? 1. ☐ Yes   2. ☐ No

IF YOU ANSWERED YES TO THE LAST QUESTION, PLEASE GO ON TO QUESTION 11 AND FINISH THIS QUESTIONNAIRE. IF NO, YOU ARE FINISHED WITH THE QUESTIONNAIRE. THANK YOU.

11) On the diagram, shade in the areas where you feel pain. Put an X on the area that hurts the most.

12) Please rate your pain by circling the one number that best describes your pain at its worst in the last week.
   0   1   2   3   4   5   6   7   8   9   10
   No   Pain as bad as
   Pain   you can imagine

13) Please rate your pain by circling the one number that best describes your pain at its least in the last week.
   0   1   2   3   4   5   6   7   8   9   10
   No   Pain as bad as
   Pain   you can imagine

14) Please rate your pain by circling the one number that best describes your pain on the average.
   0   1   2   3   4   5   6   7   8   9   10
   No   Pain as bad as
   Pain   you can imagine

Fig. 6a.1 Brief pain inventory. Reproduced with permission from Doyle et al. (2005) *The Oxford Textbook of Palliative Medicine*, 3rd edn. Oxford: Oxford University Press.

15) Please rate your pain by circling the one number that tells how much pain you have right now.

    0   1   2   3   4   5   6   7   8   9   10
No   Pain as bad as
Pain   you can imagine

16) What kinds of things make your pain feel better (for example, head, medicine, rest)?

_____

17) What kinds of things make your pain worse (for example, walking, standing, lifting)?

_____

18) What treatments or medications are you receiving for your pain?

_____

19) In the last week, how much relief have pain treatments or medications provided? Please circle the one percentage that most shows how much relief you have received.

0% 10%   20%   30%   40% -50%   60%   70%   80%   90%   100%
No   Complete
Relief   Relief

20) If you take pain medication, how many hours does it take before the pain returns?
- ☐ 1. Pain medication doesn't help at all
- ☐ 2. One hour
- ☐ 3. Two hours
- ☐ 4. Three hours
- ☐ 5. Four hours
- ☐ 6. Five to twelve hours
- ☐ 7. More than twelve hours
- ☐ 8. I do not take pain medication

21) Circle the appropriate answer for each item.
I believe my pain is due to:

☐ Yes ☐ No 1. The effects of treatment (for example, medication, surgery, radiation, prosthetic device).

☐ Yes ☐ No 2. My primary disease (meaning the disease currently being treated and evaluated).

☐ Yes ☐ No 3. A medical condition unrelated to primary disease (for example, arthritis).

22) For each of the following words, check yes or no if that adjective applies to your pain.

Aching	☐ Yes	☐ No	Exhausting	☐ Yes	☐ No
Throbbing	☐ Yes	☐ No	Tiring	☐ Yes	☐ No
Shooting	☐ Yes	☐ No	Penetrating	☐ Yes	☐ No
Stabbing	☐ Yes	☐ No	Nagging	☐ Yes	☐ No
Gnawing	☐ Yes	☐ No	Numb	☐ Yes	☐ No
Sharp	☐ Yes	☐ No	Miserable	☐ Yes	☐ No
Tender	☐ Yes	☐ No	Unbearable	☐ Yes	☐ No
Burning	☐ Yes	☐ No			

23) Circle the one number that describes how, during the past week, pain has interfered with your:

A. General Activity

    0   1   2   3   4   5   6   7   8   9   10
Does not   Completely
Interfere   interferes

B. Mood

    0   1   2   3   4   5   6   7   8   9   10
Does not   Completely
Interfere   interferes

C. Walking ability

    0   1   2   3   4   5   6   7   8   9   10
Does not   Completely
Interfere   interferes

D. Normal work (includes both work outside the home and housework)

    0   1   2   3   4   5   6   7   8   9   10
Does not   Completely
Interfere   interferes

E. Relations with other people

    0   1   2   3   4   5   6   7   8   9   10
Does not   Completely
Interfere   interferes

F. Sleep

    0   1   2   3   4   5   6   7   8   9   10
Does not   Completely
Interfere   interferes

G. Enjoyment of life

    0   1   2   3   4   5   6   7   8   9   10
Does not   Completely
Interfere   interferes

Pain Research Group, Department of Neurology, University of Wisconsin-Madison

Pain and function

Surveys across different cultures show that the relationship between pain and physical performance is non-linear. Impairment in function becomes markedly worse above a pain severity rating of four on a ten point scale. This suggests that we have the capacity to deal with a certain amount of pain but once this capacity is exhausted, function quickly becomes impaired.[4]

This has important implications in the management of pain, as reducing some of the secondary effects of pain, such as anxiety or financial worries, may decrease the overall experience of pain to a point where function is markedly improved. Improvement of function can have a very positive effect reducing the experience of pain and restoring morale; some of the symptom control success achieved in inpatient palliative care units must be attributed to a reduction in secondary pain effects.

The pain threshold will vary from person to person and within the individual. It also varies according to multiple physical and psychosocial factors which are constantly changing. Models that help us understand pain need to take account of this constantly changing nature of pain perception. Such a model understands pain perception as a 'plastic phenomenon' which is constantly in flux.

This is supported by the growing understanding of the rapidly altering neurochemical environment of the central and peripheral nervous system. Changes in concentrations of neurotransmitters and of neuroreceptors impact on the transmission of painful stimuli.

Tom had been admitted to the hospice for symptom control from his local area hospital. Despite receiving nearly 1000 mg of diamorphine subcutaneously per day he persisted in scoring his pain at 8 or above.

Tom was a self made man of 55 who had built up a chain of shoe shops after leaving school at 16. When his oesophageal carcinoma was diagnosed he had a chain of shops all over the area.

He was not expecting his diagnosis of cancer and the news that curative intervention was not possible came as a devastating blow to a man used to controlling his own life and business.

Suddenly his life had been invaded and his inner resources for dealing with the situation overrun.

One week later Tom went home from the hospice requiring MST 20 mg b.d. and diazepam 5mg nocte to control his symptoms.

Tom achieved his improved pain control by having his underlying anxiety addressed and treated, and by gaining back some control over his life, the lack of which had caused him deep anguish.

'The space and peace in the hospice gave me time to get my head around things'.

---

4 Serlin R. C., Mendoza T. R., Nakamura Y., Edwards K. R., Cleeland C. S. (1995) When is cancer pain mild, moderate or severe? Grading pain severity by its interference with function. *Pain*, 61, 2: 277–84.

Pain classification

Pain is traditionally classified into four different modalities:

1 Physical,
2 Psychosocial,
3 Emotional, and
4 Spiritual.

It is imperative that patients' anxieties and frequent misconceptions related to these factors are explored. Pain will not be adequately controlled unless patients feel a degree of control over their situation. To ignore such psychological aspects of care may often be the reason for seemingly intractable pain. Having prescribed analgesics, the patient's pain should be under constant supervision and the response to treatment reviewed *regularly*.

Having identified the *cause* of the pain, it is useful to *classify* the pain into predominantly *nociceptive* or *neuropathic* categories in order to determine the correct management.

Nociceptive pain

This refers to pain resulting from stimulation of peripheral nerves transmitted by an undamaged nervous system. Pain impulses enter the spinal cord through the dorsal horn, where they ascend to higher centres in the brain. Inhibitory impulses block transmission at the dorsal horn in the spinal cord, preventing further transmission of the pain impulse. It is usually opioid responsive.

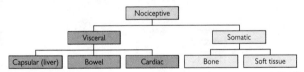

Fig. 6a.2 Nocioceptive pain

Neuropathic pain

Neuropathic pain refers to pain arising from damage in the peripheral or central nervous system. Clinically it may present with hyperalgesia and allodynia, with patients describing sensations such as burning or stabbing. It may be only partially opioid responsive.

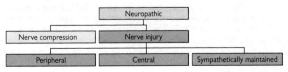

Fig. 6a.3 Neuropathic pain

Peripheral pain
Peripheral neuropathic pain is caused by damage within the peripheral nervous system. There is often an associated area of altered sensation around the site of nerve injury.

Central pain
Central pain refers to neuropathic pain caused by damage within the central nervous system. There is usually an area of altered sensation incorporating the area of pain. A cerebrovascular accident or spinal cord damage may be associated with central pain.

Sympathetically-maintained pain
Sympathetically-maintained pain is due to sympathetic nerve injury. Essential features are pain (often burning) and sensory disorder related to a vascular as opposed to neural distribution. In patients with cancer such pain is more common in the lower limbs, and is usually associated with disease in the pelvis.

Such pain is also associated with reduced sweating and dry shiny skin within the affected area.

Practical pain control

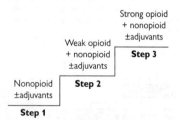

Fig. 6a.4 The analgesic ladder[5]

Step 1: Non opioid ± adjuvants
Start treatment with paracetamol 1g every 4 h REGULARLY (Max. daily dose 4g). If this is not adequate in 24 h, stop and proceed to step 2.

Step 2: Weak opioid + non opioid ± adjuvants
Start treatment with a combined preparation of paracetamol with codeine or dihydrocodeine. Use of dextropropoxyphene and paracetamol (co-proxamol) is being phased out in the UK in 2005. Many combined preparations are available and are some of the most widely used medicines in the community. NB Studies have shown that there is no additional analgesic benefit from preparations which contain only 8mg of codeine combined with paracetamol as opposed to paracetamol alone. It is important to stipulate the dose of codeine required in the preparation e.g. 'paracetamol 500mg/codeine 30mg'. Patients need also to be clearly advised to take these tablets regularly and not to assess efficacy after only a couple of doses.

5 World Health Organization (1996) *Cancer pain relief: with a guide to opioid availability.* 2nd edition. Geneva: WHO.

Step 3: Strong opioid + non opioid ± adjuvants

Two tablets of co-codamol contain 60mg of codeine which is already approximately equi-analgesic to oral morphine 5mg every 4h. (See conversion table). If changing to morphine, it will therefore be necessary to use a minimum of morphine 5mg but 10mg may be needed. Caution should be exercised in patients who are elderly or in renal failure, since active morphine metabolites are excreted by the kidney. The formulation of morphine may be immediate release (i/r) tablets or solution, depending on patient preference. If the pain seems responsive to opioids and there are no undue side-effects, continue to titrate the dose upwards by no more than 30–50 per cent every 24 h until pain is controlled. It is not necessary to wake the patient at night to give medication, but if pain during the night or first thing in the morning is a problem, it may be helpful to increase the last evening dose by 50 per cent.

Step 4: Adjuvant drug (co-analgesic)

This is a drug which is not an analgesic in its prime function but in combination with an analgesic can enhance pain control.

Examples of use of adjuvant drugs			
Corticosteroid:	pain caused by oedema	Night sedative:	when lack of sleep is decreasing pain threshold
Antidepressant:	neuropathic pain		
Anticonvulsant:	neuropathic pain	Anxiolytic:	when anxiety is contributing to pain
Muscle relaxant:	muscle cramp pain		
Antispasmodic:	bowel colic	Antidepressant:	when depressed mood is contributing to pain
NSAID:	inflammatory pain		
Antibiotic:	infection pain		

Breakthrough pain

Breakthrough pain is a flare in pain of rapid onset, moderate to severe intensity and of short duration. It may be precipitated by activity but it can also happen spontaneously. If pain starts to occur regularly before the next dose is due, this is probably an indication to increase the regular background dose.

- Analyse and avoid precipitating activities if possible. Predict pain and give analgesia 20 minutes prior to activity e.g. prior to changing dressings or movement

Treatment options to consider:
- Immediate release oral morphine or other opioid according to background analgesia (or diamorphine SC/ i/v if unable to swallow) at 50–100 per cent of the equivalent regular background 4 h dose
- Oral transmucosal fentanyl citrate lozenges (OTFC) or other fentanyl-like drugs
- Midazolam 2.5–5mg SC/lorazepam 0.5mg sublingually to allay anxiety
- NSAID SC e.g. parecoxib 40mg

Other therapies include:
- Visualization techniques, hypnotherapy, reassurance and a calm professional manner, distraction etc.

NB Nitrous oxide gas (Entonox) inhalation is now rarely used prior to painful procedures. For this means of analgesia to be effective, the patient needs to be able to inhale deeply, whilst holding the mask to the face. It is therefore not very useful with the weak , infirm or older patient. It *must* be administered with the demand valve and this *must* be held to the face by the patient alone. If the patient is made drowsy by the Entonox, the mask automatically falls away from the face and the patient breathes air again and recovers, before there is any risk of losing protective reflexes. Entonox should *never* be used on patients who have any air where it should not be e.g. pneumothorax, or pneumoperitoneum. Nitrous oxide rapidly enters these areas, causing potentially dangerous expansion.

Opioid-resistant cancer pain

Pseudo-resistant?
- Underdosing
- Poor alimentary absorption of opioid (rare, except where there is an ileostomy)
- Poor alimentary intake because of vomiting
- Ignoring psychological aspects of patient care

Semi-resistant?
- Bone pain
- Raised intracranial pressure
- Nerve trunk compression
- Neuropathic pain
- Activity-related pain

Resistant?
- Muscle spasm
- Abdominal cramps
- Spiritual pain (🔲 Chapter 9)

As stressed earlier, patients with chronic unremitting pain from a deteriorating condition are particularly at risk of spiritual pain which needs to be addressed. Referral for psychological/spiritual support is important, and/or use of a complementary therapist. Using Hay's seven model assessment[6], 'spiritual pain' can be broken down into:
- Spiritual suffering—interpersonal or intra-psychic anguish
- Inner resource deficiency—diminished spiritual capacity
- Belief system problem—lack or loss of personal meaning system
- Religious request—a specifically expressed religious need

---

6 Hay M. W. (1989) Principles in building spiritual assessment tools. *The American Journal of Hospice Care*, **6**: 25–31.

Opioid analgesic therapy

Paracetamol and weak opioids

Codeine

Five to ten per cent of caucasians are CYP2D6 poor-metabolizers, an hepatic enzyme necessary to convert codeine to morphine. These patients will not obtain equivalent analgesia using codeine-containing analgesics. This bioactivation is markedly inhibited by antipsychotics (chlorpromazine, haloperidol, levomepromazine, and thioridazine), metoclopramide, and tricyclic antidepressants (amitriptyline etc.). If hepatic metabolism is decreased in patients taking these drugs, or with liver disease, the analgesic action of codeine may also be compromised.

Co-proxamol

Systematic reviews suggest that co-proxamol (dextropropoxyphene and paracetamol) is no more effective as an analgesic than paracetamol alone. Dextropropoxyphene has a longer elimination half-life than paracetamol and will therefore accumulate to higher blood levels during repeated dosing.

Compound analgesics containing sub-therapeutic doses of opioids should not be used for pain control in cancer patients.[7] The UK Committee of Safety of Medicines decided in January 2005 to withdraw co-proxamol use in the UK over a 12 month period because of its efficacy and safety profile.

Morphine

> We are all strong enough to bear the misfortunes of others.
> Duc de la Rochefoucauld 1613–80: *Maximes* (1678)

Morphine is the strong opioid of first choice for moderate to severe cancer pain. Alternative opioids may be as effective, and are appropriate for certain patients.

Starting a patient on morphine

- Start with immediate release (i/r) morphine liquid or tablets
  - Adult, not pain controlled on regular weak opioids: 10mg 4-h morphine
  - Elderly, cachectic, or not taking regular weak opioids: 5mg 4-h morphine
  - Very elderly and frail: 2.5mg 4-h morphine
- Although 4-h morphine gives greatest flexibility for initial dose titration, patients with less severe pain, difficulties with compliance and especially outpatients, can be started on 12-h modified release (m/r) morphine:
  - Adult, not pain controlled on regular weak opioids: 15–30mg 12-h morphine m/r
  - Very elderly and frail: 10mg 12-h morphine m/r
- Always prescribe a laxative concurrently
- Consider prescribing a regular antiemetic for those with a history of nausea/vomiting, e.g. haloperidol 1.5mg nocte: this can usually be stopped after a week. If not prescribed prophylactically, warn the patient to report any nausea so that an antiemetic can be prescribed as soon as possible
- Explain to patients that any drowsiness will usually wear off after a few days

[7] Scottish Intercollegiate Guidelines Network (2000) *Control of pain in patients with cancer.* Edinburgh: SIGN.

- Advise patients not to drive, for at least one week after starting morphine, or after any increase in dose. Patients should continue to avoid driving even after this time of drowsiness persists

Titrating dose of morphine
- Increase the dose as needed by increments of 25–50 per cent rather than by a fixed amount. The increment percentage tends to decrease a little as the dose increases e.g.
  5–10–15–20–30–40–60–80–100–130–160–200mg. There is no pre-set maximum dose of opioids as long as increasing the dose gives further analgesia. Very few patients will require more than 600mg daily
- When pain is reasonably well controlled consider converting to modified release morphine 12-h for convenience of b.d. administration

Morphine preparations
Morphine (immediate release, 4-h)
- Mixture 10mg/5ml *(Oramorph/Sevredol)*
- Mixture 20mg/ml *(Oramorph concentrated/Sevredol concentrated)*
- Tabs. 10, 20, 50mg—scored Tabs. *(Sevredol)*

Morphine Unit Dose Vials
- Vials. 10, 30, 100mg all in individual 5ml vials *(Oramorph Unit Dose Vials)*

Morphine preparations, (modified release, 12-h)
MST and *Zomorph* can be used interchangeably.
MST Continus (Morphine m/r)
- Tabs. m/r 5, 10, 15, 30, 60, 100, 200mg
- Susp. 20, 30, 60, 100, 200mg
  Sachets to prepare Susp.

Zomorph caps. (Morphine m/r)
- caps. m/r 10, 30, 60, 100, 200mg
  Can be broken and administered via a **NG/PEG** tube, or sprinkled on food. Bioequivalent to *MST*

Morphine preparations—modified release (24-h)
MXL (Morphine m/r)
- caps. m/r 30, 60, 90, 120, 150, 200mg

Morcap m/r (Morphine m/r)
- caps. m/r 20, 50, 100mg
May not be bioequivalent to MST

Morphine preparations—rectal (4-h)
Morphine Supps.
- Supps. 10mg 15mg 20mg, 30mg
- Equianalgesic dose by oral and rectal routes

Converting to 12-h morphine
Divide daily morphine intake by half to give 12-h dose (e.g. morphine 10mg 4-h → 30mg morphine m/r 12-h).

Ensure the patient has access to immediate release morphine for breakthrough pain. A dose of morphine of 50–100% of the 4-h dose equivalent may be taken for breakthrough pain.

Diamorphine

Diamorphine is more soluble in water than morphine, and is commonly used as the injectable strong opioid in a syringe driver for subcutaneous infusion.

To convert from oral morphine to SC diamorphine, divide the total dose of oral morphine by 3

e.g. 10mg 4-h morphine

$\cong$ 60mg oral morphine in 24h

$\cong$ 20mg diamorphine by CSCI over 24h

e.g. morphine 3mg p.o. $\cong$ Diamorphine 1mg by SC injection

Increments in dose should be between 25–50 per cent as for oral morphine. Additional SC doses for 'breakthrough' pain should be 50–100 per cent of the equivalent 4-h dose.

> If vomiting or no longer able to swallow medication, convert to a subcutaneous infusion of diamorphine via a syringe driver by dividing the 24-h total dose of oral morphine by three.

Breakthrough doses

Use 50–100 per cent of the equivalent 4-h dose currently being used e.g.

A. for a patient on morphine m/r 270mg 12-h:

$\cong$ 540mg oral morphine in 24h

$\cong$ 90mg morphine p.o. 4-h

i.e. use breakthrough dose 45–90mg morphine p.o. 4-h p.r.n.

B. for a patient on 180mg diamorphine SC in 24h

$\cong$ 30mg diamorphine SC 4-h

i.e. use breakthrough dose of 15–30mg diamorphine SC 4-h

Intravenous use for pain emergencies

Various different protocols have been described for intravenous titration of opioids for severe pain 'emergencies'.

- monitor respiratory rate and conscious level regularly
- draw up diamorphine diluted to 10ml with water
  - If opioid naive dilute 5mg of diamorphine in 10ml of water
  - If on regular opioid use equivalent 4-h dose based on previous opioid use in last 24h (see 'Breakthrough doses' above) diluted in 10ml water
- give appropriate diamorphine dilution i/v at 1ml/minute (total over 10 minutes)
- stop if pain <5/10 or toxicity develops
- repeat the above after a further 10–20 minutes if required
- calculate the total dose of diamorphine administered and multiply by 6
- start maintenance infusion with CSCI, or regular oral morphine equivalent dose over 24h

> NB It is unusual to give diamorphine intravenously in a hospice setting. Subcutaneous administration is most commonly used (takes 10 to 20 minutes to work) unless the pain is very severe and immediate relief is needed.

> Diamorphine preparations
> Inj. 5mg, 10mg, 30mg, 100mg, 500mg

Alternative strong opioids

A number of alternative strong opioid analgesics are available which have their place in palliative care:

Table 6a.2a Alternative strong opioids

Morphine and similar drugs	Morphine
	Diamorphine
	Hydromorphone
	Oxycodone
Fentanyl and similar drugs	Fentanyl
	Alfentanil
	Sufentanil
Methadone	Methadone
Intermediate weak–strong opioid	Tramadol
Other opioids occasionally used	Buprenorphine
Not recommended	Pethidine

Differences between these drugs are not fully understood, but include patient factors and drug factors. In clinical practice they may be divided into:

Morphine-like opioids

Oxycodone and hydromorphone, like morphine and diamorphine, are available in a wide range of doses in immediate (4-h) and modified release oral preparations. They can be used by CSCI.

Although there may be small intrinsic differences between the side-effect profiles of these drugs (e.g. oxycodone and hydromorphone may cause less toxicity than morphine in patients with renal failure, but neuroexcitatory side-effects are still reported), inter-individual variability seems to be a greater factor in determining the clinical picture. Substituting one opioid for another may reduce side-effects in up to 75 per cent of selected individuals.

Fentanyl and its analogues

Fentanyl and its analogues (alfentanil, sufentanil and remifentanil) are *selective* μ receptor agonists, unlike morphine. They may cause less sedation, cognitive impairment and constipation than morphine-like drugs in some patients. They are largely inactive orally because of high first-pass hepatic metabolism, but can be used by transdermal patch, oral lozenge (buccal absorption) or CSCI.

Fentanyl does not appear to accumulate and cause toxicity in renal failure.

Methadone

Methadone is an agonist at the μ- and δ-opioid receptors, and also an NMDA receptor antagonist and monoamine reuptake inhibitor. These actions make it a useful treatment for neuropathic and other pain states not fully responsive to morphine. However, it has a long and variable elimination half-life, making it difficult to use safely, and should be reserved for neuropathic, ischaemic or inflammatory pain, or use as a third- or fourth-line opioid.

Tramadol

Tramadol may be classed somewhere between the weak and strong opioids. It has additional pharmacological actions to its opioid effects. It is not classed as a 'controlled drug' which has some practical prescribing advantages.

Tramadol is a synthetic analogue of codeine that binds to μ-opioid receptors and also inhibits norepinephrine and serotonin reuptake. It is rapidly and extensively absorbed after oral doses and is metabolized in the liver. Analgesia begins within one hour and starts to peak in two h. In studies comparing equianalgesic doses of oral tramadol (up to 300 mg/day) and oral morphine for moderate cancer pain, constipation, nausea, neuropsychological symptoms, and pruritus were reported more frequently with morphine. Slow release formulations have also been shown to provide effective relief of moderate cancer pain.

Tramadol preparations

- caps. 50mg; Sachets effervescent powder 50mg; Sol. Tabs 50mg
- Tabs. m/r (12-h) 75mg, 100mg, 150mg, 200mg
- caps. m/r (12-h) 50mg, 100mg, 150mg, 200mg
- Tabs. m/r (24-h) 150mg, 200mg, 300mg, 400mg

Starting dose: 50mg q.d.s. p.o. or 100mg b.d. p.o. (12-h m/r)
  Inj. 100mg/2ml

Buprenorphine

For many years palliative care physicians have been concerned about the use of buprenorphine because of potential problems encountered when patients taking regular morphine were given buprenorphine with consequent exacerbation of pain. Although buprenorphine is a very potent analgesic that strongly binds to opioid receptors displacing other opioids, it is a less effective analgesic.

The introduction of buprenorphine patches has caused such opinions to be revisited. Other opioids can be used in conjunction with buprenorphine patches if pain breaks through.

Side-effects of buprenorphine are similar to those of other strong opioids. Care needs to be taken with patients who are sweating heavily to ensure that the patch is sticking well to the skin.

- For opioid naïve patients the starting dose recommended by the manufacturers is 35mcg/h
- No more than two patches should ever be applied at the one time
- The maximum dose is 140 mcg/h
- The patch should be changed every three days

Buprenorphine preparations

- Patch strength 35, 52.5, 70 mcg/h
Applied every three days. Packs of 5 patches:

- Tabs. (sublingual) 200mcg

Other opioid analgesics

Pethidine has a short duration of action, and, when given regularly, active metabolites accumulate and can cause convulsions. It causes more dysphoria than morphine and is best avoided in palliative care.

Indications for starting with an opioid other than morphine:

- Patient choice
- Subacute/partial intestinal obstruction. A less constipating opioid such as fentanyl may be appropriate
- Patient reluctant to take 'morphine' despite appropriate counselling
- Patient reluctant to take oral medication regularly
- Renal failure

Indications for changing to alternative opioids

This practice is known as opioid rotation or opioid substitution.

- Patient choice
- Unacceptable side-effects with current opioid
- Renal failure
- Route of administration needs to be changed from oral as cannot swallow

Choice of alternative opioid

Rationale

- Hydromorphone, oxycodone and fentanyl are useful alternatives to morphine and diamorphine
- Methadone is difficult to use safely, and should be reserved for neuropathic, ischaemic or inflammatory pain, or used as third- or fourth-line opioid under specialist supervision
- Few strong opioids other than morphine have the range of doses and preparations needed to be suitable for routine use in cancer pain
- There is little to choose between oxycodone and hydromorphone, but oxycodone is chosen in preference because:
  - a liquid immediate release preparation is available
  - an injectable form is readily available in the UK
  - doses are simpler to calculate
  - there is less variation in the reported equianalgesic ratios
  - the manufacturer's recommended conversion of 7.5:1 for morphine to hydromorphone is higher than the more commonly used ratio of 5:1. This makes the tablet doses of 1.3mg even more complicated
- Fentanyl may cause less side-effects in some individuals (sedation, cognitive impairment, constipation, myoclonus and pruritus)
- Transdermal patch or CSCI are the only methods of administering fentanyl regularly for chronic pain as fentanyl has a short half life

Dose titration for unstable pain should not be attempted using a fentanyl patch

Oxycodone

Oxycodone is a strong opioid analgesic similar to morphine. It is available in 4-h immediate- release, and 12-h release preparations. It is a useful, though more expensive, alternative opioid in selected patients who develop side effects with morphine. The receptor affinity of oxycodone is not fully clear. It is partially metabolized to potent oxymorphone. Oxycodone is approximately 1.5–2 times as potent as morphine orally.

Side-effects

The side-effects are similar to morphine though vomiting, itch, and drowsiness may be less common in some individuals.[8]

Indications

Alternative opioid when morphine causes unacceptable side-effects.

Using oxycodone

Oxycodone should be used in the same way as morphine (remember to prescribe a laxative).

Comparison with morphine

In comparative studies with morphine, there are inconsistent reports of side-effect profiles. More vomiting has been reported with morphine, whereas constipation was more common with oxycodone. Other studies have shown no difference.

When selectively substituting morphine for oxycodone in patients with side-effects, improvements in almost all side-effects have been reported: less nausea, hallucinations, drowsiness, sweating and pruritus, but especially confusion/delirium. These reports do not necessarily reflect an overall difference between the drugs, but may reflect inter-individual variation.

Hepatic metabolism

Oxymorphone, a potent analgesic metabolite of oxycodone, is formed by the hepatic enzyme CYP2D6, which is under polymorphic genetic control. The rôle of oxymorphone in the analgesic effect of oxycodone is not yet clear. Oxycodone conversion to oxymorphone may be important for analgesic effect in some patients, and genetically 'poor-metabolizers' may not obtain the expected analgesia from oxycodone.

Synergy between opioids

In animal models, a combination of sub-analgesic doses of oxycodone and morphine showed synergy producing analgesia.

Oxycodone
- caps. 5mg, 10mg, 20mg (*OxyNorm*)
- caps. m/r (12-h) 10mg, 20mg, 40mg, 80mg (*OxyContin*)
- Liquid 5mg/5ml, 10mg/1ml

Manufacturers recommended conversion from oral morphine to oxycodone: divide morphine dose by 2.
- Injection: 10mg/ml 1ml and 2ml Amp

Manufacturers recommended conversion from oral oxycodone to subcutaneous oxycodone: divide dose by 2.

---

8 Heiskanen T, and Kalso E. (1997) Controlled-release oxycodone and morphine in cancer related pain. *Pain*, **73**: 37–45.

Hydromorphone

Hydromorphone is a strong opioid analgesic very similar to morphine, although it is a more selective μ-receptor agonist. It is used widely in North America as an alternative to diamorphine, which is not available. It is available in 4-h immediate release, and 12-h modified release preparations, but the injection is not routinely available in the UK.

It is a useful alternative opioid in selected patients who develop side effects with morphine. Hydromorphone has been used successfully and without toxicity in renal failure, but it has also been reported to cause neuro-excitatory effects in some patients (☐ see renal failure later).

Indications

- Alternative opioid if morphine causes unacceptable side-effects, especially—
  - Opioid-induced pruritus

Using hydromorphone

- Hydromorphone should be used in the same way as morphine (remember to prescribe a laxative)
- The capsules can be broken open and sprinkled on soft cold foods

Cough and dyspnoea

Information about the efficacy of alternative opioids for symptoms other than pain is limited. Hydromorphone may help cough and dyspnoea in lower doses than those used for analgesia.

Conversion ratios with other opioids

Conversion ratios between hydromorphone and other strong opioid analgesics seem more variable and uncertain than for other opioids, perhaps representing greater variability in metabolism and bioavailability (10–65 per cent) between individuals.

- When converting from oral morphine to oral hydromorphone, the manufacturers recommend a ratio of 7.5:1 (i.e. morphine 10mg ≈ hydromorphone 1.3mg)
- It is suggested that the lowest potency ratio is used for any conversion, with the expectation of titrating up the dose rapidly if needed

Side-effects

Hydromorphone and morphine generally have the same side-effects. Pruritus, nausea and vomiting, sedation and cognitive impairment, which may be less common with hydromorphone. There may also be individual variation in side-effect profile between patients.

Drug preparations-Hydromorphone

- caps. 1.3mg, 2.6mg (*Palladone*)
- caps. m/r (12-h) 2mg, 4mg, 8mg, 16mg, 24mg (*Palladone SR*)

Manufacturers recommended conversion from oral morphine: divide morphine dose by 7.5

- Inj. 10mg/1ml 20mg/1ml 50mg/1ml
  Injections available in UK as a special order from Martindale. See BNF for contact details.

Fentanyl

Fentanyl is a selective μ-receptor agonist (morphine acts on μ and κ receptors). It has been promoted as causing less constipation, sedation, and cognitive impairment than oral opioids. Fentanyl may be associated with a slightly higher incidence of nausea than morphine.

As it has inactive metabolites and is metabolized mainly in the liver, it is less likely to cause adverse effects in uraemic patients.

As it is more selective than morphine, fentanyl will not relieve pain that is resistant to morphine, but may help patients with morphine-responsive pain who develop intolerable side-effects to morphine.

Fentanyl is available as a transdermal patch, oral lozenge (buccal absorption), or can be given CSCI. CSCI is better than a patch for establishing effective blood levels rapidly, and should be used when speed is important, or when more flexibility is desired.

Converting a patient from morphine to fentanyl can lead to a modified withdrawal syndrome of shivering, diarrhoea, bowel cramps, sweating and restlessness, even though pain relief is maintained. These symptoms can be relieved with morphine given p.r.n. for a few days.

Fentanyl toxicity may be clinically more subtle than morphine toxicity and may present as vagueness, drowsiness or 'not feeling well'.

Indications

Alternative opioid when morphine causes unacceptable side-effects.
- Starting a strong opioid in a patient with:
  - a history of subacute bowel obstruction (less constipating than morphine)
  - renal failure (which can lead to myoclonus or confusion with morphine due to metabolite accumulation)
  - biliary colic/obstructed bile duct (see additional notes below)
- Patient acceptability/compliance

Transdermal fentanyl patch—only when pain is stable
- Start with 25mcg/h, or convert dose from morphine
- It takes 12–24h to achieve therapeutic blood levels, and approximately 72h to reach steady-state:
  - CSCI of fentanyl or alfentanil will achieve more rapid blood levels
- If converting from morphine, give last dose of 12-h modified release morphine when applying patch except when accumulation of opioids in renal failure has occurred
- If converting from morphine, remember the possibility of withdrawal symptoms and use immediate release morphine p.r.n. until symptoms settle
- Up to 25 per cent of patients need a patch change every 48h
- Use either oral morphine or oral transmucosal fentanyl for breakthrough pain
- Fever may increase drug absorption due to vasodilation
- Sweating may decrease drug absorption because it prevents the patch from sticking to the skin
- After removal of the patch, blood levels decrease by only 50 per cent in 18h

- Mild to moderate skin erythema or pruritus in the location of the patch have been reported in <5 per cent of patients

Fentanyl patches

Absorption rate from a fentanyl transdermal patch is roughly proportional to the surface area in contact with the skin. Various techniques have been used to allow only half of the area to contact with the skin—to approximate to a 12.5mcg/hour dose delivery. Tegaderm or Opsite dressings, with the fentanyl patch placed half on skin/half over the dressing, have been used, but note that these dressings are semipermeable. Others have folded the patch in half and covered with adhesive tape. *Although the delivered analgesic effect may theoretically be less, the side-effect profile does not alter. Neither method is recommended by the manufacturers.*

Some patients develop itching and irritation at the site of transdermal patches—reports suggest that spraying the skin with aerosol corticosteroid spray may be effective (use beclometasone dipropionate aerosol inhaler 50mcg/dose).

Subcutaneous fentanyl

- Calculate dose as equivalent to transdermal patch e.g. 25mcg/h = 600mcg/24h; for convenience (and considering the widely variable absorption from a patch) use 500mcg/24h CSCI as equivalent to a 25mcg/h patch
- Large volumes are needed for high doses: consider substituting alfentanil (see next section)
- Compatible with most commonly used drugs in palliative care

Oral transmucosal fentanyl citrate (OTFC)

Fentanyl lozenges (on a stick) are rapidly absorbed through the buccal mucosa, leading to onset of pain relief within 5–10 minutes. The maximum effect is reached within 20–40 minutes with a duration of action of 1–3h. Bioavailability is about 50 per cent. One comparative study suggests they may give better results than immediate release oral morphine.

Indication

Breakthrough pain in patients on regular strong opioid therapy.

Use

The optimal dose is determined by titration, and cannot be predicted by a patient's regular dose of opioid. Approximately 25 per cent of patients fail to obtain relief even at the highest dose, or have unacceptable adverse effects.

- Lozenge should be placed in the mouth and sucked, constantly moving it from one cheek to the other
- Should not be chewed
- Water can be used to moisten the mouth beforehand
- The lozenge should be consumed within 15min
- Partially consumed lozenges should be dissolved under hot running water, and the handle disposed out of reach of children

Dose titration

- Initial dose is 200mcg, regardless of dose of regular opioid. This dose is probably approx. equivalent to morphine 2mg i/v
- A second lozenge of the same strength can be used if pain is not relieved after 15 minutes
- No more than two lozenges should be used to treat any individual pain episode
- Continue with this dose for a further 2–3 episodes of breakthrough pain, allowing the second lozenge when necessary
- If pain still not controlled, increase to the next higher dose lozenge
- Continue to titrate in this manner until dose is found that provides adequate analgesia with minimum adverse effects
- No more than four doses per day should be used (regular strong opioid dose should be increased)

Inflammatory and neuropathic pain

A few observations suggest that fentanyl (and similar analogues) may be less effective than morphine for inflammatory or neuropathic pain. This may be explained by the additional effects of morphine (e.g. at kappa or delta receptors).

Dose equivalence

Manufacturer's recommended dose conversion from oral morphine to transdermal fentanyl patch is based on a ratio of 150:1 (i.e. 15 mg morphine p.o 4-h $\cong$ 25mcg/h patch). Manufacturers information sheets should be consulted.

Bile duct obstruction

Many opioid μ-receptor agonists, including morphine and diamorphine, have been shown to increase the common bile duct pressure. Fentanyl or sufentanil have no discernable effect on common bile duct diameter and may be preferable.

Topical use of fentanyl

Fentanyl has been used topically for painful skin ulcers.

Drug preparations-Fentanyl

- Patches 25, 50, 75, 100mcg/h (*Durogesic*)
  Starting dose: (25mcg/h) patch every 3 days
- Inj. 50mcg/1ml, 100mcg/2ml, 500mcg/10ml
  Starting dose: 500mcg/24h CSCI
- Lozenge with applicator 200, 400, 600, 800, 1200, 1600mcg (*Actiq*)
  Starting dose: 200mcg lozenge regardless of regular opioid dose

Alfentanil

Alfentanil is a selective μ-receptor opioid agonist, similar to fentanyl. It is mainly metabolized in the liver to inactive compounds. It has been given by CSCI in a syringe driver, and appears to mix with most other commonly used drugs in palliative care. It should be diluted with water.

Compared to fentanyl, an equianalgesic dose can be used in a much smaller volume, making CSCI of large doses possible. It is thus a useful substitute for fentanyl if CSCI use is desired.

Alfentanil is rapidly eliminated and elimination appears unaffected by renal failure. Its onset is more rapid than for fentanyl.

Its short-lasting effect means it has been used for incident pain (dressing change), but should not be used for breakthrough pain as it quickly wears off.

Drug preparations-Alfentanil

• Inj. 1mg/2ml, 5mg/10ml, 5mg/1ml

Starting dose: 500mcg/24hCSCI (equivalent to diamorphine 5mg CSCI)

Sufentanil

Sufentanil is a synthetic opioid very similar to fentanyl, but with more rapid onset and shorter duration of action. It can be used as an alternative to alfentanil if the fentanyl dose necessitates too large a volume for the portable syringe driver in use. It has also been used sublingually. The clinically-derived sufentanil to fentanyl relative potency is approximately 20:1.

Methadone

Methadone is a strong opioid analgesic, with several non-opioid actions. It differs from morphine/diamorphine in a number of ways:

- δ-opioid receptor agonist
- NMDA receptor antagonist
- serotonin re-uptake inhibitor
- long and variable elimination half-life
- potential for numerous and complex drug interactions
- inactive metabolites (lower toxicity in renal failure)

The first three of these actions may help account for reports of its effectiveness in managing neuropathic pain.

The pharmacology of methadone is complex and very variable, so it must be used with specialist supervision. The commonest mistake is to underestimate its duration of action, since up to 10 days may be required to reach steady state plasma levels. The greatest tendency to accumulate the drug is in the elderly or those with liver failure.

Drug interactions

Methadone metabolism is increased by a number of other drugs, which when started could cause opioid withdrawal symptoms. Other interactions which inhibit metabolism can lead to overdose and toxicity.

Table 6a.3 Interactions which interfere with methadone metabolism

Decrease methadone levels	Increase methadone levels
Phenytoin	Fluconazole
Phenobarbitalno	SSRIs
Carbamazepine (not sodium valproate or gabapentin)	
Rifampicin	

Subcutaneous methadone

Subcutaneous methadone has been used but there is a problem with skin reactions, partly because methadone in solution is acidic. If necessary to use, dilute as much as possible. In conversion of oral to subcutaneous or intravenous dosing, halve the dose of methadone.

Use of methadone

Indications

- Pain only partially responsive to morphine e.g. inflammatory, ischaemic or neuropathic pain
- Alternative opioid when side-effects develop with morphine (or other opioid)
- Renal failure
- Morphine tolerance—patients requiring ever increasing doses of morphine with no overall improvement in pain
- Use with special caution in the elderly, COPD or asthma

Guidelines for use

Note: Patients are rarely started on methadone for pain outside a specialist unit.

The efficacy of methadone in comparison with morphine increases with chronic dosing and with higher dose. This is in part due to a long elimination half-life, and in part due to its non-opioid action. Many studies have shown the difficulty in converting doses between opioids and methadone. Several guidelines have been published.

Morley and Makin guidelines are most commonly used in the UK, and are recommended for general use, and especially for patients switching opioid because of lack of effect.

Guidelines (Morley and Makin 1998 Pain Reviews)

- Stop all other opioids abruptly, i.e. do *not* reduce gradually
- Loading dose of methadone. 1/10 of the 24h p.o. morphine or equivalent up to a maximum of 30mg
- This same dose can be given as needed but not more frequently than 3-h
- On day six, add the total dose of methadone given in last 48h, divide by four, and give at 12-h intervals, with provision for a similar or smaller dose q3h as required
- Subsequent dose changes are by percentage increments as for morphine, every 4–6 days. [example 10mg b.d. → 15mg b.d.; 30mg b.d. → 40mg b.d.]
- Re-assess carefully as accumulation can occur up to 10 days after methadone begun or dose changed

Side-effects

All the typical opioid side-effects can be expected, although hallucinations and myoclonus are rare. Compared to morphine, methadone may cause less constipation, sedation and nausea. Methadone causes histamine release and can exacerbate asthma. It also has an antidiuretic effect.

Drug preparations-Methadone
- Mixture 10mg/ml
- Mixture 1mg/ml
- Tabs. 5mg; Linctus 2mg/5ml (for cough)

Topical opioids

Opioids can act peripherally as analgesics, and there are a number of reports of their use on ulcerated skin, relieving pain and possibly inflammation. Morphine and diamorphine have been used most commonly, but fentanyl has also been reported. There have been no reports of systemic toxicity, and standard doses have been used, regardless of doses of systemic opioids taken simultaneously.

Morphine or diamorphine 10mg may be mixed with sterile aqueous gel, a hydrocolloid gel (e.g. intrasite), or metronidazole gel, as appropriate. Apply once daily, and increase frequency if needed up to three times daily.

Summary

1 Subcutaneous diamorphine is 3 times as potent as oral
  morphine.
2 Subcutaneous oxycodone is twice as potent as oral oxycodone.
3 Transdermal Fentanyl patches deliver 25,50,75 or 100mcg/h over
  three days.

  Peak plasma concentrations are achieved after 12–24h and a depot
  remains in the skin for some 24h after the patch is removed.
  Breakthrough doses of opioid will be necessary during the first 24h of
  application. One in ten patients who have had their pain controlled by
  morphine may experience a withdrawal reaction when converted to
  fentanyl. They may require oral morphine on a p.r.n. basis to manage
  the withdrawal symptoms for a day or two.
  A reduction of laxative may be necessary when converting from morphine to fentanyl.
4 Transdermal Buprenorphine delivers 35, 52.5 and 70 mcg/h over
  three days. No more than 140 mcg/h (two patches) should be used.
  Opioids other than buprenorphine can be used for breakthrough
  pain.
5 Transdermal Fentanyl and Buprenorphine should only be used where
  opioid requirements are stable.
6 Oral Transmucosal Fentanyl Lozenges (OTFC). For breakthrough
  pain in patients already on regular strong opioid therapy for chronic
  pain. Start titration at lowest dose (200 mcg) regardless of
  background opioid dose.
7 Topical opioids have been mixed with both metronidazole and
  hydrocolloid gels for the pain of skin wounds.

Table 6a.4 Equivalent opioid doses for step two and step three of the analgesic ladder

Opioid	Oral medication					
	Step 2 mild to moderate pain	Step 3 moderate to severe pain				
Codeine	30–60mg q.d.s.	Not applicable				
Morphine i/r	2.5–5mg 4-h	10mg 4-h	20mg 4-h	30mg 4-h	40mg 4-h	60mg 4-h
Morphine m/r	5–15mg b.d.	30mg b.d.	60mg b.d.	90mg b.d.	120mg b.d.	180mg b.d.
Oxycodone i/r	1.5–3mg 4-6 h	5mg 4-h	10mg 4-h	15mg 4-h	20mg 4-h	30mg 4-h
Oxycodone m/r	5mg b.d.	10–20mg b.d.	30mg b.d.	40–50mg b.d.	60mg b.d.	90mg b.d.
Hydromorphone i/r	Not applicable	1.3mg 4-h	2.6mg 4-h	3.9mg 4-h	5.2mg 4-h	6.5mg 4-h
Hydromorphone m/r	Not applicable	4mg b.d.	8mg b.d.	12mg b.d.	16mg b.d.	20mg b.d.
Tramadol i/r	50mg 4h	Not applicable				
Tramadol m/r	100–150mg b.d.	Not applicable				
Approximate 24 h oral morphine	**10–30mg**	**60mg**	**120mg**	**180mg**	**240mg**	**360mg**

In all opioid conversions there is uncertainty. It is safer to err on the side of underestimating analgesic requirements when converting between opioids but ensure that the patient has ready access to appropriate breakthrough analgesia. If in doubt about a conversion seek specialist advice if you are unfamiliar with the particular opioid.

Table 6a.5 Equivalent opioid doses for step two and step three of the analgesic ladder

| Opioid | Transdermal medication | | | |
	Step 2 mild to moderate pain	Step 3 moderate to severe pain		
Fentanyl	Not applicable	25 mcg/h every three days	50 mcg/h ever three days	75 mcg/h every three days	100 mcg/h every three days
Buprenorphine	35 mcg/h every three days	52.5 mcg/h every three days	70 mcg/h every three days	2×70 mcg/h every three days	Not applicable
Approximate 24 h oral morphine	15mg	60mg	120mg	180mg	240mg	360mg

In all opioid conversions there is uncertainty. It is safer to err on the side of underestimating analgesic requirement when converting between opioids but ensure that the patient has ready access to appropriate breakthrough analgesia. If in doubt about a conversion always seek specialist advice if you are unfamiliar with the particular opioid.

Table 6a.6 Equivalent opioid doses for step two and step three of the analgesic ladder

Opioid	Subcutaneous medication					
	Step 2 mild to moderate pain	Step 3 moderate to severe pain				
Alfentanil CSCI (24h)	0.5–1mg 24h	2mg 24h	4mg 24h	6mg 24h	8mg 24h	12mg 24h
Diamorphine SC 24h p.r.n.		2.5–5mg 4-h	5–7.5mg 4-h	10mg 4-h	15mg 4-h	20mg 4-h
Diamorphine CSCI (24h)	5–10mg 24h	20mg 24h	40mg 24h	60mg	80mg	120mg
Morphine SC (4h p.r.n.)	2.5mg	5mg	10mg	15mg	20mg	30mg
Morphine CSCI (24h)	15mg	30mg	60mg	90mg	120mg	180mg
Oxycodone SC (4h p.r.n.)		2.5mg 4-h	5mg 4-h	7.5mg 4-h	10mg 4-h	15mg 4-h
*Oxycodone CSCI (24h)	5mg 24h	15–20mg 24h	30mg 24h	50mg 24h	60mg 24h	90mg 24h
Approximate 24 h oral morphine	**30mg**	**60mg**	**120mg**	**180mg**	**240mg**	**360mg**

In all opioid conversions there is uncertainty. It is a safer to err on the side of underestimating analgesic requirement when converting between opioid but ensure that the patient has ready access to appropriate breakthrough analgesia. If in doubt about a conversion seek specialist advice if you are unfamiliar with the particular opioid.

* The manufacturer of oxycodone states clearly that the conversion factor between oxycodone SC and diamorphine SC is 1:1. While most clinicians are comfortable with this ratio when converting from oxycodone SC to *diamorphine* SC, when converting from *diamorphine* SC to oxycodone SC some would advocate a 2:1 ratio with provision for breakthrough medication. As in every dose conversion the clinician must assess each individual patient and clinical situation.

Opioid side-effects and toxicity

> Thou hast the keys of Paradise,
> Oh just, subtle, and mighty opium!

Thomas De Quincey 1785–1859: *Confessions of an English Opium Eater* (1822)

Patients should be warned of the possible side-effects of morphine such as nausea and drowsiness, which are usually short-lived, and are not often a problem. If drowsiness continues after a few days other possible causes e.g. uraemia, hypercalcaemia or toxicity from other medication, should be excluded—otherwise seek advice. Constipation is predictable and most patients need prophylactic laxatives.

If unacceptable toxicity occurs, reduce morphine dose. The patient may need to miss several doses and restart at a lower dose.

Warning signs of morphine toxicity
- Drowsiness
- Hallucinations (auditory or visual)
- Confusion
- Vomiting
- Myoclonus
- Pin point pupils

Always ensure opioid doses are carefully titrated ('fine-tuned') to maximize analgesia and minimize side-effects.

Opioid toxicity may be increased by:
- dehydration or renal failure
- other change in disease status e.g. hepatic function, weight loss
- pain relieved by other methods
- co-administration of amitriptyline increases the bioavailability of morphine

General management
A number of different approaches may be used to manage persistent opioid-related side-effects:
- treat the side-effect
- use an alternative opioid
- use an alternative analgesic method, such as spinal opioids, which may cause less systemic or central side-effects

Drowsiness and cognitive impairment
Initial mild drowsiness on initiating opioid therapy will often abate over a few days as the body adjusts. It is often appropriate to continue opioid and wait for the drowsiness to wear off.

For persistent drowsiness or subtler cognitive impairment:
- Parenteral rehydration, if appropriate, may help neuropsychiatric toxicity (e.g. hallucinations, sedation, myoclonus)

- Alternative opioid
- Psychostimulants have been used to combat sedation in specialist units

Hallucinations or delirium
- Parenteral rehydration, if appropriate
- Alternative opioid
- Antipsychotic e.g. haloperidol 3–5mg nocte or by CSCI

Myoclonus
Consider renal failure—renal failure alone can cause myoclonus, but also causes opioid metabolites to accumulate, thereby increasing the risk of opioid toxicity. Myoclonus may be more likely in patients also taking anti-depressants , antipsychotics or NSAIDs. Consider the following:
- Parenteral rehydration, if appropriate
- Review other medication which may exacerbate myoclonus
- Alternative opioid
- Clonazepam 2–4mg/24h. Diazepam or midazolam are probably less effective than clonazepam but may be appropriate if sedation is also desirable
- Gabapentin 600–1200mg/24h in divided doses

Constipation
- Constipation can usually be treated acceptably with laxatives
- Fentanyl may cause less constipation than morphine

Increase in generalized pain
Hyperalgesia and allodynia have been reported with high dose opioids. It is usually associated with myoclonus, and an increase in the opioid dose may lead to worsening of the pain. Substitution of an alternative opioid often resolves the symptoms. Alternatively, reduction of dose and the addition of an alternative co-analgesic may be useful.

Nausea and vomiting
Initial nausea may wear off after a week and usually responds to:
- Haloperidol 1.5mg nocte
- Metoclopramide (for opioid-induced gastric stasis)
- Cyclizine or 5-HT$_3$ antagonists
- Alternative opioid

Sweating
- Alternative opioid
- Exclude other causes of sweating
- Antimuscarinic drugs

Pruritus (itching)
More common with spinal than with systemic opioids.
- Alternative opioid
- If unsuccessful, treat opioid induced pruritus with 5-HT$_3$ antagonists such as ondansetron

Respiratory depression/sedation

Reduction of the dose is usually all that is required immediately. Infusion by a syringe driver should be temporarily stopped to allow plasma levels to decrease, before restarting at a lower dose

Naloxone

- Naloxone is only indicated if significant respiratory depression is present; acute opioid withdrawal symptoms and pain can be severe in patients who have been on long-term opioids Naloxone has a half-life of 5–20 minutes. As the half-life of most opioids is longer than this, it is important to continue assessment of the patient and give naloxone at further intervals if necessary

Indications for naloxone:

- respiratory rate <8 breaths/min, or
- <10–12 breaths/min, difficult to rouse and clinically cyanosed, or
- <10–12 breaths/min, difficult to rouse and SaO_2 <90 per cent on pulse oximeter

Method of use of naloxone

- Dilute naloxone 0.4mg vial in 10ml 0.9% sodium chloride
- Use an i/v cannula or butterfly
- Administer 0.5ml i/v every 2 minutes until respiratory status satisfactory
- Repeat further doses as needed

Neuropathic pain

Neuropathic pain: Pain which is transmitted by a damaged nervous system, and which is usually only partially opioid sensitive.

Up to 40 per cent of cancer-related pain may have a neuropathic mechanism involved. Neuropathic pain may be difficult to control. A wide variety of treatments may be needed:

Management

Table 6a.7 Examples of treatments used for patients with neuropathic pain

Opioids	Ketamine
Antidepressants (tricyclic)	Spinal (epidural and intrathecal)
Anticonvulsants	Methadone
NSAID trial	Lidocaine patch/infusion
TENS	
Accupuncture	Neurolytic procedures e.g. coeliac plexus block, cordotomy
Radiotherapy	Capsaicin
Corticosteroids	

Remember that most cancer pains which seem to be predominantly neuropathic will also probably have a nociceptive *opioid responsive* element. i.e. try WHO analgesic ladder first.

Classes of drugs used in neuropathic pain

Opioid analgesics

Opioids may be effective in both cancer-related and non-malignant neuropathic pain. Opioids other than morphine/diamorphine have been shown to be effective including tramadol, fentanyl, and oxycodone.

Opioids are used in cancer-related neuropathic pain as:

- many patients will have a different, coexisting nociceptive pain
- there may be a nociceptive element to the pain
- opioids alone may control a third of neuropathic pains, and partially control a further third

If the pain seems to be resistant to first-line opioid (or opioid toxicity is a problem):

- an alternative opioid analgesic may be tried for better tolerance
- medication can be given to counteract side-effects (e.g. psychostimulants for drowsiness)
- the pain may be morphine-resistant

Methadone can be considered different from the other opioids with respect to neuropathic pain. It can either be tried as an alternative to a first-line opioid, or introduced later, when other options have failed which is more usual. See p. 196.

Tricyclic Antidepressants

The mechanism of analgesic action is principally by facilitation of descending inhibitory pain pathways.

e.g.   amitriptyline 25–100mg
       dosulepin 25–100mg

Note that amitriptyline can increase the bioavailability of morphine leading to opioid side-effects.

- Start with amitriptyline 25mg (10mg in the elderly) nocte
- If no response by day five, increase the dose (or, according to clinical circumstances, consider changing to anticonvulsant)
- Some patients do not see benefit until after 4–6 weeks of treatment, and/or doses of up to 50mg/day
  - severity of pain and the patient's prognosis will dictate how long to persevere with antidepressants
  - many patients do not tolerate amitriptyline especially in higher doses, therefore consider changing to dosulepin
- Use lofepramine for frail, elderly, or those already suffering antimuscarinic side-effects from other drugs:
  - start at 70mg nocte
  - may increase to 70mg b.d. on day 5–7

Lower doses of tricyclic antidepressants than those commonly required in depressive illness are reported to be effective in neuropathic pain, and faster responses are to be expected.[9] Other less sedating tricyclic antidepressants (e.g. imipramine) may be more useful for certain patients. Newer antidepressants are being used,[10] but their rôle is as yet unclear and there is growing concern about withdrawal reactions and cardiotoxicity, particularly with venlafaxine. Mirtazapine is a noradrenergic and specific serotonergic antidepressant (NaSSA); there are a few reports of its use in neuropathic pain. Topical tricyclics such as doxepin cream have also been tried.

Amitriptyline

- Tabs. 10mg, 25mg, 50mg
- Syrup 25mg/5ml, 50mg/5ml

Starting dose: 25mg nocte p.o.

Dosulepin

- caps. 25mg
- Tabs. 75mg (Prothiaden)

Starting dose: 25mg nocte p.o.

Lofepramine

- Tabs. 70mg
- Susp. 70mg/5ml

Starting dose: 70mg nocte p.o.

Doxepin

- Cream 5% 30g

Starting dose: Apply t.d.s to q.d.s., maximum 12g daily

---

9 McQuay H. J. (1996) A systematic review of antidepressants in neuropathic. *Pain* **68**: 217–27.

10 Pernia A., Mico J. A., Calderon E., Torres L. M. (2000) Venlafaxine for the treatment of neuropathic pain (letter). *Journal of Pain and Symptom Management*, **19, 6**: 408–10.

Anticonvulsants[11]

e.g. sodium valproate 100–600mg b.d.
     gabapentin 100–600mg t.d.s.
     carbamazepine 100–400mg b.d.

Anticonvulsants have for a long time been considered better than tricyclic antidepressants for lancinating or paroxysmal pain, but evidence from studies does not support this.

There is little to choose overall between antidepressants and anticonvulsants for neuropathic pain in terms of efficacy or adverse effects.

There is little data to compare anticonvulsants in terms of efficacy, although in one trial comparing the efficacy of different anticonvulsants for lancinating pain, the results suggested that clonazepam was superior to phenytoin, sodium valproate and carbamazepine.[12]

- **Carbamazepine** has been used most extensively, but is often tolerated poorly by elderly, frail or ill patients. It has numerous drug interactions and tends to result in more side-effects, particularly when used in combination with other drugs. Doses should be built up slowly to minimize adverse effects
- **Sodium Valproate** has therefore been recommended by many in palliative care, but more data on its efficacy is needed
- **Clonazepam** has been used in cancer-related pain and has the advantage of subcutaneous administration
- **Lamotrigine** has had mixed results
- **Gabapentin** is the only drug licenced for all types of neuropathic pain. Trials have shown it to be effective in non-malignant and cancer-related pain. It appears to be well tolerated in palliative care patients. Doses up to 2.4g/24h have been used successfully
- Pregabalin has recently been introduced and is thought to work in a similar way to Gabapentin. It is unclear if patients who are unresponsive to Gabapentin may gain benefit from Pregabalin apart from its simpler dose regime (Pregabalin—for neuropathic pain November 2004, www.druginfozone.org)

Unlike the antidepressants, anticonvulsants are pharmacologically diverse in their actions, and there is good theoretical reason to try alternative anticonvulsants if one is ineffective.

All anticonvulsants are used in their typical 'anticonvulsant' doses.
- Start with gabapentin: day one—300mg nocte, day two—300mg b.d., day three—300mg t.d.s.
- If no response by day five, either increase dose in 300mg increments every few days (maximum 1800–2400mg/day), use an alternative anticonvulsant, or move on to another method:
- Some patients do not see full benefit from anticonvulsants until after 4–6 weeks of treatment
- The severity of pain and the patient's prognosis will dictate how long to persevere with gabapentin, or with anticonvulsants in general

11 McQuay H. J. (1995) Anticonvulsant drugs for management of pain: a systematic review. *BMJ,* **311**: 1047–52.

12 9. Swerdlow M., Cundill J. G. (1981) Anticonvulsant drugs used in the treatment of lancinating pain. A comparison. *Anaesthesia* **36, 12**: 1129–32.

Gabapentin
- caps. 100mg, 300mg, 400mg
- Tabs. 600mg 800mg

Starting dose; Day 1—300mg nocte, day 2—300mg b.d., day 3—300mg t.d.s. p.o.

Usual maintenance: 0.9–1.2g/24h. Maximum recommended dose 1.8g/24h, but doses up to 2.4g/24h (and even higher) have been used.

Sodium valproate
- Tabs. 200mg, 500mg
- Syrup 200mg/5ml

Starting dose; 200mg t.d.s. p.o. or 500mg nocte p.o.

Increase 200mg/day at 3-day intervals. Usual maintenance 1–2g/24h. Max. 2.5g/24h in divided doses. Supps. are available as special orders.

Carbamazepine
- Tabs. 100mg, 200mg, 400mg
- Liquid 100mg/5ml
- Supps. 125mg, 250mg

Starting dose; 100mg b.d. p.o.

Increase from initial dose by increments of 200mg every week. Usual maintenance dose 0.8–1.2 g/24h in two divided doses. Max. 1.6–2g/24h. Equivalent rectal dosage: 125mg PR ≅ 100mg p.o.

Carbamazepine levels are increased (risk of toxicity) by dextro-propoxyphene (co-proxamol), clarithromycin, erythromycin, fluoxetine, fluvoxamine.

Clonazepam
- Tabs. 500mcg, 2mg
- Inj. 1mg/1ml

Starting dose; 1mg nocte for 4 nights

Increase gradually to usual maintenance dose 4–8mg/24h. Oral solutions in various strengths are available from several sources.

Pregabalin
- Caps. 25mg, 50mg, 75mg, 100mg, 150mg, 200mg, 300mg

Starting dose; 75mg b.d.

Increase after three days to 150mg b.d.

Increase after seven days to 300mg b.d.

Corticosteroids

Corticosteroids (usually dexamethasone) may help cancer-related neuropathic pain, either by reducing inflammatory sensitisation of nerves, or by reducing oedema which may cause pressure on nerves. A high initial dose is used to achieve rapid results (dexamethasone 8mg/day will work in 1–3 days); the dose should then be rapidly reduced to the minimum that maintains benefit.

Although long-term corticosteroids may be best avoided, they can sometimes buy useful time whilst allowing other methods (e.g. radiotherapy or antidepressants) time to work.

- Hydrocortisone has a high mineralocorticoid effect
- Dexamethasone has a relatively high equivalent corticosteroid dose per tablet and less mineralocorticoid effects than prednisolone, or methylprednisolone with consequently less problems with fluid retention
- Prednisolone causes less proximal myopathy than dexamethasone.[13]

If steroids are not helpful for pain within five days, consider stopping

Table 6a.8 Relative anti-inflammatory steroid doses (approximate)

Steroid	Administration	Equivalent dose
Dexamethasone	Oral/SC	2mg
Prednisolone	Oral/Rectal	15mg
Hydrocortisone	Oral/i/m/i/v	60mg
Methylprednisolone	Oral/i/m/i/v	12mg

NSAIDs

NSAIDs are sometimes effective in cancer-related neuropathic pain, either because there is mixed nociceptive pain or because they reduce inflammatory sensitization of nerves. NSAIDs exert an anti-inflammatory action by inhibiting prostaglandin synthesis.

There is considerable variation in individual patient tolerance and response. Pain relief starts soon but an anti-inflammatory effect may take a few weeks. The main differences between NSAIDs are in the incidence and type of side-effect, and efficacy should be weighed against the possible side-effects. NSAIDs vary in their selectivity for inhibiting different types of cyclo-oxygenase; selective inhibition of cyclo-oxygenase-2 (e.g. celecoxib) improves gastrointestinal tolerance but significant cardiac side-effects have created recent concerns and lead to the withdrawal of some preparations, most notably rofecoxib (vioxx). Ibuprofen has fewer side-effects than other non-selective NSAIDs.

e.g. ibuprofen 200–400mg t.d.s. p.o.
diclofenac 50mg t.d.s. (can be used p.o. SC or Supps.)
celecoxib up to 200mg b.d. p.o.
naproxen 250–500mg b.d. (p.o. or PR)
ketorolac 10–30mg SC every 4–6 h p.r.n. Max. 90mg daily (max. 60mg for elderly). Max. duration 2 days
parecoxib 40mg, then 20–40mg every 6–12 h p.r.n. Max. 80mg daily (max. 40mg for elderly).

13 Kingdon R. T. *et al.* (1998) *Handbook for pain management.* London: Saunders.

Elderly patients or those with a past history of peptic ulceration may be more at risk from side-effects. A proton pump inhibitor such as lansoprazole has been shown to reduce this risk.

Aspirin causes long acting inhibition of platelet coagulability and its unique cardiovascular protective effect makes joint prescribing of low dose aspirin and a non selective NSAID appropriate for patients in need of aspirin prophylaxis. However, the reduction in gastrointestinal side-effect risks gained by use of a selective COX2 inhibitor is obviated if given with low dose aspirin.

Risk factors for GI bleed with NSAID

- Age ≥ 75
- Corticosteroids
- Aspirin
- Anticoagulant
- Platelets < 50x10^9/t
- Dyspepsia on NSAIDs now or in the past
- Peptic ulceration/ bleed in last year

Other drugs

Topical lidocaine (Lignocaine)

Topical lidocaine may be useful for superficial localized areas of pain such as fungating wounds for short periods of time.[14] A combination of lidocaine gel with diamorphine may also help pain. Prolonged use may lead to skin sensitization. A lidocaine 5 per cent patch has been shown to reduce pain and allodynia from post herpetic neuralgia. Up to three patches for periods of up to 24 h seems to be safe. An adequate trial over several weeks may be required. Mild to moderate skin redness, rash or irritation may occur. While the systemically absorbed dose from topical lidocaine will be small care should be exercised with patients susceptible to cardiac problems.

Oral flecainide and mexiletine

These medications should only be used **under specialist supervision and are rarely used in palliative care**.

Infusions of lidocaine (lignocaine) have been claimed as effective in neuropathic pain, and have been used long-term over many weeks.

As a continuous infusion is not always acceptable, oral drugs with similar sodium-channel blocking properties have been used (flecainide and mexiletine).

A positive response to lidocaine infusion may predict a response to mexiletine, and possibly therefore flecainide.

That neuropathic pain is particularly challenging to treat is illustrated by the very large number of strategies which have been tried to a greater or lesser extent.

- Hypomagnesaemia should be looked for and corrected
- Baclofen may specifically help paroxysmal pain; up to 60mg daily has been used
- Levomepromazine appears to have intrinsic analgesic activity. The sedative/anxiolytic effect may also benefit distressed patients
- Clonidine is used extensively in spinal infusions. Given by mouth, its tolerance is limited by hypotension and sedation. Doses of 25mcg t.d.s. increasing to 100 mcg t.d.s. have been used
- Capsaicin cream has proved useful in neuropathic pain, especially post herpetic neuralgia. The application of the cream can itself cause stinging which can be relieved by the use of Emla cream applied prior to the capsaicin. Capsaicin is a derivative of chilli pepper and must be applied with gloves five times a day. The pain may increase to start with but perseverance may provide relief. Studies suggest its mode of action is mediated by reducing the amount of substance P available for neurotransmission
- Cannabinoids may have a place in neuropathic pain, or pain associated with muscle spasm

---

Capsaicin
- Cream 0.075% 45g (Axsain)
Starting dose: Apply topically 3–4 times daily
Clonidine
- Tabs. 25mg. Tabs. 100mg, 300mg
- caps. m/r 250mg
Starting dose: Neuropathic pain 25mg t.d.s. p.o. increasing to 100 mg t.d.s.
Baclofen
- Tabs. 10mg; Liquid 5mg/5ml
Starting dose: 5mg t.d.s. p.o.

---

14 Back I. N., Finlay I. (1995) Analgesic effect of topical opioids on painful skin ulcers. *Journal of Pain and Symptom Management*, **10, 7**: 493.

N-methyl-D-aspartate (NMDA) receptors

The NMDA receptor is thought to be involved in the development of the 'wind-up' phenomenon of neuropathic pain. Ketamine and methodone are NMDA antagonists which may explain their efficacy in neuropathic pain.

The site of action of opioid analgesics is closely related to the NMDA receptor, and anecdotal reports suggest that opioid analgesics may be needed for NMDA receptor antagonists to work.

> Wind up is the phenomenon of central sensitization when the experience of unchanged chronic pain stimulation worsens as nerve fibres become 'trained' to deliver pain signals better.

Ketamine

Ketamine is a dissociative anaesthetic with strong analgesic properties. Its analgesic effect may be partly due to NMDA receptor blocking and may be useful clinically in sub-anaesthetic doses for treating neuropathic, inflammatory or ischaemic pain. In higher doses approaching anaesthetic doses, it may be useful for treating terminal uncontrolled overwhelming pain.

It has been used byp.o., CSCI and i/v routes, and in a very wide range of doses.

- CSCI in doses of 50–360mg/24h ± a loading dose of 10mg SC
- p.o. starting doses between 2mg and 25mg t.d.s. have been used, and up to 50mg q.d.s. or 240mg/day
- i/v bolus doses of 0.1–0.5mg/kg (approx. 5–25mg)

Dysphoric effects including hallucinations are reported quite commonly in higher doses. They are more common in anxious patients, and small doses of benzodiazepines may help. Anaesthetic experience suggests pre-treatment may help reduce the incidence.

Neuropathic pain

Use oral route if possible:
- Diazepam 2mg p.o. 2 h before first dose then 2mg nocte for 3 days
- Start ketamine 10mg q.d.s. p.o.
- Increase by 10mg increments once or twice daily, up to 50mg q.d.s. as appropriate

If parenteral route appropriate:
- Ketamine 10mg SC stat. may be given if indicated for severe pain
- Start infusion of ketamine 50–100mg/24h CSCI
- Add midazolam 5mg/24h CSCI to reduce dysphoric effects, or higher dose if patient is very anxious
- Increase ketamine dose by 50–100mg increments as indicated to maximum 500mg/24h CSCI

Oral versus Parenteral doses

Ketamine is effective orally and in view of the wide dose ranges used, it is difficult to assess the potency ratio. It undergoes first-pass hepatic metabolism to an active metabolite, and one study suggests it may be more potent given orally than parenterally. In general, equivalent daily doses should initially be used when changing route.

Ketamine for procedures

Ketamine can be used as an analgesic to allow patients to be positioned for epidural or certain procedures (e.g. dressing changes). It carries a high incidence of dysphoric effects at these doses.

- Ketamine 0.5mg/kg by slow i/v injection (for 50kg man=25mg), or
- Ketamine 1.5mg/kg i/m (for 50kg man=75mg)
- Pre-treatment with a benzodiazepine to reduce the incidence of dysphoric effects:
  - midazolam 2.5mg SC given 30 min before, or
  - midazolam 1-3mg slow i/v immediately before
  (N.B. Anaesthetic dose for 50kg man is 50–150mg i/v over 1 min or 300–600mg i/m)

Terminal overwhelming pain

- Give ketamine 25–50mg slow i/v or SC for immediate effect if needed
- Midazolam 5mg SC stat
- Start ketamine 300–600mg/24h CSCI
- Add midazolam at least 20mg/24h to prevent hallucinations
- Increase ketamine to a maximum of 1,200mg/24h CSCI (up to 3.2g/24h have been given)

Methadone (📖 see p. 220)

Table 6a.9 Efficacy of drugs for neuropathic pain (NNT)[15]

	Diabetic neuropathy	Postherpetic neuralgia
Oxycodone	2.7	2.5
Tramadol	3.4	
Tricyclic antidepressants	2.4	2.3
SSRIs	6.7	
All antidepressants	3.4	2.1
Carbamazepine	3.3	
Gabapentin	3.7	3.2
All anticonvulsants	2.7	3.2
Mexiletine	10.0	
Baclofen	1.4	
Capsaicin	5.9	5.3

NNT is the number of patients who have to be treated for one to achieve the specified level of benefit, in this case benefit in terms of pain relief.

15 Sindrup S. H. and Jensen T. S. (1999) Efficacy of pharmacological treatments of neuropathic pain: an update and effect related to mechanism of drug action. *Pain*, **83**: 389–400.

Table 6a.10 Examples of treatments used for patients with neuropathic pain

Opioids	Ketamine
Antidepressants (tricyclic)	Spinal (epidural and intrathecal)
Anticonvulsants	Methadone
NSAID trial	Lidocaine patch/infusion
TENS Accupuncture	Neurolytic procedures e.g. coeliac plexus block, cordotomy
Radiotherapy	Capsaicin
Corticosteroids	

Treatment of other causes of poorly controlled pain

Malignant bone pain

- Radiotherapy—around 50 per cent will experience less pain within two weeks and 85 per cent within four weeks of treatment. In around 5 per cent a 'pain flare' is described with the pain worsening in the first few days after treatment before settling
- NSAID e.g. diclofenac 50mg t.d.s.
- Strong opioids (morphine)
- Corticosteroids
- Bisphosphonates

Bisphosphonates

Bisphosphonates have a rôle in a long-term strategy to reduce skeletal complications, including pain, from bone metastases of any origin (most data available for myeloma, breast and prostate cancer). Bisphosphonates may also have a rôle in the 'acute' management of metastatic bone pain. Patients may experience a 'flu-like reaction post treatment. Doses may need to be altered in renal failure.

Treatment

Bisphosphonates

- Analgesic effect should be expected within 14 days. Disodium pamidronate, sodium clodronate, and ibandronic acid need to be given every three to four weeks, but zoledronic acid has a longer duration of action (four to six weeks)
- It is not clear for how long bisphosphonates should be continued. The rôle of oral bisphosphonates has yet to be clarified in patients with metastatic bone disease

Treat

- Zoledronic acid 4mg i/v over 15 minutes. Calcium levels must be watched closely as hypocalcaemia may need treatment with calcium and vitamin D supplements
- Disodium pamidronate 90mg i/v infusion diluted to 500ml in sodium chloride 0.9 per cent (minimum 375ml), infuse over 2–4h
- Sodium clodronate i/v infusion 1500mg (can exceptionally be given SC)
- Ibandronic acid 6mg i/v every 3–4 weeks. (2–4mg for hypercalcaemia.)

Radiotherapy

- Radionuclides such as strontium are absorbed at areas of high bone turnover. They may take 12 weeks to have full effect and 80 per cent will experience pain relief. External beam hemi-body irradiation is an alternative for multiple-site bone pain

Surgery

- Surgical techniques. The pain of bone metastases may respond to local infiltration or intra-lesional injection with depot corticosteroid ± local anaesthetic. Consideration should be given to prophylactic pinning of osteolytic metastases in long bones. Vertebroplasty, in which injection of acrylic cement is administered percutaneously, into unstable fractures of the vertebrae may be worth considering if the patient is relatively well. Spinal or epidural anaesthetic blocks may also be needed

Bisphosphonates and bone pain

Disodium pamidronate
- Inj. 15mg, 30mg 90mg (dry powder for reconstitution)

Sodium clodronate
- Inj. 300mg/5ml 300mg/10ml

Starting dose: 800mg or 520mg b.d. p.o.

Zoledronic acid
- Inj. 4mg

Ibandronic acid
- Inj. 6mg
- p.o. 50mg daily

Treatment of poorly controlled pain

Pain	Possible co-analgesics
Headache due to cerebral oedema	dexamethasone
Painful wounds	metronidazole
Intestinal colic	hyoscine butylbromide or hydrobromide (Kwells)
Gastric mucosa	lansoprazole
Gastric distension	asilone + domperidone
Skeletal muscle spasm	baclofen/diazepam
Cardiac pain	nitrates/nifedipine
Oesophageal spasm	nitrates/nifedipine

Renal impairment/renal failure[16,17]

Palliative care teams may be involved in the care of patients with different degrees of renal failure. Many drugs and their metabolites accumulate in uraemic patients and cause significant side-effects.

Degree of Renal Impairment

	GFR	Serum Creatinine
Mild	20–50ml/min	150–300 mmol/l
Moderate	10–20ml/min	300–700 mmol/l
Severe	<10ml/min	>700 mmol/l

Drugs in renal failure

- Metabolites of morphine accumulate in renal failure and can cause neurotoxic side-effects such as myoclonus and confusion
- Oxycodone and hydromorphone have active metabolites which are renally excreted, and their value in renal failure is less clear. However, case reports suggest they *may* be better than morphine, at least in individual patients switched from morphine because of problems with metabolite accumulation. In health, there is a large reserve of renal function, urea and creatinine remaining at normal values until there is a reduction of 50–60 per cent in glomerular filtration rate
- Paracetamol is safe in renal failure but should be reduced to 3g every 24 h if the patient has severe renal impairment. Paracetamol is dialysed out by haemodialysis but not by peritoneal dialysis

Factors associated with altered handling of drugs in renal failure

- Loss of plasma protein binding capacity occurs due to uraemia itself, which may be relevant for drugs which are highly protein-bound such as diazepam
- Changes in hydration may affect the distribution of drugs in the body causing overdosage
- Oral absorption of drugs may be reduced because of vomiting, diarrhoea and gastrointestinal oedema
- Increased permeability of the blood brain barrier in uraemia may exaggerate the unwanted central nervous system effects associated with certain drugs

- Codeine and Dihydrocodeine can both cause prolonged narcosis but can be used if necessary in a combined preparation with paracetamol (e.g.co-codamol/co-dydramol) in reduced doses. There is an increase in the CNS side effects of weak opioids in renal failure
- Co-proxamol should be used with caution in patients with severe renal impairment
- Diamorphine is metabolized to morphine which is itself metabolized to morphine-3-glucuronide (M3G) and morphine-6-glucuronide (M6G). Accumulation of M3G may cause clinical excitation or agitation

16 Kirkham S. R., Pugh R. (1995) Opioid analgesia in uraemic patients. *Lancet*, **345**, 8958: 1185.

17 Farrell A., Rich A. (2000) Analgesic use in patients with renal failure. *Eur J Pall Care*, **7, 6**: 201-5.

Accumulation of M6G, the useful analgesic metabolite, may account for symptoms of drowsiness, nausea and vomiting, respiratory depression and even coma. Haemodialysis may produce significant falls in morphine concentration leading to pain during or shortly after dialysis. The complex nature of opioid usage in renal failure requires that, particularly in the opioid naïve, very small doses are used and then only with the ready availability of naloxone. For similar reasons the use of long-acting preparations should be avoided. Opioids which do not have active metabolites may be more suitable for patients in renal failure than morphine or diamorphine. (Alfenanil or fentanyl.)

- Fentanyl is mainly metabolized in the liver to inactive metabolites and it has a short half-life, making it a useful drug in renal impairment
- Alfentanil is a short acting opioid metabolized by the liver to inactive compounds. It is 10 times more potent than diamorphine when given subcutaneously and there are some case studies showing less agitation when changed from diamorphine
- Twenty per cent of methadone is excreted unchanged in urine. With its long half-life the dose should be reduced in renal impairment.
- Hydromorphone has been used in patients with renal failure even though it is metabolized to a metabolite which can potentially accumulate causing neuroexcitatation and cognitive impairment
- Oxycodone is 90 per cent metabolized in the liver. In severe renal impairment, it is contra-indicated because the 10 per cent which is normally excreted unchanged in the urine, may then accumulate. For patients with mild or moderate renal failure, oxycodone can be used with caution, so long as the dose is titrated up slowly
- NSAIDS should be avoided, if possible, in patients with any degree of renal impairment, though this counsel of perfection may not necessarily be appropriate in the palliative care setting. Where appropriate, sulindac is the NSAID of choice as it is reported to have renal sparing effects. These effects are lost with doses above 100mg twice daily. In patients with total renal failure on dialysis NSAIDs should not be forgotten if kidney protection is no longer an issue.

Table 6a.11 Commonly used palliative care medication in different degrees of renal failure

Drug	Mild Creat. 150–300mmol/l GFR 20–50ml/min	Moderate Creat. 300–700mmol/l GFR 20–50ml/min	Severe Creat. >700mmol/l GFR <10ml/min
Analgesics			
Paracetamol	ND	ND	500mg–1g every 8 h
NSAIDs	Avoid if possible	Avoid if possible	Avoid
Weak opioids			
Co-codamol,	ND	6 Tabs. in 24h	4 Tabs. in 24h
Co-dydramol	ND	6 Tabs. in 24h	4 Tabs. in 24h
Co-proxamol	ND		
Tramadol	ND	50–100mg every 12h	50mg every 12h
Strong opioids			
Morphine	75% of ND	2.5–5mg every 6–8 h**	1.25–2.5 every 6–8 h*
Oxycodone	Start at a low dose and titrate slowly	Avoid	
Diamorphine	75% of ND**	2.5mg SC every 6 h**	2.5mg SC every 8 h*
Hydromorphone	ND**	1.3mg every 6–8 h**	1.3mg every 8 h*
Methadone	ND**	ND**	50% of ND
Fentanyl	ND**	75% of ND**	50% of ND
Alfentanil	ND**	ND**	ND**

Antiemetics		
Metoclopramide	ND	75% of ND	50% of ND

Antiemetics			
Metoclopramide	ND	75% of ND	50% of ND
Haloperidol	ND but avoid repeated dosing as haloperidol may then accumulate.		
Cyclizine	ND	ND	ND
Levomepromazine	ND	ND	ND
Domperidone	ND	ND	ND
Ondansetron	ND	ND	ND
Anticholinergics			
Hyoscine butylbromide	ND	ND	ND
Hyoscine hydrobromide	ND	ND	ND
Central nervous system			
Baclofen	Max. 5mg o.d.	Max. 5mg o.d.	Max. 5mg o.d.
Benzodiazepines	Start with very small doses. Increased cerebral sensitivity		
Gabapentin	300mg b.d.	300mg o.d.	ND on alternate days
Amitriptyline	ND	ND	
Fluoxetine	ND	ND	ND
Citalopram	ND	ND	No information available
Mirtazapine	15mg o.d.	15mg o.d.	15mg
Paroxetine	20mg o.d.	20mg o.d.	20mg o.d.

** Titrate

ND normal dose

From: Bunn R, Ashley C. (1999) *The Renal Drug Handbook*. Oxford: Radcliffe Medical Press

With thanks to the Renal Pharmacists at the Belfast City Hospital Pharmacy Department.

Anaesthetic procedures in palliative care

Presently she cast a drug into the wine of which they drank, to lull all pain and anger and bring forgetfulness of every sorrow

Homer's Odyssey

Introduction

The majority of patients with cancer can have their pain needs met by following the WHO three-step analgesic ladder. For the minority of patients who do not gain satisfactory pain relief, a 'fourth step' (interventional pain management) can be useful in helping to control pain, maintain psychomotor performance and improve quality of life.

As with all interventions, patient selection is vital for success. General selection criteria include:

- Patient competent/consented
- Patient compliant
- Absence of systemic infection
- Absence of specific allergy
- Absence of significant coagulopathy
- Adequate support for post-procedural care and maintenance

Patients with palliative care needs are often debilitated, have limited mobility and have a limited life span. It is therefore imperative that measures to alleviate their pain are minimally disruptive. Many spinal procedures can easily be done at the bedside, while more involved interventions such as chemical neurolysis necessitate radiological guidance, usually in a hospital setting. With this in mind, patients should be selected for procedures acceptable to them and appropriate to their level of disability.

Intrathecal and epidural (neuraxial) techniques

Direct delivery of opioids to the spinal cord via epidural and intrathecal techniques has become increasingly popular in recent decades, and has proven an effective and reversible way to provide profound analgesia with reduced systemic side-effects. Intrathecal opioids bind to the mu and kappa opioid receptors in the substantia gelatinosa of the spinal cord. This is achieved to a lesser extent with epidural opioids, which exert a simultaneous systemic and intrathecal effect (10 per cent and 90 per cent respectively).

Common indications for the use of neuraxial techniques:

- Unacceptable side-effects despite successful analgesia with systemic opioids
- Unsuccessful analgesia despite escalating doses and use of sequential opioids
- Intolerable neuropathic pain which may be amenable to spinal adjuvants
- Sympathetically mediated pain amenable to sympathetic blockade
- Incident pain which may benefit from numbness (local anaesthetic)

Possible contra-indications to neuraxial techniques (risk-benefit decision):
- Platelet count of <20 × 10^9/l with clinical symptoms of poor clotting
- Full anti-coagulation or INR>1.5
- Active infection with concurrent septicaemia
- Concurrent chemotherapy likely to cause neutropenia
- Occlusion of epidural space by tumour at the site of catheter tip placement (epidural catheters only)
- Allergy or unmanageable side-effects from anticipated treatment
- Psychosocial issues that make technique untenable
- Inadequate professional support to resolve ongoing problems

There is a growing body of evidence favouring intrathecal over epidural administration of opioids in the palliative setting.

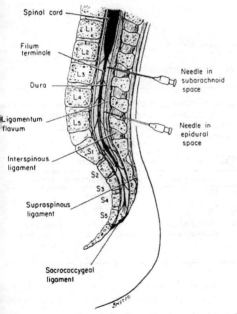

Fig. 6a.5 Schematic diagram of lumbosacral anatomy showing needle placement for lumbar subarachnoid, and epidural spaces.

Table 6a.12 Comparing the two routes of administration

Factors	Intrathecal	Epidural
Infection rate	Same as epidural	Same as intrathecal
Pain relief	Better for long-term	Good only for short-term
Dose	Lower (10–20% of epidural dose)	Higher
Pump refills	Less frequent	More frequent (higher volumes)
Side-effects	Fewer	More
Technical difficulty	Easier to place, less likely to become displaced	Potentially more difficult, and catheter may migrate
Long-term complications	Less (approx. 5%)	More (approx. 55%)
Catheter occlusion and fibrosis	Minimal	Higher frequency (leading to loss of analgesia/pain on injection)
Epidural metastases	Less affected	More affected (may compromise drug delivery)
Overall advantage	Effective analgesia with fewer complications	

Catheters may be externalized through the skin at the puncture site or may be tunnelled subcutaneously away from the spine. Alternatively, a totally implantable pump system may be employed if the patient has a life expectancy of several months.

Table 6a.13 Comparison of continuous versus bolus techniques

Factor	Continuous	Intermittent bolus
Dose escalation	Higher	Lower
Analgesic quality	Better	Fair
Local anaesthetic combinations	Minimal motor or haemodynamic complications	Higher risk of motor or haemodynamic complications (Not recommended for intraspinal administration)

Ideally, the continuous infusion technique should be used, with a familiar delivery system e.g. standard Graseby syringe pump delivering the infusion solution over 24 h.

Technical complications of neuraxial catheters

1 Mechanical problems
2 Skin breakdown at insertion site
3 Infection-local/catheter infection/epidural abscess/meningitis/systemic infection
4 CSF leak, causing headache
5 CSF seroma
6 Haematoma
7 Catheter dislodgement, occlusion or migration
8 Nerve damage (rare but possible).

Adverse effects attributable to spinal opioids

1 Minor sedation (opioid dose excessive)
2 Urinary retention (commonest in males in first 24 h)
3 Persistent nausea
4 Pruritus
5 Respiratory depression (may be severe and insidious if opioid-naïve)
6 Hyperalgesia (at higher doses)
7 Myoclonus (higher doses, indicating toxicity)
8 Constipation.

Management of adverse affects

1 Sedation: reduce dose of opioid
2 Urinary retention: usually requires once-only catheterization
3 Nausea: regular antiemetic
4 Pruritus:
   • consider adding spinal bupivacaine
   • i/v ondansetron 8mg has been shown to be effective
   • i/v nalbuphine may be effective
5 Respiratory depression: (R.R. less than 8/minute or excessive drowsiness)
   • naloxone 100–400mcg
   • stop intrathecal infusion
   • reduce infusion dose
6 Hyperalgesia:
   • reduce opioid dose
   • consider addition of adjuvant agent
7 Myoclonus:
   • reduce opioid dose
   • check renal function
   • encourage rehydration
   • Consider low dose benzodiazepine therapy (myoclonus may not be opioid dose-dependent)
8 Constipation: regular laxatives from the outset of therapy.

Choice of drug: Opioids, local anaesthetics, clonidine

Opioids

Morphine is one of the least lipid soluble opioids available, and when given in the spinal space, it has the slowest rate of uptake into the surrounding vasculature, which gives it a longer and primarily spinal site of action. Intrathecal morphine is regarded as 100 times more potent than a systemically given dose. Data from postoperative pain studies suggest that morphine is twice as potent as diamorphine by the intrathecal route. Intrathecal morphine should be preservative free.

Diamorphine can be administered intrathecally, with a potency ratio of 1:100 (intrathecal:systemic). Diamorphine should be reconstituted in sodium chloride 0.9 per cent. Alternatives to morphine and diamorphine are used less frequently. **Hydromorphone** is an effective and affordable option for the morphine-intolerant patient. The potency of intrathecal hydromorphone is five times that of morphine. Of the lipophilic drugs, both **fentanyl** and **sufentanil** are used. Greater lipid solubility may be an advantage for rapid onset of action, but rapid systemic absorption means shorter duration of action with less dose-sparing effect when compared to systemic administration. There is no published data on dose equivalences.

Typical dosing schedule

- If opioid-naïve, start with intrathecal diamorphine 0.5–1mg/24h or epidural diamorphine 2.5–5mg/24h
- If the patient is established on a systemic opioid, the following regimen may be used to minimize the withdrawal phenomenon during route conversion
  - Give half of the systemic opioid by the established route
  - Convert the remaining half dose to equivalent dose of diamorphine, and then divide by 100 to get the intrathecal dose
- Add 2ml of 0.5 per cent bupivacaine to diamorphine
- Add sodium chloride 0.9% up to total of 10ml
- Infuse solution over 24 h
- After 24 h, reduce the systemic dose by 50 per cent again and titrate upwards the intrathecal dose (usually in increments of 10–30 per cent)
- Attempt to discontinue the systemic opioid by day two (may not always be possible)

Local anaesthetics

Local anaesthetic agents are sodium channel blockers and are unique in their ability to block nerve impulses conducted proximally (pain relief) and impulses conducted distally (motor blockade). The conduction blockade produced is both painless and reversible.

Side-effects of local anaesthetics

- Postural or overt hypotension—sympathetic block
- Numbness—sensory block
- Leg weakness—motor block
- Altered proprioception in low doses, even when motor weakness is not apparent
- Urinary retention
- 'Total spinal'—this potentially catastrophic event can occur if a large dose of local anaesthetic is delivered to the subarachnoid space

erroneously. A profound drop in blood pressure is accompanied by motor paralysis of the lower limbs, spreading to the upper limbs and respiratory muscles and ultimately the brain. Both cardiovascular and ventilatory support are required until the local anaesthetic effects wear off

Table 6a.14 The most frequently used local anaesthetic agents

Agent	Lidocaine	Bupivacaine	Ropivacaine
Onset	Rapid	Slower	Similar to bupivacaine
Duration	Short (h)	2–3 times longer than lidocaine	Slightly longer than bupivacaine
Typical dosage	2ml 2% over 24 h	2ml 0.5% over 24 h	2ml 0.75% over 24 h
Advantages	Rapid onset and offset Synergism with opioids	Synergism with opioids	May preferentially block sensory nerves Two-thirds as potent as bupivacaine Synergism with opioids

Spinal adjuvants
Clonidine
Clonidine is an α-2adrenergic agonist and appears to act at the level of the spinal cord. It acts synergistically with opioids but is also a powerful analgesic when used alone in the management of neuropathic pain. It is a lipophilic compound and its spinal effect may be more pronounced with intrathecal rather than epidural administration. The dose of clonidine is often limited by the appearance of side-effects such as sedation, hypotension and bradycardia. Nausea, pruritus and urinary retention have also been reported. Starting doses range from 10–20mcg/24h and should be titrated for analgesic effect and minimal side-effects. Doses above 150 mcg/24h should not be necessary.

Other analgesics have been tried as intrathecal agents, including midazolam, ketamine, octreotide, calcium channel blockers and neostigmine. As yet, there is no convincing body of evidence to support their use.

Guidelines for percutaneous intrathecal catheter insertion
- Patient consent
- Nurse assistant present
- Adequate space for aseptic trolley
- Patient in sitting or lateral position, with their head and knees curled toward their abdomen
- Skin asepsis (eg. chlorhexidine)
- Local anaesthetic infiltration of skin at chosen level of insertion
- 18G Tuohy needle inserted into spinal space, piercing the dura, until CSF is free-flowing
- Aseptic epidural catheter inserted to 15cm, and free-flow of CSF confirmed
- Catheter secured and dressing applied to insertion site (one which allows daily visual inspection)

- An antibacterial filter should be connected and may remain attached for up to a month
- Connection made to infusion pump or syringe driver

Follow-up care

- All staff involved in aftercare of the patient should be familiar with the possible side-effects and complications listed, and should be vigilant for signs of infection or problems developing
- The catheter insertion site should be inspected on a daily basis
- A pain chart should be kept initially until the analgesia is considered sufficient
- If the patient is being discharged to the community, there should be liaison with the key members of the primary care team (GP, district nurse and community specialist palliative care nurse) prior to discharge and written guidelines should accompany the patient home
- Patients should not be discharged home until dose escalation have been stabilized

Chemical neurolysis for cancer pain

Neurolysis of nerves by chemical means is indicated for patients with limited life expectancy. The use of neurolytic techniques has diminished over recent years due to advancements in spinal analgesia and increased life expectancies in cancer patients. However, neurolysis should be considered in the following circumstances:

- the pain is severe, intractable and has failed to respond to other measures
- the nociceptive pathway is readily identified and related to a peripheral nerve pathway or sympathetic chain
- a trial block of local anaesthetic has been successful
- the effects of the local anaesthetic block are acceptable to the patient

The goals of neurolysis include reduction in pain, and reduction in the need for other pharmacotherapy. Neurolysis is rarely permanent and pain returns as a consequence of regrowth of neural structures or disease progression in the treated area. When used centrally, there is a risk of motor paralysis and sphincter weakness, which are generally unacceptable to most patients. For that reason, patients should be fully consented by the practitioner prior to the procedure.

Neurolytic agents

Alcohol and phenol are the two most commonly used agents.
Effects of alcohol:

- Burning sensation upon injection along the distribution of the nerve, followed by warm numbness
- Pain relief increases over a few days and is maximal by one week
- Alcohol is hypobaric, hence the patient should be able to tolerate a position that allows the alcohol solution to float upwards to the affected nerve root

Effects of phenol:

- Following injection, an initial local anaesthetic effect subsides to neurolysis which may take 3–7 days to become apparent
- Density and duration of block is felt to be less than that of alcohol
- Since phenol is hyperbaric, the patient should be able to tolerate a position that allows the phenol to sink down to the nerve roots

Visceral cancer pain is often produced by a combination of visceral afferent stimulation, as well as somatic and neuropathic elements. The sympathetic chain carries much nociceptive information, and blockade of the sympathetic chain may improve both visceral and sympathetically-mediated pain. Visceral cancer pain can often be alleviated by a combination of oral medication and neurolytic blockade of the sympathetic axis. Since neurolytic techniques have a narrow risk/benefit ratio, they should only be performed by experienced pain clinicians in appropriate surroundings.

Coeliac plexus block

The coeliac plexus is responsible for transmission of nociceptive information from the entire abdominal contents, excluding the descending colon and pelvic structures. It has been successfully used to combat pain from pancreatic cancer and other upper abdominal viscera. For an experienced operator it is a relatively safe and simple technique, performed under CT guidance. Patients referred for this procedure should be able to tolerate lying on an X-ray table, and should have no coagulopathy or local infection.

Possible complications include:
- Orthostatic hypotension (may persist for days)
- Backache at the site of needle insertion (if backache and hypotension persist, observe serial haematocrit measurements to rule out retroperitoneal haemorrhage haematoma)
- Diarrhoea
- Abdominal aortic dissection
- Paraplegia and motor paralysis (rare)

Superior hypogastric block

The superior hypogastric sympathetic ganglion transmits nociceptive information from the pelvis, excluding the distal Fallopian tubes and ovaries. It has been successfully used to manage pain of pelvic origin, other than ovarian pain. Neurological complications have not been reported with this block.

Ganglion of impar block

This ganglion marks the end of the sympathetic chains and is situated at the sacrococcygeal junction. Visceral pain in the perineal area has been successfully treated with neurolytic blockage of this ganglion. These patients often present with a vague, poorly localized perineal pain, accompanied by burning or urgency, and oral medication alone is often inadequate. No complications have been reported with this block.

Other neurolytic blocks

Pleural phenol block

Insertion of an epidural catheter into the pleural space and infusion of local anaesthetic or phenol has been described in the management of visceral pain associated with oesophageal cancer and rib invasion by bony metastases.

It is a relatively simple technique with few complications. These include:
- Pneumothorax (avoid bilateral blocks)
- Phrenic nerve palsy
- Trauma to local structures caused by the needle, catheter or as a consequence of the phenol injection

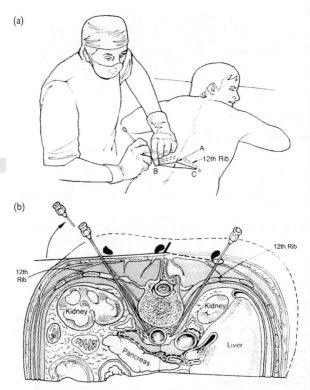

Fig. 6a.6 (a) Positioning for coeliac plexus block; (b) Deep anatomy showing placement of needles for coeliac placement block

Saddle block

This is a modified low spinal technique where phenol is injected into the CSF in the lumbar area, with the intention of causing chemical neurolysis of the low sacral nerve roots that serve the perineum and perianal area. It is useful for patients complaining of pain in the 'saddle' area, but carries the potential risk of sphincter compromise (<10 per cent).

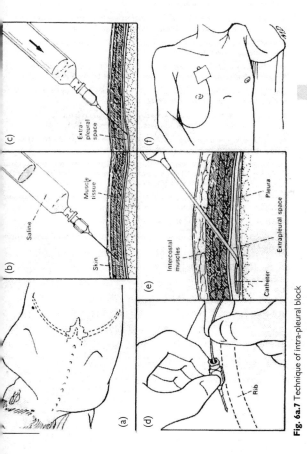

Fig. 6a.7 Technique of intra-pleural block

Further reading

Borgeat A., Stirnemann H. R. (1999) Ondansetron is effective to treat spinal or epidural morphine-induced pruritus. *Anesthesiology*, **90**: 432–6.

Buchheit T., Rauck R. (1999) Subarachnoid techniques for cancer pain therapy: When, Why and How? *Current Pain and Headache Reports*, **3, 3**: 198–205.

Cohen S. E., Ratner E. F., Kreitzman T. R. *et al.* (1992) Nalbuphine is better than naloxone for treatment of side effects after epidural morphine. *Anesth Analg*, **75**: 747–52.

de Leon-Casasola O. (2000) Critical evaluation of chemical neurolysis of the sympathetic axis for cancer pain. *Cancer Control*, **7, 2**: 142–8.

Hill D. A. (2003) Peripheral nerve blocks: practical aspects. In H. Breivik *et al.* (eds.) *Clinical Pain Management, Practical Applications and Procedures*, pp. 197–232. London: Arnold.

Lema M. J., Myers D. P., de Leon-Casasola. (1992) Interpleural phenol therapy for the treatment chronic oesophageal cancer pain. *Rge Anesth*, **17**: 166–70.

Mercadante S. (1999) Neuraxial techniques for cancer pain: an opinion about unresolved therapeutic dilemmas (review). *Regional Anesthesia and Pain Medicine*, **24, 1**: 74–83.

Miguel R. (2000) Interventional Treatment of Cancer Pain: the fourth step in the World Health Organization analgesic ladder? *Cancer Control*, **7, 2**: 149–56.

Schnitzer T. J., Burmester G. R., Mysler E. *et al.* (2004) Comparison of lumiracoxib with naproxen and ibuprofin in the Therapeutic Arthritis Research and Gastrointestinal Event Trial (TARGET), reduction in ulcer complications. *Lancet*, **364**: 665–74.

Simpson K. H., Russon L. (2000) The use of intrathecal drug delivery systems in pain management. *CME Bulletin Palliative Medicine*, **2**: 17–20.

Twycross R. *et al.* (2003) Itch. *QJM*, **96**: 7–26.

Zeppetella G. *et al.* (2004) Topical opioids for painful skin ulcers—do they work? *European Journal of Palliative Care*, **11**: 93–6.

Other non-pharmacological pain interventions

A range of techniques and expertise exists complementing the pharmacological and interventional approaches, which have dominated the module thus far.

These techniques are not just an adjunct to medication but point to the centrality of holistic patient-centred care. Not all approaches will be appropriate for every patient, but for some traditional medicine has little to offer either.

Table 6a.16 Complementary therapies and other non-pharmacological interventions

Complementary therapies	Other non-pharmacological interventions
Acupuncture	Positioning
Reflexology	Catheterization
Aromatherapy	Reassurance
Art therapy	Good communication
Music therapy	Diversional therapy
Touch therapy	TENS
	Splinting of a fractured limb
	Psychological support

📕 See also Chapter 11.

Pain and difficulties in communication

High prevalence of pain in the elderly population is a recognized reality. Almost half of those who die from cancer are over 75 years old. One study showed that 40–80 per cent of elderly in institutions are in pain. There is evidence that many patients suffering from some form of dementia receive no pain relief at all, despite the presence of a concomitant, potentially painful illness.

The reason for this lies in the difficulty in assessing those with communication difficulties. Additionally, the elderly often minimize their pain making even more difficult to evaluate. The patient's unusual behaviour and return to normal with adequate analgesia, may be the only indication of pain.

There have been various attempts to evaluate pain in such circumstances. The DOLOPLUS[19] was developed in 1993. It is based on observations of the behaviour of patients in ten different situations that could be associated with pain. The pain is classified into somatic, psychomotor and psychosocial aspects and scores are allocated. A collective score level confirms the presence of pain.

19 (2001) Lefebvre-Chapiro, S. and the DOLOPLUS group. (2001) The DOLOPLUS 2 scale-evaluating pain in the elderly. *European Journal of Palliative Care*, **8**, 5: 191–4

examples of unusual behaviour indicating pain[20]

verbal expression e.g.
crying when touched
shouting
becoming very quiet
swearing
grunting
talking without making sense

facial expression e.g.
grimacing/wincing
closing eyes
worried expression

behavioural expression e.g.
jumping on touch
hand pointing to body area
increasing confusion
rocking/shaking
not eating
staying in bed/chair
withdrawn/no expression
grumpy mood

physical expression e.g.
cold
pale
clammmy
change in colour
change in vital signs if acute pain (e.g. BP, pulse)

Further reading

Back I. N., Finlay I. (1995) Analgesic effect of topical opioids on painful skin ulcers. *J Pain Symptom Manage,***10, 7**: 493.

Back P., Gibbs L., Sykes N. (2000) Diamorphine-metronidazole gel effective for treatment of painful infected leg ulcers. *J Pain Symptom Manage,* **20, 6**: 396–7.

Scottish Intercollegiate Guidelines Network (2000). *Control of pain in patients with cancer.* Edinburgh: SIGN.

Ventafridda V., Ripamonti C., De Conno F., Bianchi M., Pazuconi F., Panerai A. E. (1987) Antidepressants increase the bioavailability of morphine in cancer patients (letter). *Lancet* i: 1204.

20 Galloway S. and Turner, L. (1999) Pain assessment in older adults who are cognitively impaired. *Journal of Gerontological Nursing* **25**, 37: 34–9.

Gastrointestinal symptoms

Roast Beef, Medium, is not only a food. It is a philosophy.

Edna Ferber, *Roast Beef, Medium*, 1911

A sizeable proportion of palliative care is concerned with the management of gastrointestinal symptoms. Traditionally such symptoms have received less attention than pain management, yet the same principles apply.

Patients with pain usually show a response or a lack of response to treatment within hours. Patients with gastrointestinal symptoms may take several days to respond to interventions, and the temptation is thus to have a more lax attitude to monitoring gastrointestinal problems. In reality the doctor and nurse need to be much more attentive to these problems which deceptively cause great patient morbidity, yet may not become obvious until major management difficulties arise.

Example

Every time a patient is prescribed a strong opioid for the first time: Waiting to see if the patient will become nauseated or constipated will lead to major problems. The patient may become so sick that they refuse all morphine again. The patient may become severely constipated with serious and unpleasant consequences.
- The patient and family may lose trust in the healthcare professional. Such trust is one of the strongest tools in helping patients and it may be difficult to repair if it is shaken so fundamentally

Therefore
- Every time a strong opioid is prescribed for the first time, or the dose of a strong opioid is markedly increased, always prescribe or increase the dose of a laxative
- Antiemetics should be prescribed for the first five to ten days of a strong opioid being started or a higher dose being initiated, but after five days can, and should be, stopped as nausea due to the opioid side-effects may wear off. In practice, if patients have tolerated analgesics on step two of the analgesic ladder, they will probably not need antiemetics when changing to strong opioids

Anticipation of problems before they occur.
Ongoing assessment of treatments and their effectiveness.
Appropriate prescribing of background medication as well as medication for 'breakthrough' symptoms

Oral problems

Oral problems may affect up to 60 per cent of patients with cancer and can impact greatly on quality of life, both physically and psychologically.

Pathology and physiology

A healthy mouth is moist, clean and pain-free with an intact mucosa. Saliva is a major protector of the tissues of the mouth.

About 1500mL of saliva are produced daily by the parotid, submaxillary, sublingual and several minor salivary glands.

Saliva is composed of a serous part (alpha amylase), which initiates starch digestion, and a mucus component which acts as a lubricant. It also contains calcium, phosphate and bicarbonate which help maintain healthy teeth and other components such as mucin which protects oral tissue from chemical and mechanical trauma and infections.

The majority of oral problems seen in palliative care are related to a reduction in saliva secretion, although poor oral hygiene is also a major factor. Candidiasis and dry mouth (xerostomia) are two of the most common problems. Other problems include pain, stomatitis, mucositis, ulceration, halitosis, altered taste and hypersalivation (drooling).

During cytotoxic therapy the cells of the oral mucosa are vulnerable due to their high proliferation rate. Other treatment complications may arise due to direct stomatotoxicity or indirectly due to myelosuppressive effects. Risk factors for oral problems in patients with advanced cancer:
- Reduced oral intake
- Debility (reduced ability to perform own oral hygiene)
- Dry mouth (often aggravated by medicines, mouth breathing, oxygen therapy)
- Dehydration
- Local irradiation
- Chemotherapy
- Local tumour

General mouth care

The aim of good mouth care is to prevent problems before they arise and to control unpleasant symptoms.

Assessment:
- Assess daily for symptoms or signs of problems such as altered taste, oral pain, dry mouth, halitosis, ulcers, oral or pharyngeal candidiasis or dental problems
- Regular examination of lips, tongue, teeth and oral mucosa
- Involve local dental team if necessary
- Assess patient's ability to carry out mouth care effectively
- Encourage good oral hygiene for general well being

*An oral assessment tool may be useful. Eilers *et al.*'s oral assessment guide has been found to be appropriate for use in patients with advanced cancer.[1]

1 Eilers J., Berger A., Petersen M. (1998) Development, testing and application of the Oral Assessment Guide. *Oncol Nurse Forum*, **15**: 325–30.

Management

Basic oral care—by staff or patient if able.

Keep mouth moist—encourage regular sips of fluids/oral rinsing

Brush teeth with toothpaste or clean dentures regularly, especially after meals

Rinse mouth thoroughly and frequently with sodium chloride 0.9 per cent (helps removal of oral debris and is soothing and non-traumatic[2])

Gently clean coated tongue with a soft toothbrush or sponge

Apply moisturizing cream or white soft paraffin (petroleum jelly) to lips

Soak dentures overnight in cleansing solution

If the patient is unconscious or too unwell to carry out oral hygiene, instruct and involve family in this important area of care.

Management of oral problems[2, 3, 4]

Coated tongue/dirty mouth

In addition to basic oral care, if no candidiasis:

Use mouthwashes to remove debris e.g. cool water or sodium chloride 0.9 per cent

Gentle brushing with soft toothbrush or sponge

Pineapple (fresh or tinned) to chew—contains proteolytic enzyme ananase which cleans the mouth

Effervescent vitamin C has been used for furred tongue—place ¼ of 1g effervescent tablet on tongue and allow to dissolve; repeat up to q.d.s. for up to one week

Dry mouth (xerostomia)

Xerostomia is the subjective feeling of a dry mouth and is often associated with difficulties with speech, chewing or swallowing, the need to keep drinking and loss of taste. This is a common problem in advanced cancer and appropriate management may involve the use of both saliva stimulants and substitutes.

Causes:

Drugs e.g. antimuscarinics, antidepressants, opioids, diuretics

Candidiasis

Dehydration

Anxiety

Mouth breathing

Radiotherapy

Oxygen therapy (non-humidified)

Miller M., Kearney N. (2001) Oral care for patients with cancer: a review of the literature. *Cancer Nursing*, **24, 4**: 241–54.

Twycross R. (2001) *Symptom Management in Advanced Cancer*, 3rd edn. Oxford: Radcliffe Medical Press.

Sweeney M. P., Bagg J., Baxter W. P., Aitchison T. C. (1997) Clinical trial of a mucin-containing oral spray for treatment of xerostomia in hospice patients. *Palliative Medicine*, **11**: 225–32.

Management
- Treat underlying cause if possible e.g. infection, dehydration
- Review medication
- Basic oral care regimen (see the previous page)
- General measures (little scientific rationale[2]):
  - sipping semi-frozen drinks
  - sucking ice-chips
  - chewing pineapple pieces
  - sugar-free chewing gum
  - petroleum jelly applied to lips
  - oral sprays may be beneficial[5]

Consider saliva substitutes, especially pre-meals:
- Saliva orthana (NB pork mucin-based spray—may be no more beneficial than placebo)
- OralBalance gel
- Methylcellulose solution e.g. Glandosane spray
- Saliva stimulation
  - Pilocarpine—a parasympathomimetic agent which stimulates salivary gland secretion. (It should be avoided in bowel obstruction, glaucoma, asthma, COPD and cardiac disease)
  - Dose: Pilocarpine 5mg tablets p.o. t.d.s. Sweating is a common side-effect
  - Pilocarpine 4 per cent eye-drop solution has been used in raspberry syrup or peppermint water (2–3 drops taken orally t.d.s.—unlicensed use[6])
  - Bethanechol starting with 10mg t.d.s. with meals and increase if necessary

Painful mouth and stomatitis
Stomatitis refers to painful, inflammatory and ulcerative condition affecting the mucous membranes lining the mouth and may be caused by:
- Infection
- Ulceration
- Mucositis post radiotherapy or chemotherapy
- Iron deficiency (angular stomatitis and glossitis)
- Vitamin C deficiency (gingivitis and bleeding)
- Dry mouth

Other causes of oral pain include:
- Tumour infiltration
- Dental problems

Management
Non-drug treatment
- Treat underlying cause if possible e.g. infection
- Good oral hygiene
- Avoid foods that trigger pain e.g. acidic foods
- Avoid tobacco and alcohol
- ENT/Oncology review

5 Sweeney M. P., Bagg J., Baxter W. P., Aitchison T. C. (1997) Clinical trial of a mucin-containing oral spray for treatment of xerostomia in hospice patients. *Palliative Medicine*, **11**: 225–32.

6 Back I. N. (2001) *Palliative Medicine Handbook*, 3rd edn. Cardiff: BPM Books.

Drug treatment

Generalized oral pain
- Systemic analgesic:
- Analgesic mouthwash e.g. benzydamine hydrochloride (difflam) 10mL q.d.s. (dilute 1:1 if stings)
- Chlorhexidine 0.2 per cent (Corsodyl)—rinse mouth with 10mL for 1 minute b.d.
- Sucralfate Susp. 10mL as mouthwash 4-h
- Soluble aspirin 300—600mg q.d.s. (if no contra-indications)
- Cocaine mouthwash 2 per cent is used for mucositis in some centres

Some claim there is no evidence that benzydamine, sucralfate or chlorhexidine ease oral pain.[7]

Localized oral pain
- Topical analgesia e.g.
  - Choline salicylate oral gel (Bonjela/Teegel)—apply q.d.s.
  - Carmellose paste (orabase)—protective oral paste—apply p.r.n.
  - Lidocaine spray, gel or cream (beware pharyngeal anaesthesia and risk of aspiration)
- Systemic analgesics
  - NSAIDs e.g. diclofenac (if no contradictions)
  - Opioids—consider starting or increasing systemic opioids and monitor response
  - Consider ketamine for persistent oral neuropathic pain

Ulceration of oral mucosa

Causes include trauma (chemical or physical), recurrent aphthae, infections, cancer, nutritional deficiencies, haematinic deficiency (iron, folate, B_{12}) and drug therapy.

Management: Identify and treat cause where possible.
- Consider referral for further investigation if mouth ulcer persists
- Pain relief—as for Stomatitis

Aphthous ulcers
- Topical corticosteroids for five days e.g. Adcortyl in Orabase (triamcinolone 0.1 per cent paste) applied twice daily or Corlan lozenges (hydrocortisone) 1 q.d.s. p.o. to ulcerated area
- Tetracycline mouthwash (for resistant ulcers). Caps. 250mg—dissolve contents in water and hold in mouth for 2–3 minutes twice daily for three days. Avoid swallowing. May stain teeth[7]
- Persistent and severe ulcers may respond to thalidomide (seek specialist advice)

Infection
- Fungal—candidiasis is most common in patients with cancer
- Viral—e.g. herpes simplex
- Bacterial—e.g. coliforms or staphylococci

Predisposing factors:
- Reduced salivary flow

7 Regnard C., Hockley J. (2004) *A Guide to Symptom Relief in Palliative Care. 5th edition.* Oxford: Radcliffe Medical Press.

- Immunosuppressants
- Chemotherapy
- Antibiotics
- Poor nutritional state
- Diabetes
- Wearing dentures
- Poor oral hygiene

Candidiasis

Present in up to 80 per cent of patients.[8] (Present in normal oral flora o'
50 per cent general population.) May be asymptomatic.

Presenting features may include:

- Dry mouth
- Loss of taste
- Smooth red tongue
- Adherent white plaques on tongue or mucous membranes
- Soreness
- Dysphagia (remember oropharyngeal/oesophageal candidiasis)
- Angular cheilitis

Investigation

In palliative care swabs are not routinely taken, although it may be useful
since fungal infections may become resistant to standard treatment.

Treatment

- Specific treatments should be accompanied by good oral hygiene
- There is no clear evidence to suggest superiority of the various
  antifungal agents in this patient population
- Remember to treat dentures—soak in Nystatin or dilute Milton overnight
- Topical:
  - Nystatin Susp. 100,000 U/mL or Nystatin pastilles 100,000 U
  - Dose: 2–5mL q.d.s. p.o. or 1 pastille q.d.s. p.o. for at least five days
    (reduced activity if nystatin combined with chlorhexidine mouthwash)
  - Miconazole oral gel 25mg/mL, apply q.d.s. p.o.
  - Amphotericin lozenges 10mg, dose: 1 lozenge q.d.s.
- Systemic:
  - Ketoconazole Tabs./Susp., Dose: 200mg o.d. p.o. (watch liver function)
  - Fluconazole Tabs./Susp., Dose: 50mg o.d. p.o. for seven days

Recurrent candidiasis in patients with AIDS may require prophylactic
treatment with fluconazole 50mg daily. Concern is arising that 'azole' (i.e.
fluconazole) resistance may become a clinical problem in palliative care.[9]

Herpes simplex infection may require oral Aciclovir 200mg 4-h for one
week.

> NOTE: Systemic antifungal drugs may interact with several drugs
> metabolized by the cytochrome P450 enzymes including phenytoin,
> warfarin, sulphonylureas and midazolam. It is always best to check for
> possible interactions when co-prescribing.

8 Back I. N. (2001) *Palliative Medicine Handbook*, 3rd edn. Cardiff: BPM books.

9 Davies A., Brailsford S., Broadley K., Beighton D. (2002) Resistance amongst yeasts isolated from
the oral cavities of patients with advanced cancer. *Palliat Med*, **16**: 527–31.

Bacterial infection

Malignant ulcers or local tumour may be associated with halitosis due to anaerobic bacteria.

Treatment

- Metronidazole 400mg t.d.s. p.o. or 500mg b.d. PR × 5 days
- May be used as mouthwash if adverse effects. Metronidazole Susp. 400mg (10mL) t.d.s. and spit out[8]

Drooling

May be due to overproduction of saliva (sialorrhoea) or inability to swallow normal amounts of saliva. Drooling is common in MND (40 per cent) but uncommon in advanced cancer (except head and neck).

Causes

- Neuromuscular:
  - MND
  - CVA
  - Cerebral palsy
  - Carcinoma of pharynx
  - Parkinson's disease
  - Brain tumours
- Oral factors:
  - Ill-fitting dentures
  - Deformity post surgery e.g. oral surgery
  - Dysphagia
- Drugs:
  - Cholinesterase inhibitors
  - Cholinergic agents
  - Lithium

Management

- Non-drug treatment:
  - Head positioning
  - Suctioning
- Drug treatment:
  - Antimuscarinic drugs (if patient is able to swallow) will reduce saliva production
  - Most patients will not be able to swallow tablets or capsules, or large volumes, and a number will have PEG tube feeding
  - Drugs that do not cross the blood-brain barrier minimise the risk of sedation and other central side-effects; however they may also be poorly and unpredictably absorbed when given orally
  - Other drugs with antimuscarinic effects will reduce saliva production, e.g. amitriptyline p.o. 25mg nocte or propantheline 15mg t.d.s., but use is often limited by side-effects
  - Choice will depend on local availability and patient's circumstances

Table 6b.1 Drug treatment

Given by injection	
Glycopyrronium 0.1–0.4mg/24h CSCI	Ideal drug, but requires regular or continuous injection. Most reliable way of establishing effective symptom control rapidly.
Glycopyrronium 25–100mcg b.d. SC as needed	
Transdermal patch	
Hyoscine hydrobromide transdermal patch	Central side-effects can occur, especially in the elderly.
Given orally/PEG/sublingual	
Glycopyrronium p.o. 0.6–2mg up to t.d.s.	Solution for injection can be used but may need 3–10mL. Powder for oral solution requires pharmacy to prepare, is not routinely available, and is expensive. Titration to effective dose may take longer.
Atropine eye drops 1% 2 drops p.o./sublingual q.d.s.	Cheapest; least published experience. Central side-effects may occur, but less than hyoscine hydrobromide.

Further reading

Books

Back I. N. (2001) *Palliative Medicine Handbook*, 3rd ed. Cardiff: BPM Books.

Doyle D., Hanks G. W. C., Cherny N. (eds) (2004) *Oxford Textbook of Palliative Medicine*, 3rd edn. Oxford: Oxford University Press.

Regnard C., Hockley J. (2004) *A Guide to Symptom Relief in Palliative Care*. 5th edn. Oxford: Radcliffe Medical Press.

Twycross R. (2001) *Symptom Management in Advanced Cancer*, 3rd edn. Oxford: Radcliffe Medical Press.

Twycross R., *et al.* (2002) *Palliative Care Formulary*. 2nd edn. Oxford: Radcliffe Medical Press.

Articles

Davies A., Brailsford S., Broadley K., Beighton D. (2002) Resistance amongst yeasts isolated from the oral cavities of patients with advanced cancer. *Palliat Med*, **16**: 527–31.

Eilers J., Berger A., Petersen M. (1988) Development, testing and application of the Oral Assessment Guide. *Oncol. Nursing Forum*, **15**: 325–30.

Regnard C. (1994) Single dose fluconazole versus five-day ketoconazole in oral candidosis. *Palliat Med*, **8**: 72–3.

Sweeney M. P., Bagg J., Baxter W. P., Aitchison T. C. (1997) Clinical trial of a mucin-containing oral spray for treatment of xerostomia in hospice patients. *Palliative Medicine*, **11**: 225–32.

Reviews

Miller M. Kearney N. (2001) Oral care for patients with cancer: a review of the literature. *Cancer Nursing*, **24**, 4: 241–54.

Nausea and vomiting

> Last night we went to a Chinese dinner at six and a French dinner at nine, and I can feel the sharks' fins navigating unhappily in the Burgundy.
>
> Peter Flemming, Letter from Yunnanfu, 20 March 1938

Nausea is an unpleasant feeling of the need to vomit often accompanied by autonomic symptoms.

Vomiting is the forceful expulsion of gastric contents through the mouth.[10]

Nausea and vomiting are symptoms which can cause patients, and their relatives, deep distress. Of the two, nausea causes most misery; many patients can tolerate one or two episodes of vomiting a day while prolonged nausea is profoundly debilitating. Causes of nausea are multiple and it is important to try to analyse the likely cause so that appropriate therapy can be initiated.

Evaluation
- Distinguish between vomiting, expectoration and regurgitation
- Separately assess nausea and vomiting
- Enquire if nausea is absent for prolonged periods after vomiting or is persistent
- Review drug regimen
- If there is a likelihood of cerebral secondaries, check fundi for papilloedema (although its absence does not exclude raised intracranial pressure)
- Examine the abdomen
- Do a rectal examination if faecal impaction is a possibility
- Consider checking plasma concentrations of: creatinine, calcium, albumin, and digoxin
- Consider radiological investigations if major doubt remains about cause
- Note the content of the vomitus e.g. undigested food, bile, faeculent
- Timing of onset of nausea or vomiting
- Associated symptoms (e.g. the headaches of raised intracranial pressure are coincidental with vomiting)

Causes
Common causes of nausea and vomiting in advanced cancer include:
- Gastrointestinal, e.g. gastric stasis, intestinal obstruction
- Drugs, e.g. opioids, antibiotics, NSAIDs, iron, digoxin
- Metabolic, e.g. hypercalcaemia, renal failure
- Toxic, e.g. radiotherapy, chemotherapy, infection, paraneoplastic
- Brain metastases
- Psychosomatic factors, e.g. anxiety, fear
- Pain

Treat reversible causes
- Severe pain
- Infection
- Cough
- Hypercalcaemia
- Tense ascites

Raised intracranial pressure (using corticosteroids)
Emetogenic drugs—stop or reduce dose
Anxiety—pharmacological and psychological management

Opioid-induced nausea and vomiting

Opioids can cause nausea and vomiting through a number of different possible mechanisms. These include stimulation of the chemoreceptor trigger zone, increased vestibular sensitivity, gastric stasis or impaired intestinal motility and constipation.

Haloperidol is usually recommended as first-line for opioid-induced nausea and vomiting, however metoclopramide (for gastric stasis), cyclizine or hyoscine hydrobromide may all be effective in certain patients. 5HT₃ antagonists have also been shown to be useful but are expensive for long term use.

Non-pharmacological management of nausea and vomiting

Control of malodour from colostomy, fungating tumour or
decubitus ulcer
A calm, reassuring environment away from the sight and smell
of food
Avoid exposure to foods which precipitate nausea which may mean
transferring the patient to a single room
Small snacks, e.g. a few mouthfuls, and not large meals
If the patient is the household cook, someone else may need to take on
this rôle
Use of acupressure wrist bands, Sea Bands—These devices are helpful
to some patients, particularly those who prefer non-pharmacology
treatments

Drug management of nausea and vomiting

There are many neurotransmitter receptors involved in nausea and vomiting. These include those for histamine, acetylcholine, 5-hydroxytryptamine and dopamine located in varying concentrations largely in the vomiting centre and the chemoreceptor trigger zone in the mid brain.

In simple terms, neural impulses from a variety of emetic stimuli are relayed to these sites in the brain stem, triggering the vomiting reflex. A single antiemetic may be adequate to suppress symptoms, but if there are different causes for the vomiting in the same patient, it may be necessary to combine drugs. For instance, if the cause of vomiting is thought to be raised intracranial pressure and uraemia, it may be necessary to combine e.g. cyclizine and haloperidol.

Levomepromazine antagonises several receptors and may thus be a useful single alternative at a dose of 6.25mg o.d. or b.d. orally, doses higher than this causing sedation.

It may be possible to control nausea with oral medication, but persistent vomiting requires drug delivery by an alternative route such as per rectum or, more reliably, subcutaneously by means of stat doses or continuously via a syringe driver.

Twycross R. (2001) *Symptom Management in Advanced Cancer*, 3rd edn. Oxford: Radcliffe Medical Press.

Side-effects

All antiemetics have side-effects with which it is necessary to familiar.

It is very easy to overlook minor extrapyramidal effects of the dopam antagonists which thus adds to a patient's distress. For instance, haloperi and metoclopramide may cause restlessness and inability to keep s (akathisia). More marked signs include Parkinsonian effects such as stiffn and tremor. The effect can be reversed by stopping the drug. If necessar small dose of an antimuscarinic drug, such as procyclidine, can be giv Domperidone is an alternative to metoclopramide since extrapyrami problems are less.

Cyclizine and the phenothiazines (e.g. levomepromazine) are associat with anticholinergic side-effects such as dry mouth, blurring of vision a urinary retention.

5-HT$_3$ antagonists cause constipation.

Table 6b.2

Cause of vomiting	Choice of antiemetic drug
Drug or toxin induced	Haloperidol 1.5mg nocte/b.d. Levomepromazine 6.25mg (a quarter tablet). 6mg Tabs. available soon
Radiotherapy	Granisetron 1mg stat then 1mg b.d. Haloperidol 1.5–3mg nocte/b.d.
Chemotherapy	Granisetron 1mg stat then 1mg b.d. Dexamethasone 4–8mg o.d. (often as part of a chemotherapy regime) Metoclopramide 20mg q.d.s.
Metabolic e.g. hypercalcaemia	Haloperidol 1.5mg nocte/b.d. Levomepromazine 6.25mg nocte
Raised intracranial pressure	Cyclizine 50mg t.d.s./ or 150mg /24h SC. Dexamethasone 4–16mg o.m.
Bowel obstruction[11]	Cyclizine 150mg/24h p.o. or SC Hyoscine butylbromide 40–100mg/24h SC Octreotide 300–1000mcg/24h SC Ondansetron 8–24mg/24h p.o., i/v or SC
Delayed gastric emptying	Metoclopramide 10–20mg q.d.s. Domperidone 10–20mg q.d.s.
Gastric irritation	Treat gastritis e.g. proton pump inhibitor Stop gastric irritants e.g. NSAID Cyclizine 50mg t.d.s. Ondansetron 8mg b.d.

11 Baines M. J. (2000) Symptom control in advanced gastrointestinal cancer. *Eur J Gastroenterol Hepatol*, **12**: 375–9.

Management of nausea and vomiting: practical guide

Identify any causes of nausea and vomiting that can best be treated specifically e.g.

- constipation—remember to do a rectal examination
- gastritis—epigastric discomfort and tenderness
- raised intracranial pressure—neurological signs
- oropharyngeal candida
- hypercalcaemia—dehydration, confusion
- drug induced—recent introduction of morphine?
- intestinal obstruction

Choose an antiemetic based on the most likely cause of nausea and vomiting

- drug or metabolic haloperidol
- gastric stasis metoclopramide
- GI tract involvement or cerebral tumour cyclizine

If first choice drug unsuccessful or only partially successful after 24h, increase dose or use different antiemetic(s)

- nausea and vomiting in cancer is often multifactorial
- if confident that there is a single cause for the nausea and vomiting, consider increasing the dose of antiemetic (especially metoclopramide), or changing to a second-line specific antiemetic (e.g. ondansetron for drug-induced nausea)
- if not confident of cause, empirically try one of the other first-line antiemetics (metoclopramide, haloperidol, cyclizine)
- combinations of antiemetics with different actions (e.g. at different receptor sites) are often needed and can act additively
- if using more than one antiemetic, one from each class of antiemetics should be considered, see Table 6b.3
- cyclizine and haloperidol are a logical combination
- levomepromazine acts at several receptor sites, and alone may replace a previously unsuccessful combination
- levomepromazine may be useful as a non-specific second-line antiemetic for nausea and vomiting of any or unknown aetiology
- cyclizine may antagonise the prokinetic effects of metoclopramide, and they should not usually be mixed

General points

Always give antiemetics *regularly*—not p.r.n.

If vomiting is preventing drug absorption, use an alternative route e.g. CSCI

Dexamethasone 4mg daily often contributes an antiemetic effect for nausea and vomiting of unknown mechanism

Check blood urea and electrolytes, liver function tests and calcium:

- Renal failure—consider lowering the dose of opioids
- Hypercalcaemia—treat with intravenous bisphosphonates

Monitor carefully if giving prokinetic drugs (e.g. metoclopramide) in intestinal obstruction in case intestinal colic and vomiting increase.

Always reassess the patient regularly as the cause of nausea and vomiting can change with time.
- Levomepromazine tends to cause sedation at doses above 6.25mg b.d.
- Octreotide dries up gastrointestinal secretions tending towards constipation
- Granisetron and ondansetron are also associated with constipation

ANTIEMETIC LADDER

	2nd line narrow Spectrum	e.g. ondansetron
	OR combination	e.g. cyclizine + haloperidol
	OR broad spectrum	e.g. levomepromazine

Selected narrow spectrum antiemetic
- metoclopramide
- cyclizine
- haloperidol

Step 2

Step 1

± administer by **CSCI**
± dexamethasone

Antiemetic drugs

Anti-histamines

The *vomiting centre* is rich in histamine and acetylcholine receptors. Mos antihistamine drugs are also antimuscarinic.

Cyclizine is a commonly used antihistamine antiemetic. Acting at th vomiting centre, it is useful for vomiting of many causes.

Dose: 25–50mg t.d.s. orally or 100–150mg/24h CSCI.

Side-effects: antimuscarinic effects like dry mouth and drowsiness ofte abate after a few days.

Antimuscarinics

Hyoscine hydrobromide is a potent antimuscarinic. It is especiall useful if there is intestinal obstruction or colic as it reduces peristalsis.

Side-effects of dry mouth, drowsiness or confusion may be more sever than with cyclizine.

It is available as buccal tablets (Kwells), transdermal patch (Scopoderr TTS), and can be used by CSCI. 200–1200 mcg/24h CSCI.

Antipsychotics

Drugs and metabolic disturbances cause vomiting by stimulating the CTZ Antipsychotics (as potent dopamine antagonists) block this pathway an are very effective against drug or metabolic induced nausea and vomitin (e.g. opioids and renal failure).

Haloperidol. Dose: 1.5mg nocte orally (0.5–1.5mg b.d.) o 2.5–5mg/24h CSCI

Sedation and extrapyramidal effects are rare at these low doses.

Prochlorperazine is relatively more sedative but is available in bucca (Buccastem) and suppository form. Prochlorperazine cannot be given sub cutaneously as it is irritant.

Levomepromazine. Dose ranges: 6.25mg–25mg nocte or b.d. orall' or 6.25–25mg/24h CSCI. Oral bioavailability of levomepromazine i approx. 40 per cent. Use half the daily oral dose by CSCI.

A sedative, broad spectrum antiemetic which is effective in low doses Some patients show a narrow therapeutic window.

It also has antimuscarinic, antihistamine and 5-HT$_2$ antagonist effects, a well as an anxiolytic effect.

Phenothiazines and haloperidol should be avoided with amiodarone sinc there is an increased risk of ventricular arrhythmias. The low, antiemeti doses of haloperidol used in palliative care probably carry a low risk.

Prokinetic drugs/drugs altering gastric motility

Metoclopramide acts peripherally on the gut restoring normal gastri emptying. It also acts at the CTZ and thus helps drug-induced nausea Dose: 10mg–20mg q.d.s. p.o. or 30–80mg/24h CSCI.

Side-effects: extrapyramidal effects are rare, but most common in youn female patients.

Domperidone is very similar to metoclopramide but is less likely t cause extrapyramidal effects because it does not cross the blood brair barrier; it is available as suppositories.

5-HT₃ antagonists

5-HT₃ receptors are found in the chemoreceptor trigger zone. They are very effective against acute-phase chemotherapy and radiotherapy induced nausea with little to choose between ondansetron and granisetron, but their place in other situations (e.g. intestinal obstruction) is as yet uncertain.

Ondansetron has been shown to be ineffective in motion sickness, but effective at treating morphine-induced nausea and vomiting. 5-HT₃ antagonists may work synergistically with haloperidol in some cases.

In the UK, 5-HT₃ antagonists are only licensed for chemotherapy-induced and postoperative emesis.

Other drugs

Corticosteroids often have a non-specific benefit in reducing nausea and vomiting.

Additional drugs

Newer atypical antipsychotics may be expected to show antiemetic effects. Olanzapine has a similar pharmacological profile to levomepromazine and there is weak anecdotal evidence that it may be an effective antiemetic.

Risperidone has potent 5-HT₂ antagonist effects as well as being anti-dopaminergic but there is no published evidence to date of any antiemetic effect. It should be avoided in patients with cerebrovascular disease.

Table 6b.3 Receptor affinity of antiemetic drugs

Agonist/Antagonist	ACh_M Ant	H_1 Ant	5-HT₂ Ant	D_2 Ant	5-HT₃ Ant	5-HT₄ Ag
Hyoscine hydrobromide	+++					
Cyclizine	++	+++				
Haloperidol				+++ (*)		
Ondansetron					+++	
Metoclopramide				++	(+)	++
Domperidone				++		
Levomepromazine	+	+	++	+ (*)		

(*) Prokinetic effect of metoclopramide and domperidone is partly attributed to D_2 antagonism—however there is no evidence that haloperidol or other neuroleptics have prokinetic activity.

Avoid dopamine antagonists (particularly haloperidol), in patients with Parkinson's Disease.

Constipation

Constipation is characterised by difficult or painful defaecation, and is associated with infrequent bowel evacuations, and hard, small faeces.

Stool frequency varies considerably in the normal population: 45 per cent of patients are constipated on admission to a hospice. Complications of constipation include pain, bowel obstruction, overflow diarrhoea and urinary retention which cause great distress and every effort must there fore be made to avoid them.

Causes

- Disease-related
  - Immobility
  - Decreased food intake
  - Low residue diet
- Fluid depletion
  - Poor fluid intake
  - Increased fluid loss i.e. vomiting, polyuria, fever
- Weakness
  - Inability to raise intra-abdominal pressure
    - e.g. general debility   • paraplegia
  - Inability to reach toilet when urge to defaecate occurs (immobility leads to decreased peristalsis)
- Intestinal obstruction
- Medication
  - Opioids (90 per cent of patients taking opioids need laxatives)
  - Diuretics
  - Antimuscarinics
    - phenothiazines   • tricyclic antidepressants   • hyoscine derivatives
  - Serotonin inhibitors
    - ondansetron/granisetron/tropisetron
  - Somatostatin analogues
    - octreotide   • lanreotide
- Biochemical
  - Hypercalcaemia
  - Hypokalaemia
- Other
  - Embarrassment in public setting
  - Pain on defaecation e.g. fissure in ano

Complications of constipation

- Pain—colic or constant abdominal discomfort
- Intestinal obstruction
- Urinary retention or frequency
- Overflow diarrhoea
- Faecal incontinence
- Confusion or restlessness if severe

Traditionally laxatives are divided into

- Stimulants   • Bulking agents
- Osmotic agents   • Faecal softeners

In reality, these categories are arbitrary as there is much overlap between the agents. For example, an osmotic agent will act as a stimulant by decreasing the GIT transit time by increasing pressure within the bowel.

Management of constipation
- Anticipate this common problem
- Enquire about bowel function regularly
- Start prophylactic laxatives when starting opioid drugs
- Use oral laxatives in preference to rectal measures
- Use a combination of a stimulant laxative with a softener/osmotic laxative if necessary
- Titrate components to achieve optimum stool frequency and consistency

Remember also to:
- Increase fluid intake
- Increase fruit/fibre in diet
- Encourage mobility
- Get patient to toilet, if possible avoiding bed pans
- Provide privacy
- Raise toilet seat for comfort

Laxatives

Choice of laxative
- A number of laxative combinations may be equally effective
- Patient preference may dictate choice
- Mixed preparations of softener/stimulant (e.g. co-danthramer) keep medications to a minimum
- Separate softener and stimulant allows titration of components to give optimum stool frequency and consistency
- Senna has a greater tendency to cause colic than dantron-containing combination laxatives

Stimulants e.g. senna, dantron, bisacodyl
Avoid stimulant drugs if there is the possibility of intestinal obstruction. Dantron is useful with a softener such as docusate (co-danthrusate) or poloxamer (co-danthramer) for opioid-induced constipation, but may colour urine red and cause excoriation around the perineum if in contact with skin. (Dantron is only licensed for use in patients with a terminal illness.)

Osmotic agents e.g. lactulose, magnesium salts, and macrogols
In palliative care, the use of such agents is often inappropriate because of the need to drink 2–3 litres per day for the agents to function well. In addition, lactulose may be unpalatable and cause uncomfortable abdominal bloating and flatus.
  Macrogol (polyethylene glycol) in the palliative setting, particularly in intractable constipation and faecal impaction, may have a particular rôle to play.[12]

Lactulose is usually to be avoided in the palliative care setting because:
- It can increase abdominal cramps
- Its sweet taste can be hard for the palliative care patient to tolerate
- It causes flatulence
- It should be consumed with large volumes of liquid which palliative care patients are often unable to take

Faecal softeners e.g. docusate
These are useful in conjunction with a stimulant (e.g. docusate + dantron in co-danthrusate and docusate + poloxamer in co-danthramer). It may be safer to use docusate alone in resolving intestinal obstruction.

12 Culbert P., Gillett H., Ferguson A. (1998) Highly effective new oral therapy for faecal impaction. *British Journal of General Practice*, **48**: 1599–600.

Bulk-forming agents e.g. methylcellulose (Celevac), ispaghula husk (Fybogel)

Patients are rarely started on these preparations in the palliative care setting because they have been implicated in worsening constipation when used with reduced fluid intake. They are also unpalatable and may aggravate anorexia.

Rectal agents (1 glycerol suppository + 1 bisacodyl suppository)

Bisacodyl is a rectal stimulant and should be placed in direct contact with the rectal mucosa. If appropriately placed, it should stimulate an evacuation within one hour.

Glycerol is a faecal lubricant which facilitates defaecation by softening the stool.

For more severe constipation

Arachis oil enema (130mL) overnight to penetrate hard stool, soften and lubricate. Follow with high phosphate enema in the morning to stimulate bowel clearance.

Do *not* attempt *manual evacuation* of impacted stool without some form of sedation or analgesia.

In circumstances of intractable constipation, close consultation with nursing colleagues is vital if a clear strategy for managing the problem is to be achieved.

Faecal impaction

If the patient has faecal impaction, try:
- Bisacodyl suppositories (must be in contact with rectal mucosa)
- Arachis oil retention enema to soften
- Phosphate enema
- An alternative is polyethylene glycol, *movicol* taken for three days
- Manual removal (with midazolam, diamorphine, or caudal anaesthesia)
- Once successful it is imperative to start regular oral measures to prevent recurrence of the problem

Table 6b.4 Classification of commonly used laxatives

Category	Examples	Description	Comments
Osmotic Laxatives	**Lactulose Polyethylene glycol**	Osmotic laxatives are not absorbed from the gut and so retain water in the lumen by osmotic action (this action may be partial). This increase in volume will encourage peristalsis and consequent expulsion of faeces.	Can cause abdominal distension and abdominal cramps. Patients need to drink over a litre a day which may not be practical

Surfactant Laxatives	**Docusate Poloxamer**	Act to reduce surface tension and improve water penetration of the stools.	
Stimulant Laxatives	**Senna Bisacodyl**	Senna and bisacodyl both rely on bacterial transformation in the large bowel to produce active derivatives and so have little small intestinal effect.	Can cause abdominal cramps. Should be avoided in patients with intestinal obstruction.
	Dantron	Absorbed from the small bowel and undergoes first pass hepatic metabolism to glucuronide forms. These may be secreted in the bile and converted to the active drug prolonging its action	Dantron is available only combined wilh a surfactant softener e.g. Co-danthramer with poloxamer, or Co-danthrusate with docusate. Dantron-containing preps are subject to licence limitations following evidence from animal studies that in high doses it can cause tumours. It is licensed for use in analgesic induced constipation in terminally ill patients. Dantron may colour urine red. It should be avoided in patients who may be incontinent of urine or faeces, as it can cause severe rashes if it comes in contact with the skin.

Table 6b.5 Onset of action

• Bisacodyl tablet	10–12 h		• Laxoberal	10–14 h
• Bisacodyl Supps.	20–60 min		• Microlax enema	20 min
• Dantron	6–12 h		• Phosphate enema	20 min
• Docusate	24–48 h		• Senna	8–12 h
• Glycerin Supps.	1–6 h		• Sodium picosulfate	min
• Lactulose	48 h			

Diarrhoea

Diarrhoea is a less common symptom than constipation amongst patients requiring palliative care and has been defined as the passage of more than three unformed stools within a 24-h period.

As with constipation, patients can understand 'diarrhoea' in different ways and clarification of the term is always required.

Up to 10 per cent of patients admitted to hospice complain of diarrhoea. (In contrast, 27 per cent of HIV infected patients are reported as having diarrhoea).

Treatment of diarrhoea

A **cause** for the diarrhoea should be looked for prior to giving antidiarrhoeal agents. The presence of fever or blood in the stool should prompt further discussion to ensure the most appropriate treatment.

General measures

- Increase fluid intake, constant sipping
- Reassurance that most diarrhoea is self-limiting

Management

Treat or exclude any specific causes.

Table 6b.6 The most common causes of diarrhoea in the palliative care setting

1 Imbalance of laxative therapy. (Especially when laxatives have been increased to clear severe constipation.)
Diarrhoea should settle within 24 h if laxatives are stopped. Laxatives should be reintroduced at a lower dose.

2 Drugs such as antibiotics and antacids, NSAIDS or iron preparations.

3 Faecal impaction is associated with fluid stool which leaks past a faecal plug or a tumour mass.

4 Radiotherapy involving the abdomen or pelvis is likely to cause diarrhoea especially in the second or third week of therapy.

5 Malabsorption associated with:
Carcinoma of head of pancreas with insufficient pancreatic secretions thus less fat absorption and resultant steatorrhoea.
Gastrectomy resulting in poor mixing of food with pancreatic secretions and consequent resultant steatorrhoea. Vagotomy can cause increased water secretion into the colon.
Ileal resection reduces the ability of the small intestine to reabsorb bile acids. These acids increase fluid in the colon and contribute to explosive diarrhoea.

Table 6b.6 (Continued)

A resection of over 100-cm of terminal ileum will outstretch the liver's capacity to compensate for the bile salt loss, and fat malabsorption will compound the diarrhoea.

Colectomy. Immediately following surgery for a total or a near total colectomy, the water in the gut cannot be adequately absorbed. Although this tends to settle over a week, the bowel seldom returns to its pre-surgical function. The small intestine is unable to adequately compensate for the loss of this colonic water-absorbing capacity. This can lead to an ongoing daily loss of an extra 400–1000mL of gut fluid rectally.

Such patients often require an ileostomy and need an extra litre of fluid and 7g of extra salt a day with vitamin and iron supplements.

6 **Colonic or rectal tumours** can cause diarrhoea through causing partial bowel obstruction or through increased mucus secretion

7 **Rare endocrine tumours** which secrete hormones cause diarrhoea. e.g. carcinoid tumour

8 Concurrent disease such as gastrointestinal infection

9 Odd dietary habits.

Table 6b.7 Diagnostic diarrhoea patterns

Defaecation described as 'diarrhoea' happening only two or three times a day without warning suggests anal incontinence.

Profuse watery stools are characteristic of colonic diarrhoea.

Sudden onset of diarrhoea after a period of constipation raises suspicion of faecal impaction.

Alternating diarrhoea and constipation suggests poorly regulated laxative therapy or impending bowel obstruction.

Pale, fatty offensive stools (steatorrhoea) indicate malabsorption due to either pancreatic or ileal disease.

Table 6b.8 Cause management

Subacute small bowel obstruction	See intestinal obstruction
Laxatives (including self-administered magnesium-containing antacids)	Discontinue and review
Faecal impaction (with anal leakage or incontinence)	Rectal disimpaction /manual evacuation/ macrogol
Antibiotic-associated diarrhoea/ pseudomembranous colitis (recent or broad-spectrum antibiotics)	Check stool for Clostridium difficile (metronidazole 400mg t.d.s. for 7–14 days) vancomycin 125mg q.d.s.
Radiotherapy-induced	Ondansetron, aspirin, colestyramine
NSAID	Try stopping or changing NSAID
Misoprostol	Use a PPI or other alternative
Pre-existing disease e.g. Crohn's or ulcerative colitis	Corticosteroids or sulfasalazine
Ileal resection (causing bile salt diarrhoea)	Colestyramine
Steatorrhoea/fat malabsorption	Pancreatic enzymes ± PPI (reduces gastric acid destruction of enzymes)
Carcinoid syndrome	5-HT$_3$ antagonists, octreotide
Zollinger –Ellison syndrome	H$_2$ antagonist e.g. ranitidine
Non-specific profuse secretory diarrhoea	Opioids such as loperamide and codeine and morphine may be necessary. (Loperamide is not absorbed)

Somatostatin has a place in the management of severe, profuse, secretory diarrhoea, such as that associated with HIV infection when other agents have failed to work. It is best given by CSCI.

Intestinal obstruction

This most commonly occurs with carcinoma of the ovary or bowel. The obstruction may be intramural, intraluminal, or extraluminal due to surrounding peritoneal disease, and is often at multiple sites. In addition, there is often a clinical obstruction in the absence of a mechanical lesion (functional obstruction).

A plain abdominal X-ray may be helpful in excluding constipation.

If surgical intervention is inappropriate, symptomatic measures using medication are the mainstay of treatment, avoiding the standard 'drip and suck' approach, which may be distressing and is ineffective in 80% of patients.

- In the presence of advanced peritoneal disease, the most likely cause of obstruction is due to malignant tumour. The cause may also be due, however, to benign factors such as adhesions
- If the patient is fit enough, a surgical opinion should be sought and the advantages and disadvantages of laparotomy assessed
- The potential mortality and morbidity associated with surgery should be weighed against quality of life in a patient whose prognosis may only be predicted to be a few weeks or months
- If the obstruction is incomplete or mainly functional, it may resolve. It may therefore be helpful in the first place to try:

Reducing bowel wall oedema
Using: Dexamethasone 8–16mg SC before midday

The evidence for such an approach is equivocal, but if a three day trial proves beneficial and vomiting subsides it may be useful to consider continuing with reducing doses of oral steroids. Whether improvement is due to steroids or to the passage of time remains the subject of debate.

If dexamethasone is not helpful after three days it should be stopped (unless the patient has been on longer-term steroids (more than a week) in which case it should be tailed off slowly).

Stimulating gut motility
Metoclopramide 30–120mg/24h via subcutaneous infusion. Beware of any increase in gut colic and stop if obstruction is not resolving.

For complete obstruction or obstruction not resolving with the above measures in 24–48 h, focus on treating symptoms rather than the underlying cause:

- **Nausea and vomiting:**
  - cyclizine 100–150mg/24h CSCI
  - ± haloperidol 3–5mg/24h CSCI
  - or levomepromazine 6.25–25mg/24h CSCI
- **Colic:**
  - hyoscine butylbromide 40–100mg/24h CSCI (diamorphine may also be needed for background pain)
- **Diarrhoea:**
  - codeine 30–60mg p.o. every 4 h, or
  - loperamide 2–4mg p.o. every 4 h. *Use with caution if possibility of reversible obstruction*

- **Constipation:**
  - Ensure that reversible constipation is not contributing to the obstruction. Gentle rectal measures or a small dose of a faecal softener such as docusate may be used, particularly if there is no colic and obstruction is thought to be colonic and subacute. More vigorous measures should be avoided for fear of aggravating symptoms

If intestinal obstruction is still not resolving

1 *Reduce* or *encourage reabsorption of gut secretions* and reduce intestinal motility using:
  - hyoscine butylbromide (Buscopan) 40–100mg/24h CSCI
  - octreotide 300–600 mcg/24h CSCI
2 Nasogastric tube
  - *If* vomiting is not subsiding, or *if* very distressing and/or faecal, it may be necessary to use a nasogastric tube after full discussion with patient and carers. Although this is an infrequent practice in a hospice setting, and can be seen as a very undignified approach to patient care, it can bring comfort in exceptional circumstances
3 Venting gastrostomy
  - With occasional, clinically stable patients who are distressed by vomiting but who have a prognosis of at least weeks, and who are keen to resume oral intake, it *may* be an option to discuss venting gastrostomy and subcutaneous fluids.[13] In practice venting gastrostomies are rarely performed

---

13 Roila F. *et al.* (1996) Comparative studies of various antiemetic regimes. *Supportive Care in Cancer,* **4**: 270–80.

Hiccup

Definition: Spasmodic contraction of the diaphragm that causes a sudden breath in, cut off when the vocal cords snap together, creating the characteristic sound

Hiccups result from diaphragmatic spasms caused by diaphragmatic irritation, which is often associated with liver enlargement or gastric distension.

Causes
- Via vagus nerve
  - gastric distension
  - gastritis/gastro-oesophageal reflux
  - hepatic tumours
  - ascites/abdominal distension/intestinal obstruction
- Via phrenic nerve
  - diaphragmatic tumour involvement
  - mediastinal tumour
  - CNS
  - intracranial tumours, especially brainstem lesions
  - meningeal infiltration by cancer.
- Systemic
  - renal failure
  - corticosteroids
  - Addison's disease
  - hyponatraemia

Management of hiccup

Pharyngeal stimulation is effected in a number of ways. The soft palate can be massaged, the patient can try eating dry granulated sugar or holding the breath or rebreathing into a bag etc. These measures are often effective, at least temporarily. Alternatively:

1 Reduce gastric distension:
- Pro-kinetic drugs e.g.
  - metoclopramide 10mg q.d.s.
  - domperidone 10mg q.d.s.
- Gastric distension may also improve with a change to small frequent meals and using a defoaming antiflatulant with an antacid, such as activated dimeticone and aluminium hydroxide (Asilone) 5–10mL q.d.s.

2 Relax smooth muscle:
- nifedipine 5mg p.r.n. or regularly three times daily, either by mouth or sublingually, may be effective
- baclofen 5mg t.d.s. is an alternative

3 Suppress central hiccup reflex: If symptoms are severe and not responding to other measures including pharyngeal stimulation it may be necessary to give:
- chlorpromazine 25mg p.o. Intravenous administration may cause sedation and hypotension and is only used in intractable cases

4 **Suppress central irritation from intracranial tumour**: This may respond to dexamethasone (starting with high doses e.g. 16mg daily) or to an anticonvulsant e.g. phenytoin 200–300mg given at night. NB Corticosteroids can also cause hiccups—consider stopping if recently started.

Anorexia/cachexia/asthenia

Primary anorexia is the absence or loss of appetite for food.

Cachexia (📖 See Chapter 6c) is a condition of profound weight loss and catabolic loss of muscle and adipose tissue. It is often associated with primary anorexia and fatigue.

Asthenia(📖 See Chapter 6c) is characterized by:

- Fatigue or easy tiring and reduced sustainability of performance
- Generalized weakness resulting in a reduced ability to initiate movement
- Mental fatigue characterized by poor concentration, impaired memory, and emotional lability[14]

Secondary anorexia is often due to several conditions and may be reversible and should be actively sought.

- Dyspepsia
- Altered taste
- Malodour
- Nausea and vomiting
- Sore mouth
- Pain
- Biochemical
  - Hypercalcaemia
  - Uraemia
- Gastric stasis
- Constipation
- Secondary to treatment
  - Drugs
  - RT
  - CT

Early satiety (patient hungry but then feels full) occurs with small stomach, hepatomegaly and gross ascites. Anxiety and depression will contribute to loss of appetite. Patients are 'put off' by too much food and food which is unappetizing.

These symptoms which are closely interrelated occur in about 70 per cent of patients with advanced cancer particularly gastric and pancreatic cancer.

Management

1 Assess and treat any reversible causes as outlined above.
2 Involve the dietician and multidisciplinary team to maximize treatment goals.
3 Non-drug treatment:
  - Explore the patients' and carers' fears of anorexia
  - Reassure patients that it is normal to feel satisfied with less food
  - Consider if advice on food fortification/supplementation would be appropriate for this patient at this point of their illness
  - Suggest smaller helpings to allow patients to eat frequently small amounts of what they enjoy
4 Evidence-based drug treatments:
  - **Corticosteroids** e.g. dexamethasone 2–4mg o.d.
    - Appetite stimulant and may help nausea
    - May improve subjective feeling of anorexia and weakness

- Non-specific central euphoric effects
- Effects generally short lasting (weeks)
- Onset of side-effects rapid
- **Progestogens** e.g. megestrol acetate 160–800mg o.d.
  - Improves appetite, nutritional status and calorie intake
  - Take two—three weeks to produce effect
  - Associated with modest weight gain, (though not gain in lean body mass)
  - Effects may last for months
  - Increased incidence of thrombotic episodes
  - Expensive
- **Prokinetic drugs** e.g. metoclopramide 10mg q.d.s.
  - Try if early satiety, gastric stasis (many patients with malignancy have associated autonomic dysfunction)

Total parenteral nutrition (📖 See Chapter 10c)

In case of total parenteral nutrition (TPN) in the palliative care setting, some studies have shown an association with survival shortened with the introduction of TPN.

Universal benefit and efficacy have not been clearly proven with TPN and its routine use is not recommended in view of this, the practical disadvantage, and the risk of side-effects and complications.

Aggressive nutritional therapy could perhaps be justified in particular situations such as when patients are recovering from surgery or awaiting chemotherapy.

Hydration (📖 See Chapter 1)

There is often an overwhelming need for relatives and staff to give dying patients food and water but this must not be allowed to override the patients need for comfort.

Avoiding overhydration in a dying patient may improve comfort, by minimizing urinary output (and therefore the need for catheterisation) and the volume of distressing bronchial secretions. In bowel obstruction gastric secretions will be minimised, thereby reducing the frequency of vomiting and the need for a nasogastric tube. A dry mouth can be treated with local measures.

In contrast, those patients who may survive for many months but who are unable to swallow adequately may find life easier with, for instance, a percutaneous gastrostomy tube. However, when these patients are dying it is necessary to explain to the relatives why it may be helpful to reduce fluid input.

14 Woof R. (1998) Asthenia, cachexia and anorexia. In C. Faull et al. (eds) *Handbook of Palliative Care*. Oxford: Blackwell.

Ascites (📖 See Chapter 16)

The healthy adult has about 50mL transudate in the peritoneal cavity. This has a protein level of about 25 per cent of that found in plasma. Peritoneal fluid turnover is 4–5mL/h in health.

Malignant ascites

- Malignant ascites accounts for about 10 per cent of all cases of ascites and occurs in up to 50 per cent of all patients with cancer
- Malignant ascitic fluid is an exudate with a protein content of about 85 per cent of that found in plasma. This protein-rich fluid is an excellent culture medium for malignant cells and bacteria. It may also have high levels of certain enzymes
- In malignant ascites, the ascitic fluid turnover can be twenty-fold of that found in healthy individuals
- Ascites may be the presenting feature of the malignancy or be indicative of recurrence or metastatic spread. It is often indicative of end-stage disease
- It is caused by malignant peritoneal deposits, blockage of sub-diaphragmatic lymphatics and secondary sodium retention

Causes of malignant ascites

- Ovarian primary (50 per cent of cases)
- Unknown primary (20 per cent of cases)
- Stomach, colon, pancreatic primary (most of the remainder)

Non-malignant ascites

- Cardiac failure, liver failure and renal failure are common causes of non-malignant ascites, accounting for 90 per cent of cases
- The significance of this for patients with palliative care needs is that ascites should not automatically be attributed to underlying malignancy
- Management options, however, are similar for both malignant and non-malignant disease

Management

Treatment of the primary cancer, usually with chemotherapy, may be the most effective measure to reduce ascites. Analgesics and good symptom control may be all that is necessary, particularly for a patient who is bed-bound and has a short prognosis.

Diuretics may alleviate symptoms over several days. Doses must be adequate and include a combination of spironolactone (100mg b.d. and possibly higher) and a loop diuretic e.g. furosemide (40–80mg o.d.).

Patients with liver metastases are more likely to respond to diuretics; paracentesis will provide more immediate relief (see below).

A peritoneo-venous shunt could be considered and inserted under general or local anaesthesia.

Shunts comprise a multi-perforated catheter in the peritoneal cavity which joins to a one-way valve positioned subcutaneously just above the costal margin. From here ascitic fluid is drained into the superior vena cava via a tunnelled catheter which enters the external or internal jugular vein. Fluid flows through the shunt on inspiration. Patients are encouraged to pump the reservoir to keep fluid flowing through the shunt. The two commonest shunts in use (Denver and LeVeen) have similar performance profiles. Results from use of such shunts have been mixed as they are prone to blockage.

Paracentesis

General

Paracentesis is a simple procedure, which can be performed as a day case (usually only removing 2–4 litres maximum), or as an inpatient.

- In tense, symptomatic ascites there may be up to 12 litres of ascites present
- Removal of 4–6 litres is usually enough to give symptomatic relief
- Removal of more than 4–6 litres increases the risk of hypovolaemia and adverse effects, but may give symptom relief for longer until ascites re-accumulates
- For an ill, elderly patient, small volume paracentesis repeated as needed may be preferable

Indications

- Pain, discomfort, or tightness due to stretching of the abdominal wall
- Dyspnoea, usually exacerbated by exertion, due to upward pressure on the diaphragm
- Nausea, vomiting and dyspepsia due to the 'squashed stomach' syndrome
- Patients are usually symptomatic only when the abdominal wall is tensely distended. Patients who are also bothered by ankle (or generalized) oedema, may fare better with diuretic therapy

Complications of paracentesis

- After a large volume paracentesis, the compensatory large fluid shifts from circulating volume into extracellular fluid can decompensate the patient's cardiovascular system leading to hypovolaemia, and in severe cases, collapse and renal failure
- A low albumin or sodium level will exacerbate this effect
- The cannula site may continue to leak ascites after removal
- If a limited, partial paracentesis has been performed, this may rarely become a continuing leak over days to weeks. (Use colostomy bag to collect leakage)
- The patient needs to be warned about possible leaking which may otherwise cause distress
- Bowel perforation is a risk, especially if intestinal obstruction is present
- Infection is a rare complication, providing an aseptic technique is used

Investigations prior to paracentesis
- An ultrasound scan will confirm the presence of ascites, and may determine if it is 'pocketed' by tumour adhesions
- A scan should be performed if:
  - ascites is not easily clinically identified
  - there is a chance of bowel obstruction
- A serum albumin and urea and electrolytes should be taken if:
  - more than 4–6 litres is to be removed and the patient has oedema, or
  - the patient is clinically dehydrated, or
  - the patient has reacted badly to a previous paracentesis
- A platelet count and clotting screen should be measured in at risk patients

Contra-indications to paracentesis
- Local or systemic infection
- Coagulopathy—platelets <40 × 10^9 /l or INR >1.4
- Limit paracentesis to 4–6 litres maximum if:
  - Hepatic or renal failure (creatinine >250mmol/L)
  - Albumin <30g/L or sodium <125mmol/L

Follow-up care to paracentesis
- Ascites will usually re-form after a paracentesis; this can vary between one and many weeks
- Diuretics may reduce the rate of re-accumulation, or prevent it becoming as tense again
- Repeated paracentesis on an as-needed basis is appropriate management for patients with advanced cancer

The procedure of paracentesis
- The patient should be asked to pass urine before the procedure
- Blood pressure should be measured and recorded
- The patient should lie in a semi-recumbent position
- It may be helpful if the patient tilts 30 degrees towards the side of the paracentesis
- Use left iliac fossa unless local disease is present, avoiding scars and inferior epigastric artery (see Fig. 6b. 1)
- Confirm that site is dull to percussion
- Using aseptic technique, anaesthetize skin locally
- A large bore intravenous cannula or 'Bonanno' catheter can be used
- Avoid clamping the catheter if possible, since malignant ascites can be very proteinaceous and is likely to block it

Large volume paracentesis (>6 litres)
If it is intended to drain to dryness, or >6 litres:
- Stop diuretics (if used solely for ascites) 48h before procedure
- Check blood pressure and pulse every 30 minutes during paracentesis, then hourly for 6h
- Some units give plasma substitutes such as intravenous dextran 70 or gelatin infusion (e.g. Gelofusine), 150mL for every litre of ascites drained, during the paracentesis or shortly afterwards to reduce hypovolaemia

Tenesmus and tenesmoid pain

Tenesmus is the painful sensation of rectal fullness, usually caused by local rectal tumour. There may be associated spasm of smooth muscle, or neuropathic pain from lumbosacral plexus infiltration causing stabbing or more continuous pain. It may be difficult to distinguish from pudendal neuralgia.

Management
- Prevent and treat constipation
- Opioid analgesia may be helpful but not reliably
- NSAID e.g. diclofenac 50mg t.d.s.
- Radiotherapy
- Nifedipine m/r 10–20mg b.d.
- Co-analgesics as for neuropathic pain
- Amitriptyline
- Anticonvulsants
- Corticosteroids
- Lumbar sympathectomy: >80 per cent success rate
- Spinal infusion of local anaesthetic ± opioids

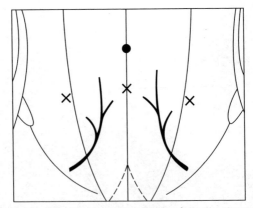

Figure 6b.1 Usual sites for paracentesis, avoiding the inferior epigastric arteries

Dyspepsia

Gastro-oesophageal reflux/oesophagitis (GORD)

Assessment
- Exclude or treat oesophageal candida
- Consider oesophageal spasm
- Avoid drugs which cause oesophagitis—potassium, NSAIDs
- Consider pain of cardiac origin

Treatment
- Raise head of bed to reduce acid reflux
- Consider paracentesis for tense ascites
- Metoclopramide 10mg t.d.s. if signs of gastric stasis or distension
- Antacid e.g. Gaviscon 10mL q.d.s. for mild symptoms
- Proton pump inhibitor (PPI) e.g. lansoprazole 30mg daily for moderate or severe symptoms; start with treatment dose then step-down after a few weeks

NSAID and steroid-related dyspepsia

Treatment of drug-related dyspepsia
- Consider stopping or reducing dose of NSAID/steroids
- PPI e.g. lansoprazole 30mg o.d. for severe symptoms or proven pathology. Start with treatment dose and reduce after four weeks. For milder symptoms start with maintenance dose (15mg) and increase later if needed
- If symptoms persist on treatment dose of PPI, and NSAID needed by the patient to control pain, consider changing to a selective COX-2 inhibitor (e.g. Celecoxib)

Indications for prophylaxis
- Prescribing NSAID with recent history of dyspepsia
- Prescribing steroids with recent history of dyspepsia
- Co-prescribing NSAID with steroids, anticoagulants, or aspirin
- Prescribing NSAID in elderly patient >70 years (less clear evidence—use judgement)

Drugs for dyspepsia
Proton pump inhibitors (PPIs)
- There is little difference in efficacy between the current PPIs available
- A single daily dose is appropriate for PPIs rather than divided doses
- Lansoprazole and omeprazole can be taken before or after food with equal efficacy

Despite the variations in dose recommendations in the product literature, omeprazole, lansoprazole and pantoprazole display similar dose-response relationships with similar potency at the same milligram dose. Daily doses of 15–20mg PPI are appropriate for maintenance therapy, prophylaxis, or less severe gastro-oesophageal reflux disease. Doses of 30–40mg daily are appropriate for treatment.

Antacids

Aluminium-containing antacids cause constipation whereas magnesium-containing antacids are laxative. Dimeticone in asilone is a defoamer, useful for gastric distension/hiccups.

Prostaglandin analogues

Misoprostol is effective at preventing NSAID-induced ulcers, but is less well tolerated than PPIs, and diarrhoea is a common side-effect. Misoprostol is available in combination with diclofenac.

H2 antagonists

H2 antagonists are less effective at acid suppression than PPIs, and are less effective clinically at healing ulcers. Ranitidine has significantly fewer drug interactions and adverse affects than cimetidine.

Gastrointestinal bleeding

Gastric bleeding and melaena

Assessment

Consider the commonest causes:

- Tumour bleeding
- Clotting disorders
- Peptic ulcer ±NSAIDs

Management considerations for gastrointestinal bleeding

- Review or stop NSAIDs, aspirin, corticosteroids, warfarin
- Commence PPI in treatment dose, e.g. lansoprazole 30mg o.d. when able to take orally
- Blood tests for clotting screen and platelets and treat if appropriate
- Consider radiotherapy referral if bleeding due to tumour
- Tranexamic acid 1–2g t.d.s. p.o. (or by slow i/v until able to take p.o.)
  - Stop if no effect after one week
  - Continue for one week after bleeding has stopped, then discontinue
  - Only continue long term (500mg t.d.s.) if bleeding recurs
  - Avoid tranexamic acid with history of thromboembolism/CVA etc.
- Small bleeds can herald a larger haemorrhage;
  - consider siting an i/v cannula to administer emergency drugs
- Intravenous high-dose PPI e.g. omeprazole 80mg i/v stat., then 8mg/h i/v infusion
- Arterial embolization
- Oral sucralfate
- Octreotide which is an accepted medical management for bleeding from oesophageal or colonic varices. Circumstantial evidence indicates that the actions of octreotide are mainly mediated by a splanchnic vasoconstrictive effect, possibly with gastric acid suppression and enhancement of platelet aggregation. It is uncertain whether it has a rôle in gastrointestinal bleeding of other aetiology
- Etamsylate

Rectal bleeding

Assessment

Consider the commonest causes:

- tumour bleeding
- clotting disorders
- pelvic infection
- haemorrhoids

NSAIDs can cause lower gastrointestinal bleeding as well as the better-documented upper GI bleeding.

Treatment
- Review or stop NSAIDs
- Treat any evidence or signs suggestive of pelvic infection
- Consider radiotherapy referral
- Blood tests for clotting screen and platelets and treat as appropriate
- Tranexamic acid 1–2g t.d.s. p.o. (or by slow i/v until able to take p.o.)
  - Stop if no effect after one week
  - Continue for one week after bleeding has stopped, then discontinue
  - Only continue long term (500mg t.d.s.) If bleeding recurs
  - Avoid tranexamic acid with history of thromboembolism/CVA etc.
- Small bleeds can herald a larger haemorrhage;
- Consider siting an i/v cannula to administer emergency drugs
- Arterial embolization
- Etamsylate
- Oral sucralfate for post-radiation proctitis applied topically

Major gastrointestinal or rectal bleeding

If patient's condition is not stable, with history of major haemorrhage or ongoing bleeding:
- Consider if the patient should be transferred to an acute medical/endoscopy unit
- Site an i/v cannula to anticipate need for emergency drugs

Treat anxiety or distress as needed:
- Midazolam 2–5mg initially by slow i/v titration (diluted 10mg in 10mL with saline)
- If no i/v access, midazolam 5–10mg SC (or i/m if shocked/vasoconstricted)

The case for proton pump inhibitors in gastrointestinal bleeding

- Acid suppression in early studies did not help in the management of acute bleeding
- It has more recently been shown that intensive therapy aimed at achieving complete acid suppression does substantially reduce the risk of recurrent bleeding after initial endoscopic treatment
- Pharmacokinetic studies have shown that a bolus of 80mg pantoprazole or omeprazole followed by immediate continuous infusion of 8mg/h will result in an intragastric pH of 7 within 20 minutes This has been continued for 72h in studies[15]

Support for patient and family

Bleeding is very frightening. Ensure that the patient and family are well supported. Ensure that drugs are readily available for sedation if necessary and that dark bed linen (to disguise the amount of blood loss) is accessible.

15 Lau JY et al. (2000). Effect of intravenous omeprazole on recurrent bleeding after endoscopic treatment of bleeding peptic ulcers. *N Eng J Med*, **343**: 310–16.

Bowel stoma care

A bowel stoma is an artificial opening, created surgically, for patients to allow faeces to leave the body by a new route through a spout or outlet on the abdomen.

The majority of stomas encountered in patients with palliative care needs have been fashioned following surgical resection for cancer or as a bypass for inoperable or recurrent cancers of the bowel or ovary causing obstruction.

Any patient with a stoma (whether newly created or created many years ago, for example in Crohn's disease) and malignant intra-abdominal disease is at risk of a number of different symptoms which need appropriate management. These include abdominal pain (constant or intermittent colic), nausea, vomiting, abdominal distension, constipation, diarrhoea and depression all of which may impact on the holistic management of the patient.

Bowel stomas are generally created from the colon (colostomy) or ileum (ileostomy). The bowel proximal to the stoma continues to function in the normal way whereas function distal to this is normally lost.

Temporary (de-functioning) stomas

These include loop ileostomies or colostomies which are usually created to protect an anastomosis or to facilitate decompression or healing in the distal bowel. The bowel loop is usually brought out onto the abdominal wall (right and left iliac fossa respectively for ileostomy and colostomy) and may be supported by a temporary rod or bridge so that it does not retract. The proximal opening allows the passage of stool which is collected in a stoma bag and the distal opening leads to the redundant section of bowel. Mucus and old faeces may be expelled through the rectum. A temporary transverse colostomy may be created at an emergency operation for bowel obstruction since it is a relatively easy procedure in a sick patient.

Permanent stomas

These are end sections of bowel which are brought to the skin surface. The potential stoma site along the path of the bowel is planned preoperatively, if possible, to allow optimal positioning of a stoma bag for the individual.

- Panproctocolectomy—a permanent ileostomy is created from the terminal ileum. The rectum and anus are removed
- Total colectomy—an ileostomy is formed and the rectal stump is retained which may be brought out onto the abdominal wall as a mucus fistula
- Abdominoperineal (A–P) excision—the rectum and anus are removed leaving a colostomy in the left iliac fossa
- Hartmann's procedure—procedure for excision of sigmoid colon or upper rectum. An end colostomy is formed and the rectal stump is closed and left in the pelvis
- Pelvic exenteration—a radical operation removing pelvic organs. A colostomy and urostomy are formed. Men are likely to become impotent. An artificial vagina can be created for a woman

Issues in stoma management

The stool consistency of a sigmoid colostomy is no different from that passed naturally in health through the anus. The stool is less formed the further proximal in the colon the colostomy is. The formation of an ileostomy or colostomy should not in itself interfere with sexual function unless the definitive surgery interfered with the pelvic nerve supply.

Stoma appliances and problems

Stoma appliances are disposable, self-adhesive and skin-friendly. The type of appliance used is determined by several factors which include the shape and position of the stoma itself, including body contours, the type of effluent, skin type and the needs of the individual such as lifestyle and ability to self care. Adequate adherence, comfort and skin protection are paramount.

Ileostomy appliances are drainable for ease of emptying semi-formed/liquid stool. Modern appliances have integral velcro-type closures. The bags are emptied several times a day and changed every 1–3 days.
Colostomy appliances may be in one piece such that the whole appliance needs removing every time the bag needs changing.
Alternatively, a two-piece appliance is used which allows the flange to remain in position for for several days, allowing the non-drainable bag to be changed as necessary, protecting the skin from the trauma of frequent changes
The flange size should be cut to fit accurately around the base of the stoma. The peristomal skin must be kept healthy and intact
A stoma usually shrinks in size during the first few months but should always retain the bright red colour, indicating a good blood supply
Checks for colour, odour, consistency and volume should be made routinely

Psychological care

Enjoyment, comfort and satisfaction with life for the patient and his/her family needs support from healthcare professionals, giving adequate time for answering questions and responding to needs. Frequently patients have a short prognosis and the stoma is a visible daily reminder of this. In addition, they may be distressed by a feeling of no longer being in control. They have to learn new skills at a time when it is important to be concentrating on other more important issues, and they may be having to adapt reluctantly to relying on others for care. Relationships with family, friends and particularly spouses may be affected.

Overactive stoma

A cause may need to be identified and treated. Diet may need to be altered until overactivity settles. Foods such as cooked white rice and stewed apple may help. Marshmallows and 'jelly babies' may help in thickening the output from an ileostomy. Extra fluids orally should be encouraged to maintain hydration, especially in hot weather. A drainable bag may be necessary temporarily for a colostomy if the output is liquid. Some medication, particularly longer-acting modified release preparations e.g. MST, enteric coated drugs and capsules, may not be absorbed adequately and are not recommended with ileostomies.

Loperamide (taken three-quarters of an hour before meals) with an ileostomy in the form of 'melts' or tablets but not capsules may be helpful. If all else fails, systemic opioids and antisecretory agents may be needed. 📖 See the section on diarrhoea, p. 258.

Constipation

A cause should be sought where possible and may include medication, particularly opioids, partial/complete bowel obstruction and dehydration. It may be necessary to instil warm arachis oil through a Foley catheter with the balloon inflated (only 5mL for a short time) to aid enema retention. The patient will usually be turned on the right side if the stoma is in the left iliac fossa to allow oil to flow across the transverse colon. The oil may cause difficulties with flange adhesion and the possibility of nut allergy should always be considered. Suppositories, phosphate and microlax micro-enemas may also be useful. As a general rule, bulking aperients such as ispaghula husk (Fybogel) are not used in palliative care.

Odour

This is rarely a problem with modern appliances which contain charcoal filters. Proprietary stoma deodorizing agents are available. A few drops of vanilla essence placed in a bowel stoma bag may help. Topical metronidazole may be helpful for offensive fungating tumours in the region of the stoma.

Bleeding

The stoma may bleed due to clotting deficiencies and fungating tumour. Wafers of kaltostat soaked in tranexamic acid or epinephrine may help with local pressure. Silver nitrate may be used for oozing granulation tissue. Bleeding from local cancer growth may abate with radiotherapy or cryotherapy.

Skin excoriation

Skin excoriation is a rare occurrence with modern appliances and good skin care. Various preparations are available to aid skin protection including pastes to make a level surface onto which an appliance can be fitted. This is particularly important with an ileostomy, when damage to the skin from digestive enzymes must be avoided.

Flatulence

Flatulence can usually be minimized by avoiding various foods and medication such as lactulose.

A diet with fibre such as porridge, root vegetables and brown bread is advised although the terminally ill may not find these foods palatable. In relatively good health, most people with stomas can eat most food although certain food such as vegetables and fruit may cause an increase in stoma activity with embarrassing flatulence and odour. Camomile tea and peppermint tea or capsules may be helpful.

Enterocutaneous fistulae

Enterocutaneous fistulae may occur in 3 per cent of patients with advanced malignant disease. Patients with gastrointestinal tumours are those who have had abdominal radiotherapy are most at risk. A dehisced wound may also need management with a stoma appliance. If the effluent is greater than 100mL per 24 h a stoma appliance will probably be needed.

Meticulous preparation of the skin will be needed prior to applying an appliance. Suction may be needed while cleansing and preparing the fistula if there is excessive exudate, or it may need to be spigotted with a balloon catheter for a while. Various pastes, fillers and skin barriers may be needed to protect the skin and ensure a good fit to the edges of the wound. The stoma appliance may need to be adapted with time to take account of the change in size of the tumour and the weight loss of the patient.

Gastrostomy

A gastrostomy is used for the purpose of feeding when the patient is unable to swallow adequately or safely such as in motor neurone disease, or with head and neck cancers. A venting gastrostomy is occasionally used in a relatively fit patient with intestinal obstruction who wants to be able to eat. In this situation, the patient is able to take nutrients by mouth but food contents are expelled through the gastrostomy.

In patients with advanced disease, the decision to insert a gastrostomy has to be judged carefully.[16] It is important to distinguish starvation, which responds to feeding, from cachexia, which does not respond to feeding alone. The latter is more likely in the presence of large tumour masses, certain tumour types or ongoing sepsis.

Types of gastrostomy

Percutaneous endoscopic gastrostomy (PEG): Inserted under sedation and local anaesthetic using a 'pull' technique. Throughout its lifetime, the PEG tube should be rotated through 360° at least twice a week to prevent adhesion formation.

Radiologically inserted gastrostomy (RIG): Inserted in the radiology department without sedation by a 'push' technique under fluoroscopic control. The tube is thinner than a PEG tube, and is held in place by its pigtail shape. It should NOT therefore be rotated, or it will dislodge.

Surgical gastrostomy: Carried out under general anaesthetic, usually when it is impossible to insert a PEG or RIG.

Care of the gastrostomy tube: The fixation plate should be maintained at 1 to 1.5cm from the abdominal exit stoma. A 50mL flush of sterile water should be used before and after every feed or administration of medication and regularly three times a day. Soda water, but not other fizzy drinks (they are too acidic) can be used to unblock stubborn blockages.

Feeding: Patients should be maintained at an angle of 30–45° during feeding and for two h after to reduce the risk of aspiration. Many centres are less keen for feeding to occur during sleep because of the aspiration risk.

Problems with gastrostomies

- Dislodgement
- Leakage: chemical digestion of surrounding skin
- Overgranulation
- Infection

16 Rabeneck L., Wray P., Petersen N. J. (1996) Long-term outcomes of patients receiving percutaneous endoscopic gastrostomy tubes. *Journal of General Internal Medicine*, **11**, 5: 287–93.

A major concern with the use of PEG and RIG tubes in the UK involves ensuring that the best possible decision about when to insert a tube is taken.

Often the clinical team which asks for a tube to be inserted is different from the team which carries out the procedure which in turn is different from the team who manage the tube once it has been inserted.

While tube insertion can play a crucial rôle for certain patients, especially where clear objectives for the intervention have been discussed and documented with the patient and family, figures show that a large percentage of patients die within weeks of tube insertion, perhaps before they have had time to gain benefit from the procedure and its management.

Further reading

Books

Doyle D., Hanks G., Cherny N. (2004) *Oxford Textbook of Palliative Medicine*. 3rd edn. Oxford: Oxford University Press.

Twycross R. (2001) *Symptom Management in Advanced Cancer*. 3rd edn. Oxford: Radcliffe Medical Press.

Watson M., Lucas C. (2003) *Adult Palliative Care Guidelines*. London: The South West London and the Surrey, West Sussex and Hampshire Cancer Networks.

Articles

Coco C., Cogliandolo S., Riccioni M. *et al.* (2000) Use of a self-expanding stent in the palliation of rectal cancer recurrences. A report of three cases. *Surgical Endoscopy*, **14, 8**: 708–11.

Potter K. (2000) Surgical oncology of the pelvis: ostomy planning and management. *Journal of Surgical Oncology*, **73, 4**: 237–42.

Baines M. J. (2000) Symptom control in advanced gastrointestinal cancer. *Eur J Gastroenterol Hepatol*, **12**: 375–9.

Culbert P., Gillett H. and Ferguson A. (1998) Highly effective new oral therapy for faecal impaction. *British Journal of General Practice*, **48**: 1599–600.

Cachexia, anorexia, and fatigue

Background

Cachexia and fatigue are common symptoms affecting patients with advanced or chronic disease. They are closely related in 70 per cent of patients with advanced cancer, particularly gastric and pancreatic cancer. Apart from marked weight loss and lethargy, there is also an association with physical, emotional and mental symptoms and loss of motivation and social contact.

'Listless, sluggish, faint, despondent, apathetic, tired, slack, indifferent, paralysed', are some of the adjectives used by patients and some describe the fatigue of advanced disease as 'pain'.

Cachexia and fatigue are multifactorial. They are seldom seen in isolation from other symptoms experienced by patients with advanced disease, thus adding to the disease burden.

Cancer has become more of a chronic rather than an acute illness, due to improvements in its management. There is an increased awareness of the suffering caused by cachexia and fatigue but they still remain poorly recognized by clinicians. Advances in management have not kept pace with that for other common symptoms in advanced disease.

Definitions

Cancer-related fatigue is defined by the National Comprehensive Cancer Network as 'a persistent, subjective sense of tiredness related to cancer or cancer treatment that interferes with usual functioning'.[1] It has further been described in terms of

Perceived energy, mental capacity, and psychological status. It rises over a continuum, ranging from tiredness to exhaustion. In contrast with the tiredness sometimes felt by the healthy individual, cancer-related fatigue is perceived as being of greater magnitude, disproportionate to activity or exertion, and not relieved by rest.[2]

Patients may describe fatigue **subjectively** in 3 dimensions:-
Physical sensations—unusual tiredness, and decreased capacity for work
Affective sensations—decreased motivation, mood and energy
Cognitive sensations—decreased concentration and mental agility

Patients may describe fatigue **objectively** as a quantifiable decrease in physical or mental performance

These two experiences of fatigue may not be related, and patients may feel fatigued without any loss of objective performance and vice versa[1]

1 Mock V. et al. (2000) NCCN Practice Guidelines for cancer-related fatigue. Oncology (Huntington), **14**: 151–61.

2 Ahlberg K. et al. (2003) Assessment and management of cancer-related fatigue in adults. Lancet; **362**: 640–50.

Cancer cachexia involves involuntary loss of weight that is not caused simply by anorexia. The syndrome includes anaemia and immunosuppression along with a number of biochemical changes indicating some systemic effects of malignancy. Cachexia is a term derived from the Greek word *kakos*, meaning bad, and *hexis*, meaning condition.

Cancer Cachexia:-

- Weight loss (usually defined as more than five percent of premorbid weight in the previous six months)
- Cancer tumours produce cytokines e.g. cachectin—tumour necrosis factor, interleukin I and VI, lipolytic hormones and proteolysis inducing factor (PIF) which cause metabolic abnormalities such as lipolysis and protein loss
- Progressive loss of lean and adipose tissue that is unrelated to anorexia
- Cannot be reversed by feeding
- Is commonly associated with **anorexia** (the absence or loss of appetite for food) and **asthenia** (a syndrome of physical fatigue, generalised weakness and mental fatigue)
- Affects over eighty percent of patients with advanced cancer and is a major contributor to cancer morbidity and mortality
- Occurs more commonly in solid tumours such as pancreas, lung, stomach, colorectal and oesophagus, but less frequently in carcinoma of the breast and prostate and haematological malignancies
- Creates a major source of distress to patients and families who often seek to reverse it by pressurising the patient to eat more
- Has a negative psychological impact due to body image changes
- Is a constant reminder to patients of underlying disease
- Decreases social interaction and support
- Decreases ability to tolerate and respond to oncological treatments

Prevalence

Fatigue

- Approaching one hundred per cent of patients treated for cancer are affected by fatigue
- Patients report fatigue more commonly when undergoing chemotherapy or radiotherapy, or in the presence of advanced malignancy

Cachexia

- More than 80 per cent of patients with advanced cancer are cachexic

Aetiology

Non-malignant causes of cachexia and fatigue all of which can also contribute to symptoms in advanced cancer.

Infection	Metabolic and electrolyte	Pharmacological toxicity
Anaemia	disorders	Cachexia due to HIV/AIDS or
Chronic hypoxia	Insomnia	progressive illness
Neurological disorders	Malnutrition	Chronic pain
Psychogenic causes	Over-exertion	Dehydration

Reversible causes of 'secondary' anorexia should be actively sought and corrected as appropriate. They include:
- Dyspepsia
- Altered taste
- Malodour
- Nausea and vomiting
- Sore mouth
- Pain
- Biochemical
  - Hypercalcaemia
  - Hyponatraemia
  - Uraemia
  - Gastric stasis
- Constipation
- Secondary to treatment
  - Drugs
  - Radiotherapy
  - Chemotherapy
- Anxiety
- Depression

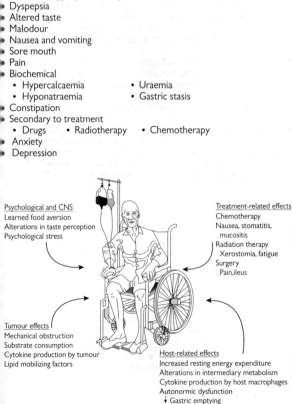

Psychological and CNS
Learned food aversion
Alterations in taste perception
Psychological stress

Treatment-related effects
Chemotherapy
Nausea, stomatitis,
mucositis
Radiation therapy
Xerostomia, fatigue
Surgery
Pain, ileus

Tumour effects
Mechanical obstruction
Substrate consumption
Cytokine production by tumour
Lipid mobilizing factors

Host-related effects
Increased resting energy expenditure
Alterations in intermediary metabolism
Cytokine production by host macrophages
Autonormic dysfunction
↓ Gastric emptying

Fig. 6c.1 Multifactorial causes of cancer fatigue and cachexia. From Bruera and Higginson, *Cachexia-anorexia in cancer patients* (1996), Oxford University Press.

Metabolic effects

The metabolic changes seen in cachexia differ from those seen in starvation. In starvation, protein is conserved, energy expenditure reduced and fatty acids and ketones become a major source of energy. This contrasts with cancer cachexia where the resting energy expenditure is *increased* and both protein and fat are inefficiently utilized, in association with increased gluconeogenesis.

The reasons behind these metabolic changes are unknown, but postulated mechanisms may include the following:

A non-specific response to the tumour or factors released by the tumour. The presence of a tumour may cause chronic stimulation of the body's inflammatory system leading to classic cachexic metabolic changes including an increase in carbohydrate, fat and protein catabolism.

- Solid tumours metabolize glucose anaerobically and thus inefficiently, increasing the resting energy expenditure of the body
- The neuroendocrine axis appears to be important in the regulation of appetite
- There is evidence of increased insulin resistance in patients with cancer and reduced glucose tolerance, perhaps caused by an imbalance of cortisol, insulin and glucagons
- An increase in protein turnover, particularly in skeletal muscle, is associated with the striking loss of lean muscle mass occurring in malignancy associated cachexia
- The acute phase response is the systemic response to inflammation or tissue damage occurring in trauma and sepsis, as well as cancer cachexia. This response appears to be mediated by cytokines. The activity of this response has been shown to correlate with the development of cachexia in patients with malignancy

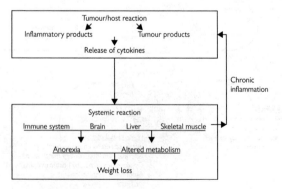

Fig. 6c.2 The systemic inflammatory response and cancer

Management

Cachexia and fatigue can often be anticipated and potentially correctable causes **actively** sought. A multidisciplinary approach maximizes the potential to improve symptoms.

National Comprehensive Cancer Network cancer related fatigue guidelines propose the following:[1]

Regular screening of patients using an instrument to evaluate degree of fatigue

For those who describe mild fatigue, the subject is discussed and education provided. For those who describe moderate or severe fatigue a fuller, *primary* assessment is required, looking in particular for the presence of:

- Pain
- Emotional distress
- Sleep disturbance
- Anaemia
- Hypothyroidism

If such primary factors are detected, they should be treated according to practice guidelines.

If primary factors are not detected a *secondary* comprehensive assessment is advocated, with referral to other healthcare professionals as appropriate, including:

- Review of medications
- Assessment of co-morbidities e.g.
  - Nutritional/metabolic evaluation
  - Assessment of activity level

If specific causes (and therefore treatment) of fatigue and weakness cannot be found, symptomatic interventions should be considered.

Non-drug interventions

- There is a large body of evidence to suggest that a moderate exercise programme can improve functional capacity, reduce fatigue and improve mood
- Nutritional advice—to eat when hungry, what is enjoyed, in frequent small amounts
- Pacing activity so that important activities can be carried out. Pacing allows gradual adaptation to lower levels of energy
- Promotion of good sleep hygiene
- Help the family: listen to their concerns and explain cachexia. They may need to find other ways of expressing love than being obsessional about quantities of food that can no longer be eaten and that will not alter prognosis

Drug interventions

Corticosteroids (i.e. dexamethasone 4mg o.d.)

- Rapid onset of benefits within 2–3 days
- Rôle is limited by the rapid onset of side-effects (proximal myopathy, fluid retention and insulin resistance) and loss of effectiveness after only a few weeks
- They do not increase lean body mass
- They may be useful to improve appetite and well-being, particularly when prognosis is limited and a fast response is needed

Progestogens (i.e. megestrol acetate 160–320mg/day; medroxyproges
terone acetate 200mg t.d.s.)
- Onset of benefit may take up to two weeks
- Clear evidence of appetite improvement but less clear evidence
  of anything other than minimal weight gain. Fluid retention may be
  a problem
- Does not increase lean body mass
- Higher doses of progestogens above 800mg/day not noted to be more
  effective than lower doses
- Comparisons between corticosteroids and progestogens show
  no survival advantage, but more side-effects are noted with
  corticosteroids

Metoclopramide
- Useful in situations where there is gastric stasis
- Prokinetic action counteracts autonomic dysfunction which
  is common in malignancy
- Reduces nausea

Erythropoietin
- For patients with anaemia, erythropoietin on a weekly basis has
  been shown to reduce fatigue
- It is unclear if the beneficial effect is due to anaemia correction or
  a direct erythropoietin effect on its receptors, which have been
  isolated in several different tissues including the brain
- Expensive treatment
- Most efficient dosage schedules still to be worked out

Future treatment possibilities

There is growing understanding as to the complex nature of the
pathophysiological basis of cachexia. Cytokine activity has been strongly
implicated in much of the recent research.

However, the processes involved remain complex, with both procata-
bolic and anticatabolic cytokine involvement, altered inflammatory
responses, neuroendocrine effects and the interactions of both tumour
and host. Drugs which interrupt the harmful catabolic effects of cytokines
are being developed, though it is unlikely that any single agent will be able
to benefit every patient with cachexia or fatigue.

The causes of cachexia and fatigue are so multifactorial that it is essential to develop individualized treatment approaches for each particular
patient. Such a strategy requires a careful clinical history and examination
in order to decide which interventions are appropriate.

As yet the therapeutic tools for such intervention are limited, but if the
current research activity bears fruit, the management of patients with
anorexia/cachexia syndrome will be transformed.

Table 6c.1 Possible mechanisms of action of established and emerging pharmacological agents in the management of cachexia

Possible mechanism	Agent
Central nervous system effects	Metoclopramide
	Corticosteroids
	Progestational agents
	Cannabinoids
	Thalidomide
Modulate immune response/reduce inflammation	Corticosteroids
	Progestational agents
	Polyunsaturated fatty acids
	Thalidomide
	Melatonin
	NSAIDs
Anabolic effect	Growth hormone/insulin growth factors
	Anabolic agents
	Beta 2 adrenergic agents
Stimulate gastrointestinal motility/increased gastric emptying	Metoclopramide

Further reading

Books

Doyle D., Hanks G., Cherny N. (2004) *Oxford Textbook of Palliative Medicine*. 3rd edn. Oxford: Oxford University Press.

Bruera E., Higginson I. (1996) *Cachexia-anorexia in cancer patients*. Oxford: Oxford University Press.

Neuenschwander H., Bruera E. (1996) *Cachexia-Anorexia in Cancer Patients*. Oxford: Oxford University Press.

Articles

Ardies C. M. (2002) Exercise, cachexia, and cancer therapy: a molecular rationale. *Nutr Cancer*, **42, 2**: 143–57.

Bruera E., Macmillan K. *et al.* (1990) A controlled trial of megestrol acetate on appetite, caloric intake, nutritional status, and other symptoms in patients with advanced cancer. *Cancer*, **66, 6**: 1279–82.

Bruera E., Neumann C. M. *et al.* (1999) Thalidomide in patients with cachexia due to terminal cancer: preliminary report. *Ann Oncol*, **10, 7**: 857–9.

Curt G. A. (2000) The impact of fatigue on patients with cancer: overview of FATIGUE 1 and 2. *Oncologist*, **5, (Suppl. 2)**: 9–12.

Inui A. (2002) Cancer anorexia-cachexia syndrome: current issues in research and management. *CA Cancer J Clin*, **52, 2**: 72–91.

MacDonald N., Easson A. M. *et al.* (2003) Understanding and managing cancer cachexia. *J Am Coll Surg*, **197, 1**: 143–61.

McMillan D. C., Watson W. S. *et al.* (2001) Albumin concentrations are primarily determined by the body cell mass and the systemic inflammatory response in cancer patients with weight loss. *Nutr Cancer*, **39, 2**: 210–3.

McMillan D. C., Wigmore S. J. *et al.* (1999) A prospective randomized study of megestrol acetate and ibuprofen in gastrointestinal cancer patients with weight loss. *Br J Cancer*, **79, 3–4**: 495–500.

Nelson K. A., Walsh D. (2002) The cancer anorexia-cachexia syndrome: a survey of the Prognostic Inflammatory and Nutritional Index (PINI) in advanced disease. *J Pain Symptom Manage*, **24, 4**: 424–8.

Stone P., Richardson A. *et al.* (2000) Cancer-related fatigue: inevitable, unimportant and untreatable? Results of a multi-centre patient survey. Cancer Fatigue Forum. *Ann Oncol*, **11, 8**: 971–5.

Tchekmedyian N. S., Hickman M. *et al.* (1992) Megestrol acetate in cancer anorexia and weight loss. *Cancer*, **69**: 1268–74.

Toomey D., Redmond H. P. *et al.* (1995) Mechanisms mediating cancer cachexia. *Cancer*, **76, 12**: 2418–26.

Willox J. C., Corr J. *et al.* (1984) Prednisolone as an appetite stimulant in patients with cancer. *Br Med J (Clin Res Ed)*, **288, 6410**: 27.

Wolfe G. (2000) Fatigue: the most important consideration for the patient with cancer. *Caring*, **19, 4**: 46–7.

Sweating and fever

Definition

- Sweating (diaphoresis) is the secretion of fluid onto the skin surface to aid cooling
- Hyperhidrosis is the production of large volumes of sweat
- Sweating is a normal phenomenon in the regulation of body temperature, but in illness can be a troublesome and distressing symptom
- Severity of sweating can change with climate, and perception of the symptom may differ with varying cultural norms

Measurement tools include:

- Symptom diary
- Three grade
- Severity scale (Quigley and Baines 1997[1])
- Six point rating scale (Deaner 2000[2])

To date, none of these tools have been validated nor have their reliabilities been tested.

Causes (common):

- Tumour burden (Chang 1988[3])
- Sepsis
- Lymphoma (neoplastic fever)
- Disseminated malignancy esp. hepatic and renal metastases (neoplastic fever)
- Sex hormone insufficiency due to cancer treatment, especially breast cancer (tamoxifen, induction of menopause by chemotherapy or radiotherapy) and prostate cancer (gonadorelin analogues)

Causes (less common)

- Endocrine disturbance e.g. hypoglycaemia, hyperthyroidism
- Thermoregulation in response to increase in temperature, exertion or nutrition
- Weakness
- Hypoxia
- Severe pain (infarction, fracture)
- Fear and anxiety
- Medication e.g. opioids (rare), antidepressants, ethanol
- Drug reactions; blood products (transfusion reaction)
- Neuropathy (diabetic, autonomic); autoimmune disease, idiopathic

1 Quigley C. S., Baines M. (1997) Descriptive epidemiology of sweating in a hospice population. *Journal of Palliative Care.* **13**: 22–6.

2 Deaner P.B. (2000) The use of thalidomide in the management of severe sweating in patients with advanced malignancy: trial report. *Palliative Medicine.* **14**: 429–31.

3 Chang J. C. (1988) Antipyretic effect of naproxen and corticosteroids on neoplastic fever. *J Pain and Symptom Management,* **3**: 141–4.

Management
- Exclude reversible cause(s) and treat if appropriate
- Supportive measures:
  - decreasing ambient temperature
  - lowering humidity
  - increasing airflow around patient (fan)
  - clothing (modern synthetic materials, e.g. Gore-Tex, allow evaporation)

Pharmacological measures
- Sepsis:
  - Antibiotics if appropriate
  - Paracetamol 1gram p.o./PR qds (effective in palliating sepsis induced sweating)
- Neoplastic fever:
  - Naproxen 250–500mg p.o. b.d. can relieve neoplastic fever for 10–14 days; once stopped, fever recurs in 66 per cent of patients[3]
  - Patients may benefit from switching to an alternative NSAID[4]
  - Corticosteroid therapy with dexamethasone has been shown to reduce symptoms, independently of NSAIDs. However, there is no agreement on starting dose. Suggestion:
    - Start dexamethasone at 1–2mg o.d. and titrate to effect (or to corticosteroid side-effects)
- Sex hormone insufficiency:
  - Venlafaxine 37.5mg p.o. o.d. is effective as is clonidine 0.3–0.4mg p.o. nocte
  - Higher doses of venlafaxine may be required, though this drug can also *cause* sweating[5]
  - Diethylstilboestrol 1–3mg p.o. o.d. improves symptoms in men but risk of thromboembolic events is increased
  - Progestogen therapy is effective in women but has a high side-effect profile
- Non specific treatments:
  - antimuscarinic therapy can block parasympathetic mediated sweating e.g. propantheline p.o. 15mg nocte
  - drugs used for other antimuscarinic effects such as glycopyrronium may also help
  - thalidomide 100mg p.o. nocte[2] has been used in the hospice setting with some effect, though controlled studies are still required
  - Other drugs of reported benefit include:
    - Cimetidine (for opioid induced sweats)
    - Beta-blockers
    - Calcium channel blockers (e.g. diltiazem)
    - Benzodiazepines
    - Olanzapine

4 Tsavaris N., Zinelis A. *et al.* (1990) A randomised trial of the effect of three non-steroid anti-inflammatory agents in ameliorating cancer induced fever. *J of Int Med*, **228**: 451–5.

5 Loprinzi C. L., Barton D. L. *et al.* (2001) Management of hot flashes in breast cancer survivors. *Lancet Oncol*, **2, 4**: 199–204.

Further reading

Books

Back I. (2001) *Palliative Medicine Handbook.* BPM Books: Cardiff.

Doyle D., Hanks G., Cherny N., Calman K. (2004) *Oxford Textbook of Palliative Medicine.* Oxford: Oxford University Press.

Watson M., Lucas C. (2003) *Adult Palliative Care Guidelines.* London: The South West London and the Surrey, West Sussex and Hampshire Cancer Networks.

Articles

Chang J. C. (1988) Antipyretic effect of naproxen and corticosteroids on neoplastic fever. *Pain and Symptom Management,* **3**: 141–4.

Chang J. C. (1989) Neoplastic fever: a proposal for diagnosis. *Arch Int Med,* **149**: 1728–30.

Loprinzi C. L., Barton D. L. *et al.* (2001) Management of hot flashes in breast cancer survivors. *Lancet Oncol,* **2, 4**: 199–204.

Miller J. I., Ahmann R. D. (1992) Treatment of castration induced menopausal symptoms with low dose diethylstilboestrol in men with advanced prostate cancer. *Urology,* **40, 6**: 499–502.

Quigley C. S., Baines M. (1997) Descriptive epidemiology of sweating in a hospice population. *J Pall Care,* **13, 1**: 22–6.

Respiratory symptoms

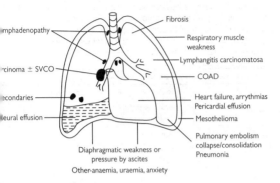

Fibrosis

mphadenopathy

Respiratory muscle weakness

rcinoma ± SVCO

Lymphangitis carcinomatosa

COAD

econdaries

Heart failure, arrythmias
Pericardial effusion

leural effusion

Mesothelioma

Pulmonary embolism
collapse/consolidation
Pneumonia

Diaphragmatic weakness or
pressure by ascites

Other-anaemia, uraemia, anxiety

g. 6e.1 Causes of breathlessness

▸reathlessness[1]

- Breathlessness is common in palliative care (the prevalence is 40–80 per cent in some series)
- Breathlessness is common in patients with cancer
- The pathophysiology of breathlessness is complicated and not fully understood
- Normal breathing is maintained by regular rhythmical activity in the respiratory centre in the brain stem. This is stimulated by *mechanical receptors* (stretch receptors in the airways, lung parenchyma, intercostal muscles and diaphragm) and by hypoxia and high levels of CO_2 (detected by *chemoreceptors* in the aortic and carotid bodies and in the medulla)
- In malignant lung disease, breathlessness is usually due to distortion and stimulation of the mechanical receptors, and blood gases are often normal
- Fatigue, muscle weakness (often due to cachexia or steroid myopathy), phrenic nerve palsy and restrictive chest wall tumours are common problems in cancer that can cause or exacerbate breathlessness
- Muscle weakness, fatigue and anxiety are the predominant factors correlating with breathlessness in cancer

Bruera E. (2000) The frequency and correlates of dyspnoea in patients with advanced cancer. ›ain Symptom Manage, **19**: 357–62.

Management

Look for reversible causes of breathlessness
- Do not assume that breathlessness is directly caused by cancer
- Reversible causes of breathlessness, such as congestive heart failure, an exacerbation of chronic obstructive airways disease, cardiac arrhythmia anaemia, pleural/pericardial effusions, bronchial infection and pulmonary emboli, should be treated appropriately
- Breathlessness due to lung cancer per se, can be alleviated in a high proportion of patients with radiotherapy or chemotherapy

Consider causes that may best be treated specifically:	
Lung tumour	Radiotherapy (**RT**) or Chemotherapy
Bronchospasm	Bronchodilators
	Corticosteroids
Infection	Antibiotics
Pleural effusion	Pleural tap
	Pleurodesis
Anaemia	Blood transfusion
	Iron
	Erythropoetin
Lymphangitis carcinomatosa	Can only be diagnosed on X-ray, and even this may not be diagnostic; suspect when consistent severe breathlessness at rest or on exertion, and widespread fine crepitations in lungs
	Corticosteroids
	Diuretics??
	Bronchodilators
Large airway obstruction	Diagnosed clinically by difficulty on breathing in, and inspiratory stridor
	RT
	Stent
	Laser treatment
	Brachytherapy
	Corticosteroids
SVC obstruction	Dilated veins over upper chest and neck, swollen face, neck and arms
	RT

Symptomatic treatment of breathlessness

General management

Relaxation techniques, physiotherapy in the form of percussion, postur drainage or breathing exercises may all be very helpful. Directing a stream air over the face can reduce the sensation of breathlessness. Explanation an patient confidence that the awareness of breathing will be reduced by th drugs, and that he or she can feel more in control, is essentia Breathlessness clinics, where a multidisciplinary team approach is used t

lp breathless patients using a full range of routine and alternative thera-
es, are available
Breathlessness tends to cause at least as much (if not more) concern
among healthcare professionals than other common distressing
symptoms such as pain
A calm, positive, logical approach can do much to alleviate the
distress of the patient and their family as well as other members
of the healthcare team
Occasionally breathlessness is very difficult to control despite general
measures and medication, especially in the terminal situation
Sedation may then be necessary to alleviate patient and family distress

edication

onchodilators

en in the absence of obvious 'wheeze', there may be an element of
versible bronchoconstriction.
Try:

- Salbutamol 2.5–5mg 6 h via nebuliser, or 2 puffs q.d.s. via spacer
  device. (Beware of increased anxiety, tremor and tachycardia if used
  regularly)
- Ipratropium bromide 250–500 mcg 6 h via nebuliser, or 2 puffs q.d.s.
  via spacer device
- Sodium chloride 0.9 per cent via a nebuliser. (May help liquidize
  tenacious secretions)

orticosteroids

eroids are thought to reduce the oedema associated with tumour.
reathlessness may improve if due to multiple lung metastases, stridor due
 tracheal obstruction, SVCO and lymphangitis carcinomatosa. Benefit
ould be apparent within seven days.
Try:

- Dexamethasone 4–8mg p.o. daily, for a one week trial. If there
  is no improvement, **stop**

heophyllines

nese can significantly reduce the sensation of breathlessness in the absence
f any bronchodilator effect.
Try:

- Theophylline m/r 200mg b.d. (uniphyllin continus)
- Aminophylline m/r 225–450mg b.d. (phyllocontin continus)
- Aminophylline can also be given by i/v infusion. (see the *BNF*)

The half-life of theophylline may be *increased* in hepatic impairment,
heart failure and with certain drugs including cimetidine, ciprofloxacin,
and erythromycin
The half-life is *decreased* in smokers, heavy drinkers and by phenytoin,
carbamazepine and barbiturates

opioids

Morphine reduces inappropriate and excessive respiratory drive
and substantially reduces the ventilatory response to hypoxia and
hypercapnia. By slowing respiration, breathing may be made more
efficient, and the sensation of breathlessness reduced.

Morphine does not cause CO_2 retention if used appropriately, and useful in patients with cancer and with terminal respiratory failure due chronic obstructive airways disease.

- Try:
  - oral morphine 2.5mg p.o. p.r.n. or regularly 4-h if dyspnoea is continuous

The dose may be escalated if well tolerated but doses above 10–20 4-h are unlikely to produce further benefit. Morphine modified relea (MST) seems to be less effective for breathlessness than immediate relea morphine preparations given 4-h. Nebulised morphine is probably no mo useful than nebulised saline, which has some benefit.

Benzodiazepines

Panic with hyperventilation and the fear of suffocation may worsen breat lessness.

- Try:
  - diazepam 2–5mg b.d. and p.r.n.
- Benzodiazepines with shorter half-lives (such as lorazepam or midazolam) can be useful in crisis situations, but there is then a risk of reactive agitation and anxiety as the effect wears off quickly
  - lorazepam 1–2mg p.r.n. (works fast and is well absorbed sublinguall
  - midazolam 5–10mg SC or buccal stat

Oxygen

Oxygen may help breathlessness (or confusion) in patients who are hypoxic either at rest or on exertion. It may help other breathles patients (with a normal PaO_2) because of the effect of facial or nasa cooling, or as a placebo.

Hypoxic respiratory drive usually only starts with $PaO_2 < 8kPa$ (rough) equivalent to an oxygen saturation (SaO_2) of 90%); hypoxic drive is ofte not significant until $PaO_2 < 5.3kPa$ (approx. SaO_2 75%). Most breathles cancer patients are not hypoxic to this degree and will not benefit from oxygen physiologically. It is difficult to predict those patients who wi perceive benefit from oxygen purely from their oxygen saturation.

It is best to avoid *unnecessary* dependency on oxygen, which can limi mobility, may become a barrier between patient and family, and is expen sive and inconvenient in the community. Much dependency is caused by injudicious use, leading to habit.

Assessment

If available, a pulse oximeter should be used, and patients with a $SaO_2 \leq 90\%$ (after exertion if appropriate) *should* be offered a trial o oxygen. Those with an $SaO_2 > 90\%$ (or if pulse oximeter not available) *may* be offered a trial if desired.

Trial of oxygen

A trial of oxygen for a fixed period e.g. 15–30 minutes is recommended After this time the patient should be reassessed, and a decision made as to its benefit. (If it is agreed that it has not helped, the oxygen cylinder mask may be discontinued). Explanation of the rationale for lack of benefit from oxygen, and offer of alternative strategies, such as a fan, open windows etc. will help.

Domiciliary oxygen

Intermittent or continuous domiciliary oxygen can be prescribed for palliation of breathlessness in patients with cancer. An oxygen concentrator is generally more cost-effective for patients requiring oxygen more than 8 h/day, unless it is only very short term. The 1,360l size of cylinder is the one usually dispensed in the community and at 2l/min this gives about 11 h of use. Warn families about smoking! (Less of a problem with a concentrator.)

Oxygen concentration

Method	Flow rate	% O$_2$delivered
Nasal cannulae	1l/min	24%
	2l/min	28%
Ventimask	2l/min	24%
	6l/min	35%

Patients with severe COPD who are chronically hypoxic should not be given more than 28% oxygen unless properly monitored for respiratory depression. Many patients with carcinoma of the bronchus also have COPD.

Flow rates of <4l/min via nasal cannulae do not require humidification.

The costs of initiating oxygen therapy are considerable in financial, social, psychological, logistical and safety terms. It should not be undertaken lightly and only after a full discussion of the cost benefits have been explored.

Cannabinoids

Nabilone 0.1–0.2mg orally four times a day may be given for patients who are continually breathlessness, anxious and who do not tolerate other conventional respiratory sedatives. Sedation and dysphoria may occur with higher doses. It is unsuitable for patients with atrial fibrillation or heart failure.

Breathlessness symptomatic treatments summary

Trial of oxygen if patient is hypoxic SaO$_2$ <90%

Massage, aromatherapy or other relaxation methods

Advise patient on non-drug measures:
  position—sitting upright rather than lying
  cool air from fan or open window

Consider a trial of bronchodilators e.g. nebulised salbutamol 2.5mg q.d.s. Bronchospasm is not always associated with wheeze, and bronchodilators can improve breathlessness without measurable changes in lung function; a therapeutic trial is appropriate for any patient with advanced cancer. Other drug measures include steroids, opioids, and benzodiazepines.

Non-pharmacological management of breathlessness

A non-pharmacological approach to breathlessness in lung cancer works well alongside existing medical treatment. This approach may also be helpful to patients suffering from breathlessness due to end-stage non-malignant disease.

Exploring the patient's experience of breathlessness

An essential prerequisite to managing breathlessness involves understand
what it means to be that person in that particular situation.

- The patient is asked to describe his/her breathlessness experience
- Open acknowledgement of the feelings of 'terror' associated with breathlessness is encouraged
- The patient is helped gently to confront fears of suffocation, choking, not being able to get another breath, or dying during an episode of acute breathlessness. Reassurance is offered that these fears are unlikely to be realized
- The patient's exercise tolerance is ascertained and he/she is asked to identify things which either trigger or alleviate breathlessness
- The impact of breathlessness on the patient's daily life is explored and he/she is assisted in coping with and adjusting to the loss of rôles and activities. It is important to be aware of the extent to which depression may be a component of breathlessness
- Time is given to talk sensitively and at the patient's pace about the disease and associated feelings

Teaching skills to assist the patient in managing breathlessness

The patient is offered an educational programme, consisting of a numb
of skills and strategies, to manage breathlessness. The programme
dependent on a partnership and therapeutic working relationship betwe
the patient and professional, and has three main aims:

1 **To enable efficient and effective breathing, where possible**.
Breathing re-training is a core part of this approach. This involves
teaching the patient to use diaphragmatic breathing exercises as a
controlled breathing technique when they feel breathless (as opposed
the tendency to breathe rapidly using the upper respiratory,
accessory muscles, which tire easily leading to inefficient lung aeration)
Diaphragmatic breathing exercises involve a combination of:
   - pursed lip breathing which promotes control, slows the respiratory rate, increases tidal volume and decreases the possibility of airway collapse
   - controlled breathing with the diaphragm, or lower chest which help to improve function and breaks the pattern of upper chest breathin

2 **To enable the patient to feel in control by reducing anxiety
   and panic**. The effect of tension and anxiety versus the effect of
   relaxation on breathlessness, and the concept of the mind–body link are
   fully discussed with the patient. Relaxation and distraction techniques ar
   taught with the purpose of reducing residual tension, and for use when
   anxiety and panic are exacerbating breathlessness.

3 **To enable the patient to adjust and conserve energy for
   activities which are important to them**. Pacing, prioritizing and
   problem-solving in relation to activity are explored with the patient.
   Advice is offered on managing activities of daily living such as:
   - washing/showering/bathing
   - dressing and undressing
   - bending
   - climbing stairs
   - talking on the telephone
   - making love
   - carrying shopping/heavy objects
   - gardening

goal-setting for learning breathing techniques, in relation to activity,
encouraged. It is important that this is realistic and achievable. The patient
given both verbal and written information focusing on the skills taught.

Other non-pharmacological measures

A draught of air from a fan, or open window may be helpful to some
patients

Massaging the patient's back during an episode of respiratory panic can
encourage muscular relaxation and may be comforting to someone
experiencing an attack of breathlessness

Positioning of the patient in bed is important. The upright position uses
gravity to assist in lung expansion and to reduce pressure from the
abdomen on the diaphragm. Lying high on one side can be helpful to
the patient with copious secretions by preventing aspiration. Getting
the patient to sit in a good position assists relaxation of the upper
chest muscles and encourages freer use of the diaphragm. The patient
can achieve this by sitting forward and resting the arms on the thighs.
The wrists should be relaxed

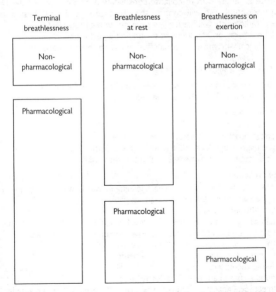

Fig. 6e.2 The relative contributions of pharmacological and non-pharmacoligical
approaches for the management of breathlessness in patients with cancer according
to the severity of the breathlessness and the patient's prognosis. From J. Corner
et al. (1997) *The Palliative Management of Breathlessness*. London: European
Congress for Palliative Care

Pleural aspiration (thoracocentesis)

General

Aspiration of a pleural effusion can give symptomatic relief from dyspnoea. A pleural effusion large enough to cause dyspnoea will be detectable clinically. Aspiration of 300–500mL fluid will usually give some symptomatic improvement, but up to 1.5 litres may be aspirated in some cases.

Complications

Haemothorax can occur, either from damage to the lung or from vascular pleural tumour. Pneumothorax can occur due to puncture of the lung. A significant pneumothorax is unlikely after an uncomplicated aspiration if simple precautions are taken. A routine check X-ray after aspiration is not essential in a palliative care setting.

If a small i/v cannula is used for aspiration as opposed to a large-bore chest drain, very little air can enter through the cannula if reasonable care is taken. Aspiration of a very large effusion that is causing the heart and mediastinum to be displaced may cause cardiovascular embarrassment.

Infection is a rare complication, providing an aseptic technique is used.

Investigations

A chest X-ray will show a pleural effusion, but it can be difficult to differentiate an effusion from collapse/consolidation or a mixture of the two. An ultrasound scan will confirm the presence of a pleural effusion, and many radiologists will mark a site for aspiration if requested.

Chest X-ray or ultrasound scan should be performed if:
- A clinically-diagnosed pleural effusion has not been confirmed radiologically
- The clinical signs are not straightforward

Platelet count and a clotting screen should be checked if the patient has any symptoms of bleeding or unexplained bruising.

Contra-indications
- local skin infection
- coagulopathy—platelets <40 or INR >1.4
- the presence of local pleural tumour is a relative contra-indication, as tumour cells may be 'seeded' in the chest wall

The procedure
- The patient should sit on a chair, leaning forward, resting the head on folded arms on a pillow on a bedside table
- Use the site marked by ultrasound scan, OR
- Choose a point in the posterior chest wall, medial to the angle of the scapula, one intercostal space below the upper limit of dullness to percussion. The mid-axillary line can also be used
- Confirm that the site is dull to percussion
- Avoid the inferior border of the rib above since the neurovascular bundle runs in a groove inferior to the rib
- Inject local anaesthetic into the skin over the area. When the area is anaesthetized, it is helpful to advance the needle until pleural fluid is obtained which will confirm the depth of the pleural fluid beneath the skin surface and confirm a suitable site for aspiration, thereby minimizing the risk of complications

- Introduce a large-bore i/v cannula with syringe attached until fluid is just obtained, then advance a further 0.5–1cm to ensure that the cannula is in the pleural space
- Asking the patient to exhale against pursed lips (to increase intrathoracic pressure), remove the metal trochar or needle and immediately attach a 50/60mL syringe via a three-way tap
- Aspirate fluid 50mL at a time, until:
  - 1 litre has drained (1500mL maximum),
  - or the patient starts to cough,
  - or giddiness, light-headedness or chest discomfort occur
- Remove the cannula, having asked the patient to take a breath, and immediately seal with flexible collodion BP, and cover with a dressing

Further reading

Books

Ahmedzai S. (1998) Palliation of respiratory symptoms. In D. H. Doyle et al. (eds) *Textbook of Palliative Medicine*, 2nd edn, pp. 583–616. Oxford: Oxford University Press.

Davis C. L. (1998) Breathlessness, cough and other respiratory problems. In M. Fallon, B. O'Neill (eds.) *ABC of Palliative Care*, pp. 8–11. London: BMJ Books.

Wilcock A. (1997) Dyspnoea. In P. Kaye (ed.) *Tutorials in Palliative Medicine*, pp. 227–49. Northampton: EPL Publications.

Articles

Booth S., Kelly M. J., Cox N. P., Adams L., Guz A. (1996) Does oxygen help dyspnoea in patients with cancer? *American Journal of Respiratory and Critical Care Medicine* **153, 5**: 1515–18.

Bredin M., Corner J., Krishnasamy M., Plant H., Bailey C., A'Hern, R. (1999) Multicentre randomised controlled trial of nursing intervention for breathlessness in patients with lung cancer. *British Medical Journal*, **318**: 901–4.

Bruera E. et al. (1990) Effects of morphine on the dyspnoea of terminal cancer patients. *Journal of Pain and Symptom Management*, **5**: 341–4.

Connolly M., O'Neill, J, (1999) Teaching a research-based approach to the management of breathlessness in patients with lung cancer. *European Journal of Cancer Care*, **8**: 30–6.

Reuben D. B., Mor V. M. (1986) Dyspnoea in terminally ill cancer patients. *Chest*, **89, 2**: 234–6.

Ripamonti C. (1999) Management of dyspnea (sic) in advanced cancer patients. *Supportive Care in Cancer*, **7, 4**: 233–43.

van der Molen B. (1995) Dyspnoea: a study of measurement instruments for the assessment of dyspnoea and their application for patients with advanced cancer. *Journal of Advanced Nursing*, **22, 5**: 948–56.

Cough

Cough may be present in up to 50 per cent of patients with termir cancer and in up to 80 per cent of patients with lung cancer. It occurs as result of mechanical and chemical irritation of receptors in the respirato tracts. The cough reflex involves afferent nerve input to the medulla a efferents to the respiratory muscles. The causes are similar to tho causing shortness of breath.

Prolonged bouts of coughing are exhausting and frightening, especially associated with dyspnoea and haemoptysis, and can also lead to vomitin

Management

This will depend on the cause of the coughing, which may or may not reversible, and the clinical status of the patient. The glottis has to clo briefly in order to generate sufficient intrathoracic pressure to exp sputum, which may not be possible if there is paralysis of one vocal cor as can occur in carcinoma of the left upper lung. Coughing in this situatio becomes less effificient and may become physically tiring. Active interve tion, such as drainage of a pleural effusion, may be appropriate for patier with a relatively long prognosis, whereas comfort and relief of sympton would be the therapeutic aim for patients in the terminal phase.

The palliation of distressing cough should follow the same general pri ciples as for dyspnoea, remembering that reversible underlying caus should be sought and treated where possible and appropriate.

Symptomatic management of cough

The main distinction to be made is between a productive, wet cough a a dry cough.

Productive/wet cough

Promotion of an easy, effective cough to clear the mucus should be the ai unless the patient is dying, and too weak to expectorate. Antibiotics may appropriate, even in very ill patients, as symptomatic treatment for cough.

For patients still able to cough effectively with help:

- Nebulised sodium chloride 0.9 per cent 2.5mL q.d.s. and p.r.n.
  - May help to loosen tenacious mucus and aid expectoration, but patients must be capable of swallowing the large amounts of sputum/liquid that may collect. The evidence for using drugs which aim to reduce the viscosity of mucus, such as carbocysteine (500–750 t.d.s. p.o.) is weak, but they do have some effect on reducing the number of exacerbations of COPD and the length of the episode. Again, patients must be able to swallow well, as the production of copious amounts of secretions may be triggered

Bronchospasm should be treated with nebulised salbutamol.

Patients who are not imminently terminal may benefit from standa vibration, percussion and postural drainage, to help clear sputum, from t physiotherapist. Weaker patients are helped by explanations and beir shown breathing techniques.

For chronic persistent infection causing cough, nebulised gentamicin ca be considered.

Antitussives should ideally be avoided, but may be helpful at night to a sleep (📖 see below for choice).

For patients who are dying and too weak to cough:

Antimuscarinics and cough suppressants should be used. Occasionally bronchorrhoea (voluminous amounts of clear frothy sputum which occurs in 6 per cent of cases of alveolar cell cancer of lung and 9 per cent of other lung cancers), may be very debilitating. Radiotherapy should be considered, but other suggested symptomatic treatments are largely *anecdotal*;

- Antimuscarinic drugs (e.g. ipratropium (nebulised) or glycopyrronium (SC) or hyoscine (SC))
- Cough suppressants (see below—usually diamorphine CSCI if patient is dying)
- Corticosteroids p.o.
- Macrolide antibiotics (erythromycin, clarithromycin)
- Nebulised furosemide 20mg q.d.s.

Dry cough

A dry cough should be suppressed, once measures have been taken to exclude or treat an underlying reversible cause.

- Nebulised sodium chloride 0.9 per cent 2.5mL q.d.s. may be helpful, by reducing the irritation of dry airways (breathing oxygen or mouth-breathing) and helping loosen the normal bronchial secretions

Cough suppressants

If it is not possible to reverse the cause of the cough or appropriate to continue to encourage expectoration, cough suppressants will be needed.

1 Peripheral suppressants:
- As an alternative to relieving the cause of the cough or to aiding expectoration, it may be more appropriate to aim for cough suppression, particularly in a patient who is terminally ill. Local anaesthetics block cough receptors in the carina and bronchioles and may therefore be useful in endobronchial malignancy. Bupivacaine (5mL of 0.25 per cent t.d.s.) and lidocaine (5mL of 0.2 per cent t.d.s.) have been used via ultrasonic nebulisers with effect. Pharyngeal anaesthesia occurs and food and drink should be avoided for an hour or so after treatment to avoid aspiration. The first dose should be given as an inpatient in case of reflex bronchospasm

Cause	Treatment
Pharyngeal irritation	Simple linctus
Bronchial irritation	Nebulised bupivacaine

2 Central suppressants:
- Pholcodine 10mL t.d.s. is non-analgesic, causes less sedation and constipation than analgesic opioids and should be tried first for patients not already on opioids
- Codeine 30mg q.d.s. and increased if needed to 60mg q.d.s. may be useful or alternatively morphine 5mg 4-h p.o., or diamorphine 5–10mg/24h CSCI, as appropriate. The dose should be titrated as for pain until either it is successful or side-effects intervene. If a patient is already taking opioids, a dose increment or two should be tried, but there is little evidence supporting the use of high

doses of opioids for cough. Nebulised morphine has been tried but may not be much more effective than nebulised sodium chloride 0.9 per cent

- The efficacy of hydromorphone, oxycodone and fentanyl is not well described
- Methadone is a little more potent than morphine and may be more useful. The long duration of action means that a single dose may be given. A trial should be considered if the patient cannot tolerate morphine in low doses (e.g. <10mg 4-h). The usual starting dose is methadone 2mg (2mL of 1mg/mL solution)
- Inhaled sodium cromoglycate 10mg q.d.s. has been used for cough in lung cancer, usually acting within 48 h

Diazepam may also be needed to relieve anxiety and distress and as central cough depressant.

	Comparable antitussive dose
Pholcodine	10mg
Dextromethorphan	10–15mg
Dextropropoxyphene	10–12.5mg
Codeine	15mg
Dihydrocodeine	15mg
Morphine	2.5–5mg
Methadone	2mg
Benzonatate	100mg

Haloperidol and antitussives
Studies on experimental models have shown that pre-treatment with haloperidol markedly reduces the antitussive effect of pentazocine and dextromethorphan. Haloperidol is a potent sigma-ligand and it is suggested that the antitussive effect is mediated by sigma-sites. Clinical relevance is unknown, but a trial of an antiemetic other than haloperidol may be worth trying if a patient has intractable cough resistant to antitussives.

Oncological measures
As a generalization, palliative radiotherapy (for non-small cell lung tumours) and chemotherapy (for small cell lung tumours and metastatic lung disease) is good palliative treatment. Cough may be relieved in up to 80 per cent of patients.

Antibiotics
Chest infections commonly occur in the last few days of life. It may be inappropriate to treat relatively asymptomatic bronchopneumonia. However, infected chest secretions may be copious and more effectively treated with antibiotics than with symptomatic measures alone. Frequently patients have had several prior courses of antibiotics, in which case a short course of a broad spectrum antibiotic may be justified. Offensive sputum suggestive of anaerobic infection may respond to metronidazole.

Nebulised gentamicin is used quite frequently in cystic fibrosis. Purulent secretions colonized with gram negative organisms can be treated with nebulised gentamicin 80mg b.d.–t.d.s. with a significant reduction in the volume of secretions. Negligible systemic absorption has been shown.

Anecdotally, massive terminal haemoptysis is associated with anaerobic smelling foetor.

Further reading

Doyle D. H., Hanks G. W. C., McDonald N. (1998) *Oxford Textbook of Palliative Medicine*. 3rd edn. Oxford: Oxford University Press.

Zylicz Z., Krajnik M. (2004) The use of antitussive drugs in terminally ill patients. *Europ J Pall Care.* 1: 225–9.

Skin problems in palliative care

A man's illness is his private territory and, no matter how much he loves you and how close you are, you stay an outsider. You are healthy.

Lauren Bacall, *By Myself*, 1978

Wound care in cancer

Skin infiltration with subsequent ulceration or fungating wounds can be distressing. A small metastatic skin nodule is a visual reminder of disease progression and a fungating carcinoma with malodour, discharge and bleeding add to the misery of advanced and uncontrolled metastatic disease.

Loco-regional skin involvement (e.g. breast fungation) should be distinguished from generalized skin metastases which imply very late disease. Local extension of malignant tumour leads to embolization of blood and lymphatic vessels, compromising tissue viability. Infarction of the tumour leads to necrosis with subsequent infection, particularly anaerobic.

The ideal aim is complete healing through either local or systemic treatment, which may involve surgery, radiotherapy, hormonal manipulation or chemotherapy. If such treatment is inappropriate, then care is directed to the minimisation of:

- pain
- infection
- bleeding
- odour
- psychological trauma

Treatment should be realistic and acceptable to the patient and carers. The primary aim is the promotion of comfort (as opposed to healing) and the enhancement of quality of life, which may hitherto have been severely impaired.

Following assessment of the problems, choose a dressing regime to meet the needs of the patient. Be prepared to change and experiment since there are no rights or wrongs. The aim is to contain problems and improve quality of life.

Continually re-evaluate

There are numerous commercially available products: alginates, hydrocolloids, hydrogels, semi-permeable films, cavity foams, desloughing agents and charcoals. All may have a place in the management of chronic wounds. The health professional must keep abreast of the merits of established and newer products. The simplest products may be the best and the most cost-effective.

The criteria are comfort, acceptability, and availability.

Choosing a wound care regime
Consider:-
- Pain
- Exudate
- Necrotic tissue
- Bleeding
- Comfort
- Odour
- Infection
- Cosmesis
- Patient Lifestyle
- Psychological Effects

Pain
Ensure that pain is caused neither by infection nor the dressing itself. Try to stick to simple regimes, limiting the frequency of dressing changes. Non-stick and sealed dressings may be useful. Prior to applying the dressing, use short-acting analgesia, or relaxation techniques after discussing the options with the patient.

Exudate
Use dressings with high absorbency and further packing on top in addition to plastic pads to protect clothing. Change the top layer as often as necessary, avoiding frequent changes of dressings placed directly over the wound. Protect the surrounding good skin with Cavilon TM barrier cream or, if skin is broken, use Cavilon TM no-sting barrier film spray.

Necrotic tissue
Surgical debridement may be necessary to remove dead tissue and larvae therapy may also be appropriate.

Bleeding
Gauze soaked in adrenaline 1:1000 or sucralfate liquid or alternatively kaltostat may be used over bleeding points. Gentle removal of dressing with normal saline spray, Steripods or irrigation using a syringe containing warm sodium chloride 0.9 per cent prevents trauma at dressing changes. Kaltostat becomes a jelly-like substance and can be easily lifted off using forceps or gloved fingers. Sorbsan dressings become liquefied and can be washed off with sodium chloride 0.9 per cent. It is preferable to use dressings that can be left in place for a few days to prevent frequent dressing changes—these include the alginates kaltostat, sorbsan and sorbsan plus.

Odour
Use systemic or topical metronidazole but consider limiting to seven days use, as aerobes may increase in numbers on removal of natural competition of anaerobic bacteria. Charcoal dressings are useful and the wound should be sealed. Disguise the smell with deodorizers used sparingly on top of the dressing.

Infection
This is usually chronic and localized. The wound should be cleaned with sodium chloride 0.9 per cent or preferably under running water in the shower or the bath. If the surrounding areas are inflamed, especially if there is spreading inflammation, not just a red rim, antibiotic(s) should be used

e commonest organisms grown in fungating, cancerous wounds and in
essure sore areas include coliforms, anaerobes, staphylococcus aureus
d group G beta-haemolytic streptococcus. Staphylococcus aureus is
obably the commonest pathogen.

Antibiotics such as flucloxacillin or, failing this, trimethoprim or
ythromycin should cover most common infections, but metronidazole
ay be needed for anaerobic infections and topical metronidazole gel is
rticularly useful for eradicating the associated noxious smell. Methicillin-
sistant Staphylococcus aureus (MRSA) is difficult to eradicate. It may
t necessarily result in morbidity to the patient, but there is clearly
transmission risk to other immunocompromised individuals. Present
idelines for inpatients suggest isolation of patients who are MRSA
fected or colonized and the observance of strict 'standard' isolation
ecautions.

Remember that agents such as cephalosporins, which cover a wider
ectrum of bacterial infections, increase the risk of Clostridium difficile
arrhoea.

omfort

trial and error, a combination of dressings and top packing that is most
mfortable for the individual patient will be needed.

osmesis

ne best cosmetic effect possible should be achieved, in order to boost
onfidence.

festyle

atients may need different regimes for different occasions. For social
ccasions, avoid bulky unsightly dressings. Large sheet hydrocolloids may
e more appropriate. Daily relaxing baths, perfumes and cosmetics should
e encouraged to promote well-being and confidence. Use minimal skin
rapping by fixing dressings with vests, cling film, netelast or incontinence
ds (which may be more comfortable).

sychological effects

ttention to detail and, in particular, ensuring leakproof/odourproof
ppliances and giving information and explanation will lessen the sense of
plation and enhance confidence and morale.

urther reading

ooks

rocott P., Dealey C. (2004) In D. H. Doyle et al. (eds) Textbook of Palliative Medicine, pp. 628–40.
d edn. Oxford: Oxford University Press.

ll C. (1998) Skin problems in palliative care: nursing aspects.

Pruritus (itch)

Pruritus may be defined as 'an unpleasant sensation that provokes desire to scratch'. The prevalence is 27 per cent with the common cance and 80 per cent in the presence of cholestasis.

Pathogenesis of pruritus

This is complex and not fully elucidated, but it is known that both cent and peripheral mechanisms are involved. A number of mediators includ serotonin, neuropeptides, cytokines, prostaglandins and growth facto are being studied to generate future treatment options.

Complications of pruritus

- Excoriation +/− secondary infection
- Lack of sleep, social unacceptability, interference with daily functionin
- Depressive symptoms in up to one third of patients with generalized pruritus

Medical history assessment of the pruritic patient

- Generalised or localised itch
- Drug history
- Exacerbating factors
- Previous medical history

Causes of pruritus in patients with cancer

These can be divided into general causes of pruritus (which occur in t healthy population as well as those with cancer) and those specifically relat to malignancy. In either case pruritus may be localized or generalized.

Senile itch

This is experienced by 50–70 per cent of those over the age of 70 yea The majority have xerosis and skin atrophy, in others the cause unknown. It is best treated with general measures (see below) and t application of emollient cream.

Iatrogenic itch

The following drugs are common causes: opioids, aspirin, amfetamin and drugs that can cause cholestasis such as erythromycin, hormor treatment and phenothiazines.

Iron deficiency

This can cause pruritus with or without anaemia, and responds to ir replacement.

Hormonal itch

Pruritus occurs in up to 11 per cent of patients with thyrotoxicos particularly long-term untreated Graves' disease, and less commonly hypothyroidism. The link between diabetes mellitus and pruritus controversial.

Management of pruritus

Removal of causative agents (e.g. drugs) and the appropriate investigatio and treatment of underlying disease are essential first-line measure Management can be divided into *general* and *cause-specific*.

Evidence for the use of different systemic agents in the treatment pruritus is limited, but specific drugs may be useful for specific situations outlined below.

General management

For intact skin

Ensure that the skin is not dry

Discontinue using soap

Use emulsifying ointment or aqueous cream as a soap substitute, or add oilatum to bath water

Avoid hot baths

Dry skin gently by patting with soft towel (not rubbing)

Apply aqueous cream or alternative emollient ('moisturizer') to the skin after a bath or shower each evening

Avoid overheating (wear light clothes) and sweating day and night (may need an antimuscarinic agent)

Use sedatives, such as benzodiazepines, to help improve associated anxiety and insomnia

Discourage scratching; keep nails short; allow gentle rubbing; wear cotton gloves at night

Avoid exacerbating factors such as heat, dehydration, anxiety and boredom

Avoid alcohol and spicy foods which may worsen itch

Consider behavioural treatments and hypnotherapy, which may help ease associated psychological issues and break the cycle of itching and scratching

Consider TENS and acupuncture

For macerated skin

Dry the skin and protect from excessive moisture

Use a hair dryer on cool setting

Apply surgical spirit to assist evaporation

Apply a wet compress t.d.s. and allow it to dry out completely

If infected, use an antifungal solution e.g. clotrimazole

If very inflamed, use 1 per cent hydrocortisone solution for 2–3 days

Avoid adsorbent powders e.g. starch, talc, zinc oxide which may form a hard abrasive coating on the skin and be abrasive

Cause-specific management

Itchy skin rashes and insect bites

One–two per cent menthol in aqueous cream or oily calamine lotion with .5 per cent phenol (which can be enhanced up to 1 per cent) may be useful. Antihistamine creams should be used when the cause of itch is thought to be histamine-related, e.g. acute drug rash. Prolonged topical use, however, may lead to contact dermatitis, which is best treated with 1 per cent hydrocortisone until it has settled.

Paraneoplastic itch

Cancer per se is an infrequent, but important, cause of generalized pruritus (paraneoplastic itch), the mechanism for which is unknown. Pruritus is particularly associated with haematological malignancies such as Hodgkin's lymphoma and polycythaemia rubra vera.

Treatment of an underlying lymphoma with steroids (dexamethasone 4–8mg o.d. or prednisolone 30–60 o.d.) may be helpful. There is some evidence that paroxetine 5–20mg o.d. (see below), mirtazepine 7.5–15mg o.n. or cimetidine 800mg a day (or other H_2 receptor antagonists) may be effective (see below). Thalidomide may also be useful but its association with teratogenicity and peripheral nerve damage may be difficult to manage.

Cimetidine, an H_2 receptor antagonist, has been shown to be helpful in itch associated with lymphoma and polycythaemia rubra vera. This is not thought to be a direct antihistaminic effect as it has little effect on itching caused by histamine, but is thought to be related to its inhibitory action on liver enzymes which are involved in the synthesis of endogenous opioids, and possibly other agents, causing pruritus.

Paroxetine, a selective serotonin reuptake inhibitor (SSRI) antidepressant, has been shown to relieve itch in a case series of patients with advanced cancer with paraneoplastic and opioid-induced itch probably due to downregulation of $5-HT_3$ receptors, but side-effects (nausea, vomiting and sedation) may limit its use.

Opioid-induced pruritus

Itch is a well recognized side-effect of opioids and a switch to an alternative opioid (or stopping if possible) may be helpful.

Ondansetron has been shown to be useful in opioid-induced itch at traditional antiemetic doses, although most studies pertain to its success in treating the pruritus associated with opioids given by infusion into the epidural/spinal area. Opioid antagonists are theoretically useful in reducing pruritus but may reverse the essential analgesic effects.

Cholestasis

In palliative care, cholestasis (causing itch) occurs most commonly due to obstruction of the common bile duct from primary or secondary tumour involving the pancreas and biliary tree. (It may also occur as a result of gall stones, drugs or intrahepatic disease.) Stenting of the common bile duct and relief of jaundice should relieve the itch and dexamethasone may be of some help. Drug treatment may include an opioid antagonist (e.g. naltrexone 12.5–25.0mg o.d.) which may be helpful if the patient is not taking opioids for pain relief or an androgen (e.g. methyltestosterone 25mg SL o.d., or danazol 200mg o.d.–t.d.s.). Alternatively, rifampicin 75mg o.d.–150mg b.d. may be used or colestyramine (unpalatable and not effective in complete biliary obstruction) or charcoal which is equally unpalatable.

Renal failure

The pathogenesis of pruritus in renal failure has not been fully defined, but is thought to be multifactorial. Pruritus may be localized (in 70 per cent) or generalized, and is more common in patients receiving dialysis than those who are not. Ultraviolet light/phototherapy may be helpful. Opioid antagonists such as naltrexone may be effective but cannot be used in patients already receiving opioids because of the risk of reversing analgesia. Ondansetron, mirtazepine and thalidomide have been shown to be effective for generalized itch, whereas topical capsaicin cream can be effective for localized itch.

Further reading

Books

Doyle D. H., Hanks G. W. C., McDonald N. (2004) *Oxford Textbook of Palliative Medicine*. 3rd edn. Oxford: Oxford University Press.

Articles

Borgeat A., Stirnemann H. R. (1999) Ondansetron is effective to treat spinal or epidural morphine-induced pruritus. *Anesthesiology*, **90**: 432–6.

Breneman D. L., Cardone J. S., Blumsack R. F. *et al.* (1992) Topical capsaicin for treatment of hemodialysis-related pruritus. *J Am Acad Dermatol*, **26**: 91–4.

Connolly C. S., Kantor G. R., Menduke H. (1995) Hepatobiliary pruritus: What are effective treatments? *J Am Acad Dermatol*, **33**: 801–5.

Daly B. M., Shuster S. (2000) Antipruritic action of thalidomide. *Acta Dermato-vener*, **80, 1**: 24–5.

Ibata T., Izumi H., Aizawa H. *et al.* (1998) Effects of nitrazepam on nocturnal scratching in adults with atopic dermatitis: a double blind placebo-controlled crossover study. *Br J Dermatol*, **138, 4**: 631–4.

Krajnik M., Zylicz Z. (2001) Understanding pruritus in systemic disease. *J Pain Symptom Manage*, **21, 2**: 151–68.

Sheehan-Dare R. A., Henderson M. J., Cotterill J. A. (1990) Anxiety and depression in patients with chronic urticaria and generalized pruritus. *Br J Dermatol*, **123, 6**: 769–74.

Zylicz Z., Smits C., Krajnik M. (1998) Paroxetine for pruritus in advanced cancer. *J Pain Symptom Manage*, **16**: 121–4.

Lymphoedema

Lymphoedema is a collection of excessive interstitial fluid with a high protein content and is associated with chronic inflammation and fibrosis. It may occur in any part of the body, generally in a limb. It is progressive and may become a grossly debilitating condition. Acute inflammation and trauma cause a rapid increase in swelling. In patients with cancer, lymphoedema is usually due to blockage of lymphatic vessels and glands by malignancy or by fibrosis as a result of previous radiotherapy or surgery.

The aim of treatment is to prevent complications developing, and to achieve maximum improvement and long-term control. Success requires full patient cooperation and treatment strategies devised by the physiotherapist or lymphoedema nurse may include the following:

- Explanation, information and encouragement
- Scrupulous skin care
- Avoidance of trauma, such as sunburn, or venepuncture to minimize infection risks

Massage

- *Manual lymphatic drainage* is a very gentle form of massage used to encourage lymph flow from areas of congestion to areas of normal lymphatic drainage
- *Simple lymphatic drainage* is taught to patients and their carers and, paradoxically, involves very gentle, slow massage beginning from areas of healthy lymphatic drainage towards areas of lymphatic obstruction, 'opening up' the drainage channels

Additional management

- Compression stockings and sleeves can give support and help to prevent fluid accumulating. These may be extremely effective within 24–48 h in patients suffering from lymphorrhoea
- Exercises which should be gentle but performed regularly within compression hosiery
- Compression pumps and intensive low compression bandaging may also be needed for slowly resolving oedema

Contra-indications to compression include local extensive cutaneous metastases, truncal oedema (since fluid from a limb may be diverted to an already congested area), infection or venous thrombosis. Various drugs which influence capillary protein flux and filtration and reduce protein viscosity in interstitial spaces are currently under evaluation but are not in regular use.

Chronic lymphoedema leads to changes in both subcutaneous tissue and skin which make them vulnerable to infection

- Careful hygiene reduces the risk of infection and moisturizing skin creams should be liberally applied to prevent drying and cracking. Any suggestion of impending infection requires prompt treatment with antibiotics
- Diuretics are of limited value in the treatment of lymphoedema, unless the swelling has deteriorated since the prescription of a NSAID or systemic corticosteroid or there is a cardiac or venous component

Further reading

Doyle D. H., Hanks G. W. C., Cherny N. (2004) *Oxford Textbook of Palliative Medicine*. 3rd edn. Oxford: Oxford University Press.

Portenoy R. K., Thaler H. T., Kornblith A. B. *et al.* (1994) Symptom prevalence, characteristics and distress in a cancer population. *Quality of Life Research*, **3**: 183–9.

Twycross, R., Jenns K., Todds J. (2000) *Lymphoedema*. Oxford: Radcliffe Medical Press.

Genito-urinary problems

Anatomy and physiology of the bladder and micturition

Patients with palliative care needs may suffer a variety of symptoms attributable to dysfunction of the urinary system. In order to focus treatment appropriately, it is helpful to understand the basic anatomy and physiology.

Bladder wall

- Made up of detrusor muscle, which is a smooth muscle with an adventitial outer covering together with a supporting inner submucosa for a specialized transitional cell epithelium
- Detrusor muscle forms a functional syncytium with relatively indistinct muscle layers. The outer and inner layers of muscle bundles tend to be longitudinal in orientation with a middle layer circularly orientated
- Bladder emptying is accompanied by detrusor contraction
- The trigone is a smooth, sensitive triangular area at the base of the bladder with apices formed by the ureteric orifices and the internal urinary meatus or bladder neck

Sphincter active urethra

- The distal sphincter mechanism is situated just beneath the prostate in males and in the distal half of the urethra in females. There is a smooth muscle component and a striated muscle component within the wall of the urethra
- The striated muscle component, the intrinsic rhabdosphincter, is the most important component for maintaining continence
- The striated sphincter contains fatigue-resistant, slow-twitch fibres that are responsible for passive urinary control. Voluntary contraction of the levator ani musculature is responsible for active continence

Nerve supply of bladder and urethra

- Micturition is partly a reflex and partly a voluntary act
- Parasympathetic nerve fibres in the anterior sacral roots of S2 to S4 are the principle motor supply to the detrusor muscle. Parasympathetic (cholinergic) nerve stimulation results in bladder contraction and bladder neck sphincter relaxation, allowing micturition
- Smooth muscle in the region of the bladder neck and prostate is regulated by sympathetic fibres from the hypogastric plexus arising from T11 to L2. Sympathetic stimulation relaxes the detrusor muscle (beta-adrenoceptors) and contracts the bladder neck sphincter, preventing micturition. The rôle of the sympathetic nervous system in the female is less exact
- The functional innervation of urethral smooth muscle is adrenergic

- Somatic innervation comes from S2 to S4 as the pudendal nerve to the striated muscle of the sphincter
- The neurovascular bundles running alongside the prostate carry the autonomic innervation of the sphincter active urethra as well as the cavernous nerves responsible for erections. It is these nerves which may be damaged during radical prostatectomy with resulting erectile dysfunction

Clinical relevance of nerve supply

Anticholinergic drugs, including hyoscine and tricyclic antidepressants, cause urinary retention by causing relaxation of the detrusor muscle and contraction of the bladder neck mechanism. Alpha blockers (including doxazosin and tamsulosin) increase urinary flow in bladder outflow obstruction by relaxing the smooth muscle of the bladder neck and prostate.

Pain

Bladder pain is referred to the hypogastric (suprapubic) region of the abdomen.

Blood supply of the bladder

The bladder has a considerable blood supply from the vesical arteries and from branches of the anterior division of the internal iliac arteries. This facilitates reconstructive surgery of the bladder but makes the management of haemorrhagic cystitis difficult.

Bladder pain

Bladder discomfort or pain presents in the hypogastric (suprapubic) area and may be associated with other symptoms such as dysuria, frequency, nocturia and urgency as well as urine retention and/or incontinence. If the trigone is affected the pain may radiate to the tip of the penis. Pain may be constant (e.g. urinary tract infection) or intermittent (e.g. bladder spasm). It may vary in intensity from a dull ache (e.g. urinary tract infection) to acute disabling pain (e.g. acute obstructive pathology causing retention of urine).

Commonest causes of bladder pain in palliative care

- Urinary tract infection (UTI)
  - Bacterial (see later) including tuberculous cystitis
  - Fungal (immunocompromised patients)
  - Urethritis
  - Genital herpes
  - Vaginitis
- Anatomical
  - Pelvic mass
  - Urethral obstruction
  - Cystocoele
- Neoplastic
  - Bladder cancer
  - Urethral cancer
- Foreign body
  - Urethral or suprapubic catheter (usually comfortable unless infected or blocked)
  - Bladder calculus

- Bladder instability
  - Bladder spasm may be idiopathic or more commonly due to contraction around the balloon of an indwelling catheter, blood clots, tumour and infection
- Inflammatory
  - Radiotherapy
  - Chemotherapy—cyclophosphamide
  - Intravesical chemotherapy or immunotherapy for bladder cancer
  - Interstitial and eosinophilic cystitis
  - Amyloid

Treatment of bladder pain/irritability

Treat reversible causes.

Non-drug management

Regular toileting, good fluid intake (which may be difficult for the terminally ill), avoiding caffeine and alcohol, drinking real cranberry juice (although evidence is limited).

Drug management

- Antimuscarinic drugs may be helpful but should be avoided in significant bladder outflow obstruction or urinary retention
- Antispasmodics
  - Oxybutinin 2.5–5mg b.d.–q.d.s. (also has a topical anaesthetic effect on the bladder mucosa and can be given intravesically as 5mg in 30mL o.d. to t.d.s.). Modified preparations available
  - Tolterodine 2mg b.d. (better tolerated than oxybutinin, use lower dose if hepatic impairment). Modified release preparations available
  - Propiverine hydrochloride 15mg o.d.–t.d.s.
  - Trospium chloride 20mg b.d.
- Tricyclic antidepressants
  - Amitriptyline 25–50mg o.n.
  - Imipramine 25–50mg
- NSAIDs may be useful
- Corticosteroids may reduce tumour-related inflammation of the bladder and thereby improve bladder comfort
- Local anaesthetic and opioids can be used intravesically. Lidocaine 2 per cent (diluted in sodium chloride 0.9 per cent) can be instilled through an indwelling catheter, which should then be clamped for 20 minutes to 1 hour. Bupivacaine 0.5 per cent can be combined with morphine 10–20mg and instilled t.d.s. through an indwelling catheter which should be clamped for 30 minutes[1]

Terminal situation

- Antimuscarinics can be given CSCI: hyoscine butylbromide 60–120mg over 24h glycopyrronium 0.2–0.4mg over 24h

---

[1] McCoubrie R., Jeffrey D. (2003) Intravesical diamorphine for bladder spasm. *Journal of Pain and Symptom Management*, **25**: 1–2.

Urinary tract infection (UTI)

UTI is common in palliative care patients and presentation may be non-specific. The clinical picture may vary from asymptomatic to severe symptoms to septicaemia.

Presentation: Dysuria, incontinence, urinary retention, haematuria supra-pubic pain, loin pain, pyrexia of unknown origin, confusion.

Risk factors: Low urinary output (dehydration), bladder dysfunction (outlet obstruction, neuropathic bladder), catheterization, atrophic vaginitis renal calculi, diabetes mellitus, immune impairment, vesical fistulae.

Pathogens: *E. coli* commonest, also *Strep. faecalis, Proteus, Klebsiella Pseudomonas.*

Management: Bedside testing for protein, blood, leucocytes and nitrates (any or all may be positive). UTI unlikely if all bedside tests negative. MSU for culture: clinical diagnosis and positive bedside testing sufficient to start treatment in most patients. Catheter *in situ*—do not treat unless symptomatic or undergoing re-catheterization/instrumentation. Encourage increased fluid intake.

- Antibiotic regime:
  - Trimethoprim 200mg b.d. for three days effective in most uncomplicated infections
  - Other regimes:
  - Ciprofloxacin 250–500mg b.d. p.o./i/v, co-amoxiclav 375mg t.d.s. p.o./i/v, cephalexin, 250mg q.d.s. p.o., cefuroxime 125–250mg b.d. p.o./i/v.
  - Recurrent symptomatic UTI (proven on MSU):
  - Prophylaxis with trimethoprim 200mg o.d. or nitrofurantoin 50–100mg nocte

Renal pain

Renal pain is characteristically a dull ache in the loin caused by capsule distension, irritation or obstruction.

Causes

- Infection—pyelonephritis, abscess
- Haematoma (trauma)
- Infarct
- Tumour—renal cell carcinoma, transitional cell carcinoma, oncocytoma, bleed into angiomyolipoma
- Hydronephrosis

Diagnosis

Urine culture, ultrasound scan, CT scan (MRI may be useful if contrast contra-indicated).

Management

Treat underlying cause if possible, consider dexamethasone 8–16mg for enlarging tumour, analgesics (WHO ladder).

Ureteric colic

Ureteric colic is a severe constant pain, usually located to the loin and may radiate to the ipsilateral groin and testicle. Its onset is typically over 15 to 20 minutes building to an intense plateau of pain with fluctuations in intensity but never disappearing, as for example in small bowel colic

It relates to acute ureteric obstruction, and depending on the cause may abate with a similar time course to its onset. The patient will become agitated, unable to settle and roll around in agony, unlike the patient with peritonitis who lies still.

Causes

Calculus, tumour, clot, renal papillae, fungal infection.

Treatment

NSAIDs will inhibit the renal response to acute urinary obstruction (*avoid with impaired renal function*) and opioid analgesia may also help. Treating tumour-related oedema with dexamethasone 8–16mg may be useful. Anticholinergics (e.g. hyoscine butylbromide) play no rôle in the management of acute ureteric colic.

Pelvic pain

Can be highly problematic and multifactorial. Assessment needs a logical and thorough approach.

1 Consider which structures may be the site of pain:
  - GU tract:
    - Males: Ureters, bladder, prostate, urethra, penis, testes
    - Females: Ureters, bladder, urethra, ovaries, uterus and fallopian tubes, vagina
  - Perineum
  - GI tract: Distal colon, rectum, anus
  - Bones: Sacrum, pelvis
2 Consider pathological process leading to pain:
  - Cancer—can be nociceptive (visceral or somatic), musculoskeletal or neuropathic and due to the tumour itself/local invasion/ metastases/extrinsic compression of nearby structures
  - Concurrent non-cancer disease (e.g. UTI)
  - Iatrogenic (caused by cancer treatment or non-cancer treatment, e.g. radiotherapy, surgery, constipation)
3 Treat underlying cause—but also consider:
  - Medical treatment
    - Specific to the cause (e.g. antibiotics for infection)
    - Symptomatic: Follow WHO ladder, adjuvant analgesia as appropriate to type of pain
    - Consider dexamethasone 8–16mg daily for extrinsic compression from tumour as a 3 day trial
  - Surgery: e.g. stabilization of fractures such as neck of femur
  - Oncological treatment: Palliative chemotherapy or radiotherapy, hormone therapy (hormone sensitive tumours)
  - Anaesthetic analgesic interventions: Interruption of the pre-sacral sympathetic nerve supply may help pelvic pain. A caudal or lumbar epidural may be useful. Neurolytic techniques may result in lower limb paralysis and double incontinence[2]
  - Non-physical treatments: Complementary therapies, psychological support, spiritual input, social support

---

2 Wilsey N., Ashford N., Dolin S., (2002) Presacral neurolytic block for relief of pain from pelvic cancer. *Palliative Medicine*, **16**: 441–4.

Urinary retention

Urinary retention is common in palliative care patients and should always be considered in those showing non-specific symptoms such as confusion restlessness and agitation. Patients presenting with retention often have a previous history of urological difficulties. Risk factors for retention include drugs (such as opioids, anticholinergics), constipation, poor mobility and inadequate toileting facilities and should be avoided as far as possible.

Causes

Local
- Urinary tract infection
- Benign prostatic hypertrophy (BPH)
- Pelvic tumours (any)—primary or secondary
- Constipation
- Urethral stricture—rare, since usually presents with bad lower urinary tract symptoms first
- Haematuria with clot retention

Drugs
- Tricyclic antidepressants
- Phenothiazines
- Opioids
- Anti-cholinergics e.g. oxybutinin, hyoscine, glycopyrronium
- Alpha agonists (contained in some proprietary cough medicines)

Neurological
- Spinal cord compression
- Pre-sacral plexopathy
- Intrathecal/epidural anaesthesia

Debility
- Immobility/weakness
- Decreased conscious level

Acute obstruction

Symptoms: hesitancy and poor urinary stream, post micturition dribbling early morning frequency and nocturia. Subacute symptoms may have been present previously but may be of sudden onset.

Diagnosis
- Severe lower abdominal pain
- Intense desire to urinate
- Anxiety/irritability—may be the only symptom in terminal or unconscious patient
- Distended, tense bladder: Tender to palpation, increases desire to urinate, dull to percussion
- >500mL on catheterization in presence of symptoms

Chronic obstruction

Symptoms: classic and cardinal symptom is nocturnal enuresis. The onset is often slow and insidious, and is often missed or misdiagnosed as incontinence.

Diagnosis
- Dribbling incontinence
- Large, non-tender bladder (low pressure chronic retention)
- Percussion dull (may extend to above umbilicus)
- High residual volume (>300mL) post micturition. (May be otherwise symptomless). Acute on chronic volumes may be >800mL on catheterization

Complications
- Urinary infection (📖 see also infection as cause in acute obstruction, p. 324) and bladder stones
- Hydronephrosis and post renal failure (high pressure chronic retention)
- Constipation refractory to laxatives
- Agitation, confusion
- Post-catheterization diuresis: due to released pressure on renal cortex and osmotic effects of high urinary urea. A record should be kept of urine output and if excessive, intravenous fluid should be replaced accordingly, with measurement of serum biochemistry. It is no longer good practice to clamp catheters to allow slow drainage

Treatment
Acute retention
- Immediate catheterization with 16–18Fr gauge urethra catheter
- Antibiotic cover e.g. gentamicin 120mg stat (well tolerated and safe as single dose even in renal failure). Ciprofloxacin is a possible alternative
- Catheter should be left in if the patient is in agreement. There are risks of bacteraemia when catheters are both inserted and removed. In the terminally ill, this will prevent risk of further retention and aid in nursing management
- Measure residual volume
- Rectal examination in male and vaginal examination in female as appropriate

If it is not possible to pass a urethral catheter, a suprapubic catheter will be needed. In a hospice setting in the terminally ill, a Bonanno catheter can be used. It should be inserted in the midline away from scars, two finger breadths above the symphysis pubis. This is a short term measure and the catheter should be changed by a urologist to a more appropriate tube if appropriate for the patient. A suprapubic catheter is contra-indicated with clot retention.

Chronic retention
- catheterization—as above
- fluid balance and monitor electrolytes Na^+ and K^+
- consider IVI.

Clot retention
- This should ideally be managed by the urologists who will use a stiff 22 Fr catheter and may need to use an introducer. In a hospice setting with a terminally ill patient a 22 Fr catheter should be tried.

Treat underlying cause as appropriate for the patient
- Laxatives for constipation
- Treat UTI
- Review medication and reduce or stop drugs causing retention (if possible)
- Clot retention—stop anticoagulants and correct bleeding diathesis if possible. NB Tranexamic acid should be used with caution since it might exacerbate the situation
- Consider and treat spinal cord compression. Investigate/treat pelvic tumour (surgery, radiotherapy or chemotherapy according to type)
- Urethral stent e.g. in patients too unwell for surgery
- Debilitated patient—regular toileting, use commode rather than bedpan (women), sit/stand at edge of bed (men), privacy—anxiety will inhibit micturition

Further investigations (unnecessary if patient is in terminal decline)
- CSU for culture and sensitivity
- Urea and electrolytes, creatinine—uraemia not improving after catheterisation may indicate other cause e.g. NSAID nephropathy or a high obstruction not corrected by catheterization
- Consider urinary imaging: IVU, USS, cystoscopy if patient is well and corrective treatment is contemplated

Choice of catheter

Size 16Fr is the smallest useful size in adults, smaller sizes tending to curl in the urethra. A 22Fr gauge will be needed for clot retention. The French (Fr) gauge is the circumference of the catheter in mm. Silastic catheters are most appropriate.

Ureteric obstruction

This may be unilateral or bilateral and is caused, in palliative care, largely by pelvic tumours, e.g. carcinoma of the cervix in women and carcinoma of the prostate in men. A reduction in urine volume, abdominal pain and/or serial blood tests of deteriorating renal function alert the team to the possibility of bilateral obstruction and impending renal failure. Renal ultrasound will confirm the diagnosis of ureteric obstruction due to tumour and rule out other contributing factors.

Obstructing stones are best diagnosed on plain abdominal X-ray. In the presence of ureteric obstruction, cystoscopy and retrograde pyelograms can be carried out which should outline the level/s and cause of obstruction. An indwelling ureteric stent can then be passed under cystoscopic control if there appears to be reasonable potential for regaining function. If this is not possible a percutaneous nephrostomy could be considered under ultrasound guidance. This can sometimes be replaced by antegrade insertion of ureteric stents. In some circumstances, antegrade ureteric insertion into an ileal conduit may be appropriate. With modern equipment and techniques, long-term nephrostomies are a possible option but this needs very careful discussion with patients who may already be suffering from pelvic pain, fistulae or other tumour related problems. They may not want artificial prolongation of life at the expense of relentlessly distressing symptoms.

In palliative care this discussion with the patient and family is crucial in guiding the patient to the correct management for them. Clearly if restoration of renal function with reasonable quality of life and minimal symptoms and disruption to life is a possibility, interventional management will be in the patient's best interests. On the other hand, if the patient is in the terminal phase of cancer with a known large pelvic mass that is already causing pain and debility, the patient might not wish to undergo procedures that might not be successful and that, if technically successful, might prolong life for a short time but with the added burden of further discomfort. This is the choice of the patient and should be discussed adequately with him/her.

Urinary incontinence

This is a distressing symptom for patients, affecting their lives physically, psychologically, socially and sexually. Patients may become isolated from family and friends as they try to maintain their own personal hygiene, fearing to lose their dignity in public. A good history is essential and may indicate that the cause is simply an inability to mobilize and reach the toilet in time. Pelvic disease in a female patient may result in a vesicovaginal fistula leading to constant urinary drainage through the vagina.

Total urethral incontinence

This type of incontinence is relatively common for patients with advanced malignant disease. Uncontrollable loss of urine occurs secondary to local incompetence of the urethral sphincter (due to direct tumour invasion or previous surgical intervention) or central loss of sphincter control (due to confusion or dementia).

Treatment includes regular toileting for central loss of control to allow continence to be regained. Females will need a urethral catheter. A male sheath catheter can be tried first but these are often problematic since they may be difficult to fit securely and twist easily.

Neurological incontinence

Loss of neurological bladder control may be due to damage to the sacral plexus or spinal cord/cauda equina compression. A hypotonic neuropathic bladder may result in overflow incontinence and a reflex/automatic bladder empties automatically. Patients who are well, willing and dextrous enough may be taught intermittent self-catheterization. Other patients will require long-term catheters. Anticholinergics may help.

Overflow incontinence

This is associated with obstruction of the bladder outlet or a poorly contractile floppy bladder. Small volumes of 'overflow' urine may be passed without control. A palpable, distended bladder alerts the clinician to overflow incontinence, although a large distended but floppy bladder, particularly in a patient with other abdominal pathology, may be difficult to diagnose. Permanent catheterization will probably be necessary. Definitive treatment may be possible if the patient is well enough and if the obstruction is amenable to surgery or other intervention such as an intraurethral stent.

Urge incontinence

A sudden urge to urinate and subsequent urinary loss may be particularly distressing for patients with poor mobility who are unable to reach the toilet in time. The causes include all factors that contribute to an irritable bladder. The underlying cause should be treated and anticholinergic agents may help. Patients may be able to manage timed voiding.

Stress incontinence

Involuntary urethral loss of urine with increased intra-abdominal pressure from coughing, sneezing, laughing, jumping or even walking in severe cases in the absence of bladder contraction may occur. It is more common in multiparous women and is associated with poor urethral support and reduced pelvic floor tone. Support prostheses (e.g. ring pessary) and urethral inserts may be a possibility in the absence of local tumour.

Haematuria

A normal urinary tract does not usually bleed, even if the patient is on warfarin. Haematuria is a frequent presentation of urological disease. It ranges from microscopic haematuria discovered incidentally on urinalysis to frank haematuria with the passage of clots and clot retention of urine. The extent of the bleeding does not always correlate with the severity of the underlying aetiology. The bladder is a very vascular organ and will not have a chance to stop bleeding unless it is collapsed. Dantron may tint the urine pink or orange which may be confusing.

Causes:

- Tumour: Renal, ureteric, bladder, prostate (post radiotherapy or locally advanced)
- UTI
- Drug-induced—aspirin or NSAIDs do not usually cause gross haematuria in a normal urinary tract, but any bleeding associated with surgical interventions may be exacerbated. Cyclophosphamide and ifosfamide may cause haemorrhagic cystitis (see below)
- Systemic coagulation disorder—usually evidence of bruising or bleeding elsewhere. Platelets may be low due to leucoerythroblastic anaemia and marrow infiltration
- Urinary calculus

Investigations:

- Urinalysis, microscopy and urine culture
- Intravenous urography
- Ultrasound scan
- Cystourethroscopy (visualizes the bladder and urethra)

Treatment

Treat any reversible causes i.e. treat UTI and systemic coagulation disorder and stop precipitating drug.

General measures:

- Encourage oral fluids to promote a good urine output (to avoid clot retention)
- Transfusion may improve symptoms due to anaemia

- Etamsylate: (reduces bleeding by enhancing platelet adhesion). The use of tranexamic acid (prevents fibrinolysis by inhibiting plasminogen activation) is controversial. It may result in the formation of hard clots which then need to be irrigated cystoscopically; urological surgeons describe bladders lined with clot which can be difficult to manage. As ever, however, the decision must be made on an individual basis. Terminally ill patients may prefer to risk clot retention than to continue with gross haematuria and significant blood loss
- Palliative radiotherapy often reduces haematuria from a bleeding urinary tract cancer
- Instilling 1 per cent alum, formalin, 0.5–1.0 per cent silver nitrate or epsilon aminocaproic acid solutions may be tried. (Discuss with urologists)
- Internal iliac artery embolization may provide effective relief from severe bladder haemorrhage[3]
- Bleeding from the prostate may respond to finasteride 5mg o.d. (a specific inhibitor of 5 alpha-reductase which metabolizes testosterone to the more potent androgen, dihydrotestosterone) even if patients are on other drugs
- Cystectomy may be the final option in a patient able to undergo the procedure which would be most unusual in the palliative care situation

Clot retention

The principle in the management of clot retention is to evacuate bladder clots. A non-distended bladder bleeds far less than a distended bladder. A large bore 22 Fr catheter will be needed. Patients may need referral to a urologist for insertion of a 3-lumen catheter (to permit irrigation with sodium chloride 0.9 per cent and allow removal of clots) which is stiff and may need to be inserted with an introducer. Cystoscopic bladder washouts may be necessary. Percutaneous insertion of a suprapubic catheter is contra-indicated in the presence of clot retention since the catheter is of insufficient diameter to allow satisfactory irrigation; there is also the potential for seeding of bladder tumour through the percutaneous tract.

Haemorrhagic cystitis

This may require clot evacuation and irrigation, and instillation of alum. Intravesical prostaglandin E2 may be helpful. In selected fit patients, urinary diversion, cystectomy or selective embolization of the internal iliac artery may be appropriate, but this would be very rare in the palliative care population.

3 Gujral S., Bell R., Kabala J., Persad R. (1999) Internal iliac artery embolisation for intractable bladder haemorrhage in the perioperative phase. *Postgraduate Medical Journal*, **75**: 167–9.

Catheterization

Indications: Urinary retention (acute and chronic), incontinence, patients in whom toileting is problematic e.g. pathological fracture femur.

Indwelling urethral catheterization

The French scale of catheter size is measured in mm. A 16Fr silicone catheter is most commonly used in adults since smaller diameters tend to coil in the urethra. A larger size may be needed (e.g. 18Fr) if debris and infection is suspected. A size 22Fr will be needed for clot retention (see above). Long term catheters should be changed every 6 weeks to avoid blockage, encrustation and formation of stones in the catheter.

For male urethral catheterization:
- Retract foreskin to view urethral meatus
- Clean glans with sodium chloride 0.9 per cent or aqueous chlorhexidine
- Anaesthetize and lubricate with 10mL lignocaine 2 per cent gel via syringe
- Wait for a few minutes and gently pass catheter using aseptic technique. Resistance may be encountered at the level of the distal sphincter complex or bladder neck. Sphincter spasm will diminish in a few minutes. Asking the patient to cough, may facilitate passage of catheter
- A catheter introducer should only be used by experienced urological surgeons
- The female meatus may be difficult to identify and is often situated in the vaginal introitus or along the anterior vaginal wall
- Inflate catheter with required volume of water to prevent catheter dislodging

Urethral catheter problems[4]

- Trauma and false passages—refer to urological team
- Haematuria
- Infection is extremely common with long term catheterization. The incidence of UTIs is related to the duration of catheterization, bacteriuria developing at a rate of about 5 per cent per day of catheterization. Antibiotic treatment should be given if the patient is symptomatic (fever, urinary symptoms, delirium etc). Antibiotic prophylaxis should be used for catheter insertion and removal (gentamicin or ciprofloxacin) but this should be judged in relation to the individual clinical circumstances
- Bladder spasm—Caused by irritation of trigone of bladder by balloon. Often this is relieved by removing water from the balloon, although most long-term silicone catheters have only a 10mL balloon and there is the risk that the problem will not be solved and the catheter will fall out. Antispasmodics (e.g. oxybutynin) may be helpful
- Blockage may occur from debris or clots. Flushing the catheter with antiseptic (0.02 per cent chlorhexidine) or sodium chloride 0.9 per cent may relieve the situation but at the risk of encouraging further infection. This decision will depend on the particular clinical circumstances
- Bypassing is due to a blocked catheter or bladder spasm

- Paraphimosis—failure to reposition foreskin may lead to constriction causing swelling and pain of glans penis. Reduction with gentle squeezing pressure over 1/2 hour using swab soaked in 50 per cent dextrose may allow foreskin repositioning
- Undeflated balloon—if the balloon will not deflate to allow removal of the catheter, it will need deflating with a wire, usually under ultrasound control

Suprapubic catheter

A suprapubic catheter is indicated if passing a urethral catheter has failed. This may be due to a stricture, obstruction due to intrinsic or extrinsic compression or distorted anatomy of the urethral meatus due to tumour or lymphoedema. It may also be used as an alternative to a urethral catheter in a patient with an unstable bladder in whom the balloon is constantly irritating the trigone. A suprapubic catheter is contra-indicated in clot retention.

For suprapubic catheterization:

- The distended bladder is palpated suprapubically
- Patient placed with foot of bed raised
- The skin is infiltrated with lignocaine 1 per cent about two finger breadths above the pubis in the midline and urine aspirated with a 21G needle
- A suprapubic catheter is inserted using an aseptic technique. A pigtail (e.g. Bonanno) catheter may be needed as a short term measure if the patient is not well enough for transfer for the more appropriate insertion of a 16Fr silicone catheter, which should be sited by a urologist
- Caution: Midline scar, previous pelvic surgery, unsuccessful urine aspiration with needle. In these situations, the insertion should be under ultrasound control

Intermittent self catheterization[5] is unusual in patients with palliative care needs. It may be used in patients with a neuropathic bladder e.g. after spinal cord compression. Clean catheter insertion at least four times daily frees patients from indwelling urinary catheterization, gives them control, and prevents renal damage from urinary retention. Patients need to be highly motivated, have manual dexterity and be well enough to perform the task. Refer to incontinence advisor for counselling/instruction.

General management of catheters

Catheters (especially suprapubic) need skin protective agents around the base of the catheter to stop leakage spilling directly onto the skin. Secretions around the catheter site should be removed with soap and water. Over-granulated areas can be removed with silver nitrate. Meatal cleaning around urethral catheters is necessary since secretions are increased due to urothelial irritation. The secretions form crusts which, when removed, form areas of exposed damage which are prone to bacterial colonization and can then ascend into the bladder.

4 Zylicz Z., Krajnik M. (1999) Improvement of transurethral catheterization in male patients. *Palliative Medicine*, **13**: 261–2.

5 Hunt G., Oakeshott P., Whitaker R. (1996) Intermittent catheterisation: simple, safe, and effective but underused. *BMJ*, **312**: 103–7.

Genito-urinary fistulae

Fistulae (abnormal communications between two hollow viscera or viscera and body surface) are common in patients with advanced cancer, causing considerable morbidity and distress. They may be associated with previous radiotherapy and are managed where possible, and appropriate for the clinical circumstances, with bypass surgery.

General management includes:
- Meticulous skin protection—barrier creams, e.g. zinc and castor oil, sudocrem or cavilon (applied as a spray or stick protector and dries to form a protective membrane). Lutrol gel (solidifies when warmed in contact with skin, forming a protective layer) is not commercially manufactured but some hospital pharmacies may be able to prepare it
- Water absorbent pads or tampons
- Treatment of odour: Metronidazole 400mg t.d.s. may reduce odour from anaerobic infection. Charcoal dressings and charcoal placed in the room may have some effect. Masking the smell with lavender oil etc. has been tried but is often ineffective

Vesicoenteric fistulae

A fistula may develop between the bladder and any segment of bowel. The cause in palliative care is usually colonic malignancy, although diverticulitis or small bowel inflammatory disease may also be responsible. Vesicoenteric fistulae rarely occur secondary to bladder pathology. A characteristic symptom is pneumaturia (passage of gas or froth in the urine) and there may also be a foul odour to the urine, persistent urinary tract infections and the presence of faecal matter in the urine (especially with large fistulae). Cystoscopy, contrast cystography or intestinal barium studies will normally demonstrate the fistula. Ideally, the management is surgical removal of the segments of bowel and bladder, together with repair of the bowel and bladder. Otherwise a bypass procedure may be performed, a colostomy or ileostomy may provide complete relief. Some patients may be too unwell for surgery or prefer not to have a stoma.

Vesicovaginal fistulae

These are characterized by a continuous leakage of urine from the bladder into the vagina and needs to be distinguished from total urethral incontinence. Intravenous urography will identify a ureterovaginal fistula and a cystogram will identify a vesicovaginal fistula. Cystoscopy and retrograde ureterography may be helpful. Surgical excision provides the most effective solution but is often not feasible. Urinary diversion, e.g. ileal conduit, may be necessary if the patient is well enough, but this a formidable undertaking in patients who have had radiotherapy. Bilateral nephrostomy is a potential but radical alternative. As ever the advantages and disadvantages of procedures need discussing with the patient.

Sexual health in advanced disease

Patients with palliative care needs who are very ill and symptomatic may not be interested in sexual intercourse, although they may want to maintain intimacy with their partner. Discussions of sexuality issues may be very helpful for patients and their partners.

Background

- Individuals with advanced cancer may remain sexually active
- Problems may be physical, psychological or relational and are frequently multifactorial and complex
- Many sexual problems are solvable
- Patients with cancer often fear transmission of cancer (especially genito-urinary) to their partner or partners fear contracting cancer themselves
- Patients often find it difficult to ask for help and are embarrassed, fearing that professionals might see sexual difficulties as frivolous in the context of serious disease. They also assume that nothing can be done
- Healthcare professionals without specialist knowledge find it difficult to address this area since they too may be embarrassed

General Issues

- Lack of libido in both sexes can be caused by: Change in body image (surgery to /disfigurement of face, presence of stoma etc.), depression, relationship problems, hormone deficiency, drug related side-effects (see below)
- Physical problems such as breathlessness, weakness and pain may lead to difficulties, some of which may be addressed. Catheterization does not preclude sexual intercourse, a male catheter may be folded inside a condom

Issues for males:

- Impotence:
  - Drug causes (see below)
  - Disease/treatment effects: Spinal cord compression, pelvic malignancy, pelvic surgery/radiotherapy, orchidectomy, brain neoplasm
  - Concurrent disease: Diabetes, peripheral vascular disease, age-related
  - Psychological: Fear of failure to acquire or maintain erection for fear of experiencing or causing pain
- Treatment:
  - Stop or change medication
  - Discuss trial of sildenafil with urologist. Patients with psychogenic ejaculatory dysfunction, spinal cord injury, nerve-sparing prostatectomy and hypertension may get a response of approximately 80 per cent. Absolute contra-indications include the use of nitrates, liver impairment, hypotension and recent stroke or myocardial infarction (MI). Relative contra-indications include poor libido, history of priapism (may be associated with myeloma, sickle cell disease and leukaemia), bleeding disorders and active peptic ulceration

- Intercavernosal drugs (prostaglandin E), vacuum devices and prosthetic implants may very rarely be appropriate for selected patients in palliative care

Issues for females:
- Lack of libido:
  - Change in body image: disease/surgery of breast, genitals, reproductive organs. Associating gynaecological cancer with 'punishment' for previous lifestyle. Fear of pain on intercourse
- Dyspareunia:
  - Vaginal dryness: Lack of oestrogen, infection e.g. candidiasis, vaginal stenosis following radiotherapy or surgery
  - Post-pelvic surgery, pelvic tumour, pelvic infection
- Treatment:
  - Local oestrogen creams, HRT, treat infections, lubrication using KY jelly, use of vaginal dilators post-surgery/radiotherapy (needs to be started early and used persistently), encouragement of regular intercourse to maintain vaginal passage

Approach to management:
- Pre-treatment counselling, regarding sexual issues, may help to avoid problems
- Exploration of issues with open questions: e.g. 'has your disease affected the way you view yourself?'...'has it affected your relationships?'...while allowing the patient to guide the consultation into more specific areas
- General patient information literature available
- PLISSIT model framework for exploring/managing sexual problems
- Referral for further counselling with specialists who will have information/skills addressing this area. Psychosexual counsellors are available for complex situations

Drugs associated with sexual dysfunction
- Antihypertensives
  - Thiazide diuretics
  - Beta-blockers
- Psychotropic drugs
  - Phenothiazines e.g. levomepromazine
  - Butyrophenones
  - Anxiolytics and hypnotics
  - Antidepressants
- Endocrine drugs
  - Antiandrogens
  - Oestrogens
  - Gonadorelin analogues
- Other
  - Recreational drugs
  - Digoxin
  - Spironolactone
  - Ranitidine
  - Metoclopramide
  - Carbamazepine

Further reading

Books

Back I. N. (2001) *Palliative Medicine Handbook*. 3rd edition. Cardiff: BPM Books.

Norman R. W., Bailly G. (2004) Genitourinary problems in palliative medicine. In D. Doyle, G. W.C. Hanks, N. MacDonald (eds) *Oxford Textbook of Palliative Medicine*, 3rd edn, pp. 647–58. Oxford: Oxford University Press.

Tomlinson J. (ed.) (1999) *ABC of Sexual Health*. London: BMJ Books.

Twycross R., Wilcock A. (2001) *Symptom Management in Advanced Cancer*. 3rd edn. Oxford: Radcliffe Medical Press.

Articles

Gujral S., Bell R., Kabala J., Persad R. (1999) Internal iliac artery embolisation for intractable bladder haemorrhage in the perioperative phase. *Postgraduate Medical Journal*, **75**: 167–9.

Hunt G., Oakeshott P., Whitaker R. (1996) Intermittent catheterisation: simple, safe, and effective but underused. *British Medical Journal*, **312**: 103–7.

Law C. (2001) Sexual health and the respiratory patient. *Nursing Times*, **97**: NT Plus XI–XII.

Mercadante S. (1992) Treatment of diarrhoea due to enterocolic fistula with octeotide in a terminal cancer patient. *Palliative Medicine*, **6**: 257–9.

McCoubrie R., Jeffrey D. (2003) Intravesical diamorphine for bladder spasm. *Journal of Pain and Symptom Management*, **25**: 1–2.

Penson R., Gallagher J., Gioiella M., Wallace M., Borden K., *et al.* (2000) Sexuality and cancer: conversation comfort zone. *Oncologist*, **5**: 336–44.

Wilsey N., Ashford N., Dolin S. (2002) Presacral neurolytic block for the relief of pain from pelvic cancer. *Palliative Medicine*, **16**: 441–4.

Zylicz Z., Krajnik M. (1999) Improvement of transurethral catheterization in male patients. *Palliative Medicine*, **13**: 261–2.

Further reading (Chapter ...)

Palliation of head and neck cancer

Basic epidemiology and pathology

General background

Head and neck cancer makes up about 3 per cent of all cancer deaths in the UK. It is more common in men and occurs more commonly in France, Italy, Poland, Thailand, and the Indian subcontinent than in the UK. Common primary sites include the oral cavity, pharynx, larynx, paranasal sinuses and salivary glands. Presentation is commonly with pain, hoarseness, recurrent sinusitis and a 'lump' in the neck.

Prognosis

About 50 per cent of patients overall are cured while 50 per cent die of their disease, though the mortality varies widely according to site, histology, stage at diagnosis and degree of tumour differentiation. Early recurrence after primary treatment is a bad prognostic sign. Most patients who survive two years without recurrence are likely to be cured. Second primaries are common, occurring in perhaps one in eight patients, and are associated with a poor prognosis. There are two possible explanations for the high frequency of second primaries:

- **Field change:** Carcinogens produce widespread epithelial changes which easily develop into malignancy
- **Clonal expansion and migration** of malignant cells

Common aetiological factors include:

- Smoking
- Alcohol

These two factors are synergistic and are the strongest factors in the causation of head and neck squamous cell carcinomas (HNSCC).
Tumours at particular sites also have specific risk factors e.g.:

- Betel nut chewing and vitamin deficiencies for oral cancer
- Nickel, hardwood dusts for airways tumours
- Epstein–Barr virus in nasopharyngeal carcinoma
- Iron deficiency: Patterson–Brown–Kelly syndrome (iron deficiency, koilonychia, glossitis, upper oesophageal web) associated with postcricoid carcinoma
- Familial: increased risk of head and neck squamous cell carcinoma if there are two or more first degree relatives with HNSCC

Histology

Most tumours are **squamous cell carcinomas**. This has a number of implications:

- often moderately chemosensitive but not curable with chemotherapy

- tend to develop hypercalcaemia. This is usually due to the secretion of parathyroid hormone related peptide (PTHrP), which causes mobilization of calcium from bone and reduction in the excretion of calcium by the kidneys

Less common tumours include adenocarcinomas, adenoid cystic carcinomas (salivary glands), anaplastic carcinomas, lymphomas, melanomas of the mucosa and other rare tumours.

Staging

Squamous cell carcinoma tends to progress from local disease, along lymph node levels in a stepwise manner to distant disease quite late. This allows radical treatment to be staged (see below). Treatment has now improved so substantially that the cause of death is changing: whereas forty years ago, only a small proportion died of disseminated disease, as local control has improved distant metastases are the cause of death in perhaps a third of patients, and are found in many others.[1] This has obvious implications for the likely problems to be encountered and the management of the terminal phase.

The patient with head and neck cancer

> In the face of such overwhelming statistical possibilities, hypochondria has always seemed to me to be the only rational position to take on life.
> John Diamond (died of carcinoma of the base of the tongue),
> *Because Cowards Get Cancer.*

In cancer of the head and neck, both disease and treatment can cause disfigurement and major communication problems. Many of the vital functions of life such as breathing and eating are threatened, and the patient may run the risk of severe bleeding. Understandably, the psychological toll can be considerable.

Many, though far from all, patients with head and neck cancer will have a history of heavy alcohol and tobacco use, which may indicate poor coping strategies in difficult situations. It is important to obtain a psychiatric history, as past events may predict the reaction to new problems. Those with a history of heavy alcohol intake may also have poor family and social networks to fall back upon and sometimes very damaged close relationships. This must be kept in mind in assessment, rehabilitation and discharge planning, in order to provide adequate psychosocial support for the patient and their family.

- **Adjustment reactions:** can occur around the time of surgery or other treatment as well as when function alters rapidly in advanced disease. They can take the form of anxiety, depressive reactions or mixed states. Adjustment reactions are commoner and more marked if severe disfigurement or communication problems are anticipated. They often settle with time particularly in a supportive environment, but need active management if severe
- **Depression:** has been found in over half the patients with advanced disease. Diagnosis can be more difficult in cancer as the 'classical' physical signs (anorexia, disturbed sleep and fatigue) are also prevalent in cancer itself. Counselling and antidepressants may be needed

- **Suicidal ideation risk:** is said to be considerably higher than with other cancers. A professional psychiatric assessment should be sought if the risk is judged to be significant
- **Anxiety:** may be general or related to specific fears of the airway becoming blocked, or of an impending serious bleed. Underlying fears need to be addressed and consideration given to counselling, cognitive therapy, relaxation training and/or anxiolytic medication
- **Alcohol withdrawal:** can cause confusion and agitation and benzodiazepines may be necessary

Tumour treatment: implications for the palliative phase

While these tumours may metastasise (most commonly to the lungs), they also tend to recur locally. Given the site of these tumours, local relapse may cause major palliative problems. Primary therapy is directed at maximizing local control.

Surgical treatment

Where feasible, surgical resection of the tumour offers the best chance of long term local control and cure. Surgery often involves resection of large amounts of tissue; it may be cosmetically disfiguring and cause a number of functional problems including swallowing and speech difficulties. Postoperative support and a multidisciplinary approach with input from speech therapists, dieticians and physiotherapists will be needed. Surgical treatment operates on the principle that HNSCC spreads in an orderly manner through successive lymph node groups. En bloc dissection removing the tumour, lymph nodes and intervening lymphatics should therefore give the best chance of control. The extent of disease-free margin which needs to be excised varies from tissue to tissue: if a tumour involves bone (e.g. mandible), muscle (e.g. tongue) or submucosal soft tissue and lymphatics (e.g. hypopharynx), it requires wide excision even if the tumour itself is quite small. Furthermore, excision of structures invaded by tumour may be needed. Therefore major reconstruction is frequently required involving skin, muscle, and bone with the use of flaps, as well as prostheses. This can preserve appearance and function to an impressive extent for many patients.

Another important consequence is that salvage surgery, e.g. for recurrence after radiotherapy, usually has to be quite radical to give any chance of long term benefit to the patient. It is important to be radical when a substantial improvement in prognosis, function or quality of life is the goal but also to desist when the benefits are limited compared to the severe cost to the patient. This requires addressing issues such as quality of life and body image with the patient.

The treatment of neck nodes is a central issue in such burden/benefit equations.

- Cervical nodal metastases are found in 40 per cent of patients with HNSCC at diagnosis
- Radiotherapy can 'sterilize' small neck nodes or those from certain tumours (nasopharynx, thyroid) effectively, but surgery is needed in other cases

1 Taneja C., Allen H., Koness R. J., Radie-Keane K., Wanebo H. J. (2002) Changing patterns of failure of head and neck cancer. *Arch Otolaryngol Head Neck Surg*, **128**: 324–7.

- Radical neck dissection removes all the nodes on that side, sternomastoid muscle, internal jugular vein and the spinal accessory nerve, which supplies the trapezius and sternomastoid. This is effective but disabling, and more limited forms of neck dissection are now employed when appropriate, often associated with radiotherapy or chemotherapy

Radical radiotherapy often retains function better than surgery but causes other problems, such as mucositis and subsequently dry mouth (xerostomia). Tissue fibrosis makes later salvage surgery in the face of recurrence hazardous, and occasionally damage to other structures such as the spinal cord occurs.

Radiotherapy can be delivered by *external beam or brachytherapy* (radioactive implants, such as needles in the tongue). Various fractionation regimes are used. Fractionation into a larger number of small doses reduces adverse effects, but very prolonged radiation regimes can reduce effectiveness. *Hyperfractionation*, in which several small doses are given each day, is sometimes given in the hope of better disease control. In addition radiotherapy can be given preoperatively (neo-adjuvant), postoperatively (adjuvant), or as an accompaniment to chemotherapy.

Palliative radiotherapy is used for patients with inoperable tumours or those who are unfit for surgery and may also be used as an adjunct to surgery, particularly where resection has been incomplete.

Since the need to achieve local tumour control is so important, patients are frequently treated on 'radical' radiotherapy schedules even when the treatment is palliative in intent. Such treatments are associated with a high incidence of acute toxicity including oral mucositis, odynophagia, (pain or eating) loss of taste and dry mouth. This is particularly problematic in this population of heavy smokers and drinkers. Again, input from a wide range of professionals is essential to support patients through treatment.

Radiotherapy is also used for bone pain, dysphagia or stridor from paratracheal nodes, or bleeding or infection from fungating tumours.

Chemotherapy treatment
Chemotherapy is potentially curative in some tumours, such as lymphomas, but never in HNSCC. Nevertheless, adjuvant or neo-adjuvant chemotherapy has a place alongside surgery and/or radiotherapy. Platinum-based regimes may provide some palliation in fit patients with metastatic or locally advanced disease.

Specific head and neck cancers (with emphasis on advanced disease)
Oral cavity tumours site
- anterior two-thirds of tongue
- lips
- buccal mucosa
- alveola
- hard palate
- floor of mouth
- retromolar trigone

Oral cavity tumours are the most frequent head and neck cancers. They are usually well differentiated SCC, but tumours of minor salivary gland origin are also seen. Spread is predominantly local and to nodal groups in a stepwise manner. Larger tumours are more likely to have spread and have a poor prognosis. Midline tumours metastasize quickly to deeper cervical nodes and hence further afield. Anterior tongue carcinomas have an uncanny tendency to spread or recur despite adequate primary treatment.

Oral tumours can initially be treated with surgery, with or without radical neck dissection. Radiotherapy (external beam or brachytherapy) often gives equivalent results, with less functional impairment, but causes mucositis and xerostomia. Excellent dental care is essential with radiotherapy in order to avoid dental sepsis which can contribute to osteoradionecrosis. Tumour relapse or tumours which are advanced at presentation, require extensive surgery with major reconstruction. Late disease or treatment may cause dysarthria, dysphagia if the tongue is not mobile, and local ulceration. A third of patients with tongue tumours develop multiple primaries.

Carcinoma of the sinuses

Paranasal sinus malignancies (maxillary, ethmoid, frontal, sphenoid) are commonly well differentiated squamous cell tumours. They present late, with local swelling, pain and ocular, nasal or palatal or dental symptoms depending on the site of origin. Treatment is usually surgical with extensive reconstruction for cosmesis, followed by radiotherapy.

Salivary gland tumours

Malignancy is suspected if a parotid mass is associated with facial palsy, or if a salivary gland mass is rapidly growing, hard and infiltrative.

- **Adenoid cystic carcinoma** is the commonest salivary cancer. It is slow growing and ulcerative. It is the tumour most likely to spread along perineural sheaths, which can lead to nerve palsies and neuropathic pain. It also infiltrates marrow cavities and it may be difficult to demonstrate its true extent
- **Adenocarcinomas** often have a relatively good prognosis because of their differentiation
- **Squamous cell carcinomas** are more aggressive, cause pain, and metastasize early. They are more often metastatic from another cancer than primary
- **Undifferentiated carcinomas** progress rapidly, and may mimic sarcomas
- A small proportion of **pleomorphic adenomas** become malignant

Management is usually surgical, with radiotherapy for residual or recurrent disease, high grade tumours or lymphomas. The facial nerve may be involved by tumour or sacrificed at operation.

Malignant melanoma occurs most commonly on the hard palate but also occurs on the lower jaw, lips, tongue or buccal mucosa. It is infiltrative and metastasizes early to lymph nodes. It often ulcerates and bleeds.

Carcinoma of the larynx Carcinoma of the larynx, and its recurrence, may present with voice changes, dysphagia or stridor.

- Glottic (vocal cord) carcinoma is commonest. Nodal metastases occur late, because the cords have poor vascularity and lymphatic drainage, and the main determinant of prognosis is the T stage. Initial treatment consists of radiotherapy, which preserves function, or surgery which is equally successful but may cause voice changes, although the voice is often preserved with more conservative treatment. Combined radiosurgical or radiochemotherapeutic approaches are often needed in advanced disease

- Supraglottic carcinoma presents late, with vague dysphagia, referred ear pain, or cervical lymphadenopathy. Hoarseness may signify involvement of the vocal cords or adjacent structures. Progression is by local extension (to oropharynx, especially posterior third of tongue, hypopharynx, or glottis) or lymph node spread. Treatment is commonly radical radiotherapy. Surgery may have to be radical (total laryngectomy[2]), and to be used in certain settings such as airway obstruction. Radical neck dissection may be warranted. Voice restoration has to be considered after total laryngectomy (📖 see Chapter 10e)

- Subglottic carcinomas are rare but highly invasive. Pyriform fossa tumours behave like supraglottic tumours and have a poor prognosis. Postcricoid tumours may be associated with iron deficiency (Patterson–Brown–Kelly syndrome) and invade the hypopharynx circumferentially. Radiotherapy, radical surgery and chemotherapy have a rôle in management, depending on exact site and stage

Carcinomas of the pharynx are usually squamous cell, though lymphomas are fairly common, especially in the tonsils and nasopharynx

- Nasopharyngeal carcinomas cause nasal obstruction, epistaxis, and otitis media from eustachian tube obstruction. Lower cranial nerve palsies from base of skull extension, or third, fifth and sixth nerve palsies from cavernous sinus invasion, signify advanced disease. Growth into the posterior orbit also takes place. Some varieties of nasopharyngeal carcinoma have a tendency to haematogenous spread. Radiotherapy is the treatment of choice, giving as good results as *radical* neck dissection. Radiotherapy unless meticulously planned, very occasionally causes damage to the upper spinal cord. Xerostomia is common from salivary gland irradiation. Chemotherapy is sometimes very effective. Late recurrences (over two years) can be retreated

- Oropharyngeal carcinomas (posterior tongue, soft palate, fauces, tonsils, pharyngeal wall) frequently present late. They produce dysarthria, pain and risk of aspiration. Radical radiotherapy is usual, but extensive surgery with radical neck dissection followed by radiotherapy may be indicated in locally advanced disease

- Hypopharyngeal carcinomas are uncommon but present late and have a poor prognosis. Aggressive treatment has therefore to be used judiciously

2 Ward E. C., Bishop B., Frisby J., Stevens M. (2002) Swallowing outcomes following laryngectomy and pharyngolaryngectomy. *Arch Otolaryngol Head Neck Surg*, **128**: 181–6.

Symptoms in head and neck malignancy

Pain

Pain is widely prevalent in head and neck cancers, particularly in advance disease. Diverse anatomical structures are compressed or invaded b tumour within in a small space. Thus pains are often mixed somatic (bone muscle, skin) and neuropathic. 📖 See Chapter 6a.

Sources of pain in cancer of head and neck

- Local tumour infiltration e.g. ulceration, infection
- Vascular and lymphatic occlusion producing oedema/ lymphoedema
- Bone invasion or extension of soft tissue infection causing osteomyelitis
- Nerve involvement or pressure: adenoid cystic carcinoma in particular (but to a lesser extent most head and neck tumours) can show perineural invasion and extension
- Referred pain is very common e.g. earache from most structures in the face, neck and mouth
- Treatment related e.g. chemotherapy or radiotherapy-induced mucositis

Approach to pain assessment[3]

1 Take a detailed history of pain, with special emphasis on character, exacerbating factors and accompanying dysfunction. Functional disturbances are not only clues to diagnosis but also need treatment in their own right, since they are distressing and disruptive to the patient.
2 Examine head and neck for masses and deformities.
3 Check movement of involved joints.
4 Carry out cranial nerve assessment.
5 Occasionally radiology or other tests are helpful in elucidating the cause of pain.

📖 See Table 6h.1, pp. 346–7 for specific pain syndromes.

Further pain management options

Tumour mass reduction by surgery, radiotherapy or chemotherapy is usually the best way of reducing pain.

Radiotherapy is particularly useful for bone metastases e.g. base of skul

Steroids e.g. dexamethasone 4–8mg p.o. mane may contribute to ana gesia by reducing swelling inside restricted fascial spaces. They can also be useful temporizing measure while effective doses of other agents fo neuropathic pain are being titrated upwards.

Antibiotics can relieve pain by reducing pressure due to infection tight fascial compartments, e.g. osteomyelitis.

Nerve blocks are often difficult due to the distorted anatomy followi disease or treatment.

3 Vecht C. J., Hoff A. M., Kansen P. J., de Boer M. F., Bosch D. A. (1992) Types and causes of pain in cancer of the head and neck. *Cancer*, **70,** 1: 178–84.

The key in managing pain in patients with head and neck malignancy is careful assessment and differentiating as clearly as possible the nature of the pain/pains involved

Mouth problems in head and neck cancer (☐ see Chapter 6b)

Head and neck cancer and its treatment are associated with severe oral problems. Contributory factors include:

- smoking and alcohol
- dry mouth: medication, treatment
- poor dental hygiene (made difficult by intraoral mucosal tenderness or friable tumour)
- infection and bleeding from fungating tumours
- trismus restricting mouth opening
- vitamin deficiencies associated with poor nutrition
- underlying osteomyelitis

Dry mouth (xerostomia) is extremely common and is due to:

- radiotherapy involving salivary glands
- antimuscarinic drugs, opioids
- blocked nose leading to open-mouth breathing
- dehydration, including diuretics

Xerostomia leads to many problems. Taste is diminished, appetite reduced, food becomes more difficult to swallow, and intraoral infections and dental caries become much more likely.

Management includes:[4]

- dental hygiene, ☐ see p. 238. May occasionally require specialist advice
- adequate hydration
- general measures e.g. sucking on fruit drops, pineapple chunks
- synthetic saliva e.g. saliva orthana (little evidence of effectiveness in these circumstances)
- simple sialogogues e.g. salivix tablets
- pilocarpine tablets[5] or eye drops instilled in the mouth (can induce sweating or gastrointestinal complaints)
- treating underlying causes when possible and reviewing medication

Drooling usually indicates either a problem with swallowing saliva or a mass in the mouth, such as an infected fungating tumour. It is also associated with poor lip closure, as in facial palsy.

Management:

- Antimuscarinic drugs e.g. transdermal or sublingual hyoscine, tricyclic antidepressants
- Occasionally the underlying problem may be treatable e.g. resuspension surgery with poor lip closure—rarely indicated in late stage

Seikaly H. (2003) Xerostomia prevention after head and neck cancer treatment. *Arch Otolaryngol Head Neck Surg*, **129**: 250–1.

Table 6h.1 Specific pain syndromes

Syndrome	Location/features	Causes	Notes
Shoulder syndrome	Pain in shoulder, difficulty with certain movements e.g. putting on jacket	Radical neck dissection (due to axillary nerve sacrifice/damage)	Patient can only abduct arm to 75° and flex arm to 45°
Trigeminal neuralgia-like syndrome	Lancinating, continuous/paroxysmal. Distribution of Va, Vb and/or Vc, not crossing midline, though very occasionally bilateral	Middle/posterior fossa tumours Base of skull metastases Meningeal metastases	Trigger areas on activities such as chewing, talking, breeze of air May be accompanied by neurological signs +/- diplopia, dysarthria, dysphagia, headache
Glossopharyngeal neuralgia	Severe unilateral paroxysmal pain in throat or beneath the angle of the jaw, may radiate to ear, often precipitated by swallowing	Meningeal metastases Disease around jugular foramen Local disease around the base of tongue or oropharynx	Occasionally associated with syncope or postural hypotension.
Jugular foramen syndrome	Pain occiput to vertex, ipsilateral shoulder or neck	Base of skull metastases Meningeal metastases	Horner's syndrome, lower cranial nerve signs +/- local tenderness Worse on head movement

Clivus syndrome	Vertex of head, worse on head flexion +/- VIn.–XIIn cranial nerve signs	Base of skull metastases Meningeal metastases	
Orbital syndrome	Retro-orbital/frontal headache	Orbital metastases Meningeal metastases Metastases around sella turcica, with sphenoid bone or cavernous sinus invasion	+/- diplopia, visual loss, proptosis, extraocular nerve palsies
Sphenoid sinus metastases	Bifrontal headache radiating to both temples, intermittent retro-orbital pain	Base of skull metastases: sphenoid sinus tumour Meningeal metastases	+/- nasal stuffiness, diplopia, VIn. Palsy
Occipital condyle invasion	Severe occipital pain exacerbated by movement	Occipital condyle invasion	+/- XIIn. Palsy

Sticky, viscous saliva is a much commoner problem than appreciated, and is more troubling than the actual volume of saliva.
- It is a frequent complication of radiotherapy, as serous salivary glands are more sensitive to its effects than the mucous glands
- Unfortunately antimuscarinics, in addition to reducing the volume of saliva, also render it more viscous
- Beta-blockers can make saliva less viscous

Antibiotics for intraoral infections and frequent meticulous oral hygiene appear to help. It is important to ensure adequate hydration

Mucositis usually follows radiotherapy or chemotherapy with certain agents e.g. 5-fluorouracil, methotrexate or cyclophosphamide. There are reports of reduction of mucositis by treating intraoral infections, suggesting that bacteria and fungi play a rôle in its genesis.[6] Treatment usually requires a combination of analgesics and topically applied local anaesthetic or anti-inflammatory agents. Benzydamine, an anti-inflammatory with local anaesthetic properties, is often used as a mouthwash and has been claimed to reduce the duration of mucositis. Sucralfate may also be useful, but a recent Cochrane review shows that neither of these two drugs nor chlorhexidine are significantly effective. On the other hand, allopurinol and vitamin E appear to be useful,[7] although the evidence is again weak.

Tracheostomy

A tracheostomy is a surgical opening in the anterior wall of the trachea for providing a patent airway.

Tracheal stoma—post laryngectomy

Patients may have a permanent tracheal stoma if they have had a laryngectomy (e.g. for carcinoma of the larynx). In this case the tracheal cartilages are brought to the surface of the skin and sutured to the neck as an end tracheostomy. The rigidity of the cartilage should keep the stoma open and a tracheostomy tube will not normally be needed. Since there is no connection between the trachea and pharynx, there is no risk of aspiration and the patient may eat safely (provided that any voice prosthesis, if used is safely *in situ*—see later). Apart from removing the function of speech laryngectomy also removes the function of the nose, which normally provides heat and humidity to the inhaled air, filters the air and increases breathing resistance. An artificial heat and moisture exchanger 'nose' may be applied over the stoma to redress these problems reducing mucus coughing and psychosocial problems; air enters and exits through side openings of this device which can therefore easily be covered by clothing. The 'nose' may also have a valve that can be digitally occluded to improve maximum phonation time and dynamic voice range. A small number of patients with a stoma may need a tube or a button device to maintain patency of the stoma.

Tracheal stoma (without laryngectomy)

Patients may have a temporary tracheal stoma, either fashioned as a emergency or as a more elective procedure while waiting for a definitive surgical procedure. The patient will have a tube and in the palliative care setting, there may be no plans or possibilities of reversing the stoma and recreating a natural airway, usually because of persistent tumour in the upper airways. In this case, the trachea and upper airways are still intact, albeit probably partially obstructed. If the larynx is not adequately protected on swallowing, there is the potential for aspiration of pharyngeal contents into the lungs and a cuffed tube may be required. An outer tube remains *in situ* for a variable length of time according to the particular circumstances; a silver tube may remain *in situ* indefinitely. A non-metal tube will be used during a course of radiotherapy to the neck to avoid excessive radiation skin reactions and also during MRI scanning.

Types of tube

There are a variety of tracheostomy tubes all suited for different specific purposes. Cuffed tubes are usually used in theatre or for an emergency situation, the aim of the cuff being to prevent air escaping around the tube during mechanical ventilation and to reduce the risk of aspiration.

However, prolonged cuff inflation causes ischaemic damage to the tracheal wall. Prevention requires frequent pressure checks and periods of cuff deflation. Apart from some high aspiration-risk patients (in whom cuffs should be inflated for oral intake), all patients seen in general wards, palliative care settings or the home environment are almost certain to have *uncuffed* tubes.

Essential warnings about cuffed tracheal tubes

1 For resuscitation, the cuff must be inflated for bag ventilation to be effective. In most palliative care patients, of course, resuscitation may be inappropriate.

2 If the tracheostomy is occluded e.g. by secretions or a decannulation cap, and the balloon is inflated, the airway will be totally blocked and the patient will suffocate. Open the cap, deflate the balloon or remove the tracheostomy tube immediately.

Voice prosthesis

Patients with a laryngectomy may have a voice prosthesis. This is a one-way silicon valve that slots into a surgically created fistula connecting the trachea to the pharynx. Air is expelled from the lungs, up through the trachea, and then passes through the valve into the pharynx. When the patient wants to speak, the airflow causes the pharyngeal muscles to vibrate producing the voice. Since it is a one-way valve, pharyngeal contents should not be able to pass through the valve and cause aspiration.

Johnson J. T., Ferretti G. A., Nethery W. J., Valdez I. H., Fox P. C., Ng D., Muscoplat C. C., Gallagher S. C. (1993) Oral pilocarpine for post-irradiation xerostomia in patients with head and neck cancer. *New England Journal of Medicine*, **329, 6**: 390–95.

Spijkervet F. K. L., van Saene H. K. F., van Saene J. J. M., Panders A. K., Vermey A., Mehta D. M. (1990) Mucositis prevention by selective elimination of oral flora in irradiated head and neck cancer patients. *Journal of Oral Pathology and Medicine*, **19**: 486–9.

Clarkson J. E., Worthington H. V., Eden O. B. (2004) Interventions for treating oral candidiasis for patients with cancer receiving treatment. *The Cochrane Database of Systematic Reviews*, **1**.

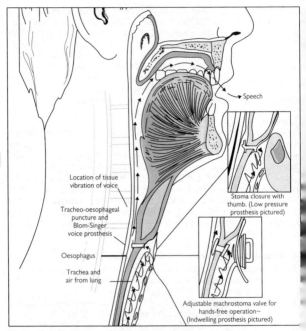

Figure 6h.1 Tracheo-oesophageal voice prosthesis

Care of voice prosthesis

The valve should be cleaned gently every day using a specialized brush and flush applicator to remove debris. Some patients are troubled by candida and may need frequent valve changes but others may be able to leave the valve in for 6 to 8 weeks. The valve will need to be changed if leaking occurs through the valve (which will be obvious if the patient coughs on eating or drinking) or if there is leakage around the valve or if the patient finds that voice cannot be generated. The valve is usually left *in situ* during a course of radiotherapy. Occasionally the prosthesis, which is normally held in place with a silicon retention collar, is dislodged accidentally on coughing or during cleaning. In this situation the patient should lie down and an introducer (which the patient should have) or, alternatively, a size 14 Foley catheter should be inserted into the fistula while a replacement prosthesis is being organized, this prevents aspiration through the fistula into the lungs and stops the fistula closing.

uidance for trachesotomy care

Good communication and patience. The patient knows his/her own tracheostomy better than anyone else!

Find out the type of stoma i.e. Post laryngectomy or not

Find out the type of tube e.g. cuffed/uncuffed, fenestrated/unfenestrated, disposable inner tube, speaking valve

Check for risk of interference with tube function. Obese or fatigued patients who have difficulty extending the neck are at risk of occluding tubes and posture/position needs to be checked. Water must not enter the stoma and patients need to fix an adhesive covering before showering

Most tubes now have a removeable inner tube which almost always prolongs the life of the outer tube, which will need changing at about 30 days (instead of 7–14 days with a single lumen tube). It also allows easy cleaning which reduces the risk of occlusion and infection. The inner tube should be removed, inspected for encrustation and cleaned regularly at least once a day, the timing depending on the needs of the individual. It should be cleaned with liquid detergent and hot running water and pipe brushes, cleaners or sponges should be avoided. If secretions are thick or crusted the inner tube should be cleaned with sodium bicarbonate first and then with hot running water

Changing the outer tube (usually at about 30 days if used with inner cannula). Make sure that the replacement outer tube is the same size as the one to be replaced and that a smaller sized tube and tracheal dilator are available if necessary, since a stoma may close over. Some tubes have a lock to ensure that the inner tube cannot be displaced and a click should be expected as the inner tube is reinserted into the outer tube

Suctioning—A suction catheter, that is no bigger than half the size of the tube, should not be inserted to more than one-third of its length, should not make the patient cough and should not be used for longer than a few seconds. Suction pressure should be no more than 100–120mm/Hg (13.5 and 20kPa). A sterile technique should be used and the catheter and gloves disposed after single use. If suctioning through a fenestrated tube, ensure there is a non-fenestrated inner cannula *in situ* to avoid sucking the tracheal mucosa into the fenestrations

Avoiding infections—clean stoma site with normal saline using aseptic technique and ensure area is clean and dry before applying any dressings

Humidification should be used with oxygen or air. Encourage patient to wear a bib sprayed hourly with water, particularly if they do not have a heat/humidifier exchanger. Regular normal saline nebulisers (via the tracheal stoma) may be needed to keep the mucosa healthy

Secretions. Any change in the colour or odour of secretions may need antibiotic treatment. Forceps may be needed to remove thick encrusted plugs of mucus

Signs of problems with tracheostomy

- Stridor
- Bleeding
- Increasing thickness and volume of sputum
- Difficulty expectorating

If these develop, consult specialist ear, nose and throat teams and/or speech and language therapist.

Swallowing problems specific to patients with head and neck cancer[8]

Swallowing requires:

- good lip closure: prevents food leakage
- teeth: break food down
- mobile tongue: crushes bolus and pushes it back into pharynx
- saliva: lubrication
- an intact palate
- functioning cheek musculature to avoid food collecting in gingival sulcus
- intact oral and pharyngeal musculature and innervation (cranial nerves V, VII, IX, X, XI, XII)

Remember innervation:

- lingual nerve (V), supplies sensation
- chorda tympani (VII) supplies taste to anterior two-thirds of the tongue
- glossopharyngeal (IX) supplies sensation and taste to posterior third of the tongue
- hypoglossal (XII) supplies tongue musculature

A tongue lacking sensation produces more long-term swallowing difficulties than a tongue with restricted mobility. Obstruction by a mass or dysfunction (muscle dysfunction, nerve damage), pain, dry mouth or tooth loss all contribute to dysphagia.

Improving swallowing: Perhaps the commonest cause of difficult swallowing is dry mouth— see Chapter 6b)

Manoeuvres to help improve swallowing

- chilled food helps re-educate lost sensation e.g. after surgery
- encouraging the patient to chew or even just manipulate the bolus in the mouth for a few seconds facilitates initiation of the swallow reflex
- alternating temperature, taste and texture of food in a meal keeps awareness of the swallowing process high
- carbonated drinks increase sensation of the liquid bolus
- placement of food boluses in parts of the mouth where sensation is still intact
- viscous boluses e.g. thickened liquids and purées, permit poorly coordinated muscles to mount a more effective swallow than thin liquids
- head or body tilting in the appropriate direction can utilise gravity in the swallowing process or protect the airway

the patient at risk of aspiration?

ints include:
Wet or gurgling noises with breathing: fluid in the airways
Altered voice during eating: food on vocal folds
Cough associated with swallowing
Fatigue during a meal: leads to prolonged meal times
Lower cranial nerve palsies
Aspiration pneumonia

eek a speech and language therapy (SALT) assessment if appropriate,
onsidering the patient's clinical state.

educing risk of aspiration

The patient should not eat unattended.
The patient should eat sitting up. Tilting the body or head may be
useful, the direction depending on the exact disability.
Avoid distractions during meals.
Consider thickening fluids (e.g. Thick n'Easy) if thin fluids cause
coughing, or other ways of increasing bolus viscosity.
Techniques that may reduce aspiration depend on the particular situation:
• Turning head towards the paralysed side of the face or tongue
  encourages the passage of food down the competent side
• Flexing neck while eating
• Double swallowing
• Supraglottic or super-supraglottic swallow: a SALT will teach
  these techniques

Gastrostomy

A gastrostomy is used for feeding when it is necessary to bypass the
mouth. In head and neck cancer this happens with dysphagia, severe oral
ain, or in some cases of chronic aspiration.

Nasogastric tubes

Nasogastric tubes can be used for feeding for up to four weeks, but
eyond that, gastrostomies are preferable.
In the normal course of events, poor nutritional status parallels disease
rogression. With aggressive feeding through a gastrostomy, a patient may
emain surprisingly well for a time only to be more aware of the gradual
isintegration of their body through infected fungating wounds, total
ysphagia with excessive dribbling, bleeding, pain and other symptoms.
he pros and cons of ongoing management should be discussed regularly
ith patients.

Kendall K. (1997) Dysphagia in head and neck surgery patients. In R. Leonard, K. Kendall K (eds)
ysphagia Assessment and Treatment Planning: A team approach, pp. 19–27. San Diego, CA:
ngular Publishing Group.

Communication problems

Head and neck cancer and its treatment impair communication in various ways:

- dysarthria e.g. tongue fixed by tumour
- laryngectomy
- recurrent laryngeal nerve palsies
- loss of facial expression: VII palsy, facial disfigurement
- kissing: tumour/body image problems
- reception of communication by others: hearing or visual impairment

Studies show that up to 92 per cent of patients with head and neck cancer have difficulties with speech. This has been found in surveys to be the single most important correlation with quality of life after treatment.

Production and articulation of speech

The vocal cords produce sound which is then modified by the action of tongue, lips and mouth to produce intelligible speech. For example good lip closure is needed to say 'p' or 'b' while a mobile tongue is necessary to produce 't' and 's'. Thus problems with any part of this apparatus can produce difficulties with intelligible speech.

Laryngectomy

This produces the most profound speech deficit, as the production of sound is removed. Various techniques have been developed to address this:[9]

- oesophageal speech is produced by swallowing air and then expelling it while mouthing the necessary sounds. Various techniques can be taught by a speech therapist. Only 25–50 per cent of patients master this technique, and it is useless in noisy environments or communicating from any distance
- Speaking valves e.g. Blom-Singer valve: an opening is made between the airway and oesophagus, and a valve is fitted which allows oesophageal air to be used to produce sound. Fluency rates of 70–90 per cent have been reported. However, the dynamics of sound production may change again if there is major local disease recurrence
- Electrolarynx: this produces clear intelligible words, although in an 'electronic' voice. It occupies one of the patient's hands to keep it against the neck while talking

Recurrent laryngeal nerve palsy

This causes hoarseness if unilateral which sometimes worsens as the day wears on.

- Bilateral nerve palsy reduces the voice to a whisper
- The recurrent laryngeal nerves are motor to the intrinsic muscles of the larynx and also supply sensory fibres to the mucosa below the level of the vocal folds. Therefore in bilateral palsy the sphincter effect of the vocal folds during swallowing is lost and aspiration can result. The aspiration will not be noticed by the patient due to the sensory loss, and the risk of aspiration pneumonia is high
- Bilateral abductor paralysis can also produce stridor which needs urgent attention

Techniques for treating vocal fold palsies

Behavioural techniques and biofeedback may be taught by speech therapists

Injection of Teflon, fat or collagen into a paralysed vocal fold

More invasive techniques (thyroplasty, arytenoid adduction, reinnervation, vocal cord lateralisation) are very rarely indicated in patients with advanced disease

Patients who aspirate from bilateral vocal fold paralysis are temporarily helped by vocal fold injection. More extensive surgery is unlikely to be indicated in this patient group with end-stage illness

Articulation difficulties result from:

tongue problems: glossectomy, tumour

facial palsy

dry mouth

poor lip closure

poor control of jaw movement: e.g. V nerve palsy

defect in palate (excision) or teeth

other lower cranial nerve palsies: base of skull metastases

How to communicate with patients with articulation problems

(Remember to involve the speech therapist)

- Choose a quiet place where you can hear better
- Sit in a position where you can see the patient talk. Make sure there is enough light to see properly
- Sit close enough to hear
- Take time to get 'tuned in'
- Encourage use of gestures which give useful clues to the meaning
- If necessary, remind patient to keep sentences short and uncomplicated
- Encourage the patient to articulate each syllable clearly but not to overarticulate
- Learn lip reading
- Encourage the family to participate
- Be aware of range of procedures on offer

Remember Lack of fluency does not just result in loss of ability to speak. Patients are often embarrassed into reducing their communication so that the *content* of speech also becomes poorer and deals only with the concrete. These patients need time to express their deeper thoughts, and utilization of alternative means of communication. Also think about non-verbal expression: e.g. art therapy, which can often express feelings better than words.

Blalock D. (1997) Speech rehabilitation after treatment of laryngeal carcinoma. *Otolaryngologic Clinics of North America*, **30, 2**: 179–88.

Infection and fistulae

Local infection has devastating consequences in advanced tumours:
- septicaemia
- cancer wound extension
- pain—from inflammation, pressure build-up within fascial spaces, erosion into adjacent tissues, maceration e.g. of skin by exudates
- fistula formation
- vascular erosion: catastrophic bleeds
- cachexia in unchecked sepsis
- thick saliva—heavy intraoral exudate makes speech and breathing difficult
  - Osteomyelitis, particularly in the jaw, is common and produces discharging sinuses, pain, and tooth loss. Necrosis may be particularly extensive in irradiated bone
  - Base of skull infections spread via the *retropharyngeal space* to the anterior mediastinum, (the cervical vertebrae are protected by thick fascia). Such infections are, however, commonly caused by tuberculosis
  - Submental space infections (Ludwig's angina) cause pain, high fever, trismus and hypersalivation. Floor of the mouth swelling occasionally causes respiratory obstruction

Treatment
- Most infections are caused by anaerobic bacteria, and Gram positive cocci which are commensals in the mouth. Gram negative organisms are less frequent
- Options include metronidazole and a penicillin, or clindamycin (concentrates in bone but associated with pseudomembranous colitis), or a third generation cephalosporin
- Antibiotics have an indispensable rôle in analgesia and reduction of intraoral exudates enabling the patient to communicate and breathe easily, often for the first time in months
- The conditions which encourage the infection in the first place usually persist, and continuous prophylactic low dose antibiotics may be worth considering. There is little trial evidence for this, but clinical experience suggests that it is an effective ongoing symptomatic measure

Fistulae

Once formed, fistulae remain patent because:
- The wound is continuously discharging exudate that is usually infected, e.g. bone sequestrate in chronic osteomyelitis
- The chemical composition of the exudate prevents healing—e.g. saliva

In palliative care there is usually an untreatable deep necrotic tumour but treatable situations such as drainable abscesses and osteomyeliti should be considered. Exudate or saliva bathing the great vessels continu ously (e.g. fistulae between oropharynx and skin), will increase the risk c catastrophic bleeding. This should be avoided by:
- Dressings
- Drying up saliva—see p. 345
- Continuous antibiotics

Applying a silicone elastomer plug to fit a fistula associated with a large wound. Unfortunately, malignant fistulae enlarge, so this plug will need to be renewed regularly. Such plugs are only used in single, clean, open cavities. Plugging complex cavities impedes drainage, extending deep infection and encouraging new fistulae to form where they can drain freely

Specific pain problems in patients with head and neck cancer

- **Neuropathic pain** affecting the head and neck and radiating to the upper arm is not uncommon. This can be the result of direct compression of nerves by the tumour or a result of treatment. There may be associated hypersensitivity of the skin and oral mucosa, which may be so severe that the patient is unable to tolerate even a light breeze or chewing soft food. The pain syndromes are often complex and only partially respond to opioids. Adjuvant analgesia in the form of antidepressant and/or anticonvulsant medication is usually needed. Specialist advice is frequently needed to maintain symptom control, especially as compliance with medication may be a problem

- **Dysphagia** due to direct compression of a tumour mass or lymphadenopathy often means that feeding gastrostomies are needed to maintain nutrition and to allow the administration of medication, as the oral route may no longer be available. There may be ethical dilemmas, particularly with regard to the administration of feeds in the last days of life

- **Other problems** The tumour or the surgery performed often adversely affects a patient's *body image* in a site which is hard to hide from public view. Patients often become *socially isolated* as they feel disfigured and become reluctant to go out and socialize. *Depression* is a common feature. Relationship problems are not uncommon

- **Difficulties with articulation and speech production** are common. The quality of the voice may change significantly and make the patient self-conscious. All these problems need the regular input of specialist speech and language therapists. Communication aids may be needed after major surgery to enable a patient to express their needs and preferences

- **Fungating and malodorous tumours** can cause considerable distress. Radiotherapy may help in some cases, especially where there is bleeding. Topical antibiotics may help along with regular dressings sensitively applied to maintain dignity, covering the most disfiguring parts of the tumour. Tumours are often infected with anaerobic organisms for which appropriate antibiotics including metronidazole may be appropriate. The use of deodorizers in the patient's room may help to disguise the smell of the infected tissue

- **Major haemorrhage**. Patients with progressive tumours near the large blood vessels of the neck are at risk of a sudden massive bleed. This is rare, but difficult to manage and the early involvement of specialists should be considered

Emergencies

Catastrophic bleeds (partly based on British Association of Head and Neck Oncology Nurses guidelines)[10].

These are among the most feared complications of cancer of the head and neck, although they are rare.

Risk factors

- Previous neck irradiation
- Fungating tumour invading the artery
- Postoperative: flap necrosis
- Infection
- Salivary fistula
- Systemic factors, such as malnutrition, cachexia, elderly patients

Warning signs

- Minor bleeding from wound, tracheostomy or mouth
- 'Pulsations' from artery or tracheostomy or flapsite—false aneurysm formation
- Sternal or high epigastric pain several hours before rupture of carotid
- The patient may become restless and irritable

Management

1 If the patient is thought to be at risk, discuss a plan within the multidisciplinary team. Can the risk be reduced by e.g. embolization or ligation of the implicated artery?
2 What should the patient and family be told?

> ### To tell or not to tell about potential bleeding?
> Consider:
> - Bleeds are often feared but rarely occur
> - No preparation for a very severe bleed can make it any less frightening
> - Can anything be done to reduce the risk of bleeding e.g. embolization?
> - Are there special circumstances e.g. children in the house who would be especially traumatised by a catastrophic bleed?
> - Is the patient doing anything that might increase the risk e.g. neglecting an infection in a dangerous area?
> - Warning bleeds or other severe risk factors which would indicate that a major bleed is more likely?

If the patient or family ask specifically about what might be expected, this needs to be discussed, giving information in small steps and letting them decide how much they want to know. It is also useful to ask in a general way if they have any special fears about how the patient will die, as this may bring out unspoken fears. Otherwise one needs to be careful not to raise fears of unlikely complications which are terrifying and about which little can be done.

Checklist

- Stop anticoagulants, aspirin, NSAIDs (COX-2 inhibitors may be safe)—though this will make no difference to a major bleed. Correct any platelet abnormalities if warning bleeds occur

Treat infection

Ensure the family, and staff, know who to contact in an emergency

Have emergency sedative drugs in the home: e.g. diamorphine, midazolam

Ensure all professionals involved know the plan e.g. district nurses, GP etc.

If in a hospice or hospital, nurse patient in a side room to avoid potential distress of other patients or relatives

Discreetly have available blue/green towels, gloves, apron

If there is a bleed, a senior member of staff must stay with the patient. Nothing is as reassuring as a calm human presence, nothing as frightening as panic. Call for help

Be respectful of the family's wishes about whether or not they wish to stay with the patient. Support them

Apply towels to bleeding site and absorb the bleeding if possible

Apply gentle suctioning to mouth and trachea as necessary

Give i/v or i/m midazolam e.g. 10mg, repeated in 10–15 minutes if necessary. Subcutaneous drugs are poorly absorbed in shock

Occasional families might be taught to administer rectal diazepam or buccal midazolam. Few will be calm enough to do this, and the extra responsibility may be too much for them to cope with in most cases

After the event, debrief family and staff, and point them in the direction of their normal supportive networks. Extensive counselling just after an event has actually been shown to be more likely to do harm than good

Offer family and staff (including non-clinical involved staff, such as domestics who have witnessed the incident) a chance for a follow-up meeting later to deal with any questions they might have

Tracheostomy tube obstruction

Causes

Infection

Excessive mucus production

Pressure sores

Tube displacement

Granulation tissue

Management

Call for help

Reposition patient to semi recumbent position

Ask patient to cough, use suction

Manipulate head to eliminate tube kinks

Give oxygen

Remove inner tube

Suction

Resuscitate if appropriate

If severe problems, sedate the patient

BAHNON website: *www.bahnon.org.uk*

Body image and sexuality

Slade[11] defined *body image* as the picture we have in our minds of the size, shape and form of our bodies, and our feelings concerning these characteristics and our body parts. This makes it clear that body image includes appearance but goes far beyond it; perceptual and subjective aspects of body image are deeply intertwined.

Indeed, some suffer from a deep dissatisfaction with their body, despite very minor or no disfigurement, whereas others with very major disfigurement have a very healthy self-image.

Perhaps surprisingly for some, there is little gender or age difference in the impact of appearance changes on body image. The degree to which people can be rehabilitated after facial disfigurement also does not depend on the degree of disfigurement, but correlates with perceived social support and with the degree of dysfunction.

Factors which have been associated with poor body image include:
• Poor self-esteem
• Social anxiety
• Self-consciousness
• Depressive features

Sexuality is a closely related field. One study found how, a year after head and neck surgery, marital and sexual relationships were still suffering and alcohol use (a marker of depression, particularly in men) was still high in very significant number of patients. Almost half of patients at least a year after treatment in another small study had problems with libido, arousal sexual activity; a significant minority still never or almost never kissed and held hands with their partner.

Questions about body image and sexuality feel difficult and embarrassing to raise, yet MUST be explored. Sometimes a broad question can be asked which the patient will often interpret as referring to their sexual relationship if it is preoccupying them:
• How has this affected your relationship with your wife/husband?
• What things that really matter to you do you miss?
• How did you feel about yourself after the operation?

Often a more direct approach, which tells the patient that it is all right to talk about issues of sex and intimacy, is needed:
• How did your husband/wife cope with the change in your appearance after the operation?
• What impact did it have on your sex life?
• How have you dealt with that as a couple?'

Normalizing embarrassing fears in this manner is one important step dealing with them.

Body image and sexuality depend more on perceived social support and the existence of supportive relationships than on the degree of disfigurement or disability. This again brings one back to one of the central though often unsaid, tenets of palliative care: that ultimately what matters most to people is being cared for and respected and loved.

ere is now good work showing how, after cancer treatment, social habilitation through a simple behavioural approach is effective. Medical ff play an important rôle by modelling attitudes and allowing patients to actice new behaviours in a safe environment. For example, patients can trained to prepare a number of responses for when people inevitably mment to them about their appearance, or when they walk into a pub d everyone stares.

Changing Faces, a UK charity, runs courses to help patients manage this d has published very useful educational material.[12]

The situation in advanced cancer, where appearance is rapidly worsing rather than static as after surgery, and is accompanied by generalized dily deterioration and by a shrinking social world, has not been plored properly yet.

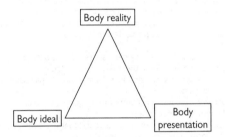

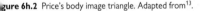

gure 6h.2 Price's body image triangle. Adapted from[13].

Price, one of the early writers about body image, presents a useful triangle body reality, body presentation and body ideal which offers a programme r working on improving body image. Thus for example, prosthetic work or constructive surgery can improve appearance or 'body reality'; makeup d choice of clothes can improve 'body presentation'; and counselling and rhaps the presentation of rôle models can tackle 'body ideal'.

Slade P. D. (1994) What is body image? *Behaviour Research and Therapy*, **32**: 497–502.

Clarke A. (2000) *Psychosocial Rehabilitation After Head and Neck Cancer—A resource for health fessionals.* London: Changing Faces. www.changingfaces.co.uk

Price B. (1990) A model for body-image care. *Journal of Advanced Nursing*, **15**: 585–93.

General medical problems in patients with head and neck cancer

When one recalls that the main risk factors for head and neck cancer are smoking and alcohol, it is not surprising that concurrent medical problems are common in these patients.

- Malignancies in other organs: these are common,[14] particularly lung, but also other smoking or alcohol-related tumours: bladder, kidney, pancreas, liver. This may both have physical consequences to the patient, for example due to metastatic disease from a distant malignancy, and have psychological morbidity. Patients are also more prone to other primary head and neck cancers
- Ischaemic heart disease: patients will be less tolerant of anaemia
- Alcohol-induced cardiomyopathies: may limit the use of some agents for neuropathic pain
- Cerebrovascular accident: if this is present in addition to neurological damage from the tumour, marked disability can result
- Chronic obstructive airways disease: airways problems from head and neck cancer can precipitate decompensation and respiratory failure
- Thromboembolic disease: may necessitate difficult decisions in continuing anticoagulation if there is a risk of bleeding. Sometimes conversion to heparin will allow more rapid control if bleeding occurs
- Alcoholic liver disease: may contribute to clotting problems or to altered handling of medication
- Nutritional deficiencies: from poor diet, dysphagia, alcohol, cachexia
- Psychiatric problems: depression, anxiety
- Substance abuse: watch out for alcohol withdrawal in particular
- **Syncope** is common among patients with cancer of the head and neck.[15] This may be carotid sinus syncope from metastatic compression or post-radiotherapy fibrosis. (Glossopharyngeal neuralgia can lead to sinus arrest, perhaps as intense glossopharyngeal nucleus stimulation overflows to the vagal nucleus leading to parasympathetic suppression of the cardiac pacemaker)

Many patients will have been on high doses of steroids for prolonged periods. In any crisis or period of physiological stress, steroids may need to be increased or restarted.

14 Crosher R., McIlroy R. (1998) The incidence of other primary tumours in patients with oral cancers in Scotland. *British Journal of Oral and Maxillofacial Surgery*, **36, 1**: 58–62.

15 MacDonald D. R., Strong E., Nielsen S., Posner J. B. (1983) Syncope from head and neck cancer *J Neuro-Oncology*, **1**: 257–67.

Further reading

Books

Close L. G., Larson D. L., Shah J. P. (1998) *Essentials of Head and Neck Oncology*. NY: Thieme.

Leonard R., Kendall K. (eds) (1997) *Dysphagia Assessment and Treatment Planning: A team approach*. San Diego, CA: Singular Publishing Group.

Watkinson J. C., Gaze M. N., Wilson J. A. (2000) *Stell and Maran's Head and Neck Surgery*, 4th edn. Oxford: Butterworth Heinemann.

Articles

Chua K. S. G., Reddy S. K., Lee M. C., Patt R. B. (1999) Pain and loss of function in head and neck cancer survivors. *Journal of Pain and Symptom Management*, **18, 3**: 193–202.

Forbes K. (1997) Palliative care in patients with cancer of the head and neck. *Clinical Otolaryngology and Allied Sciences*, **22, 2**: 117–22.

Endocrine and metabolic complications of advanced cancer

Understanding the association between endocrine and metabolic complications in advanced cancer is increasingly complex as knowledge of the processes involved at the genetic and biochemical level grows.

Malignancy produces endocrine effects in two ways:

Directly interferes with the function of endocrine glands by invasion or obstruction.

Remotely produces effects without direct local spread—paraneoplastic syndromes

Paraneoplastic syndromes are caused by:

- Tumour cells secreting hormones, cytokines and growth factors
- Normal cells secreting products in response to the presence of tumour cells (such as antibodies in the Lambert–Eaton syndrome)

Paraneoplastic syndromes

Hypercalcaemia

Cushing's syndrome

Syndrome of inappropriate antidiuresis

Hypoglycaemia (Non-islet cell)

Carcinoid syndrome

Non-paraneoplastic

Diabetes mellitus

Hypercalcaemia (📖 see Chapter 15, emergencies in palliative care)

Hypercalcaemia is the commonest life-threatening metabolic disorder associated with advanced cancer. In addition, as it is a condition which is usually amenable to treatment and untreated it is both distressing and fatal, hypercalcaemia must always be sought in patients who are deteriorating for no clear cause.

Epidemiology

Ten per cent of patients with cancer develop hypercalcaemia

Malignancy is responsible for 50 per cent of the patients with hypercalcaemia who are treated in hospital

Up to 20 per cent of patients develop hypercalcaemia without bone metastases

Most patients with hypercalcaemia of malignancy have disseminated disease—80 per cent will not survive beyond one year

The prognosis is poor with a median survival of three to four months

Table 6i.1 Clinical features of hypercalcaemia of malignancy

General	Gastrointestinal	Neurological	Cardiological
Dehydration	Anorexia	Fatigue	Bradycardia
Polydipsia	Weight loss	Lethargy	Atrial arrhythmias
Pruritus	Nausea	Confusion	Ventricular arrythmias
	Vomiting	Myopathy	Prolonged P-R interval
	Constipation	Seizures	Reduced Q-T interval
	Ileus	Psychosis	Wide T waves

Treatment

Rehydration followed by the administration of calcium-lowering agents is the mainstay of treatment. Drugs promoting hypercalcaemia (thiazide diuretics, Vitamins A and D) should be withdrawn.

The corrected serum calcium should be calculated from the formula

$$\text{Corrected calcium} = \text{measured calcium} + [(40 - \text{serum albumin g/L}) \times 0.02]$$

Intravenous fluids

Dehydration due to polyuria and vomiting is a prominent feature of acute or symptomatic hypercalcaemia. While large fluid volumes will lower serum calcium, calcium levels will seldom return to normal by rehydration alone and care to avoid fluid overload must be taken.

Rehydrating with 2–3 l/day of fluid is now accepted practice, with daily serum electrolyte measurement to prevent hypokalaemia and hyponatraemia developing. There is little evidence that there is any benefit in using diuretics in conjunction with rehydration and they should be avoided.

Corticosteroids

While steroids have been shown to inhibit osteoclastic activity and calcium absorption from the gut in vitro, their use *in vivo* is limited. They are most effective in haematological malignancies when oral prednisolone 40–100mg/day is usually effective.

Bisphosphonates

These synthetic pyrophosphate analogues reduce bone resorption by inhibiting osteoclastic activity. They are highly effective at reducing hypercalcaemia, but take 48 h to be effective. Infusions of bisphosphonate following rehydration are the mainstay of hypercalcaemia treatment.

Oral bisphosphonates have been used for maintenance therapy, but low bioavailability and gastrointestinal side-effects have limited their widespread use. Oral Ibandronic acid 50mg orally daily is increasingly used. Tablets should be swallowed whole with plenty of water while sitting/standing 30 minutes before breakfast or other medication. Many patients still receive monthly infusions as outpatients to maintain calcium levels within the normal range.

Twenty per cent of patients with hypercalcaemia of malignancy will be resistant to bisphosphonate infusion therapy.

- Disodium pamidronate 30–90mg/over 2–4 h
- Zoledronic acid 4mg over 15 minutes

Clodronate 1.5 g over 4h
Ibandronic acid 2–4 mg i/v 1–2 h

The newer more expensive zoledronic acid (4mg) has been found to achieve a normal corrected calcium in more patients, faster, and for longer (4–6 weeks).

Calcitonin

Calcitonin inhibits osteoclastic bone resorption and encourages calcium excretion. It is effective in around a third of patients and usually causes a fall in calcium within 4 h.

Doses of up to 8 IU/kg of salmon calcitonin can be used subcutaneously every 6 h. It is rarely used in palliative care.

Plicamycin (Formerly mithromycin)

This cytotoxic antibiotic blocks RNA synthesis and is toxic to osteoclasts. Given as an i/v infusion of 25mg/kg over 2 h it will produce normocalcaemia within three days in 80 per cent of patients. It is now rarely used due to its cumulative nephrotoxicity and hepatic toxicity.

Cushing's syndrome

Ectopic secretion of corticotrophin (ACTH) by non-endocrine tumours is rare

Associated pro-peptide secretion is more common producing a more complex mosaic of symptoms

Up to 20 per cent of Cushing's syndrome is caused by ectopic ACTH, often from an occult tumour

Fifty per cent of ectopic ACTH secretion is due to small cell lung carcinoma

Fifteen per cent of ectopic ACTH secretion is due to carcinoid and neural crest tumours

Long term survivors of malignancies with associated ectopic ACTH secretion will often continue to have elevated ACTH levels

Clinical features

Hypokalaemic metabolic alkalosis	Mental changes
Weak muscles	Glucose intolerance
Oedema	Weight loss
Raised blood pressure	

The more classical features of Cushing's syndrome e.g. truncal obesity moon facies and striae may suggest a benign tumour such as bronchial carcinoid or thymoma.

Investigations

Increased free urinary cortisol
Loss of diurnal variation of plasma cortisol
Failure of cortisol suppression in low dose (2mg) dexamethasone test
Failure of cortisol to suppress ACTH levels following high dose dexamethasone (2mg q.d.s. or 8mg nocte)

When the above investigations are still equivocal, more complex imaging techniques are available at specialist centres.

Treatment

The mainstay of treatment is inhibition of steroid synthesis.

Aminoglutethimide

At low doses (125mg b.d.), aminoglutethimide inhibits the enzyme arc matase which converts androgens to oestrogens, (hence its use in patient with post-menopausal breast cancer). At the higher doses (1.5–3.0g/day which are needed in Cushing's syndrome, however, aminoglutethimid blocks the production of glucocorticoids, mineralocorticoids and androger but produces unpleasant side-effects such as ataxia, sedation and rashes.

Metyrapone

250–750mg q.d.s. inhibits 11 β-hydroxylase, the final enzymatic step in steroi production, but again side-effects (nausea and vomiting) are common. In a effort to reduce drug toxicity, aminoglutethimide 250mg b.d. and metyrapon 250mg q.d.s. may be used in combination. The use of ketoconazol bromocriptine and octreotide have also been advocated in case reports.

Treatment efficacy should be monitored by measuring 24h urinar cortisol excretion. As levels return to normal, hormone replacemer therapy, as in Addison's disease, may be required, (e.g. hydrocortisone 20m at 0800 and 10mg at 1800 h with fludrocortisone 0.05–0.15mg daily).

Syndrome of inappropriate antidiuresis (SIAD)

Hyponatraemia is common in patients with advanced malignancy due t many factors including cardiac and hepatic failure, hyperglycaemia diuretics and sick cell syndrome. The presence of concentrated urine i conjunction with hypo-osmolar plasma, however, suggests abnormal fre water excretion and the presence of the syndrome of inappropriate anti diuresis. (The SIAD acronym is more appropriate than SIADH, as there i no vasopressin hormone secretion in approximately 15 per cent of cases)

The vasopressin gene codes for peptide products including arginin vasopressin (AVP) and vasopressin-specific neurophysin II (NP II). I malignancy-related SIAD, tumours secrete ectopic AVP.

SIAD is most frequently associated with small-cell lung carcinoma o carcinoid tumours but has also been noted in pancreatic, oesophagea prostatic and haematological cancers.

Causes of SIAD

- Ectopic AVP
- Infections
- Pulmonary, meningeal and cerebral
- Drugs

Morphine, phenothiazines, tricyclic antidepressants, NSAIDS, vincristine cyclophosphamide

Clinical features

Significant symptoms of hyponatraemia develop at plasma sodium leve below 125mmol/L with confusion progressing to stupor, coma an seizures. Nausea, vomiting and focal neurological signs may also develop.

The clinical features depend on both the levels of plasma sodium and th rate of decline. With gradual falls the brain cells can compensate against cere bral oedema by secreting potassium. Asymptomatic hyponatraemia sugges chronic SIAD whereas symptomatic hyponatraemia suggests acute SIAD.

Diagnosis

Essential criteria

Plasma hypo-osmolality (plasma osmolality <275 mosmol/kg H_2O and plasma sodium <135 mmol/L)

Concentrated urine (with plasma osmolality >100 mosmol/kg H_2O)

Normal plasma/extracellular fluid volume

High urinary sodium (urine sodium >20 mEq/l) on a normal salt and water intake

Exclude (i) hypothyroidism, (ii) hypoadrenalism, and (iii) diuretics

Supportive criteria

Abnormal water load test (unable to excrete ->90 per cent of a 20 mL/kg water load in 4h, and/or failure to dilute urine to osmolality -<100 mosmol/kg H_2O).

Management

Management depends on the rate of onset of symptoms and neurological complications.

Acute symptomatic hyponatraemia has a mortality of 5–8 per cent and patients will need prompt correction with intravenous hypertonic saline with meticulous monitoring, as over rapid correction can lead to central pontine myelinosis with quadriparesis and bulbar palsy.

Chronic asymptomatic hyponatraemia is best treated with fluid restriction. In effect this means reducing dietary input or urinary output to less than 500mL/day, which may take several days to produce an effect. This may not be appropriate in the terminal care setting, when patients may prefer to eat and drink what they like without strict regimes.

Drug treatments involve the use of distal nephron inhibitors preventing water reabsorption (e.g. demeclocycline) and oral osmotic diuretics (e.g. urea).

Demeclocycline (desmethylchlortetracycline) inhibits vasopressin and causes nephrogenic diabetes insipidus: 900–1200 mg/day will reverse chronic SIAD over 3–4 days and should be followed by a maintenance dose of 600–900mg/day.

Side-effects include gastrointestinal disturbances, hypersensitivity reactions and reversible nephrotoxicity.

Urea is effective in controlling SIAD by both intravenous and oral routes. Oral urea, 30g dissolved in orange juice to mask the taste, is the daily dose. (Using urea obviates the need to fluid restrict the patient.)

Non-islet cell tumour hypoglycaemia

Hypoglycaemia in malignancy is often associated with beta cell tumours which secrete insulin. More rarely, non-islet cell tumours produce hypoglycaemia by increased tumour usage of glucose, secretion of insulin-like growth factors (IGFs) (formerly somatomedins) and disruption of the balance maintaining normal homeostasis.

Increased use of glucose by tumours has been clearly documented with daily consumption sometimes reaching levels of 200g/kg per day. Hepatic glucose production may also fall, and suppression of compensatory growth hormone and glucagons also contribute to the hypoglycaemic state.

In advanced malignancy the commonest cause of hypoglycaemia is oral hypoglycaemic medication.

Epidemiology

Insulin-secreting tumours are usually large (average 2.4kg), often retroperitoneal or intrathoracic with liver invasion. The tumours may be growing over a relatively longer time course than many other cancers (often several years).

- Approximately 60 per cent are mesenchymal tumours (mesothelioma, neurofibroma, leiomyosarcoma etc.)
  - Twenty per cent are hepatoma
  - Ten per cent adrenal carcinoma
  - Ten per cent are gastrointestinal tumours

Clinical features

Hypoglycaemic symptoms often do not appear until the terminal stage of the disease. Symptoms are associated with cerebral hypoglycaemia and the associated secondary response of catecholamine secretion. Neurological features include agitation, stupor, coma and seizures, usually following exercise or fasting and occur most often in the early morning or late afternoon. Other causes of hypoglycaemia should be excluded, such as overtreatment of diabetes.

Treatment

The reversal of symptomatic hypoglycaemia initially requires intravenous glucose infusion. Central lines may be needed for hyperosmolar glucose solutions. Up to 2000 g/day of glucose may occasionally be needed. Frequent feeding, including during the night, and steroids may be helpful.

Debulking surgery, arterial embolization of tumours or chemotherapy can all have a place in the palliation of tumor related hypoglycaemia.

Carcinoid syndrome

Carcinoid tumours are a diverse group of tumours of enterochromaffin cell origin. The incidence is 1.5 per 100,000. The carcinoid syndrome develops in up to 18 per cent of patients with such tumours and these patients almost invariably have hepatic metastases.

The commonest site of origin is the appendix (25 per cent) and rectum but they have also been reported in the pancreas, lungs, thymus and gonads. Tumours may be benign but 80 per cent greater than 2cm in diameter metastasize.

Clinical features

- Flushing and diarrhoea occur in at least 75 per cent of patients
- Cardiac manifestations involving the right side of the heart are late manifestations in a third of patients
- Wheeze/right ventricular heart failure (RVF) (tricuspid valve regurgitation +/−stenosis/pulmonary valve stenosis)
- Asthma and pellagra are less common

Clinical features are mediated by several active substances secreted by tumours including:
- Numerous vasoactive amines and hormones

- Serotonin (5-HT)   5-hydroxytryptophan (5-HTP)
- Prostaglandins
- Catecholamines
- Tachykinins (Substance P, neuropeptide K)
- Histamine

Alcohol or psychological stress may precipitate symptoms.

The features of carcinoid tumours vary by their sites of origin.

Table 6i.1 Comparison of carcinoid tumours by site of origin

	Foregut	**Midgut**	**Hindgut**
Site	Resp tract, pancreas, stomach, proximal duodenum	Jejunum, ileum, appendix, Meckle's diverticulum, ascending colon	Transverse and descending colon, rectum
Tumour products	Low 5-HTP, multihormones	High 5-HTP, multihormones	Rarely 5-HTP, multihormones
Blood	5-HTP, histamine, multihormones	5-HT, rarely ACTH, multihormones	
Urine	5-HTP, 5-HT, 5-HIAA, histamine	5-HT, 5-HIAA	Rarely 5-HT or ACTH
Carcinoid syndrome	Atypical	Frequently with metastases	Rarely occurs
Metastases to bone	Common	Rare	Common

5-HIAA, 5-hydroxyindole acetic acid

'Multihormones' include tachykinins, neurotensin, enkephalin, insulin, glucagons, glicentin, VIP, Somatostatin, pancreatic polypeptide subunit of human chorionic gonadotrophin.

Diagnosis is usually established by:
1 Measuring urinary excretion of 5-hydroxyindole acetic acid (metabolite of 5-HT)
2 Platelet 5-HT levels (unaffected by diet)

Tumour localization may be achieved with somatostatin scintography or PET scanning.

Palliative debulking surgery, hepatic artery embolization, and chemotherapy may be appropriate palliative treatment for selected patients, while symptomatic treatment of diarrhoea and wheezing using more traditional agents also have a place in the management of patients with advanced carcinoid tumours.

Ketanserin has been used in some centres, ameliorating flushing in 50 per cent but only 20 per cent relief of diarrhoea. Selective 5-HT$_3$ receptor inhibitors may reduce diarrhoea.

Table 6i.2 Pharmacological management of carcinoid syndrome symptoms

Drug	Mechanism	May reduce diarrhoea	May reduce flushing	Comments
Octreotide	150–1500 mcg/day			CSCI +/– alpha interferon
Lanreotide	30mg every 7–14 days i/m			
Sandostatin LAR	20mg–30mg every 28 days Somatostatin analogues	yes	yes	First line therapy. 80% Reduced hormonal output and blocks action. Effects diminish with time. Doses need to be adjusted after three doses Very expensive
Verapamil 40–120mg t.d.s./q.d.s.	Calcium channel blocker	yes	(?)	Limited value
Cyproheptadine 4–10mg t.d.s.	5-HT$_2$ antagonism +/– Anti-histamine	yes (60%)	yes (47%)	Mean duration of response 8 months Limited value

Non-paraneoplastic complications

The incidence of hyperglycaemia in patients with cancer is higher than in the general population. Several theories to account for this have been postulated:

1 Increased gluconeogenesis
2 Increased conversion of lactate to glucose
3 Diminished glucose tolerance
4 Insulin resistance
5 Increased use of medications such as corticosteroids promoting hyperglycaemia

These changes may arise as a result of liver damage, altered glucose metabolism by tumour cells, and secretion of insulin antagonists.

Diabetes mellitus

Management of diabetes in palliative care

A limited prognosis for a patient makes *close* control of blood glucose (aimed at reducing long-term sequelae) unnecessary, thereby allowing a less invasive/interventional approach.

Changes in the patient's condition (e.g. cachexia), infection or treatment (e.g. corticosteroids) commonly alter the diabetic treatment needed—the management may have to change rapidly over time.

Aims of control

1 To prevent symptoms
   • Maintaining the blood glucose at <15mmol/L is usually sufficient to prevent symptoms of hyperglycaemia (polyuria, thirst, nausea and vomiting, feeling 'unwell', drowsiness). Hyperglycaemic patients are susceptible to infection
   • A dry mouth is commonly due to drugs (morphine or antimuscarinics) and is not a good indicator of dehydration
2 To prevent hypoglycaemia occurring
3 To minimize intervention i.e. frequency of blood sugar measurement and number of injections

Hyperglycaemia in advanced malignancy

In addition to pre-existing diabetes mellitus (including previously undiagnosed cases, which may present in the terminal stages), there are two particular causes of hyperglycaemia that may occur in patients with advanced malignancy:

• corticosteroid-induced diabetes
• insulin deficiency/resistance in pancreatic cancer

Hypoglycaemia

Common clinical changes that occur in patients with advanced malignancy, leading to reduced insulin or oral hypoglycaemic requirements in pre-existing diabetics are:

• cancer cachexia in advanced illness (reduced body mass)
• reduced food intake due to anorexia, dysphagia, 'squashed stomach' or nausea/vomiting etc.
• liver replacement by tumour causing low glycogen stores and limited gluconeogenesis

Corticosteroids

Corticosteroids are commonly used in advanced malignancy. They have a direct metabolic hyperglycaemic effect, but may also increase appetite, sometimes dramatically.

Hyperglycaemia is a dose-related effect in any patient (one in five patients on high doses will develop steroid-induced diabetes), but there is wide variability between patients in their response. The hyperglycaemia is usually asymptomatic and requires no therapy unless polyuria or polydipsia develop, in which case a short acting sulphonylurea (e.g. gliclazide) may be useful. The dose of steroids should be reduced to the minimum possible.

Treatment options for diabetes

Oral hypoglycaemic drugs

- Gliclazide is a short acting hypoglycaemic. It may be given once or twice daily at a starting dose of 40–80 mg mane
- Increase as required to a maximum total dose 160 mg b.d.
- Avoid metformin in patients with advanced cancer

Insulin

Is sensible to use only two or three insulins, such as:
- human insulin zinc suspension (mixed) (human monotard), insulin glargine long-acting half-life
- human isophane insulin (human insulatard or humulin I) medium-acting half-life
- human soluble insulin (human actrapid or humulin S) short-acting half-life

Use either:
- a single dose of human monotard daily (given at bedtime), or
- isophane insulin: two-third daily dose mane, 1/3 rd dose nocte

If converting from mixed insulin regime (e.g. isophane + human soluble insulin) to single daily human monotard:
- calculate the total daily insulin requirement
- reduce the dose by approximately 20–30 per cent to account for the conversion
- adjust the dose as necessary if blood glucose has been high or low
- give this dose once daily as human monotard

For a patient who has been uncontrolled on oral hypoglycaemics, start with human monotard 10u daily.

Insulin glargine, a human insulin analogue with a prolonged duration of action has been introduced and is given once daily in patients with type 1 diabetes.
- NICE guidelines (December 2002)
- Insulin glargine is not recommended for routine use with type 2 diabetes unless:
  - Patient requires assistance with injecting
  - Recurrent symptomatic hypoglycaemia
  - Need twice daily basal injections in addition to twice daily oral anti-diabetic drugs

Initiating treatment in new diagnosis hyperglycaemia

- Restrict diet *if overeating*: do not impose a strict diet on a patient with advanced illness. It is more important to try and achieve a regular caloric input from one day to the next
- Reduce dose of corticosteroids if appropriate
- Consider infection as a factor causing the hyperglycaemia
- Thin, cachectic patients are less likely to respond to oral hypoglycaemic drugs, and insulin should be considered early if not responding to simple measures e.g. gliclazide 80 mg o.d.
- If the patient is peripherally vasoconstricted, give insulin by i/m route, rather than SC

Sliding scale insulin regimen

Monitor blood glucose and give soluble insulin SC as indicated. 8-h if patient not eating, or before mealtimes. Adjust sliding scale dc according to response.

Fasting blood sugar mmol/L	Soluble insulin
10–14	4u
15–18	6u
19–22	8u
>22	10u

Drugs used in hyperglycaemia

Gliclazide
- Tabs. 80mg
- Dose: 80mg mane p.o.
- Blood levels increased by fluconazole and miconazole (hypoglycaemi

Human insulin soluble
- Inj. 100u/mL (human actrapid or humulin S)

Human insulin glargine
- Inj. 100u/mL (Lantus)

Human insulin isophane
- Inj. 100u/mL (human insulatard or humulin I)

Human insulin zinc suspension (mixed)
- Inj. 100u/mL (human monotard)

Drugs used in hypoglycaemia

Glucagon may be ineffective in a starved patient, as it depends adequate liver glycogen.

Glucagon
- Inj. 1mg
- Dose: 1mg i/m (<12yrs 0.5mg)
- Do not give by SC route, as the patient may be peripherally vasoconstricted

Glucose/dextrose
- Oral gel 10g (hypostop gel); Inj. 25 per cent 25mL 50 per cent 25mL
- Dose: 25mL of 50 per cent i/v or 10g p.o.

Blood sugar mmol/L	Action
1–17	Dietary advice.
	Reduce steroids if possible.
	Start gliclazide 40mg daily and increase as necessary every few days.
7–27	Start gliclazide 80mg mane if no, or mild, ketonuria.
	If moderate or severe ketonuria the patient will need insulin—start human monotard 10u nocte.
	If ketonuria and symptomatic, consider reducing blood glucose more rapidly using human soluble insulin 4–8u every 4h until glucose <17 mmol/L, or i/v regimen below.
27	Consider if admission to acute medical unit is appropriate, especially if ketonuria present.
	Use i/v regimen as below if intensive treatment appropriate, or human soluble insulin 4–8u every 4h until glucose <17 mmol/L.

Table 6i.3 Managing diabetes when vomiting or not eating

Diabetes type	Action
Oral hypoglycaemics	Reduce dose by 50% if oral intake reduced, or discontinue if no oral intake.
Insulin dependent	Insulin is required to prevent ketosis even with no oral intake.
	Use i/v regimen below if intensive control is appropriate, or use sliding scale of Human Soluble Insulin 8-h.

Table 6i.4 Managing diabetes in the terminal days

Diabetes type	Action
Oral hypoglycaemics	Discontinue when unable to take oral intake.
Insulin dependent	Insulin is required to prevent ketosis, even with no oral intake.
	1 If patient unconscious/unaware, discontinue insulin and monitoring.
	2 If the patient is still aware/conscious, several strategies may be appropriate, depending on the patients'/relatives' attitude to burden of treatment (and monitoring) and prognosis:
	• Use sliding scale soluble insulin 8-h
	• Give approximately half of the patient's recent insulin requirement as a single dose of human monotard as a single daily injection, with or without blood sugar monitoring

Further reading

Books

Back, I. (2001) *Palliative Medicine Handbook*. 3rd edn. Cardiff: BPM Books.

Doyle D., Hanks G., Cherny N., Calman K. (2004) *Oxford Textbook of Palliative Medicine*. 3rd edn Oxford: Oxford University Press.

Watson M., Lucas C. (2003) *Adult Palliative Care Guidelines*. London:
The South West London and the Surrey, West Sussex and Hampshire Cancer Networks.

Article

Poulson J. (1997) The management of diabetes in patients with advanced cancer. *Journal of Pain and Symptom Management*, 13, 6: 339–46.

Neurological problems in advanced cancer

For spinal cord compression see Chapter 15 on Emergencies in palliative care.

Brachial plexopathy

Cause

Invasion or compression by tumour, or fibrosis secondary to radiotherapy.

Clinical features

Shoulder or arm pain (suggestive of tumour), numbness or allodynia in arm or hand, muscle weakness, atrophy, Horner's syndrome.

Investigations

CT scan or MRI scan of brachial plexus.

Management

Palliative radiotherapy or chemotherapy may reduce the pain if tumour is the cause, but there is rarely an improvement in function. Otherwise, appropriate analgesia, including an agent for neuropathic pain, will be necessary.

Lumbosacral plexopathy

Cause

Invasion or compression by tumour or radiation fibrosis (rare).

Clinical features

Lumbosacral pain radiating into the legs. Leg weakness is usually unilateral and sensory dysfunction is apparent.

Investigations

CT or MRI scan of pelvis.

Management

Palliative radiotherapy or chemotherapy, if tumour is the cause, reduces pain and can occasionally improve function.

Paraneoplastic neurological syndromes

These are neurological disorders which occur in up to 7 per cent of patients with cancer

The aetiology is unclear although the production of a specific antibody may be involved

Syndromes can occur as a presenting feature, before the diagnosis of cancer is made

The commonest implicated cancers include small cell lung cancer (30 per cent), breast and ovarian cancer and lymphoma

Symptoms are usually subacute and there may be more than one syndrome in the same patient

Syndromes include:

- **Peripheral neuropathy** involving distal sensory and/or motor or autonomic nerves. Removal of tumour (which is usually SCLC, myeloma, Hodgkin's Disease, breast and gastrointestinal cancers) does not usually produce improvement in symptoms, which are usually progressive. Steroids may help
- **Cerebellar degeneration** may present rapidly, sometimes before the primary tumour becomes apparent. Response to treatment is disappointing
- **Lambert–Eaton myasthenic syndrome** is a disorder of neuromuscular transmission occuring in 3 per cent of patients with small cell lung cancer who account for 60–70 per cent of cases. It is seen occasionally with other cancers including thymoma, breast cancer and lymphoma. There is a presynaptic deficit in neuromuscular transmission caused by a reduction in the amount of acetylcholine released at the motor nerve terminal

  There is some evidence of an autoimmune aetiology, with the presence of autoantibodies to calcium channels at the neuromuscular junction. Common symptoms include proximal muscle weakness, particularly of the legs, and an associated waddling gait. Fatigue, diplopia, ptosis and dysarthria may also be a problem. Unlike classical myasthenia, weakness may be improved by repetitive activity and there is a poor response to edrophonium. It may improve with treatment of the underlying malignancy
- **Encephalomyelopathies** can affect the limbic system, brainstem and spinal cord
- **Other clinical presentations** include dementia, opsoclonus-myoclonus, limbic encephalitis (presenting rapidly with confusion, memory disturbance and agitation) and necrotizing myelopathy

Corticosteroid-induced proximal myopathy

- This can occur within a few weeks of starting dexamethasone 8–16 mg a day
- Patients experience difficulty in rising from a sitting position and in climbing stairs
- Disabling symptoms may not be readily volunteered and direct questioning may be needed. Management includes reducing the steroid dose to the minimum possible and considering a change to prednisolone, which may not cause as much muscle wasting (but is associated with more fluid retention)
- Weakness should improve in 3–4 weeks of steroid withdrawal

Drug-induced movement disorders

- Certain drugs may induce extrapyramidal symptoms and signs
- These include akathisia (motor restlessness in which the patient may frequently change position or pace up and down if able), dystonia and parkinsonism
- Implicated drugs are those which block dopamine receptors such as antipsychotics (particularly haloperidol and phenothiazines) and metoclopramide

Antidepressants and ondansetron may also cause problems
All these drugs should be avoided as far as possible in patients with Parkinson's disease

Convulsions and seizures

Common causes of seizures in palliative care include:

Brain tumour (primary or secondary)

Biochemical disturbance (e.g. severe hyponatraemia)

Previous cerebrovascular accident

Long-standing epilepsy

Isolated tonic-clonic seizures sometimes occur but rarely last more than a few minutes: treatment may not always be needed if they quickly settle and do not cause the patient distress.

Grand mal seizures should be treated promptly since it is very distressing and frightening for families to witness. Efficient management is therefore needed.

If a patient develops a grand mal seizure or status epilepticus, give:

Midazolam 5–10mg buccal/SC or slow i/v (dilute 10mg with water to 10mL) and repeat after 15 and 30 minutes if not settled. Midazolam is not licensed as an anticonvulsant, but is usually readily available in palliative care units. A number of alternative benzodiazepines can be used:

- lorazepam 4mg slow i/v or SL
- diazepam 10mg PR or diazemuls 2–10mg slow i/v
- clonazepam 1mg slow i/v (into large vein)

If the patient has not responded to a repeated dose of benzodiazepine or seizures recur, consider:

- phenobarbital 100mg SC, or 100mg in 100mL sodium chloride 0.9 per cent by slow i/v injection, over 30 mins

Repeat phenobarbital if necessary and set up syringe driver with phenobarbital 200–600mg SC over 24 h

Once seizures have been controlled, review anticonvulsant therapy.

General notes

- For patients with intracranial tumours, consider starting, or review dose, of corticosteroids
- Remember to advise the patient about restrictions on driving and to contact the DVLA
- Consider parenteral thiamine if alcohol abuse is suspected
- Consider and treat hypoglycaemia in at-risk patients
- Consider drug interactions that alter anticonvulsant levels (e.g. steroids)

Initiating anticonvulsant therapy

- It is usually appropriate to initiate anticonvulsant therapy after one seizure in patients with terminal illness
- Sodium valproate is an appropriate first line anticonvulsant for almost all types of convulsions or seizures, including focal and partial seizures, and those caused by intracranial tumours

- Aim to increase dose to lower end of quoted 'usual maintenance dose' unless side-effects occur, or the patient is frail and elderly. (Doses given below)
- Carbamazepine and phenytoin may be suitable alternatives

Patients unable to take oral medication
- Patients who are unable to take oral medication due to dysphagia, vomiting or in the terminal stages, may need anticonvulsants by another route
- The half-life of most anticonvulsants is quite long (>24h), therefore no parenteral anticonvulsant is usually needed if there is a low risk of seizures, **and only a single dose** is missed
- **The risk of seizures is higher if**:
  - patient has decreased or stopped steroids (intracranial tumours)
  - recent rise in headache or vomiting or other signs suggesting rising intracranial pressure (intracranial tumours)
  - myoclonus or other twitching is present
  - history of poor control of seizures or recent seizures
  - previously needing more than a single anticonvulsant to achieve control
- Because of the long half-life of anticonvulsants, parenteral treatment can be started at any time within 24h after the last oral dose

Choice of non-oral anticonvulsant
Choice may be determined partly by availability:

Table 6j.1 Choice of non-oral anticonvulsant

Phenobarbital CSCI or daily SC	Well-proven anticonvulsant for all types of seizures. Experience suggests it is effective in doses of 200mg/24h.
	Phenobarbital is incompatible with most other drugs in a syringe driver, therefore a second syringe driver may be necessary. Stat doses of 100mg SC or i/m can sting.
Midazolam CSCI	Midazolam is more useful as a sedative than as an anticonvulsant. Anticonvulsant efficacy of 'standard' doses is unknown, but probably requires 20–30mg/24h minimum. Unlicensed use.
	If low risk of seizures, and midazolam indicated for e.g. terminal agitation, then additional anticonvulsant probably unnecessary. If higher risk of seizures, use phenobarbital in addition.
Clonazepam CSCI	Main advantage is that clonazepam is compatible with many other drugs used in CSCI. Much less experience supporting its use in this way; doses recommended between 2–4mg/24h (4–8mg/24h if sedation acceptable or desired).
Carbamazepine or valproate suppositories	Occasionally suitable for patients well controlled on one of these drugs, who develop a temporary inability to take oral medication (e.g. vomiting and who would find rectal administration acceptable).

Phenobarbital as Anticonvulsant

- If a patient is dying, and sedation is acceptable, it is better to err on the generous side and give:
  - phenobarbital 200mg SC stat. as a loading dose
  - phenobarbital 200mg/24h by CSCI, or
  - if high risk of seizures—phenobarbital 400mg/24h by CSCI
- If needing to minimize sedation, use 100mg SC stat. as a loading dose followed by 100–200mg/24h by CSCI

Phenobarbital is compatible with diamorphine and hyoscine if given by CSCI

Management of seizures at home

Most seizures are self-limiting and require only supportive care. For more prolonged seizures occurring at home, a number of measures can be arranged in anticipation which can avoid inappropriate emergency admission to hospital.

- Diazepam rectal solution 10mg PR—administered by district nurse or carer
- Midazolam 5–10mg SC (or preferably i/m)—administered by district nurse
- Midazolam buccal 10mg/2mL can be administered by a carer if the rectal route for diazepam is unacceptable: it appears to be as effective and may be quicker-acting than rectal diazepam 10mg. Oral solution is available as a 'special' or the injectable preparation can be used

In an inpatient unit, midazolam 5–10mg SC (or preferably i/m) may be given first before treating status epilepticus as above.

Anticonvulsants

Carbamazepine and phenytoin levels are decreased (risk of fits) by corticosteroids. Carbamazepine, phenytoin and phenobarbital can reduce the efficacy of corticosteroids.

This two-way interaction is common when managing patients with cerebral tumours. Carbamazepine, phenytoin or phenobarbital plasma levels are also reduced by St John's Wort (risk of fits).

Sodium valproate
- Tabs.: 200mg, 500mg; syrup 200mg/5mL
- Dose: 200mg t.d.s. p.o.
- Increase 200mg/day at three day intervals. Usual maintenance 1–2g/24h. Max. 2.5g/24h in divided doses. Suppositories are available as special orders

Carbamazepine
- Tabs.: 100mg, 200mg, 400mg; liquid 100mg/5mL; Supps. 125mg, 250mg
- Dose: 100mg b.d. p.o.
- Increase from initial dose by increments of 200mg every week. Usual maintenance dose 0.8–1.2g/24h in two divided doses. Max. 1.6–2g/24h. Equivalent rectal dosage: 125mg PR ≅ 100mg p.o.
- Carbamazepine levels are increased (risk of toxicity) by clarithromycin, erythromycin, dextropropoxyphene (co-proxamol), fluoxetine and fluvoxamine

Phenytoin
- Caps.: 50mg, 100mg, 300mg; Susp. 30mg/5mL, 90mg/5mL
- Dose: 90mg b.d. p.o.
- Start 150–300mg daily. Usual maintenance dose: 300–400mg daily. Max. 600mg/24h. Single or two divided doses
- Phenytoin levels are increased (risk of toxicity) by clarithromycin, metronidazole, trimethoprim, fluconazole, miconazole, omeprazole, fluoxetine, fluvoxamine, aspirin, diltiazem, nifedipine and amiodarone
- Because phenytoin has a very long and variable half-life, it can take several days and even up to 3–4 weeks for changes in dosage to take complete effect: this should be borne in mind in determining the interval after dosage is altered before measuring the plasma phenytoin concentration again

Barbiturate
Phenobarbital (phenobarbitone)
- Inj: 60mg/1mL, 200mg/1mL; Tabs.: 15mg, 30mg, 60mg; elixir 15mg/5mL
- Elixir in various strengths can be made to order e.g. 10mg/mL
- Phenobarbital is a barbiturate with sedative and anticonvulsant effects. It is rarely used nowadays as a first line anticonvulsant, as it is too sedative. It can be given by CSCI, but usually needs to be given in a separate syringe driver. It can be given by daily SC or i/m injection, but the preparation is very viscous and stings on injection. *Doses: see above*

Benzodiazepines

Midazolam
- Inj: 10mg/2mL, 10mg/5mL
- Dose: 30mg/24h CSCI
- Oral solution available as special order, or use injection for buccal use
- Sedative effect markedly enhanced by itraconazole, ketoconazole and possibly fluconazole

Lorazepam
- Tabs.: 1mg, 2.5mg; Inj: 4mg/1mL
- Dilute inj. with equal volume of water or saline for i/m use

Diazepam
- Tabs.: 2mg, 5mg, 10mg; oral solution 2mg/5mL, 5mg/5mL
- Rectal tubes 5mg/2.5mL, 10mg/2.5mL; Supps. 10mg
- Inj: (emulsion) 10mg/2mL (diazemuls)—i/v use only
- Inj: (solution) 10mg/2mL—i/m use

Clonazepam
- Tabs.: 500mcg, 2mg; inj: 1mg/1mL
- Starting Dose: 1mg nocte
- Increase gradually to usual maintenance dose 4–8mg/24h. Oral solutions in various strengths are available from several sources

Further reading

Books

Back I. (2001) *Palliative Medicine Handbook*. 3rd edn. Cardiff: BPM Books.

Doyle D., Hanks G., Cherny N., Calman K. (2004) *Oxford Textbook of Palliative Medicine*. Oxford: Oxford University Press.

Watson M., Lucas C. (2003) *Adult Palliative Care Guidelines*. London: The South West London and the Surrey, West Sussex and Hampshire Cancer Networks.

Articles

Heafield M. (2000) Managing status epilepticus. *BMJ*, **320**: 953–4.

Newsom-Davis J. (1999) Paraneoplastic neurological disorders. *Journal of The Royal College of Physicians of London*, **33**: 225–7.

Sleep disorders

Sleep disorders are a frequent complication of medical illness, occurring in 50 per cent or more of those with advanced cancer, particularly where pain is a complicating factor. Night-time rest is an invaluable respite from the worries and pain of the day, allowing the patient to meet the next day with renewed energy. Despite this, it is not often taken seriously by healthcare professionals.

Human sleep is an essential, active, dynamic and complex physiological function in which stages are repeated in cyclical pattern throughout the night. There are two distinct states of sleep, non-rapid eye movement sleep (NREM) and rapid eye movement (REM). NREM sleep accounts for 75 per cent of the night, in a staged process from light to deep sleep, and is a period of relative physiological and cognitive quiescence. REM sleep, on the other hand, is characterized by muscle atonia, dreaming and autonomic variability.

The sleep–wake cycle is a component of the body's overall circadian rhythm, synchronized with other biological rhythms including temperature oscillation and cortisol and growth hormone secretion. The onset and maintenance of normal sleep patterns depend on the appropriate timing of sleep within the 24 hour circadian rhythm. Adequate physical comfort, an acceptable sleeping environment, an intact central nervous system function and relative absence of psycholological distress and psychophysiologic arousal is necessary for sleep.

The restorative functions of sleep are dependent on a well-organized and reasonably uninterrupted sleep structure. Sleep tends to be lighter with advancing age and in many medical conditions. The percentage of REM sleep, however, remains relatively constant in a healthy elderly population, but is decreased when cognitive impairment or certain other medical conditions are present.

Insomnia

Insomnia is a subjective complaint by the patient of poor sleep. This encompasses complaints of insufficient sleep, interrupted sleep, poor quality or non-restorative sleep or sleep which occurs at the wrong time in the day–night cycle. Physical, psychological and environmental factors contribute to poor sleep in medical conditions. Sleep deprivation may result in progressive fatigue, sleepiness, impairment of concentration, irritability and depression. Deep stages of NREM sleep may be critical in tissue restoration and in maintaining a healthy immune system.

Disorders of the sleep–wake cycle

A normal sleeping pattern is dependent on a well-established schedule of sleep and wakefulness. Patients who are terminally ill are prone to disturbances in the sleep–wake cycle because of frequent disruptions of nighttime sleep, an absence of usual daytime schedule demands and relative inactivity during normal waking hours. A lack of sleep at night leads to late waking and daytime napping and late settling to sleep the following night (delayed sleep phase syndrome) or early morning waking and early bedtime (advanced sleep phase syndrome). Either way, a vicious disturbed cycle then emerges. For some a rhythm disappears altogether and is replaced by a pattern of multiple shorter sleep periods interspersed with wakefulness throughout the 24 h. It must not be forgotten that coming into hospital leads to highly fragmented sleep.

Excessive daytime sleepiness

It is very common for patients receiving palliative care to complain generally of tiredness and fatigue, but this must be distinguished from sleepiness. A degree of daytime sedation can be desirable in some cases, but excessive sleepiness can be disabling leading to inactivity and poor motivation. Patients may become less capable of participating in treatment and may find it difficult to retain information and to interact socially. They may also become unnecessarily depressed, irritable and withdrawn during the important last weeks or months of life.

Causes of disturbed sleep in the terminally ill which should be actively sought and treated where appropriate

- Uncontrolled pain—contributes to lack of sleep in up to 60 per cent of patients. Sleep deprivation lowers pain thresholds
- Medication—steroids, especially if taken late in the day; bronchodilators; enervating antidepressants e.g. fluoxetine; withdrawal from sedative hypnotics or analgesia; caffeine, nicotine and alcohol may also be contributory
- Depression—at least 90 per cent of depressed patients have abnormal sleep patterns. Depression is common and it is a significant cause of sleep pathology in the terminally ill
- Bladder or bowel discomfort and incontinence
- Anxiety and fears—anxiety may be directly related to the illness or treatment and is often associated with pain. Early delirium, withdrawal from drugs and breathlessness can frequently cause anxiety. During the daytime fears are masked by distractions
- Cognitive impairment disorder—delirium is not uncommon in the terminally ill and reversible causes should be actively sought. Sleep disturbance itself may lead to delirium. Patients with dementia sleep less deeply and have reduced REM and increased awakening after sleep onset
- Patients need constant reassurance and to be nursed in a lit room to minimize disorientation. Hypnotics may aggravate the situation. Drugs such as haloperidol 0.5–2.0mg or risperidone 0.5–1.0mg may be useful, particularly if given in the early evening, to pre-empt a restless period and give adequate time for the drug to take effect before settling for the night. NB Risperidone should not be used if there is a history of cerebrovascular disease
- Nausea and vomiting
- Respiratory distress
- Psychophysiological—conditional arousal response, poor sleep hygiene
- Sleep–wake schedule disorder—disruption of normal schedule, excessive napping during the day
- Restless legs syndrome—may be associated with potentially manageable causes such as sedative hypnotic withdrawal, anaemia, uraemia, peripheral neuropathy, iron deficiency, diabetes mellitus

Management

A full assessment must be carried out to define the individual's sleep characteristics and to address all possible reversible causes. In the absence of any obviously reversible causes, the aim is to achieve enough restorative sleep to ensure daytime alertness, concentration and energy. Attention must also be given to the carer, who may have fragmented nights for weeks and months yet still has to do the daytime chores and caring.

- **Sleep hygiene** Excessive arousal in bed is a frequent cause and effect of insomnia. Anxiety is exacerbated when lying isolated in bed, mind racing with all others asleep. Patients may need to undertake a relaxing activity to turn their minds away from the pressure to fall asleep, but may not be able to get out of bed to achieve this. They may lie awake, apparently asleep, fearful of moving and waking up their exhausted carers and bedtime may become a dreaded time. A chaotic, unpredictable pattern needs to be managed by reinforcing the rest–activity sleep–wake cycle. Physical, cognitively stimulating and social activity during the day may help to strengthen the difference between day and night

- **Non-pharmacological** Cognitive behavioural treatment is the mainstay of treatment for insomnia that is due wholly or in part to heightened cognitive or physiological arousal and poor sleep hygiene. Other techniques such as hypnosis and somatic imagery training, progressive muscle relaxation, psychotherapy and complementary therapy such as aromatherapy may help

- **Pharmacological** Benzodiazepines and other drugs that act on benzodiazepine receptors such as cyclopyrrolone (zopiclone) are the standard medications of choice in the treatment of transient or short term insomnia. Hypnotic medication is used frequently in palliative care and may greatly enhance quality of life. Choice of hypnotic depends on several factors including length of time of effectiveness, rate of absorption and metabolism and potential risks or side-effects. Daytime sedation with the shorter acting hypnotics is rarely a problem. Nocturnal confusion may be induced, particularly in individuals with baseline cognitive dysfunction.

  Most are absorbed quickly reaching peak concentrations within an hour or less. The non-benzodiazepine hypnotics have a very short half-life of about 1 hour. Temazepam, lorazepam and oxazepam have intermediate half-lives ranging from 8 to 15 h in healthy adults whereas diazepam is longer acting and is cleared more slowly.

  Chloral hydrate has modest short term efficacy but is more toxic than benzodiazepines. Sedating tricyclic antidepressants (e.g. amitriptyline) are often used but are associated with anticholinergic side-effects. Trazodone is a sedating heterocyclic with milder anticholinergic side-effects and a shorter half life than most tricyclics and can be administered over a longer period of time. Chlomethiazole is sometimes used.

  Sedative hypnotics in the elderly are associated with falls, cognitive impairment and worsening of nocturnal respiratory disturbance and should be used in low doses.

Haematological aspects

Anaemia

Anaemia is defined as a haemoglobin concentration in adults of less than 13.0g/dl in men and 11.5g/dl in women. It is a common problem, occurring in over 50 per cent of patients with solid tumours and in most patients with haematological malignancies such as multiple myeloma and lymphoma.

Symptoms caused by anaemia include:
- Fatigue
- Weakness
- Breathlessness on exertion
- Impaired concentration
- Chest pain
- Exacerbation of congestive cardiac failure
- Low mood
- Loss of libido
- Anorexia

There are no specific criteria for the functional assessment of anaemia. However, randomized controlled trials of the management of anaemia in malignancy have used validated tools in assessing its effect on quality of life (QOL) e.g.
- Cancer Linear Analogue Scale (CLAS)
- Functional Assessment of Cancer Therapy-Anaemia (FACT-An)

Causes of anaemia
- Reduced red cell production due to bone marrow infiltration
  - Multiple myeloma
  - Prostate cancer
  - Breast cancer
  - Leukaemia
- Chemotherapy-induced bone marrow suppression
- Anaemia of chronic disease related to malignancy
- Malnutrition/malabsorption e.g. post gastrectomy
  - B_{12} deficiency
  - Folate deficiency
  - Iron deficiency
- Blood loss:
  - Gastrointestinal
  - Haematuria
- Chronic renal failure
- Reduced red cell survival/haemolysis:
  - Autoimmune haemolysis—lymphoproliferative disorders
  - Physical haemolysis—micro-angiopathic haemolytic anaemia (MAHA) in some adenocarcinomas

- Anaemia of chronic disorder related to malignancy—a combination of effects
  - Suppressed erythropoietin production
  - Impaired transferrin production
  - Shortened red cell survival

Management of anaemia

Investigate cause of anaemia where appropriate

Diagnostic indicators

- Reduced marrow production/bone marrow failure
  - Full blood count—pancytopenia and reduced reticulocytes
  - Bone marrow examination—may show infiltration by non-haematological cells e.g. prostatic or breast carcinoma, or hypocellular marrow post-chemotherapy
- Bleeding
  - Clinical—haematuria, melaena
  - Acute—blood count and film: normochromic, normocytic anaemia, reticulocytosis and polychromasia
  - Chronic—iron deficiency anaemia
- Malabsorption/malnutrition
  - Low serum B_{12}
  - Reduced serum or red cell folate
  - Reduced ferritin
- Haemolysis
  - Blood film: polychromasia; autoimmune—spherocytes; MAHA—red cell fragments (schistocytes); reticulocytosis
  - Autoimmune—positive direct Coombs test
  - Bilirubin—raised

Table 6l.1 Differentiation between iron deficiency anaemia and anaemia of chronic disease

	Iron deficiency anaemia	Anaemia of chronic disease
Blood film	Hypochromic microcytic	Normochromic or hypochromic
Red cell distribution Width (RDW)	Increased	Microcytic +/− Normal
Total iron binding capacity (TIBC)	High	Normal/low
Plasma iron	Low	Low
Serum ferritin	Low	Normal/raised

N.B. The two causes can co-exist

Decrease bleeding risk

- Consider discontinuation of drugs that may increase risk of bleeding e.g
  - aspirin
  - NSAIDs

- anticoagulants
- steroids
- Consider gastroprotection using:
  - proton pump inhibitors
  - H$_2$-receptor antagonists
  - prostaglandin analogues e.g. misoprostol
- Give vitamin K in liver disease-related coagulopathies as evidenced by prolonged prothrombin time (PT)
- Give tranexamic acid (antifibrinolytic agent) for mucosal bleeding. Tranexamic acid can be given topically and as a mouthwash. (Use with care in bleeding from the bladder or prostate as clot formation is enhanced and subsequent retention may become a problem.) Etamsylate may also be useful

Replace haematinic deficiencies

- Iron deficiency
  - Ferrous sulphate 200mg b.d. or t.d.s.
- Folate deficiency
  - Folic acid 5m.g. o.d.
- B$_{12}$ deficiency
  - Hydroxycobalamin 1000mcg i/m every three months

Blood transfusion

Patients who are becoming terminally ill may receive blood transfusions inappropriately. The decision to transfuse should not be made on the basis of one haemoglobin result alone, but in the context of symptoms attributable to anaemia which are adversely affecting quality of life. It is important to document the clinical effect of the transfusion which will help in discussing the merits or otherwise of further transfusions. Blood transfusion helps about 75 per cent of patients in terms of wellbeing, strength and breathlessness.

- Since 1998, all red cells have been leuco-depleted, therefore an in-line blood filter is not now required. One unit of leuco-depleted packed red cells (approximately 300mL) results in a rise in haemoglobin of 1g/dl
- The aim should be to transfuse up to 11–12g/dl but this will vary according to the individual clinical situation
- Patients at risk of pulmonary oedema should have furosemide cover (20mg p.o. or i/v with alternate units)
- Patients should be told that the beneficial effects may not be apparent for a day or two post-transfusion

Indications for blood transfusion in patients with palliative care needs

- Haemoglobin of less than 10g/dl (patients may benefit from transfusion at higher levels)
- Prognosis greater than two weeks
- Reasonable performance status (i.e. not predominantly bedbound) (ECOG > 2)
- Presence of at least two of the following symptoms:
  - breathlessness on exertion
  - weakness
  - angina
  - postural hypotension
  - worsening cardiac failure
  - worsening fatigue

Blood transfusion reactions

Acute life-threatening transfusion reactions are very rare, however, new symptoms or signs that occur during a transfusion must be taken seriously as they may herald a serious reaction. As it may not be possible to identify the cause of a severe reaction immediately, the initial supportive management should generally cover all the possible causes. These include:

- Acute haemolytic transfusion reaction
- Infusion of a bacterially contaminated unit
- Severe allergic reaction or anaphylaxis
- Fluid overload
- Transfusion-related acute lung injury (TRALI)

Acute haemolytic transfusion reaction

Incompatible Group A or B transfused red cells react with the patient's own anti-A or B antibodies. This results in acute renal failure, and can cause disseminated intravascular coagulation (DIC) The reaction can occur after only a few mls of blood have been transfused

- **Symptoms:** acute onset pain at venepuncture site, loins, chest
- **Signs:** fever, hypotension, tachycardia, oozing from venepuncture sites
- A similar picture is seen with the transfusion of bacterially contaminated red cells
- **Action:** If a severe acute reaction is suspected:
  - Stop the transfusion, keep i/v line open with sodium chloride 0.9% infusion
  - Monitor temperature, heart rate, BP, respiratory rate, urine output
  - Recheck the patient's identification, the blood unit and documentation
  - Inform the blood bank
  - Further management will depend on the patient's developing clinical picture

Major allergic reactions

Rare but life-threatening complication usually occur in the early part of a transfusion. These complications are more common with plasma-containing blood components e.g. fresh-frozen plasma (FFP) or platelets

- **Symptoms:** chest pain, breathlessness, nausea and abdominal pain
- **Signs:** hypotension, bronchospasm, periorbital and laryngeal oedema, vomiting, urticaria
- **Action:**
  - Stop transfusion
  - High concentration O_2
  - Chlorphenamine 10–20mg i/v over 1–2 minutes
  - Hydrocortisone 100–200mg i/v
  - Adrenaline 0.5–1mg (0.5–1mL of 1 in 1000) i/m
  - Salbutamol 2.5–5mg by nebuliser
  - Maintain i/v access

Fluid overload

More common in patients with a history of heart or renal disease, but any patient with advanced malignancy is susceptible. In these patients, each red cell unit should be given over 3–4h and a maximum of two units given per day. Clinical signs to be aware of:

- **Symptoms:** Breathlessness with basal crepitations
- **Signs:** BP may be raised initially, tachycardia, raised jugular venous pressure (JVP) may be present
- **Action:**
  - Stop transfusion
  - High concentration O_2
  - Furosemide 40mg i/v

Transfusion-related acute lung injury (TRALI)

Usually caused by antibodies in donor's plasma that react strongly with the patient's leucocytes.

- **Symptoms:** Rapid onset of breathlessness and dry cough
- **Signs:** Chest X-ray shows bilateral infiltrates—'white-out'

- **Action:**
  - Stop transfusion
  - Give 100 per cent O_2
  - Seek expert advice and treat as Adult Respiratory Distress Syndrome (ARDS)

Febrile non-haemolytic transfusion reaction

Affects 1–2 per cent of patients

- A rise in temperature < 1.5°C from the baseline or an urticarial rash, +/– rigors
- Usually occurs towards the end of a transfusion or up to two hours after it is finished
- Treat with paracetamol
- Give chlorphenamine 10mg p.o. or i/v for rash
- Continue transfusion at a slower rate
- Observe for any deterioration

Iron overload is not often a concern in palliative care but if 50–75 units of red cells have been given, haemosiderosis may develop causing heart and liver dysfunction or failure of pancreatic endocrine function.

Contra-indications to blood transfusion

- Patient refusal
- No symptomatic benefit from previous transfusion
- Patient moribund with life expectancy of days

Erythropoietin

- This is a hormone made by the kidney. It stimulates the production of red blood cells and is licensed for anaemia of chronic renal failure and for patients undergoing chemotherapy
- It may also be effective in improving the chronic anaemia of cancer
- An injection of 150–300 Units/Kg SC three times a week for 4–6 weeks increases the Hb significantly in 50–60 per cent of patients with cancer. The patients most likely to benefit include those with a low erythropoietin concentration, adequate bone marrow reserve and an initial good response (i.e. an increase in Hb of >1g/dl within four weeks of starting treatment)
- The maximum benefit is achieved after about two months which may be a factor limiting its usefulness in palliative care patients where prognosis is short
- Patients should be given iron supplements during erythropoietin therapy to maximize the response

Complications

- Hypertension
- Thrombosis
- Iron deficiency, if not on iron supplements

Screening of donated blood products is inevitably becoming ever more stringent and blood transfusion may become justified only for the most needy. Erythropoietin may therefore become more commonly used. It is already used where appropriate for Jehovah's Witnesses.

Bleeding and haemorrhage

Bleeding occurs in about 20 per cent of patients with advanced cancer and may contribute to death in 5 per cent. Bleeding may be directly related to the cancer itself, e.g. local bleeding from fungating tumours, or indirectly related, e.g. peptic ulceration or nose bleeds secondary to treatment with NSAIDs or thrombocytopenia respectively.

A systemic deterioration in a patient's condition may be mirrored by a decline in the haematological profile.

Obvious bleeding

- Oral mucosa or nose
- Gums
- Nasopharynx
- Haemoptysis
- Haematemesis
- Skin/muscle

Hidden bleeding

- Gastrointestinal—melaena, anaemia, (raised urea may be noted)
- Pulmonary—worsening breathlessness, pleural effusion
- Urogenital—macroscopic or microscopic haematuria
- Cerebral—headache, visual disturbance, change in neurology
- Gynaecological—vaginal bleeding

General management of bleeding

Where possible and when appropriate, attempt to correct haemostatic factors that contribute to a bleeding tendency.

Haemostatic factors that contribute to bleeding

Platelets

Thrombocytopenia due to:
- Reduced marrow production
  - marrow infiltration
  - myelosuppression following chemotherapy
- Increased consumption/utilization
  - disseminated intravascular coagulation (DIC)
  - autoimmune
- Splenic pooling
  - hypersplenism

Abnormal function as seen in:
- Acute myeloid leukaemia
- Myelodysplasia
- Myeloproliferative disorders
- Paraproteinaemias e.g. multiple myeloma
- Treatment with NSAID, aspirin
- Renal failure

Coagulation factors

High level expression of tissue factor leading to:
- Extrinsic pathway activation
- Thrombin generation
- Consumption of clotting factors
- DIC

Metastatic liver disease results in:
- Reduced synthesis of vitamin K-dependent factors

Acute DIC is uncommon and presents as a mixture of thrombosis and bleeding. The skin may develop petechiae and purpura, and gangrene may occur in areas of end circulation such as the digits, nose and ear lobes. Bleeding may occur in areas of trauma such as at venepuncture sites or as haematuria in the presence of a catheter. Treatment includes platelet infusions, FFP and cryoprecipitate.

Chronic DIC is more common and may be asymptomatic (as measured by laboratory tests) but thrombotic symptoms of DVT, PE or migratory thrombophlebitis may occur. Treatment is usually heparin (low molecular weight).

Laboratory investigations
- **D-dimers**—more specific than fibrin degradation products (FDPs). Significant increase in D-dimers + prolonged PT, reduced fibrinogen, +/– thrombocytopenia necessary for diagnosis (D-dimers also increased in infection)
- **Prothronbin Time (PT)**—less sensitive, usually prolonged in acute DIC, but may be normal in chronic DIC
- **Activated Partial Thromboplastin Time (APTT)**—Less useful, as may be normal or shortened in chronic DIC
- **Platelets**—Reduced or falling count found in acute DIC
- **Blood film**—may show red cell fragments (schistocytes)

Thrombocytopenia
Spontaneous bleeding due to thrombocytopenia is rare if the platelet count is $> 20 \times 10^9$/l but traumatic bleeding is problematic if the platelet count is less than 40×10^9/l. Sepsis will increase the bleeding tendency. If platelet function is abnormal, bleeding may occur at higher counts.
- A platelet transfusion may be considered if there is bleeding which is distressing. It will only raise the platelet count for a few days. This treatment should not be given routinely if there is no evidence of bleeding and the count is greater than 10×10^9/l. If the platelet count is less than 50×10^9/l and the patient is bleeding, platelets should be given
- A pool of platelets is derived from four units of donated blood and is approximately 300mL
- Platelets must be kept at room temperature and transfused over 30min, using a sterile administration set or a platelet infusion set. Never use an in-line filter
- The donor should be ABO compatible with the patient

It is important to anticipate which patients are likely to require platelet transfusions and to decide appropriateness prior to a crisis. The whole team should be involved in decisions concerning ongoing regular prophylactic transfusions and their withdrawal. With platelet counts of $10–20 \times 10^9$/l the risk of a major bleed is small, severe bleeding occurring mostly with counts less than 5×10^9/l

Tranexamic acid (inhibits fibrinolysis)can be used to control mucosal bleeding due to thrombocytopenia.
- 1g orally t.d.s. or slow i/v injection
- Mouthwash 1g every six hours for oral bleeding
- Topical tranexamic acid for superficial fungating tumours

On average it takes two days of therapy to slow down bleeding and four days for bleeding to stop.

Blood products

These are less commonly used in the palliative care setting and close liaison with the haematology department is essential when considering administration. The table below outlines some products and their indications.

Indications for blood products

Fresh frozen plasma (FFP)
- Disseminated intravascular coagulation
- Rapid correction of warfarin overdose
- Liver disease
- Coagulopathy due to massive blood loss

Cryoprecipitate
- In DIC when fibrinogen <1.0g/l
- For bleeding in cases of dysfibrinogenaemia

Bleeding directly related to cancer

Radiotherapy should be considered for local bleeding caused by cancer e.g. ulcerating skin tumours, lung cancer causing haemoptysis, gynaecological cancer causing vaginal bleeding and bladder/prostate cancer causing haematuria.

Specific situations

Nose bleeds
- Most nose bleeds are venous and when arising from the anterior septum can often be stopped by pressure.
- Silver nitrate caustic pencil can be applied to the bleeding point. The nose can be packed with calcium alginate rope (e.g. kaltostat) or with ribbon gauze soaked in adrenaline (epinephrine 1:1000 1mg in 1mL)
- If the bleeding is more posterior, and continues into the nasopharynx, a merocel tampon may need to be inserted for 36hours with antibiotic cover or the nose packed with gauze impregnated with bismuth iodoform paraffin paste (BIPP) for three days.
- The ENT department may need to be contacted for further management with a balloon catheter or cauterization under local anaesthetic.

Surface bleeding
The bleeding from tumour masses may respond well to radiotherapy. Other measures include the following:
Physical
- Gauze applied with pressure for 10 mins soaked in adrenaline (epinephrine) (1:1000) 1mg in 1mL or Tranexamic acid 500mg in 5mL
  - Silver nitrate sticks to bleeding points
  - Haemostatic dressings i.e. alginate e.g. kaltostat, sorbsan

Drugs
- Topical
  - Sucralfate paste 2g (two 1g tablets crushed in 5mL KY jelly)
  - Sucralfate suspension 2g in 10mL b.d. for mouth and rectum
  - Tranexamic acid 5g in 50mL warm water b.d. for rectal bleeding
  - 1 per cent alum solution for bladder
- Systemic
  - Antifibrinolytic e.g. tranexamic acid 1.5g stat and 0.5–1g b.d.–t.d.s. p.o. or slow i/v 0.5–1g t.d.s. **Do not use if DIC suspected.**
  - Haemostatic e.g. etamsylate 500mg q.d.s. (restores platelet adhesiveness).

Haemoptysis

Haemoptysis may be directly related to the underlying tumour or related to treatments or infection. A generalized clotting deficiency, seen in thrombocytopaenia, hepatic insufficiency or anticoagulation with warfarin, can also be contributory factors.

Treatments for **non-acute haemorrhage** include oncological, systemic and local measures. If radiotherapy is not appropriate, coagulation should be enhanced with oral tranexamic acid 1g t.d.s., but caution is necessary with haematuria since clots may form in the bladder, resulting in further problems The risks of encouraging hypercoagulation need to be considered carefully in patients with a history of a stroke or ischaemic heart disease.

Erosion of a major artery can cause **acute haemorrhage** which may be a rapidly terminal event. It may be possible to anticipate such an occurrence and appropriate medication and a red/green/blue towel to reduce the visual impact should be readily available. Relatives or others who witness such an event will need a great deal of support. If the haematemesis is not immediately fatal, the aim of treatment is sedation of a shocked, frightened patient.

It *may* be appropriate to have emergency medication in the home to sedate the acutely bleeding patient, but such a strategy can only be arrived at after discussion with the family, carers, and the patient's local GP, and needs to documented clearly.

Assessment
Consider the commonest causes:
- tumour bleeding
- clotting disorders
- infection
- pulmonary embolism

Treatment
- Treat any evidence or signs suggestive of infection
- Consider radiotherapy referral (not if multiple lung metastases) or brachytherapy, where the radiation sources are placed close to the tumour within the lungs
- Consider and treat other systemic causes of bleeding (📖 see Chapter 15)
- blood tests for clotting screen and platelets
- Tranexamic acid 1g t.d.s. p.o.
  - stop if no effect after 1 week
  - continue for 1 week after bleeding has stopped, then discontinue
  - continue long term (500mg t.d.s.) only if bleeding recurs and responds to second course of treatment

Small bleeds can herald a larger massive haemorrhage; *consider* siting an i/v cannula to administer emergency drugs.
- One third of patients with lung cancer develop haemoptysis, although the incidence of acute fatal bleeds is only 3 per cent of which some occur without warning

- The patient is more likely to die from suffocation secondary to the bleed than from the bleed itself. Bleeding due to cancer is most commonly from a primary carcinoma of the bronchus and a massive haemoptysis is usually from a squamous cell lung tumour lying centrally or causing cavitation. Metastases from carcinoma of the breast, colorectum, kidney and melanoma may also cause haemoptysis
- Infection in the chest and pulmonary emboli are other causes of haemoptysis

Haematemesis

The incidence is 2 per cent in patients with cancer and may be associated with cancer and/or secondary to gastroduodenal irritants such as NSAIDs. The management includes stopping NSAIDs if possible or changing to celecoxib (reduced effect on platelets) and adding a proton pump inhibitor or H2 receptor antagonist a gastroprotective agent such as sucralfate may also be useful.

Major bleeds
- If patient's condition is not stable, with history of major haemorrhage or ongoing bleeding:
- Consider if appropriate to transfer to an acute medical/endoscopy unit
- Site an Iv i/v cannula to anticipate need for emergency drugs
- Treat anxiety or distress as needed:
- Midazolam 2–5mg initially by slow i/v titration (10mg diluted to 10mL with sodium chloride 0.9%)

If no i/v access, midazolam 5–10mg SC (give i/m if shocked or vasoconstricted).

Rectal bleeding

This may be associated with local tumour (radiotherapy may be the treatment of choice to stop the bleeding) and/or radiotherapy. Bloody diarrhoea may occur acutely with pelvic radiotherapy which causes acute inflammation of the rectosigmoid mucosa, but this should be self limiting. A predsol retention enema 20mg in 100mL o.d.–b.d. or prednisolone 5mg and sucralfate 3g in 15mL b.d. may help.

Bleeding from chronic ischaemic radiation proctitis may respond to tranexamic acid, etamsylate or sucralfate suspension given rectally.

Haematuria

This may occur with carcinoma of the bladder or prostate or as a result of chronic radiation cystitis. Urine infection will aggravate the situation. Tranexamic acid or etamsylate may be useful, although there is the risk of clot formation and urinary retention. Alum 50mL of 1 per cent can be useful if retained in the bladder via a catheter for 1 hour.

Massive terminal haemorrhage

Massive terminal haemorrhage occurs as a result of a major arterial haemorrhage and usually causes death in minutes. For patients who have undergone all possible treatment options, this inevitably terminal event should be treated palliatively, the main aim being comfort for the patient and support for the family.

It is usually associated with tumour erosion into the aorta or pulmonary artery (causing haematemesis or haemoptysis) or carotid or femoral artery (causing external bleeding). If a massive haemorrhage is unexpected, the only appropriate management may be to stay with the patient and attempt to comfort any distress. It may be appropriate to warn family members of the possibility.

Major haemorrhage may be preceded by smaller bleeds. Patients may have been receiving platelets and blood products, which have now been discontinued. If major haemorrhage is anticipated, it may be appropriate to warn family members of the possibility. Appropriate drugs, already drawn up in a syringe, should be kept available at the bedside to ensure fast administration. Blue or green towels (which mask the colour of blood) should be available to help control the spread of blood.

In the event of a massive bleed, the aim of treatment will be to rapidly sedate and relieve patient distress from what will, by definition, be the terminal event. Where possible drugs should be given i/v or else by deep i/m injection.

Drug options

Midazolam

Midazolam 10mg SC, i/v or bucally will sedate most patients. Heavy alcohol drinkers and patients on regular benzodiazepines may require larger doses.

Ketamine

The effect of ketamine is more predictable in palliative care patients than benzodiazepines and opioids, since the patient is unlikely to have been taking it regularly. Ketamine 150mg–250mg i/v will rapidly sedate a patient dying from a terminal haemorrhage. If the i/m route is necessary, a larger dose of 500mg will be required.

Opioids

These are less recommended for the management of terminal haemorrhage for the following reasons:

1. As a controlled drug, nurses may not be able to leave a dose by the bedside or to check doses quickly.
2. Diamorphine needs to be dissolved, leading to further delay.
3. Variable doses will be required depending on how opioid-naïve the patient is.

Summary

- Midazolam 10–20mg i/v, SC, i/m or buccal
- Ketamine 150–250mg i/v or 500mg i/m
- Diamorphine dose will vary.

Thromboembolism

It is over 130 years since Trousseau first noticed the association between cancer and thrombosis. Patients with cancer are at high risk of developing venous thromboembolism (VTE) and the risk increases as malignancy advances. It follows that palliative care patients are extremely thrombogenic.

Studies have suggested that the incidence of deep vein thrombosis (DVT) may be as high 52 per cent (with 33 per cent of those being bilateral) in palliative care.

Thrombogenic risk

Virchow's triad describes the predisposing factors for VTE as:
1 stasis,
2 endothelial perturbation,
3 hypercoaguability.

The table below suggests some of the reasons that patients with cancer are at such high risk.

Prothrombotic risk in cancer

- **Stasis**
  - Immobility due to weakness, lethargy
  - Compression of vessels by tumour e.g. pelvic disease
  - Extrinsic compression from oedematous legs
- **Endothelial perturbation**
  - Recent surgery
  - Central venous access
  - Direct tumour invasion of vessel
- **Hypercoagulable state**
  - Dehydration
  - Tissue factor/tumour procoagulant release
  - Increased platelet activation
  - DIC
  - Cytokine-related thrombotic changes
  - Prothombotic changes from certain chemotherapeutic agents

Deep vein thrombosis (DVT)

Signs and symptoms vary depending upon the severity of DVT. It should be suspected in patients with a swollen, tender, warm, erythematous leg, although it is unreliable to make a firm clinical diagnosis on the basis of these findings alone. Some are asymptomatic whilst extreme cases may lead to vascular insufficiency and gangrene. The risk of a pulmonary embolus from a distal DVT (i.e. below knee) is low, and only about 20 per cent of calf vein thromboses progress to a proximal thrombosis.

Differential diagnosis

- Cellulitis
- Lymphoedema
- Oedema due to hypoproteinaemia
- Ruptured Baker's cyst

Diagnosis

It is not always practical to confirm the presence of a DVT if the patient is in the terminal stages of illness or to treat all patients with VTE. If a patient is not going to be anticoagulated there is little point in investigating suspected thrombus. Anticoagulation carries risks as well as benefits and these should be weighed up on an individual basis first.

- Doppler ultrasound
  - Non-invasive. No ionizing radiation. Easily repeatable
  - Can be performed at the bedside if suitable equipment available.
  - Accuracy lower for non-occlusive iliac thrombus and calf vein assessment than ascending venography
- Venography
  - Invasive. Involves ionizing radiation. Contrast media is injected into a vein on the dorsum of the foot. Low risk of allergic reaction
  - No longer the first-line investigation. Useful when Doppler is inconclusive, for example in patients with large oedematous legs or with previous deep vein thrombosis
  - Gives excellent visualisation of all the leg veins
- Light reflection rheography
  - Non-invasive
  - Can be done at bedside
  - High sensitivity but poor specificity and therefore not used greatly in clinical practice
  - Cannot localize thrombus or distinguish between intrinsic/extrinsic compression
- D-dimers
  - Use in cancer patients is limited due to high false positive rate in malignancy
- Magnetic resonance angiography
  - Non-invasive
  - Good at imaging leg vessels
  - Use in palliative care patients is yet to be evaluated

Pulmonary embolus (PE)

Evidence from *post-mortem* studies suggests that pulmonary emboli are underdiagnosed clinically in the palliative care setting.

This may be due to several factors:

- Patient not well enough for investigation
- Other lung pathologies make radiological diagnosis problematic
- Concerns over anticoagulation in some patients
- Breathlessness assumed to be due to other causes

Most PEs occur as a complication of DVT in the legs or pelvis. The risk of PE from untreated DVT is estimated at 50 per cent and the mortality rate of untreated PE at 30–40 per cent. Most deaths from PE occur in the first hour.

Signs and symptoms will vary depending upon the extent of thrombus, general condition of the patient, other respiratory/cardiovascular co-morbidity and whether chronic pulmonary emboli or an acute event has occurred.

In some patients pulmonary emboli may go unnoticed, causing mild breathlessness, whilst in more severe cases, sudden cardiovascular collapse and death occur. Features suggestive of pulmonary emboli include:

- Breathlessness and cough
- Haemoptysis
- Palpitations
- Chest pain

Clinical signs may vary and are useful if present, but absence of signs should not exclude the diagnosis if there is a strong clinical suspicion. Likewise many of the signs could be accounted for by other co-morbidities. Signs may include:

- Tachycardia
- Tachypnoea
- Atrial fibrillation
- Raised JVP
- Hypotension
- Loud P2 heart sound
- Cyanosis
- Syncope

Investigations

It is important to decide whether an investigation is going to alter management and, if so, which test would be the most appropriate and best tolerated by the patient. A balance between the test most likely to confirm the diagnosis and that with the least disruption/burden to the patient may need to be considered. Several tests that may be done in the acute setting may be less appropriate near the end-of-life.

- Arterial blood gases. Painful and unlikely to give much useful information in the setting of co-existing lung disease

- ECG
  - Majority of ECGs are normal
  - Most common abnormality is sinus tachycardia
  - $S_1Q_3T_3$ phenomenon rare
  - Atrial fibrillation may be present
- D-dimers
  - High false positive results in cancer limit their usefulness
  - Chest X-ray
  - Useful in considering other causes of breathlessness besides PE

Objective testing for PE

All imaging techniques have their limitations and different degrees of burden on the patient

- **Spiral CT**
  - First-line investigation
  - Requires large volume of i/v contrast
  - Gives assessment of pulmonary veins
  - Other chest pathologies identified
  - Can be used to assess lower limb veins and Inferior Vena Cava (IVC) at the same time
- **Ventilation/Perfusion (V/Q) scan**
  - Usually well tolerated procedure
  - Use falling due to CT and pulmonary angiography
- **Pulmonary angiography**
  - Gold standard investigation
  - Invasive
  - Complication rate 0.5 per cent, mortality 0.1 per cent
  - Limited use in palliative care population
  - Rarely used now with advent of CT pulmonary angiography
- **Magnetic resonance angiography**
  - Under evaluation
  - Limited use in palliative population

Chronic venous thrombosis

Patients with hypercoagulability related to disseminated malignancy or with cancers obstructing veins may have chronic venous thrombosis requiring warfarin and/or low molecular weight heparin (LMWH). Migratory polyphlebitis affecting superficial veins, which is largely associated with disseminated bronchogenic and adenocarcinoma, may also cause venous and arterial clotting.

Treatment of VTE

Treatment goals should be to relieve symptoms and prevent further thrombotic events.

- **DVT**
  - Consider leg elevation
  - Analgesia for swelling and tenderness (NSAIDs may interfere with the INR)
  - Compression stockings if tolerated, ease the symptoms of venous hypertension
  - Consider anticoagulation
  - Venocaval filters may prevent PE if recurrent DVTs are a problem despite anticoagulation but are associated with painful engorgement of both lower limbs
- **PE**
  - Oxygen
  - Opioids +/– benzodiazepines for breathlessness and fear
  - Consider anticoagulation

Anticoagulation in a patient with advanced malignancy should be considered carefully prior to initiation. Palliative care patients are at a high risk of haemorrhage for several reasons:

- Presence of DIC
- Consumption of clotting factors
- Platelet dysfunction/thrombocytopenia
- Tumours may be vascular
- Liver metastases

Each patient should be considered on an individual basis taking into account the following:

- Prognosis
- Bleeding risk
- Ability to control symptoms and quality of life without anticoagulation
- Perceived burden of anticoagulation
- Patient's views

Local haematology department guidelines should be sought regarding anticoagulation. Traditionally in palliative care patients were initially treated with LMWH and, depending on the clinical circumstances, considered for commencing warfarin at the same time. Once the INR is stable at a therapeutic dose, the LMWH can be discontinued.

> **Important!**
> Never commence warfarin therapy without first checking the INR or platelet count.

Warfarin in patients with cancer

Despite being the mainstay of long term anticoagulation for VTE, extreme caution should be used when recommending warfarin. Several studies have demonstrated significant increases in rates of bleeding among cancer patients on warfarin (in the order of 20 per cent). More frequent monitoring of the INR (which should be maintained between 2 to 3) is often needed in patients with cancer (i.e. every 2–3 days) to reduce the risk of bleeding.

Problems with using warfarin in patients with advanced cancer:

- High risk of bleeding. Even higher if thrombocytopenia or liver metastases
- Unpredictable metabolism of warfarin
- Interaction with other drugs
- Difficulty maintaining stable International normalized ratio (INR)
- Burden of repeated INR checks to optimize safety
- Progression of thrombus despite therapeutic INR in a proportion of patients

Rapid reversal of warfarin

Give 12–50 mL/kg FFP, 1 unit 300mL—usually 3–4 units of fresh plasma and 10mg Vitamin K by slow i/v injection.

Low molecular weight heparin in patients with cancer

Although the mainstay of treatment of VTE in patients with cancer remains long term anticoagulation with warfarin, this is likely to change. There is now level 1a evidence comparing long term LMWH with warfarin in this patient group. LMWH has been shown to reduce the recurrence of VTE from 17 per cent to 9 per cent with no statistical difference in bleeding when compared with warfarin.

LMWH may be of particular benefit in palliative care since there is no need to measure anticoagulation levels and the drug does not react with other medicines.

The progressive nature of advanced malignancy invariably heralds changing symptoms, which necessitate drug alterations. This is a particular area of risk in warfarinized patients, where drug interactions may increase the INR.

There have been concerns that the once daily injection of LMWH is too invasive, burdensome and detrimental to patients' quality of life, whilst others would argue that this is less of a burden than the alternate day INR checks that may be required to minimize the risk of warfarin-related haemorrhage.

A phenomenological study amongst palliative care patients receiving long term LMWH suggests it is an acceptable intervention and does not have an adverse impact on quality of life.

LMWH is more costly than warfarin, but this does not take into account costs of repeated blood monitoring and prolonged length of hospital stay whilst loading warfarin to therapeutic levels.

Potential benefits for LMWH
Reliable pharmacokinetics
Anticoagulant effect not altered by diet or concomitant drug use
Fast onset of action
Repeated blood test monitoring not required

At present there are no guidelines defining which patients should receive LMWH for long-term anticoagulation. Each patient should be considered individually, but the following patients should be considered for LMWH rather than warfarin:
Continued thrombosis on therapeutic warfarin
Liver metastases
Symptoms that are difficult to control adequately with regular medication
Regular INR checks considered too great a burden
Poor venous access for blood testing

VTE and brain metastases
The management of VTE in patients with brain metastases is complicated and there is no consensus. Studies comparing the use of venacaval filters with anticoagulation, show that 40 per cent of patients with filters may have further thrombotic events and 7 per cent of those anticoagulated may develop neurological deterioration from intracerebral bleeding. The role of LMWH in these patients is yet to be clarified.

Length of anticoagulation
A patient should remain anticoagulated as long as the prothrombotic risk leading to VTE persists. In cancer, the prothrombotic risk increases as disease advances and so anticoagulation should, in theory, continue indefinitely. The decision should be made taking into account the patient's views, effect of treatment, logistics of treatment and complications. As disease progresses and the bleeding tendency increases, stopping anticoagulation may be the lesser of two evils.

Table 6l.2

Target INR	Indication
2.0–2.5	DVT prophylaxis
2.5	Treatment of DVT and PE (or recurrence in patients not on warfarin)
3.5	Recurrent DVT and PE in patients receiving warfarin
	Mechanical prosthetic heart valves

Developing a good relationship with haematology colleagues

- In order to provide the best possible care for patients with end-stage haematological disease, palliative care teams need to build close working relationships with colleagues in haematology
- Historically this relationship has been challenging, as there has been lack of understanding of respective rôles
- Many patients may benefit in terms of symptom control and prolongation of life from aggressive active haematological intervention (including invasive procedures and frequent infusion of blood products even in the terminal stages. This may be difficult for palliative care teams, whose aim for dying patients is to control symptoms in the least burdensome manner
- The stereotypical prejudices inherent in both specialties are unhelpful
- It is crucial for the benefit of patients that there are good working relationships between haematology and palliative care specialists, so that patients and their families can have access and the support of both approaches, and are aware of all the issues and choices

There are reasons why palliative care involvement in haematologic. patients is challenging, as outlined below:
- There may be a misperception that palliative care teams only provide terminal care and therefore referrals should only be made when the patient is 'actively dying'
- Problems may have occurred previously with well intentioned but perhaps misguided palliative interventions, such as thrombocytopenic patients bleeding or myeloma patients developing renal failure having been started on NSAIDs
- Communication issues. The palliative care team may inadvertently question the patient's knowledge and understanding of their illness and attitude to continuation of treatment, which might overtly or covertly be seen to undermine the haematology treatment plan
- Fear that palliative care team will take over patients who have often been managed for many years by the haematology team
- It is important to fully appreciate that the haematology team may have looked after their patient through several near-death crises. Patients may have responded to previous treatments in extremis and, for instance, offering further chemotherapy may be totally appropriate
- During treatment and as disease progresses haematology patients can become very ill, very quickly. This may not be the terminal stage however as patients may respond to active support with antibiotics, fluids and blood products

n the haematology context it is often very difficult to identify when a
patient is dying.

- Haematology colleagues need to be aware that palliative care
specialists do not take over patients, or undermine their colleagues,
or use medication to shorten the lives of patients
- Palliative care teams should work alongside haematology teams,
amicably negotiating the treatment path with patients and families

Psychiatric symptoms in palliative medicine

Adjustment disorders

Adjustment disorders are defined as a maladaptive reaction to an identifiable psychosocial stressor which occurs within three months of the onset of the stressor and which does not persist for longer than six months. The symptoms are not specified, but the commonest presenting symptoms are depression and anxiety. Clinical presentations can include anger, bitterness and blaming others. A useful marker is that the patient with adjustment disorder feels bad about the situation, whereas patients with a depressive order feel bad about themselves.

Treatment

An adjustment disorder does not respond to antidepressants and generally improves as new levels of adaptation are reached. Certain interventions, such as problem-oriented psychotherapy, may be helpful. The symptoms may fluctuate in severity on a daily basis and patients can often be distracted from their distress. Beta blockers or a short course of benzodiazepines can be helpful.

Anxiety

It is normal to be anxious in certain circumstances, many of which pertain in the palliative setting. The spectrum of anxiety ranges from 'normal' through to persistent and severe anxiety. Anxiety becomes a problem when its duration and severity exceed normal expectations. It may be acute or chronic. Anxiety is common in the terminally ill for a variety of reasons, including the fear of uncontrolled symptoms and of being left alone to die.

Anxiety assessment

1 Is it severe?
2 Is it long-standing?
3 Is it alcohol withdrawal?
4 Is it situational?
5 Is it related to a specific fear?
6 Are the family anxious?[1]

Management involves assessing the patient for any reversible factors such as pain, or unfounded worries. Stimulant drugs or excessive alcohol intake or withdrawal may exacerbate the anxiety.

It is necessary to provide the time and opportunity for patients to express their worries and concerns and for these concerns to be addressed honestly and clearly. Relaxation techniques and various complementary therapies may help, as may the controlled safe atmosphere of a hospice with professional carers.

1 Kaye P. (1999) *Decision Making in Palliative Care*, pp. 34–5. Northampton: EPL Publications.

It is important for all members of the palliative care team to be aware of the 'infectious' nature of anxiety, which can distress individual members of the palliative care team and by default the whole team. These situations are often predictable, and extra effort should be made to support staff during potentially stressful situations and to avoid being driven to extreme management decisions.

Pharmacological treatment of anxiety
Benzodiazepines

These are very useful drugs but have received a bad press because of their addictive potential. They are traditionally divided between compounds which have more sedating effects and those which have more anxiolytic actions. However, there is considerable overlap on the anxiety/sedating spectrum.

They are useful to break the anxiety cycle, to restore sleep, and to reduce the suffering of the situation where a patient feels that he/she is 'losing control'. They are not a substitute for taking the time to allow a patient to ventilate fears.

- Diazepam: 1–5mg p.r.n. p.o.—diazepam has a long half-life and may therefore accumulate and be sedative. It should be possible to give it once a day at night
- Lorazepam: 1–2mg p.r.n, p.o.—lorazepam is short acting, rapidly anxiolytic and less sedating than diazepam
- Midazolam: 5–10mg p.r.n., SC or buccal—useful for emergency sedation

---

Drugs used for Anxiety

Diazepam is an appropriate first-line benzodiazepine.

Lorazepam is shorter acting, and (taken sublingually), has a faster onset of action, and is useful on a p.r.n. basis.

Midazolam can be used if a CSCI is required.

Propranolol is helpful, especially to control the somatic symptoms of anxiety e.g. tremor and palpitations.

The anxiolytic effect of buspirone develops over 1–3 weeks, and it probably has little place in palliative care.

SSRIs can be used for panic attacks if benzodiazepines are ineffective.

Diazepam

Tabs. 2mg, 5mg, 10mg; Oral solution 2mg/5mL, 5mg/5mL

Rectal tubes 5mg/2.5mL, 10mg/2.5mL; Supps. 10mg

Inj. (emulsion) 10mg/2mL (Diazemuls)—i/v use only

Inj. (solution) 10mg/2mL—i/m use

Blood levels increased by omeprazole (increased sedation).

Lorazepam

Tabs. 1mg, 2.5mg; Inj. 4mg/1 mL

Midazolam

Inj. 10mg/2mL, 10mg/5mL

Sedative effect markedly enhanced by itraconazole, ketoconazole and possibly fluconazole.

Propranolol

Tabs. 10mg, 40mg, 80mg, 160mg; Oral solution 40mg/5mL; Tabs. 80mg, 160mg

Antidepressants

Tricyclic antidepressants (TCAs) such as amitriptyline or dosulepin[2] may be useful as anxiolytics, often in 'sub-antidepressant' dosages. Selective serotonin re-uptake inhibitor (SSRI) antidepressants such as paroxetine and citalopram (must not be used <18y) are more expensive alternatives which have less reported side-effects and also have anxiolytic properties, though care must be taken to avoid enervating SSRIs such as fluoxetine, which can initially increase anxiety. Complementary therapies, e.g. aromatherapy, and massage and specific interventions, e.g. hypnosis, relaxation and imagery, may help increase the patient's sense of control.

Complex anxiety states with depression and psychosis may be more suitably treated with neuroleptics. The help of a psychiatric team may be needed.

Payne S. (1998) Depression in palliative care patients: a literature review. *International Journal of Palliative Nursing*, 4, **4**: 184–91.

Depression

Estimates of the prevalence of depression in patients vary greatly, but it probable that at least 25 per cent may develop a significant mood disord in advanced cancer. A review of 12 articles reported a range of depress rates from 3–69 per cent. Certain types of cancer, such as pancrea cancer, are associated with an increased incidence of depression.[3] A sp trum ranging from sadness to adjustment disorder to depressive illnes recognized. There is concern that depression may be underdiagnos This may be due to a number of reasons including a diurnal variation symptoms such that it may be missed, social 'cover-up', or presentat with physical symptoms. One of the main difficulties is distinguish depression from appropriate sadness at the end-of-life.

In the physically *healthy* population, depression is diagnosed if patie have a persistent low mood and a least four of the following sympto which are present most of the day for the preceding two weeks:

1 Diminished interest or pleasure in all or almost all activities
2 Psychomotor retardation or agitation
3 Feelings of worthlessness or excessive and inappropriate guilt
4 Diminished ability to concentrate and think
5 Recurrent thoughts of death and suicide
6 Fatigue and loss of energy
7 Significant weight loss or gain
8 Insomnia or hypersomnia

In patients with advanced cancer, symptoms 6–8 are almost universal, a it is doubtful whether physical symptoms should be included at all wh diagnosing depression in the terminally ill.

Atypical presentations of depression

- irritability
- agitation and anxiety symptoms
- histrionic behaviour
- hypochondriasis
- psychotic features (delusions, paranoia) that are mood-congruent e.g. content of delusions consistent with depressive thoughts

Pharmacological treatment of depression

There is little information concerning the effectiveness of antidepressa medication in terminally ill patients. There is, however, a body of eviden showing that under treatment is common, with patients being prescrib antidepressants within the final six weeks of life, allowing little time therapeutic benefit. Psychostimulants, which have a faster onset of acti than classical antidepressants, are very rarely used in this terminal situati despite some evidence of benefit. Being younger and having breast canc increase the chance of being prescribed antidepressants.[4]

Think list

- Corticosteroids—may help mild depression and low mood by improving sense of well-being, but can also induce psychosis or depression in others. Starting low dose dexamethasone e.g. 4mg daily

or a week followed by 2mg daily for a week can elevate a patient's
mood whilst awaiting a response to antidepressants
psychostimulants (methylphenidate or dexamfetamine)
ECT (electro-convulsive therapy)—response can be very rapid; very
occasionally appropriate e.g. severe depression developing during
chemotherapy
pathological crying may respond to citalopram

Tricyclic antidepressants (TCAs)

Tricyclic antidepressants may take several weeks to lift depression.
Amitriptyline and dosulepin are relatively sedative in comparison with
imipramine and lofepramine. They all have antimuscarinic properties to
greater or lesser degrees and therefore may be associated with symptoms
such as hypotension, dry mouth and difficulty in micturition. Doses should
gradually be increased to avoid unnecessary side-effects.

Selective serotonin re-uptake inhibitors

e.g. Citalopram 20mg o.d.
Sertraline 50mg o.d.
Fluoxetine 20mg o.d.

These drugs are less sedative than tricyclic antidepressants and have few
antimuscarinic effects, low cardiotoxicity and may have a faster onset of
action than the TCAs.

SSRIs may cause nausea, vomiting and headaches and extrapyramidal reactions can occur occasionally. Gastrointestinal side-effects are dose-related.
There is little to choose between the SSRIs, but fluoxetine has a slower onset
of action and may cause more agitation than other SSRIs: it is therefore not
recommended as first line particularly in patients who are agitated.

SSRIs may increase the risk of GI bleeding, especially in patients taking
NSAIDs
serious reactions may develop with MAOIs and selegiline (serotonin
syndrome)
increased serotonergic effects are seen with St John's Wort, which
should be avoided
fluoxetine and fluvoxamine increase the blood levels of
carbamazepine and phenytoin (risk of toxicity)

Use an SSRI unless other treatment is specifically indicated:
Dose escalation is not usually needed, so more rapid control of
symptoms may be possible
The side-effects of SSRIs are generally better tolerated than TCAs in
ill patients with cancer

A trial of at least three weeks, and preferably six or more, is needed to
properly assess response to an antidepressant. Discontinuation symptoms
(withdrawal) will not usually occur if stopped within six weeks of starting.

Doyle D. H., Hanks, G. W. C., Cherny, N. (2004) *Oxford Textbook of Palliative Medicine*. 3rd edn.
Oxford: Oxford University Press.

Lloyd-Williams M., Friedman T., Rudd N. (1999) A survey of antidepressant prescribing in the
terminally ill. *Palliative Medicine*, **13**: 243–8.

Antidepressant discontinuation syndromes occur with both TCAs SSRIs.

SSRI discontinuation symptoms include dizziness, light-headedn insomnia, fatigue, anxiety/agitation, nausea, headache, and sensory dist bance. SSRIs should be withdrawn gradually when possible, using altern day dosing if needed.

Symptoms of withdrawal are more common with paroxetine (sh half-life), and least common with fluoxetine (half-life of weeks).

Paroxetine
- Tabs. 20mg; liquid 20mg/10mL
- Dose 20mg mane p.o.—increase by weekly increments of 10mg as necessary to max. 50mg o.d.

Citalopram
- Tabs. 10, 20, 40mg; oral drops 40mg/mL
- Dose: 20mg mane p.o.; max. 60mg o.d.

Sertraline
- Tabs. 50, 100mg
- Dose 50mg mane p.o.; max. 200mg o.d.

Other antidepressant drugs

Venlafaxine is a serotonin and noradrenaline re-uptake inhibitor (SNRI causes less side-effects than the SSRIs. The slow release capsules preferable to use as they seem to be better tolerated. Mirtazepine noradrenergic and specific serotoninergic antidepressant (NaSSA) and useful if there is marked anxiety/agitation. At lower doses the antihis minic effect predominates producing sedation, which is reduced w higher doses when the noradrenergic transmission increases.

Venlafaxine
- Tabs. 37.5, 50, 75mg
- Dose: 37.5mg b.d. p.o. increased to 75mg b.d.
- Caps. m/r 75, 150mg
- Dose: 75mg o.d. p.o. increased to 150mg o.d.
- Dose should be increased gradually to the usual dose 150mg, and higher according to response; maximum 375mg daily (225mg if m/r)

Mirtazepine
- Tabs. (scored) 30mg
- Dose: 15mg nocte p.o. increased to 30mg nocte
- Dose should be increased gradually to usual dose 30mg, and higher according to response; maximum 45mg daily

Tricyclics and tetracyclics

The original tricyclics antidepressants (amitriptyline, imipramine etc.) used in low doses as co-analgesics, but they are poorly tolerated due side-effects in antidepressant doses and it is advisable to commence SSRI and avoid TCAs for the treatment of depression in patie with advanced cancer. Dosulepin is a good first-line antidepressa whilst lofepramine has a lower incidence of side-effects and therefore useful in the elderly. Usual treatment dose of most TCAs 150mg/day (perhaps less in elderly); lofepramine dose is 140–210mg/d

Higher doses are associated with worse side-effects e.g. dry mouth, sedation, prostatism etc.

Tricyclic antidepressants used concomitantly with amiodarone increase the risk of ventricular arrhythmias and should be avoided.

Dosulepin

Caps. 25mg; Tabs. 75mg
Dose 50–75mg nocte p.o.

Lofepramine

Tabs. 70mg
Dose 70mg o.d.—b.d. p.o.

St John's Wort

A number of patients may be taking St John's Wort as an antidepressant. It is not a licensed medication, and has a number of significant drug interactions:

Increases serotonergic effects with SSRIs; therefore avoid
Reduces anticoagulant effect of warfarin
Reduces plasma levels of carbamazepine, phenytoin, phenobarbital
(risk of fits)
Reduces plasma levels of digoxin

Screening for depression

There are no universally accepted criteria for diagnosing depression in the terminally ill. In patients with advanced cancer, many of the symptoms of depression, e.g. changes in appetite, energy levels and sleep pattern, are common and there is still considerable controversy as to whether these physical symptoms should be included. Depressed mood, irritability, loss of interest in anything, feelings of worthlessness and lack of hope for the future are more important in this population.

Rating scales to measure depression are increasingly used. Such tools are not diagnostic and can only serve to indicate whether a patient has particular psychiatric symptoms suggestive of a diagnosis of depression. The decision should then be taken whether to treat for depression or to refer the patient for further assessment. The majority of rating scales consist of a number of symptoms or feelings. Patients indicate their own response and the person administering the scale calculates the scores.

Several instruments have been developed which define a threshold score for the predictability of depression. However, a defined cut-off threshold suitable for patients with early cancer or those receiving treatment may not be valid for patients with advanced metastatic disease receiving palliative care. Recent work has suggested that a scale developed for use in the post-natal period (the Edinburgh Depression Scale) may be useful for screening in palliative care. It does not include somatic symptoms but does include symptoms such as sadness, feelings of helplessness and thoughts of self harm which may be particularly discriminatory in the palliative care population. Each item is scored from 0–3—the most negative response scoring highest. A cut-off threshold of 13 has sensitivity and specificy of approximately 80 per cent.

e Edinburgh Depression Scale

ease UNDERLINE the answer which comes close to how you have felt
THE PAST 7 DAYS, not just how you feel today

**have been able to laugh and
ee the funny side of things:**
As much as I always could
Not quite so much now
Definitely not so much now
Not at all

**have looked forward with
enjoyment to things:**
As much as I ever did
Rather less than I used to
Definitely less than I used to
Hardly at all

**have blamed myself
unnecessarily when things
vent wrong:**
Yes, most of the time
Yes, some of the time
Not very often
No, never

**have been anxious or
worried for no good
reason:**
No, not at all
Hardly ever
Yes, sometimes
Yes, very often

**get a sort of frightened
feeling as if something awful
s about to happen:**
Very definitely and quite badly
Yes, but not too badly
A little, but it doesn't worry me
Not at all

**Things have been getting
on top of me:**
Most of the time and I haven't
been able to cope at all
Yes, sometimes I haven't been
coping as well as usual
No, most of the time I have
coped quite well
No, I have been coping as
well as ever

**I have been so unhappy that
I have had difficulty sleeping:**
Yes, most of the time
Yes, quite often
Not very often
No, not at all

I have felt sad or miserable:
Yes, most of the time
Yes, quite often
Not very often
No, not at all

**I have been so unhappy,
I have been crying:**
Yes, most of the time
Yes, quite often
Only occasionally
No, never

**The thought of harming
myself has occurred to me:**
Yes, quite often
Sometimes
Hardly ever
Never

Confusional states

Delirium: An etiologically, non-specific, global, cerebral dysfunction characterised by concurrent disturbance of level of consciousness, attention, thinking, perception, memory, psychomotor behaviour, emotion and sleep-wake cycle.

An acute confusional state (or delirium) is associated with men clouding, leading to a disturbance of comprehension which is charact ized by decreased attention, disorientation and cognitive impairment w poor short-term memory and concentration.

The prevalence of delirium may be as high as 85 per cent for hospitaliz terminally ill patients and is particularly common in elderly patients mov from a familiar environment. It may be exacerbated by deafness and po vision.

While delirium is normally understood as a reversible process, the may not be time for it to improve in terminally ill patients. Occasiona irreversible processes such as multiple organ failure cause delirium.

The diagnosis may be obvious with a rapid onset of altered behavic and incoherent rambling speech. The symptoms may fluctuate and the may be insight. Severe delirium can progress to psychotic features w hallucinations and delusions.

The differential diagnosis includes dementia, which is a more chro condition, is not associated with mental clouding and is irreversible.

It may be appropriate, if done sensitively, to carry out a simplified mi mental score test to help management and to monitor clinical progress.

Mini-mental score

A test devised for the serial testing of cognitive mental state on a neuros riatric ward. A score of 20 or less was found in patients with dement delirium, schizophrenia or affective disorder.[5]

Instructions for administration	Max score
Orientation	
What is the date (year) (season) (date) (day) (month)?	5
Ask for the date. Then ask specifically for parts omitted, e.g., 'Can you also tell me what season it is?' One point for each correct.	
Where are we: (state) (county) (town) (hospital) (floor)	5
Ask in turn 'Can you tell me the name of this hospital? (town, county, etc.). One point for each correct.	
Registration	
Ask the patient if you may test his memory. Say the names of three unrelated objects, clearly and slowly, about one second for each. After you have said all three, ask him to repeat them. This first repetition determines his score (0–3; 1 point for each correct answer), but keep saying them until he can repeat all three, up to six trials. If he does not eventually learn all three, recall cannot be meaningfully tested. Count trials and record.	3
Attention and calculation	
Serial 7's. Ask the patient to begin with 100 and count backwards by 7. Stop after five subtractions (93, 86, 79, 72, 65). Score the total number of correct answers. 1 point for each correct. If the patient cannot or will not perform this task, ask him to spell the word 'world' backwards. Score the number of letters in correct order e.g. dlrow = 5, dlorw = 3.	5
Recall	
Ask the patient if he can recall the three words you previously asked him to remember.	3
Score 0–3. Give 1 point for each correct.	
Language	
Naming: Name a pencil, and watch.	2
Show the patient a wrist watch and ask him what it is. Repeat for pencil. Score 0–2.	
Repetition: Ask the patient to repeat the sentence after you: 'No ifs, ands or buts.' Allow only one trial. Score 0 or 1.	1
Three-stage command: 'Take a piece of paper in your right hand, fold it in half, and put it on the floor'.Give the patient a piece of plain blank paper and repeat the command. Score 1 point for each part correctly executed.	3
Reading: Read and obey the following: 'CLOSE YOUR EYES'	1
On a blank piece of paper print the sentence 'Close your eyes', in letters large enough for the patient to see clearly. Ask him to read it and do what it says. Score 1 point only if he actually closes his eyes.	
Writing: Give the patient a blank piece of paper and ask him to write a sentence for you. Do not dictate a sentence, it is to be written spontaneously. It must contain a subject and verb and be sensible. Correct grammar and punctuation are not necessary.	1
Copying: On a clean piece of paper, draw intersecting pentagons, each side about 1 in., and ask him to copy it exactly as it is. All 10 angles must be present and two must intersect to score 1 point. Tremor and rotation are ignored.	1
TOTAL SCORE	
(Max. 30)	

5 Folstein M. F., Folstein S. E., McHugh P. R. (1975) 'Mini-Mental State': a practical method for grading the cognitive state of patients for the clinician. *J Psychiatr Res*, **12**: 189–98.

Delirium and confusion

Treat reversible **cause** of confusion if possible.
  Consider:
- hypercalcaemia
- hypoglycaemia
- hyponatraemia
- renal failure
- liver failure
- drug-related causes
  - opioids
  - corticosteroids AND withdrawal
  - alcohol withdrawal
  - benzodiazepine AND withdrawal
  - SSRI withdrawal
  - nicotine withdrawal
  - digoxin
  - lithium
- NB benzodiazepines and phenothiazines accumulate in liver failure and opioids in renal failure
- cerebral tumour, primary or secondary
- CVA or Transient Ischaemic Attack (TIA)
- anxiety/depression
- infection
- hypoxia
- disorientation of move to hospital (in pre-existing dementia)
- thiamine (vitamin B_1) deficiency
- non-convulsive status epilepticus

The cause is often multifactorial, and symptoms such as pain or those associated with constipation or urinary retention may aggravate confusion

Prescribing for delirium and confusional states
- Drugs should only be prescribed if necessary
- Night sedation should be given only after an attempt to remove other causes of insomnia such as fear, noisy and unfamiliar surroundings, unrelieved pain, nocturia and stimulant medication such as steroids
- Reassurance and helping to orientate the patient and alleviate fear may be all that is required. The patient and family should be comforted by being told that the patient is not 'going mad', but that this is a temporary setback which is hopefully reversible. Daytime sedation should only be necessary if the patient is very distressed and not amenable to reassurance or is a danger to themselves or others
- Doses should be adjusted according to age and general condition, level of disturbance, and likely tolerance
- Antipsychotics are considered to be the drugs of choice for delirium, haloperidol being the most commonly used
- The risk of extrapyramidal side-effects (EPSE) is greatest in the elderly, and with the older antipsychotics such as haloperidol and chlorpromazine; newer drugs such as risperidone, olanzapine and promazine are better tolerated but may not be adequate if rapid control is needed of an acutely disturbed patient (Risperidone and olanzapine are associated with an increased risk of stroke in elderly patients with dementia.)

- Chlorpromazine and levomepromazine are more sedative than haloperidol
- Benzodiazepines carry a risk of paradoxical agitation (disinhibition with worsening of behavioural disturbance) especially in the elderly. Used in conjunction with haloperidol, lorazepam improves the control of the acutely disturbed patient, but used alone is less effective than antipsychotics in delirium
- Most antipsychotics decrease the convulsive threshold, and may increase the risk of convulsions in susceptible patients, but the actual risk is undetermined

Benzodiazepines in agitation and restlessness

Although antipsychotics are considered the treatment of choice for delirium, agitation and restlessness in the patient with advanced cancer may often be primarily an anxiety state, with secondary cognitive impairment or clouded consciousness. In this condition, benzodiazepines may be more effective than antipsychotics. A knowledge of the previous psychological state of the patient is vital in determining this.

Alcohol withdrawal

The best treatment for alcohol withdrawal in palliative care is usually alcohol if the patient is able to swallow. In practice, patients who have been deteriorating over months have usually gradually reduced their alcohol intake.

Clomethiazole ± benzodiazepines are the usual drug treatments. Alcohol withdrawal has also been treated with 10–20mL absolute alcohol made up to 50mL with saline/24h i/v using a syringe driver, but this type of management is rarely necessary in the palliative setting.

Wernicke's encephalopathy (thiamine/vitamin B_1 deficiency) may be more common than anticipated in the terminally ill. The diagnosis can be confirmed by red blood cell (RBC) transketolase estimation. The diagnosis should be considered in any patient with a history of alcohol misuse who develops unexplained:

- ophthalmoplegia
- nystagmus
- ataxia (not due to intoxication)
- acute confusion (not due to intoxication)
- memory disturbance
- seizures
- coma/unconsciousness

A presumptive diagnosis of Wernicke's encephalopathy should prompt treatment with high-dose parenteral B-complex vitamins.

Antipsychotics

Haloperidol

- Caps. 0.5mg; Tabs. 1.5mg, 5mg; liquid 2mg/mL; inj. 5mg/1mL
- (Indomethacin given with haloperidol can cause severe drowsiness.)

Levomepromazine (methotrimeprazine)

- Tabs. 6mg 25mg; susp. 25mg/5/mL; inj. 25mg/1mL (nozinan)
- Dose 12.5mg nocte or b.d. p.o.; 12.5mg/24h CSCI
- 6mg Tabs. available on a named patient basis only

- Oral bioavailability of levomepromazine is approx. 40 per cent. Use half the daily oral dose by CSCI
- Avoid concurrent use with mono amine oxidase inhibitors (MAOIs)

Promazine
- Tabs. 25mg, 50mg; liquid 25mg/5mL, 50mg/5mL; inj. 50mg/1mL

Risperidone
- Tabs. 0.5mg, 1mg, 2mg, 3mg, 4mg, 6mg; liquid 1mg/1mL
- Avoid in patients with cerebrovascular disease

Olanzapine
- Tabs. 2.5mg, 5mg, 7.5mg, 10mg; dispersible 5mg, 10mg, 15mg
- Dispersible tablets can be placed on the tongue to dissolve/disperse
- Avoid in patients with cerebrovascular disease

Thioridazine and droperidol
Thioridazine has had its licence for treating agitation in the elderly removed because of the risk of cardiac arrhythmias, and should not be prescribed except under guidance from a psychiatrist.

Droperidol has been withdrawn for the same reason (prolonged QT intervals).

Benzodiazepines
Lorazepam
Lorazepam is shorter acting than diazepam, and is therefore safer in repeated doses; it can be given SC or sublingually for more rapid effect and in uncooperative patients.
- Tabs. 1mg, 2.5mg; inj. 4mg/1mL
- Dilute inj. with equal volume of water or saline for i/m use

Diazepam
- Tabs. 2mg, 5mg, 10mg; syrup 2mg/5mL; rectal soln. 5mg/2.5mL, 10mg/2.5mL
- Supps. 10mg
- Blood levels increased by omeprazole (increased sedation)

Midazolam
- Inj. 10mg/2mL, 10mg/5mL
- Dose: 20–30mg/24h *CSCI* (max. 100mg/24h)
- Sedative effect markedly enhanced by itraconazole, ketoconazole and possibly fluconazole

Vitamin B preparations
Pabrinex (vitamins B and C)
- Inj. Pair of ampoules containing 10mL
- Dose: 1 pair of ampoules daily for three days—for acute and severe vitamin B deficiency states
- Serious allergic reaction may rarely occur on i/v administration (probably <1 in 250,000, compared to incidence of 1–10 per cent allergy with penicillin). Inject slowly over 10 minutes

Table 6m.1 Treatment of delirium and confusion with antipsychotics when no reversible causes diagnosed

Presentation	Non-elderly	Elderly
Confusion ± drowsiness, or where sedation undesirable/unnecessary	Non-sedative antipsychotic Haloperidol 1.5–3mg nocte or b.d. SC/CSCI (Risperidone 0.5–1mg b.d.)	Non-sedative antipsychotic with lower risk of extrapyramidal side-effects (EPSE) Risperidone 0.5mg nocte or b.d. p.o Haloperidol 0.5–1mg nocte SC/CSCI.
Agitated confusion where sedative effects desired; mild—moderate agitation	Sedative antipsychotic Levomepromazine 25–50mg SC/CSCI/p.o. (Chlorpromazine 25–50mg b.d.–q.d.s. p.o.)	Sedative antipsychotic with lower risk of EPSE Promazine 25mg nocte or up to q.d.s. p.o. Levomepromazine 12.5–25mg/24h CSCI (Olanzapine 2.5mg nocte p.o.)
Acutely disturbed, violent or aggressive; at risk to themselves or others. Antipsychotic with proven safety record in repeated high doses for rapid titration; suitable for parenteral use*	Haloperidol 5mg SC/i/m ± lorazepam 1–2mg SC/i/m repeated after 20–30 minutes.	Haloperidol 2.5mg SC/i/m ± lorazepam 0.5–1 mg SC/i/m repeated after 30 minutes

* Risperidone and olanzapine must be avoided in patients with a history of cerebrovascular disease.

Equivalent doses of antipsychotic and benzodiazepine medication

Occasionally patients are taking antipsychotic drugs or benzodiazepines on a long term basis. The approximate equivalent doses are outlined below although, as ever, doses should be based on an overall assessment of the patient's individual needs. Switching antipsychotics or benzodiazepines, while not recommended, is sometimes required in the palliative care setting especially if the previous oral route is no longer available.

Table 6m.2 Benzodiazepine drug equivalence (an approximate guide)

Antipsychotic drug equivalence			
Antipsychotic drug	**Approximate equivalent daily dose**		
Chlorpromazine	100mg		
Haloperidol	2–3mg		
Levomepromazine	25–50mg		
Pimozide	2mg		
Risperidone	0.5–1mg		
Trifluoperazine	5mg		
	Equivalent dose anxiolytic/sedative	**Approximate duration of action**	**Approximate subcutaneous dose over 24 h**
Diazepam	5mg p.o. or PR	3 h to 4 days	N/A
Clonazepam	0.25mg p.o.	6–24 h	1mg
Midazolam	2.5mg SC	15mins to 4 h	10mg
Lorazepam	0.5mg p.o.	7–8 h	N/A
Temazepam	10mg p.o.	7–8 h	N/A

Psychostimulants

Potential uses for psychostimulants:
- Depression
- Opioid -induced sedation or cognitive impairment
- Fatigue
- Cognitive impairment due to brain tumours
- Hypoactive delirium
- Hiccups

Psychostimulants for depression

Psychostimulants have been shown to be effective in depression in medically ill patients including the terminally ill, although they do not seem to be effective in primary depression. They are rarely prescribed for depression in the UK. They are useful because of their rapid onset, and are generally well tolerated. The beneficial effects of these drugs are reported to occur within 36–48 h. Drug habituation is generally not a problem.

Methylphenidate appears to have been used more widely, but dexamfetamine is equally effective.

Doses of methylphenidate as low as 1.25mg daily have been used successfully in patients over 90 years old. Methylphenidate (average dose after titration 30mg daily) is as effective as imipramine 150mg o.d. in significantly reducing depressive and anxiety symptoms.

Psychostimulants have been used as adjuvants to reduce opioid-induced sedation and potentiate analgesia. It is not known whether this is due to a reduction in opioid-induced sedation, thus allowing dose escalation of the opioid, or to a direct potentiation of opioid analgesia.

Side-effects of psychostimulant drugs including agitation, dysphoria, insomnia, nightmares and hypomania have been reported.

Methylphenidate
- Tabs. 5, 10, 20mg
- Dose: 5mg b.d. p.o. (8.00am and 12 noon); increase every few days up to 30mg b.d. according to response

Dexamfetamine sulphate
- Tabs. 5mg
- Dose 5mg b.d. p.o. (8.00am and 12 noon); increase every few days up to 30mg b.d. according to response

Terminal restlessness/anguish (📖 see Chapter 13)

Spiritual distress (📖 see Chapter 9)

At the time of referral and transition to the palliative/terminal phase of illness, many patients have an increased spiritual awareness. The conce of these patients are often based on the existential questions:

- Who am I?
- What am I?
- Will I be remembered?
- How will I be remembered?

Patients experiencing emotional suffering often have 'Soul pain', but t may go unrecognized.

The integration of spiritual care into the palliative care team is therefo vital, to ensure that patients have the opportunity to disclose and disc these concerns, which can cause great emotional distress. However, t spiritual needs are often not included in the assessment of quality of life terminally ill patients, and may not be identified by health professionals.

Suicide

Depression is increased in patients with terminal cancer and the incider of suicide and thoughts of self harm are increased in depressed patien The incidence of suicide is therefore more common than previou believed.

Patients with cancer have twice the risk of committing suicide as t general population. Factors such as depression, advancing disease a hopelessness increase the risk of suicide. Other risk factors include act suicidal thoughts, uncontrolled pain, exhaustion and fatigue, past suici attempts, substance abuse, recent bereavement, poor social support a family history of suicide. It is also thought that certain sites of cancer, oropharyngeal, lung, gastrointestinal, urogenital and breast, may increa the risk of suicide.

Patients with cancer tend to commit suicide by overdose of analgesia sedative drugs. Many doctors believe that by inquiring about suici intent, they may precipitate a suicide. Contrary to this belief, talking a sharing his/her thoughts of self harm permits the patient to descri his/her feelings.

Suicidal ideation must not, however, be confused with patients wl request death to be hastened—these patients may also be depressed, b may have other underlying fears e.g. of a painful or undignified dea 📖 see also the chapter on Euthanasia.

The initial assessment and evaluation of a patient with suicidal ideati should include the following:

1 Establish rapport and empathic approach
2 Assess the patient's understanding of illness and symptoms
3 Assess mental status
4 Assess other factors, e.g. poor pain control

5 Assess external support system
6 Establish prior psychiatric history
7 Obtain family history
8 Record past suicide attempts or threats
9 Assess suicide thinking and plans
10 Formulate treatment plan

patients may require initial close supervision on a one to one basis. Careful attention should be paid to pain relief and relief of other distressing symptoms. It may be necessary to commence neuroleptic medication initially in addition to antidepressant medication. A psychiatric opinion should be obtained.

The patient's family and the palliative care team itself may require a lot of support.

Further reading

Books

Chochinov H. and Breitbart W. (eds) (2000) *Handbook of Psychiatry in Palliative Medicine*. Oxford: Oxford University Press.

Doyle D. H., Hanks G. W. C., Cherny N. (2004) *Oxford Textbook of Palliative Medicine*. 3rd edn. Oxford: Oxford University Press.

Kaye P. (1999) *Decision-making in Palliative Care*, pp. 34–5. Northampton: EPL Publications.

Kearney M. (2000) *A Place of Healing: Working with suffering in living and dying*. Oxford: Oxford University Press.

Lloyd-Williams M. (2003) *Psychosocial Issues in Palliative Care*. Oxford: Oxford University Press.

Articles

Ahronheim J., Morrison R., Baskin S., Morris J., Meier D. (1996) Treatment of the dying in the acute care hospital: Advanced dementia and metastatic cancer. *Archives of Internal Medicine*, **156**: 2094–100.

Breitbart W., Jacobsen P. B. (1996) Psychiatric symptom management in terminal care. *Clinics in Geriatric Medicine*, **12, 2**: 329–47.

Cox J., Holden J., Sagovsky R. (1987) Detection of postnatal depression: Development of the 10-item Edinburgh Postnatal Depression Scale. *British Journal of Psychiatry*, **150**: 782–6.

Folstein G. A., Folstein S. E., McHugh P. R. (1975) Mini Mental State. *Journal of Psychiatric Research*, 12: 189–98.

Kovach C., Weissman D., Griffie J., Matson S., Muchka S. (1999) Assessment and treatment of discomfort for people with late stage dementia. *Journal of Pain and Symptom Management*, **8**: 412–19.

Lloyd-Williams M., Friedman T., Rudd N. (1999) A survey of antidepressant prescribing in the terminally ill. *Palliative Medicine*, **13**: 243–8.

Lloyd-Williams M., Payne S. (2002) Can multidisciplinary guidelines improve the palliation of symptoms in the terminal phase of Dementia. *Int J of Palliative Nursing*, **8**: 370–5.

Chapter 7

Paediatric palliative care

There can be no Doubt that a perfect Cure of the Diseases of Children is as much desired by all, as any thing else whatsoever in the whole art of Physick.

Walter Harris, 1698

Who needs paediatric palliative care?

The emergence of a new specialty

- Advances in the treatment of life-threatening neonatal and paediatric conditions have dramatically improved survival rates over recent years
- One of the most striking reductions in mortality has been achieved for children with malignant conditions, although there remain certain forms of cancer for which the prognosis remains extremely poor
- Similarly, there is a range of non-malignant conditions which continue to be life-limiting, despite the advances outlined above
- The patient population in paediatric palliative care is quite different from that encountered in adult practice. Approximately 40–50 per cent of children with palliative care needs have a malignancy
- The remainder have a variety of conditions including congenital abnormalities and neurodegenerative disorders
- Modern pharmacological and technical approaches now make it possible for some children, who would previously not have survived at all, to live longer, sometimes into adulthood. Many of these children have long illness trajectories which see them deteriorate slowly and inexorably toward a state of high dependency and disability
- It can be difficult to identify a point where treatment becomes exclusively palliative, and this presents a major challenge to service providers
- Many conditions are rare and the prognosis is often unpredictable, the child could die at any time or may live a number of years. These children often have multiple symptoms, requiring frequent medical intervention, in addition to complex psychological needs
- The parents and siblings of these children also need support in adjusting to the diagnosis and ongoing care of the child

Specialist paediatric palliative care services have recently been established in a number of centres throughout the world and focus variably on the three main care settings: home, hospice and hospital. Families will generally move between the various settings according to need but it has become clear that where home care is offered as a realistic option, most families will wish to care for their child at home. Children's home care teams and outreach nurses are becoming more common and are often able to take on a palliative care rôle providing support for children with life-limiting diseases and their families in their own homes.

In addition, children's hospices are also being established, providing an option for respite and terminal care. Specialist palliative care services for children in hospitals are not as widely available away from major centres, although adult palliative care teams are available for advice in many hospitals.

Much of the introductory material for this chapter has been produced by the Royal Children's Hospital, Melbourne Paediatric Palliative Care team.

The box below is taken from *A Guide to the Development of Children's Palliative Care Services* and lists numerous conditions that may affect the child in palliative care.[2]

---

1 Conditions for which curative treatment is possible but may fail. e.g. leukaemia.
2 Diseases where premature death is likely but intensive treatments may prolong good quality life e.g. cystic fibrosis, muscular dystrophy.
3 Progressive conditions where treatment is exclusively palliative and may extend for many years e.g. mucopolysaccharidoses, other neurodegenerative conditions.
4 Conditions, often with neurological impairment, causing weakness and susceptibility to complications e.g. non progressive CNS disease.

Background

Children in the terminal phase of illness are known to suffer significantly from inadequate recognition and treatment of symptoms, aggressive attempts at cure, fear and sadness. A child's death is experienced as a profound loss by parents, siblings, extended family and the wider community. Bereaved parents suffer intense grief and may be at increased risk of death themselves from both natural and unnatural causes.[1]

For those living in developed nations, child mortality has fallen to such an extent that the death of a child seems an utterly unnatural and devastating affront. It is now so uncommon as to create a sense of alienation for families who are caring for a dying child or whose child has died. This increases the importance of support for the family throughout the child's illness, from diagnosis and treatment through terminal care, to bereavement.

Prevalence of UK paediatric palliative care needs[2]

In a district of 250,000 people with a population of 50,000 children aged <19yrs, in one year:
- 5 are likely to die from a life-limiting condition of which 2 would be from cancer, 1 from heart disease and 2 from other life-limiting conditions.
- At the same time about 50 children would be suffering from a life-limiting condition and, of these, about half would have palliative care needs.[1]

---

1 Li J., Precht D. H., Mortensen P. B., Olsen J. (2003) Mortality in parents after death of a child in Denmark: a nationwide follow-up study. *Lancet*, **361**: 363–7.

2 Association for Children with Life-threatening or Terminal Conditions and their Families and the Royal College of Paediatrics and Child Health (2003) *A Guide to the Development of Children's Palliative Care Services*. 2nd edn. London: ACT.

Provision of paediatric palliative care

The provision of paediatric palliative care is patchy and the structure of specialist teams variable. Before thinking about service provision, it may be helpful to consider what and who surrounds a family in this situation.

A large number of agencies and individuals may be involved in supporting children and families and although this is appropriate, there is the potential for confusion, intrusion and replication of services. It is often helpful to nominate a *key worker* who can coordinate the various services involved and act as a first point of call for families. Through effective communication, including regular meetings, a comprehensive management plan can be created for the child in question. It is important that all the professionals involved are supported themselves, as this can be a demanding and unfamiliar area of practice. A specialist paediatric palliative care team can support the agencies and individuals involved in caring for the family. Such a team may include some or all of the following:

- Paediatric palliative care nurses (who may provide advice in both hospital and community settings)
- A specialist palliative care paediatrician
- Social worker
- Psychologist and or psychiatrist
- Chaplain

Sometimes, advice and support are needed from other teams or professionals with special expertise or knowledge regarding a particular condition. This is often necessary in cases where children have very rare conditions.

Differences between paediatric and adult palliative care

Developmental factors

An understanding of developmental issues is essential to the management of a child with palliative care needs. Infants and young children are completely dependent on the adults in their lives for care and protection. They also depend on others to make decisions on their behalf.

As children grow and develop, their capacity to care and decide for themselves increases. Indeed, the emergence of autonomy is a central developmental task of adolescence. In this way, care that is appropriate for a child of 11 may be inappropriate two years later as the need for independence, privacy and greater control grows. This can be difficult for both parents and healthcare professionals to accept. The natural desire to protect a child who is experiencing a devastating illness can lead to that child feeling stifled.

The relationship between development and illness is bidirectional. That is, the changing developmental status of the child influences the way in which they experience illness, and illness, in turn, influences the child's development. Chronic illness can delay development but the life experience it brings may also make a child seem old beyond their years.

The child's developmental level will influence all aspects of palliative care, but the following issues are worth highlighting:

- Communication of wishes, fears and symptoms
- Understanding of illness and death
- Assessment of symptoms
- Management of symptoms
- Decision-making
- Importance of play as a means of understanding the world
- Importance of kindergarten and school

Approach to consultation

Developmental level and cognitive ability will vary widely and are not necessarily related to age, so an appraisal of the child's level of understanding will need to be made early in the consultation. While not unique to the paediatric setting, the child and family's previous experience with medical procedures and staff will strongly influence their attitude to professionals. Honest communication and the development of trust early in the course of the illness will provide a solid foundation on which to face the challenges of palliative care. Conversely, long-term intense treatment involving repeated hospitalization and painful procedures may make a child wary of health professionals. Consultation and communication style therefore need to be highly flexible and adapted to each individual child and their family. A great deal of patience may be required.

Physiology/pharmacokinetics

These change as the child grows and develops. Neonates have a higher relative volume of distribution and lower clearance than adults, so the half-life of many drugs is prolonged. Conversely, infants and young children may metabolize certain drugs more quickly than adults. Children over six months of age, for example, may need higher doses of morphine than expected for their size.

Differences in family structure and function

Parents are socially and biologically invested with the responsibility of caring for and protecting their child. Consequently, the development of fatal illness in the child leads many parents to feel they have failed in this important rôle. Denial is a common reaction and despite advice to the contrary, parents may feel compelled to try everything and do anything to find a cure. This can be a difficult time for the child, the family, and the staff caring for them. Staff may feel the child is being subjected to overly burdensome treatment and may also worry that the child is not able to talk about the reality of what is happening. Maintaining hope and a supportive presence while advocating strongly for the child's needs are important elements in managing such situations. A 'hope for the best, prepare for the worst' approach is often helpful.

Whilst the management of the patient is foremost, involving the family in decisions and information sharing is extremely important. Families will often have a great deal of knowledge about their child's medical condition and in the case of a child with a rare disease, often know more about it than some professionals. In addition many parents will have already been heavily involved in treatment decisions, and will expect this level of involvement to continue.

The structure of families in the UK may now include the natural parents, step-parents, partners, foster parents and siblings not directly related to the child. Organizing effective communication amongst these groups is sometimes challenging but is extremely important, particularly towards the end-of-life.

Siblings require special consideration in paediatric palliative care. They are almost universally distressed, but often feel unable to share this with their parents. Negative outcomes such as developmental regression, school failure and behavioural problems may be seen if the needs of siblings are not adequately addressed (□ see Chapter 14).

School

The centre of a child's day-to-day life is school, and disruption of this routine can add to a child's sense of isolation and substantiate their feelings of being 'different' from their friends. Peer groups can be an enormous source of support for a child living with a life-limiting disease. For these reasons children often remain in school during treatment and even as death approaches. Keeping schools informed (with the permission of the parents/child) is important so that practical arrangements regarding the support required in school and flexibility of school hours can be discussed. Medical staff can facilitate school attendance by scheduling elective and semi-elective treatments appropriately. For example, the child with bone marrow suppression who really wants to be at school for art on Tuesdays might benefit from having their regular blood transfusion on Monday. As death approaches, the school staff may need support. A plan for supporting staff and pupils through bereavement may also be helpful.

Illness trajectory

This will vary with the particular diagnosis. Often the palliative phase of care in children is much longer than for adults. Indeed, it may extend from the time of diagnosis. There is also commonly a great deal of uncertainty surrounding the prognosis. Children in advanced states of disability and dependence are at high risk of dying from complications like respiratory infections but also have the potential to live many years. Families can find this extremely difficult to cope with, and they may experience negative thoughts and feelings about their situation and about their child.

Physical and emotional exhaustion, as well as concern for the child's suffering, may see them wishing it would all be over. Parents often feel alone with these thoughts, believing they are too terrible to share. The protracted nature of many illness trajectories presents challenges in planning support for the child and their family in terms of both symptom management and psychological support.

Ethical issues in paediatric palliative care

Medical ethics involves the application of ethical principles to medical practice and research.

As in adult palliative care, the most widely used framework for ethical decision-making involves the process of balancing four key principles:

1 **Autonomy**—the right to self-determination
2 **Non-maleficence**—the need to avoid harm
3 **Beneficence**—the ability to do good
4 **Justice**

In palliative care most dilemmas relate to end-of-life situations. In paediatric palliative care the inability of the child to act autonomously adds an extra dimension to the decision-making process.

Autonomy

- In order to act autonomously, one must act with intention and understanding and without controlling influences
- To act autonomously, individuals must demonstrate an understanding of their situation and the implications of their decisions
- They must also be able to communicate their decisions

Children represent a continuum in this regard, from the non-verbal infant to the adolescent striving for self-determination. A child's ability to make informed choices depends on his/her developmental level and life experience. For example, an eight-year-old child with a chronic illness may through his/her own experience and those of fellow patients be better positioned to participate in decision-making than an older child with no previous medical history.

Children may be able to make some decisions about their medical care even where major decisions are made by others. They may, for example, make choices regarding pain control and venepuncture sites. Empowering children in this way gives them a sense of control that impacts positively on their experience of care. Furthermore, even if not deemed sufficiently competent to act autonomously, a child's preferences and insights may guide decision-making by others and should be sought actively.

Decision-making in the palliative care setting requires

- The ability to understand one's illness in physiological terms and to conceptualize death as an irreversible phenomenon
- The capacity to reason and consider future implications (formal operations stage of cognitive development)
- The ability to act autonomously and not acquiesce to the authority of doctors and parents.[3]

The Royal College of Paediatrics and Child Health (UK) describes four levels of child involvement in decision-making:

1 Being informed
2 Being consulted
3 Having views taken into account in decision-making
4 Being respected as the main decision-maker[4]

Age is not necessarily a good measure of capacity although an arbitrary distinction is drawn for legal purposes.

Competence

Even young children have a right to be informed regarding decisions which affect their future. Both the Royal College of Paediatrics and Child Health and the American Academy of Pediatrics advocate strongly for the participation of children in decision-making to the extent that their ability allows.

Competence is assessed according to
- Cognitive ability. This may be reflected in young patients' ability to provide a clinical history as well as their understanding of the condition, treatment options and the consequences of choosing one option over another. Other factors to consider include level of schooling, verbal skills and demonstrated capacity to make decisions
- Presence or absence of disturbed thinking (eg. in the setting of psychiatric disorder)

Treatment should be discussed with parents and the child if appropriate, and ideally both will have an understanding of what is involved. Where this is not the case, providing more time for families to think about issues may help. In extreme circumstances a court of law can be asked to decide what is best.

Decision-making regarding life-sustaining treatment

Doctors, children and informed parents share the decision; with doctors taking the lead in judging the clinical factors and parents the lead in determining best interests more generally.'[5]

Decisions are made on the grounds of benefits/burdens proportionality. In order to justify a particular intervention, the expected benefits of that intervention must outweigh the burdens.

End-of-life decision-making is a collaborative process. It should involve the child (where possible), the family, and all the health professionals involved in providing care to the child. An important underlying principle of the process is open communication between staff and families.

.. 'physicians should do more than offer a 'menu' of choices—they should recommend what they believe is the best option for the patient under the circumstances and give any reasons, based on medical, experiential, or moral factors, for such judgements.'[6]

3 Leikin S. (1989) A proposal concerning decisions to forgo life-sustaining treatment for young people. *J Pediatrics*, **115**: 17–22.

4 Royal College of Paediatrics and Child Health (1997) *Withholding or Withdrawing Life-Saving Treatment in Children: a framework for practice.* London: RCPCH.

5 British Medical Association (2001) *Withholding and Withdrawing Life-prolonging Medical Treatment. Guidance for decision-making.* 2nd edn. London: BMJ Books.

6 American Academy of Paediatrics (1994) Guidelines on forgoing life-sustaining medical treatment. *Pediatrics*, **93**: 532–6.

The Royal College of Paediatrics and Child Health outlines five circum stances under which withholding or withdrawing curative medica treatment may be considered:

- The child has been diagnosed as brain dead according to standard criteria
- Permanent vegetative state. These children have 'a permanent and irreversible lack of awareness of themselves and their surroundings an no ability to interact at any level with those around them'[6]
- 'No chance situation': life-sustaining treatment simply delays death without providing other benefits in terms of relief of suffering
- 'No purpose' situation: the child may be able to survive with treatment but the degree of mental or physical impairment would be so great tha it would be unreasonable to ask the child to bear it
- The 'unbearable' situation. In the face of progressive, irreversible illness the burden of further treatment is more than can be borne

A practical approach to decision-making[7]—questions to be answered

- Is this intervention going to cure the disease?
- Is this intervention going to prevent progression of the disease?
- What impact will the intervention have on the child's quality of life?
- Will the intervention improve the child's symptoms?
- Will the intervention make the child feel worse?
- How long will the child feel worse for?
- What will happen without the intervention?
- How will the intervention change the outcome?

Disagreement

Society invests parents with the responsibility of acting on behalf of the children. There are occasions however, where parents insist on what sta may view as inappropriate treatment. Conversely, parents may refus treatment that is of potential benefit to the child. It is important that th best interests of the child are advocated for and that decision-making shared between the family and the healthcare team.

Families often need time to absorb and process difficult informatio and decision-making should be viewed as a process not an event. Mos disagreements can usually be resolved by regular open and hones communication. Where conflict can not be resolved, it may be helpful t request a second opinion from an independent practitioner. It may also b beneficial to include other family members or cultural and religiou leaders from the local community. In extreme circumstances wher agreement can not be reached despite the above interventions, it may b necessary to seek legal judgement.

Advance directives

Where children have an existing condition, gradual or sudden deteriora tion may be anticipated. It is helpful for health professionals to assis families in planning for crises so that interventions considered unhelpful t the child are not initiated. Written documentation in the medical recor as well as a letter for the family to have with them is required.

Advance directives should record:
- What has been discussed
- Who was present
- What decisions were made
- What the child and family's wishes are regarding various interventions
- Who should be called in case of crisis

Provision of hydration and nutrition
- Food and fluid should always be offered if the child is able to take it by mouth
- Most authors consider the provision of nutrition and hydration by artificial means to be a medical intervention subject to the same benefits/burdens assessment as any other
- The insertion of tubes into the gastrointestinal tract carries with it the burdens of discomfort and the potential for complications, and therefore needs to be justified on the grounds of the benefits it may provide to the patient
- Some argue, however, that the provision of food and fluid constitutes a basic component of humane care and can never be withdrawn or withheld
- In the paediatric setting, this concept is extended by the centrality of feeding to the parental rôle and the vulnerability of infants and small children
- Children in the terminal phase of illness will naturally cease eating and drinking as their requirements decrease, and it is not necessary in these circumstances to provide fluid and nutrition by artificial means

The situation faced by the family and staff is more problematic for children who have been kept alive for long periods prior to deterioration by gastrostomy or central venous feeding. Ethically there may be no difference between withdrawing treatment and not initiating potentially life saving treatment. Emotionally, however, it is often difficult for families not to feel guilty if they believe that by stopping artificial nutrition they are hastening their child's death. The effect of the provision or omission of artificial hydration and nutrition on the timing of death is uncertain. However, it is worth noting that dehydration may contribute to opioid toxicity, delirium and constipation and may require correction to alleviate these distressing clinical symptoms.

Medical ethics in different cultures
It is important to understand the limitations of Western ethics. The beliefs, values and conceptual frameworks used by other cultures must be considered when making decisions with families. The most appropriate source of information is the family itself, as there will be considerable variability within cultural groups.

7 Frager G. (1997) Palliative care and terminal care of children. *Child Adolescent Psychiatr Clin North Am*, **6**: 889–909.

Psychosocial needs in paediatric palliative care

Physical, emotional and spiritual needs cannot be addressed in isolation as each affects the other. For example, a child's pain can heighten parental anxiety and family distress may adversely affect pain control. A multidisciplinary approach to palliative care is required and there is therefore the potential for a large number of individuals and services to become involved in the care of the child. Coordination of these professionals and the services each is providing is essential to avoid the replication or omission of services, or disempowerment of the family. This can be achieved with regular communication between team members and the appointment of a key worker for each child. This person may be a general practitioner, paediatrician, nurse or an allied health worker.

Providing emotional and psychological support for the sick child is as essential as providing relief of physical symptoms.

Communicating with children about death and dying

A child can live through anything so long as he or she is told the truth and is allowed to share with loved ones the natural feelings people have when they are suffering..

Herbert, 1997[8]

Parents may instinctively want to protect their children from 'bad news'. However, children very often know a great deal about their illness and prognosis. Children may not reveal what they know for fear of upsetting their parents, who then falsely assume their child knows very little. Children are very sensitive to discrepancies between verbal and non-verbal information. They readily sense distress in those around them and may feel anxious and isolated as a result. They may also generate fantasies to explain unusual behaviour in their parents (eg. 'I have been bad' or 'Mummy and Daddy don't love me any more'). These notions may be more frightening than death and dying to a young child. This is particularly true of younger children, who are naturally egocentric and believe that the world revolves around them, and hence, personalize other people's emotional and behavioural reactions.

- Parents' reluctance to talk to their child about dying usually stems from an erroneous belief that their child's concept of death is similar to that of an adult's, and their consequent desire to protect them from emotional pain
- Younger childrens' greatest fear is usually around immobility and separation from loved ones during their illness and after. Opening up discussions about death can help allay these fears and provide reassurance to the child

- School-aged children frequently have worries about experiencing pain and can be greatly reassured by discussions about pain control. They may also ask questions about what will happen after their death, and can receive great comfort from religious or family beliefs about what will happen to them
- Just as parents and siblings need to plan the time they have left with the sick child in order to build memories and have as few regrets as possible, the dying child may also wish to prioritize the time left to do special activities or spend time with loved ones

Children very often ask staff questions about their illness and prognosis. When confronted by a difficult question, staff may be uncertain as to how best to respond. Questions often come unexpectedly, when the staff member is especially busy or distracted. Children generally know the answer to the question before they ask it. In this way the child who asks 'Am I dying?', may already know the answer. What they seek is a person who can be trusted to speak honestly with them. Responding with a question such as 'What makes you ask me that?' or 'What is it that makes you think you are going to die?' may elicit information on which to base a response. The real question may be something completely different. Of course children, just like adults, are very individual in how they respond, and while some children may ask plenty of questions and request lots of information, other children may wish to hear limited information. It is important to be guided by the child, and also to remind them that they can ask questions whenever they wish.

Herbert, M. (1996) *Supporting Bereaved and Dying Children and their Parents*. Leicester: BPS Books.

Supporting the sick child

These ideas mirror the supportive measures used in adult palliative care.

- Listen
  - Ask the child how he/she would like to be supported
  - Find out exactly what it is the child wants to know
  - Let the child set the pace
- Allow the child to make choices where possible
- Explain things in simple language appropriate to the child's development and cognitive ability
- Wherever possible answer questions honestly
- Answer the question that is being asked. Try not to burden the child with too much unsolicited information
- Children may find it easier to talk while drawing or doing some other activity. They may also find it helpful to talk in an abstract way eg. about a character in a story or during play with dolls
- Artwork, play, story writing, music and other creative activities may provide an outlet for emotion
- Normalize feelings of fear, anger and sadness
- Try not to dismiss a child's beliefs unless they are potentially damaging
- Model and encourage expression of emotion. Children need to know they can express their feelings without alienating those around them
- Provide physical contact and comfort
- Maintain routine to the greatest extent possible
- Involve the child's friends in visits. If this is not possible, encourage letters, photos, email, videos etc. Discourage social isolation but allow time for privacy

Recruit the child's school teacher to help—this may be helpful even where children are not able to attend school.[9]

9 Herbert, M. (1996) *Supporting Bereaved and Dying Children and their Parents.* Leicester: BPS Books.

Supporting parents

Communicating difficult information to parents

The way in which difficult information is communicated is important a[n]
sets the stage for the working relationship between professionals a[n]
family. Health professionals need to be aware of how their own feelings
anxiety, sadness and impotence may influence this process. Most paren[t]
desire a realistic appraisal of their child's condition delivered empathica[lly]
and with a sense of hope. Realistic hope can be offered in terms
ongoing support from the team, attention to symptoms and help to max[i]
mize the child's quality of life. In situations where the family is pursui[ng]
curative treatment, hope can be maintained by 'hoping for the best b[ut]
preparing for the worst'.

How should difficult news be delivered?

- Empathically
- In person, face-to-face
- Allow plenty of time
- Establish what the parents know or suspect e.g. 'How do you think
  things are going?'
- Allow the family to set the pace
- Respect silence and do not feel compelled to fill it
- Allow expression of emotion
- Avoid being evasive
- Offer to help inform other family members e.g. siblings, grandparents
- Offer to meet again soon

What information should be given?

- Honest accurate information devoid of technical jargon
- Try to determine what the family wish to know e.g. 'Are you the
  sort of person who likes to know everything or just the basic
  information?'
- Simple language—there will be time later to explore details
- Avoid ambiguous language such as 'we might lose the battle' or
  'he's passed away'. The words death or dying should be used

A brief outline of the expected disease course should be given a[nd]
expected symptoms mentioned. It may also be helpful for some families [to]
understand what can be done for these symptoms. Many parents have n[ot]
experienced the death of a relative or friend and may be frightened at t[he]
prospect of seeing someone die. Information about the bodily chang[es]
that accompany death may be helpful, and it is possible to be very rea[s]
suring about the process as, for most children who are managed careful[ly]
it is very peaceful. Families may be worried about pain and distress or [a]
final dramatic event. In most cases, however, the terminal phase is characte[r]
ized by the progressive shut down of the various organ systems.

Parental reaction to bad news

Parents are often so shocked on being told that their child is dying, even[if]
this is confirmation of their own suspicions, that they can not assimila[te]

ny other information at that moment. It is important to slow the process
own, provide multiple opportunities to speak with the family, repeat
formation where necessary and provide written information. Following
he initial shock, parents may feel confused and overwhelmed. They may
e frightened that they will not be able to cope with the child's physical
are or be able to control their emotions. Parents also experience feelings
f uncertainty. They may have difficulty making sense of what is happening
nd are unsure of what to do first.

Denial occurs occasionally. For some parents it may be an adaptive
efence and does not always need to be 'broken down'. In fact, great
aution should be exercised in confronting denial. Where denial is
mpairing optimal care and family functioning, however, it may be helpful to
ently challenge inconsistencies and explore underlying concerns. Asking a
uestion like, 'Is there ever a time even for a few seconds where you worry
ings might not turn out the way you hope?' may provide a window of
pportunity for the parent to work through the issues confronting them.

Anger may arise from fear and confusion, often as an expression of
espair. Parents feel an enormous loss of power and control in their lives.
heir sense of justice is rocked. The struggle to understand, make sense of
e situation and control emotions can produce anger. This may be
irected at staff. In managing angry parents, it is important:

To acknowledge the anger e.g. 'I can see you're very angry'
Not to take it personally
Not to be defensive
To allow ventilation of the anger 'Can you tell me more about what
you're feeling?'
Not to dismiss the complaint or try and explain the situation logically
To set limits 'I can see you are angry and I am willing to speak with you
about it but I can not let you damage property/threaten me etc.'

uilt is another common reaction amongst parents of dying children.
hey may feel that they failed to recognize and respond effectively to the
ymptoms of the child's illness. They may feel responsible because the
lness is inherited. They may experience 'survivor guilt', believing that chil-
ren are not supposed to die before their parents. They may believe that
eir action or inaction somehow triggered the illness. Parents may exter-
alize these feelings and blame others. Staff members occasionally find
emselves unfairly blamed for a child's illness or death. This may feel
urtful, but it is important not to become defensive or allow this to impact
n the care of the child. Any inclination to label the family as 'bad' should
lso be avoided.

What parents need to know

xplaining to parents that children often ask questions about their illness
nd prognosis provides a key opportunity for them to consider how they
ight deal with these themselves.

Planning in advance is helpful and a team approach, with parents forming
art of the team, essential. Parents bring particular knowledge of their
hild as a unique individual. Staff bring knowledge of the literature in this
rea and experience with other families in similar circumstances.

Families need to know that:

- Children are generally more aware of their prognosis than those around them believe
- If a child does not ask questions or speak about his/her illness it does not mean that he/she is oblivious or indifferent. Children often protec parents by feigning ignorance— 'mutual pretence'
- The anxiety generated by misinformation is potentially more harmful than any arising from the truth. Children may have all sorts of worries and fantasies, many of which an adult might not expect. What will happen to the cat? Will my school friends forget me? Will somebody be with me? Are mummy and daddy breaking up? Are mummy and daddy cross with me? Did I get sick because I was bad? Will it hurt? To a young child, abandonment and withdrawal of their parent's love may be more frightening than the notion of death because they have not ye acquired a full understanding of death. An environment of honesty provides the child with opportunities to share these worries. They need to feel they can trust those around them
- A dying child may be better able to cope with news of their impending death than their parents
- They are important rôle models. Children look to their parents for cues regarding the appropriate way of reacting to a given situation. While courage and calm will help reassure a child, it is also reasonable for parents to show their sadness. It is helpful for children to understand why their parents are upset so that they do not make incorrect assumptions. An honest explanation may be reassuring

In extreme cases where parents still insist that information is withheld but th child is clearly distressed by this approach, the health professional's duty is the child.

While, in general, honesty is the best approach, it is important recognize that not all children benefit from detailed information and n all parents feel able to communicate openly with their child. The be interests of the child are what is important. Cultural factors also requi careful consideration.

Parents' needs and the rôle of the health professional

Information: Parents generally want information so that they know what to expect. They may also want to discuss treatment options and plans for symptom control. Parents say that full information allows them to make decisions and helps them plan for the remaining time they have with their child. In general, it is best to be open and honest as a trusting relationship between parents and healthcare workers provides a solid foundation for the challenges of palliative care. It is also helpful to regularly check that families are not being overwhelmed with too much information (e.g. 'I know this is a lot of information for you to hear all at once. We can talk in more detail a little bit later on if you would prefer').

Time to be listened to: Many parents want to discuss their situation with the many healthcare workers involved in their child's care. They may need to speak about their concerns, fears, hopes, and expectations on numerous occasions to clarify and make sense of a world gone awry. The healthcare worker (whether it be a paediatrician, social worker, or nurse) needs to provide time and opportunities for parents to share these concerns. By listening to the concerns of parents, providing guidance, affirming their skills and resources and staying with them, staff can make a major difference to how a family copes. It is important to remember that some parents do not wish to have such discussions and individual coping styles should be respected.

Control: Parents talk of losing control of their lives. The healthcare worker can assist parents to regain a sense of control by providing them with information, including them in discussions regarding care, allowing them to decide who is allowed to visit and when, and so on. Making decisions for (rather than with) a family can be deskilling and destructive. Parents need to be viewed as competent partners in their child's care.

Emotional support: Parents with a sick child grieve for the 'normal' child they no longer have. With this grief comes a range of strong feelings and emotions which add to the task of caring. Parents need acknowledgement, compassion, empathy and non-judgemental understanding. Spiritual support may or may not be part of a family's support system when the child becomes sick. The child's illness may cause parents to question their faith, renew their faith or explore new avenues. Spirituality includes, but is not restricted to, religion. Local clergy, ministers of all faiths and other spiritual leaders are available to help during this confusing time.

Amidst major changes to their routines and view of the world, families may try to hang on to some sense of normality. Health professionals can facilitate this by scheduling treatment around important activities and school attendance, and encouraging the family to maintain routines and activities.

Practical support: Parents need advice and guidance from various professionals in order to learn what is available to help them. Most parents would not know where to begin if they have not had any previous experience. Liaison between the hospital and community team is a helpful step.

Medical equipment may be required as part of the child's care, either routinely or in an emergency. It is possible to have equipment items on loan from a hospital or community agency such as a palliative care service. Health professionals including social workers, occupational therapists and physiotherapists may be needed to make assessments of the child and family's needs.

Sibling needs

The needs of siblings are very similar to those of the dying child.[10]

Relationships within families and communication patterns are important factors in determining how siblings react to a brother or sister's illness. It may be easier for children to adapt to having a sick sibling in a family where it is usual to discuss matters openly and to share feelings and emotions.

Physical symptoms may develop such as nausea, vomiting, diarrhoea, constipation, headache and aching limbs. Symptoms similar to those experienced by the sick sibling may also be reported. Behavioural changes may occur including unusual aggression, temper tantrums or withdrawal from family or friends, rudeness, bullying and demanding attention. Regression in the form of thumb-sucking, enuresis, toileting problems or school refusal may occur. Sleeping problems include a fear of the dark, nightmares, waking in the night and wanting to sleep in the parents' bed. Older children and adolescents may withdraw completely or indulge in risk-taking behaviour.

It is important to note that some siblings will not experience any of the above.

Information—parents should be encouraged to be honest with siblings and to provide them with information at a level appropriate to their developmental stage. This might include facts about the illness, what treatment is being given, and what to expect. They may need reassurance that they and their parents are not likely to become ill and that nothing they did or said caused the illness. Siblings may have concerns regarding their own health and if they are reporting symptoms may benefit from the reassurance of a thorough physical examination by their doctor.

Routine

Whilst difficult to maintain at a time of such upheaval, familiar routines are important for a child's sense of security. This includes going to school, continuing with extracurricular activities and maintaining contact with his/her own peer group. Siblings may need to know that it is acceptable to have fun.

Emotional support—Siblings may try to protect their parents from added distress by not burdening them with their own worries. Many are known to suffer in silence. Unexpressed emotion may manifest as school failure, behavioural problems and physical symptoms. Siblings may also try to excel at school to 'cheer their parents up'. Feelings of resentment, jealousy, isolation, fear, guilt, anger and despair need to be explored, acknowledged and normalized. It is helpful if parents are able to dedicate special time to be with their well children. Some parents may need permission to do this as they feel guilty if they leave the sick child's side.

Contact with the sick child—Regular visits to the sick child in hospital allow siblings to see what is happening for themselves. It is important however that they are adequately prepared for what they might see e.g. 'John is very sleepy. He might not be able to talk to you but he will know you are there. He has medicine running into his body through a tube in his arm...this doesn't hurt etc.' In the rare circumstance where siblings cannot visit, regular updates, videos and photos can be helpful. Siblings can feel included by sending drawings, favourite toys, photos and videos to their brother or sister.

Inclusion in the care of the sick child—Siblings may benefit from the opportunity to be included in the care of the sick child and in the family's experience. Children can help by taking a drink to the child, changing the channel on the TV, reading a story, playing games, and taking the cat in to visit.

School—It is helpful if the sibling's school teachers are kept informed (with the family's permission) of the sick child's condition. Schools can also help by identifying one person to whom the sibling can go if they need help.

10 Goldman A. (1994) *Care of the Dying Child.* Oxford: Oxford University Press.

Community-based care

Most children who need palliative care will be looked after in, and by, their local community. It makes sense then that the community team is involved from early in the child's illness so that relationships are well established by the time the child's care needs increase. Resources available to families may include:

- General practitioner who will often know the child and family
- Community-based paediatrician
- Palliative care services
- Paediatric palliative care services
- Domiciliary nursing
- Respite
- Children's hospices
- Counselling
- Religious groups
- Family and friends
- Community agencies (which may offer family support and financial assistance)

Since children will often move between hospital and community settings, it is important that there is a collaborative approach to care and communication flows easily and appropriately. The use of a key worker can facilitate such communication.

The nature of the care available in a particular situation will vary a great deal depending on the particular community services available. Services are changing rapidly and it is important to check on current service availablity before planning community care. Non-evidence-based optimism or pessimism about the community service availability can cause much needless distress for the child and family.

Bereavement (📖 see Chapter 14)

Death and dying

- Most adult palliative care programmes become involved with patients towards the end-of-life
- In contrast children's programmes aim to identify children close to the time of diagnosis and provide services and support to the family as they progress through the disease process and eventual death
- Most children and their families wish to spend as much time at home as possible, and many hope to be able to care for their child during the terminal phase provided adequate support is available
- Some families will find this task extremely difficult and will wish to return to a hospital or hospice environment close to the time of death
- This should not be viewed as a failure of home care

The dying process

Taken from *A Practical Guide to Paediatric Oncology Palliative Care*, Royal Children's Hospital, Brisbane, 1999.

The actual dying process is usually an orderly and undramatic progressive series of physical changes which are not medical emergencies requiring invasive interventions. Parents need to know that these physical changes are a normal part of the dying process. It is very important that families are well supported at this time. If the child is dying at home, 24-hour support from experienced staff who they know and trust can make an enormous difference. Home visits by the GP, domiciliary nurse and oncology liaison nurse where appropriate, to assist with managing the child's symptoms, are greatly appreciated by the family. This is a very emotional and difficult time for the whole family.

Restlessness and agitation

Generally the child will spend an increasing amount of time sleeping, in part due to progressive disease and changes in the body's metabolism, but this may also be due to progressive anaemia or sedation from opioids required for pain relief.

Some children remain alert and responsive until the moment of death. Others may become confused, semiconscious or unconscious for several hours or days. Restlessness and agitation during the terminal phase is not uncommon and may be due to increasing pain, hypoxia, nausea, fear and anxiety. Agitation may be the child's only way of communicating distress. A calm peaceful environment and the presence of parents and family will assist in relieving the child's anxiety. Speech may become increasingly difficult to understand and words confused. Even though the child may not be able to communicate, they may be aware of people around them. Hearing may well be the last sense to be lost and the family should be encouraged to talk to the dying child. They may like to play their child's favourite music, read stories or just sit with and touch their child so the child knows they are not alone.

If agitation continues additional drugs may be needed (see medication section 'Agitation' and 'Terminal restlessness' pages for drugs and doses). Treatment is directed at inducing a degree of sedation appropriate for the individual child. At this stage oral medications may not be tolerated and alternative routes of medication are essential.

A continuous subcutaneous infusion of opioid and e.g. midazolam in a syringe driver is effective in controlling pain, agitation and restlessness. For the child dying at home it is important that the treating hospital/hospice has dispensed (or made provision for the general practitioner to organize) a home care pack containing drugs that may be required in the terminal phase of care. This ensures drugs are available in the home if and when the child requires them. Without a home care pack there may be a consider-able delay in getting drugs required for symptom relief.

Doses of medication should be recorded for parents on a treatment sheet. Occasionally haloperidol is required when the benzodiazepines are unsuccessful. Regular monitoring of effectiveness of medication is essen-tial. Additional drugs can be added to the syringe driver if needed.

Noisy/rattly breathing

Excessive secretions or difficulty in clearing pharyngeal secretions will lead to noisy breathing. Generally this occurs during the terminal phase of the child's illness and is associated with a diminished conscious state. It can also be problematic for children with neurodegenerative diseases or brain-stem lesions where swallowing is impaired. Positioning on the side or slightly head down will allow some postural drainage and this may be all that is required. Reassurance and explanation to the family is essential as the noise of the gurgling can be very distressing to the family, while the child is usually unaware and untroubled by the noise and sensation.

Anticholinergic drugs can be used to reduce the production of secretions, and a portable suction machine at home may be of benefit for children with chronic conditions or those who are unconscious (see medication section 'Noisy breathing' for drugs and doses).

Incontinence

There may be a relaxation of the muscles of the gastrointestinal and urinary tracts, resulting in incontinence of stool and urine. It is important to discuss with parents this possibility and how they wish to manage incontinence. If the child is close to death parents are often reluctant for a catheter to be inserted to drain urine and may choose to use incontinence pads or disposable incontinence draw sheets. It is important for the family that their child's dignity is respected. Disposable draw sheets are also useful for incontinence diarrhoea.

Eye changes

The pupils of a dying person become fixed and dilated. The eyes may become sunken or bulging and glazed. Eye secretions can be removed with a warm damp cloth. If eyes are bulging, which can occur with neurob-lastoma, the cornea should be protected and lubricated.

Circulatory and respiratory changes

As the heart slows and the heartbeat becomes irregular, circulation of blood is decreased to the extremities. The child's hands, feet and face may be cold, pale and cyanotic. The child may also sweat profusely and feel damp to touch. Parents may wish to change their child's clothes and keep them warm with a blanket. Respiration may be rapid, shallow and irregular then may slow with periods of apnoea (Cheyne–Stokes breathing). This breathing pattern is distressing for parents and siblings to witness, and they need reassurance that it is a normal part of the dying process and that it is not distressing to the dying child.

It is important to inform parents that when death occurs the child may again be incontinent of urine and stool. There may also be ooze from the mouth and nose, particularly if they roll their child to undress and wash him/her. Parents who are not prepared will be distressed when this occurs.

In our efforts to achieve a peaceful death for the child, it is essential that symptoms are closely monitored and that there is ongoing assessment of effectiveness of therapeutic interventions. Early detection of symptoms and appropriate intervention is crucial to achieve a pain-free and peaceful death for the child.

Staff support

The death of a child is a relatively unusual event and the modern paediatrician is more familiar with cure and prevention than with death and dying. While advances in medicine have lead to happier outcomes for the majority of children, there remains a group for whom cure is impossible. The relative infrequency with which death occurs in childhood has implications for those caring for this group of children. Staff may feel a sense of failure and impotence. A lack of exposure to dying children may leave them feeling ill-equipped to support a child and family through this phase of their care. They may also have become very attached to the child and family and experience their own grief. All of these responses are normal but in the absence of adequate self-awareness and support, health professionals may, over time, become 'burnt out'.

Burn-out is 'the progressive loss of idealism, energy and purpose experienced by people in the helping professions as a result of the conditions of their work'.[11] This may manifest as excessive cynicism, a loss of interest in work and a sense of 'going through the motions'. Other features include fatigue, difficulty concentrating, depression, anxiety, insomnia, irritability and the inappropriate use of drugs or alcohol. The consequences for families are significant as staff affected in this way may:

- avoid families or blame them for difficult situations
- be unable to help families define treatment goals and make optimal decisions
- experience physical signs of stress when seeing families

The quality of care may be compromised and families may become disenchanted with the health professional and seek help elsewhere, sometimes from inappropriate sources.

Risk factors

There are a number of risk factors for the development of behaviours and responses which may impact upon patient care and these can be categorised in the following way:

- Clinician-related
  - Identification with the family or situation
  - Unresolved loss and grief in own past
  - Fear of death and disability
  - Psychiatric disorder
  - Inability to tolerate uncertainty
- Family-related
  - Anger, depression
  - Uncooperative families
  - Family member is a health professional
  - Complex or dysfunctional family dynamics
  - Well known to staff (e.g. friends, relatives, colleagues)
  - Intractable pain or difficult symptoms
- Situation-related
  - Family member/s are friends or relatives of the clinician
  - Uncertainty/ambiguity
- Disagreement about goals of care
  - Patient/clinician
  - Team
- Protracted hospitalization[12]

While it is common for health professionals to experience emotions such as anger and sadness in the course of clinical care, it is important that these do not result in behaviours which could compromise the quality of that care. Recognition of the emotion helps control it to some extent as does accepting the normality of experiencing emotion. It may also be helpful to seek out a trusted colleague to whom you can talk.

1 Edelwich J., Brodsky A. (1980) *Burn-out: Stages of disillusionment in the helping professions.* New York: Human Sciences PR.

2 Meier D. E., Back A. L., Morrison S. (2001) The inner life of physicians and care of the seriously ill. *JAMA*, **286**: 3007–14.

3 Vachon M. L. S. (1995) Staff stress in hospice/palliative care: a review. *Pall Med* **9**: 91–122.

Strategies for self care

Stress amongst staff who provide palliative care for children, in any setting, is likely to be great, and the stresses involved in providing palliative care for children may affect the caregiver's ability to provide care in a sensitive and professional manner. Regular supervision and access to professional expertise by staff in areas where long-term relationships with patients and families are built up are important, and should ideally be written into job descriptions.[14]

There are a number of ways in which staff may be supported:

- Formal support through regular team meetings reduces conflict between staff members as long as open discussion is encouraged. This is dependent on the structure of the team and the quality of facilitation
- Formal support at an individual level is beneficial for some. It is particularly useful in circumstances where concerns can not be raised in the group context
- Informal peer support is generally regarded by staff as most effective[15]
- Support from family and friends
- Maintaining perspective through involvement in outside activities. Formal supervision may assist in developing the self-awareness necessary to achieve this
- Education provides staff with the skills they require to overcome feelings of impotence. In a recent survey of resident medical officers in the United Kingdom, lack of training in the breaking of bad news was identified as a serious deficiency in their education[16]

The care of the dying child presents enormous challenges but if done well, has the potential to bring lasting benefits to both the family and the health professional.

14 Association for Children with Life-threatening or Terminal Conditions and their Families and the Royal College of Paediatrics and Child Health (2003) *A Guide to the Development of Children's Palliative Care Services.* 2nd edn. London: ACT.

15 Woolley H., Stein A., Forrest G. C., Baum J. D. (1989) Staff stress and job satisfaction at a children's hospice. *Arch Dis Child,* **64**: 114–18.

16 Dent A., Condon L., Blair P., Fleming P. (1996) A study of bereavement care after a sudden and unexpected death. *Arch Dis Child,* **74**: 522–6.

The Association for Children with Life Threatening or Terminal Conditions and their Families (ACT) Charter

The diverse needs of children have led to the development of a national association, ACT (Association for the Care of Children with Life-threatening or Terminal Conditions and their Families).

As a service to such children and families ACT has developed the following charter.

1 Every child shall be treated with dignity and respect and shall be afforded privacy whatever the child's physical or intellectual ability.
2 Parents shall be acknowledged as the primary carers, and shall be centrally involved as partners in all care and decisions involving their child.
3 Every child shall be given the opportunity to participate in decisions affecting his or her care, according to age and understanding
4 Every family shall be given the opportunity of a consultation with a paediatric specialist who has a particular knowledge of the child's condition.
5 Information shall be provided for the parents, and for the child and the siblings, according to age and understanding. The needs of other relatives shall also be addressed
6 An honest and open approach shall be the basis of all communication which shall be sensitive and appropriate to age and understanding.
7 The family home shall remain the centre of caring whenever possible. All other care shall be provided by paediatric trained staff in a child-centred environment.
8 Every child shall have access to education. Efforts shall be made to engage in other childhood activities.
9 Every family shall be entitled to a named key worker who will enable the family to build up and maintain an appropriate support system.
10 Every family shall have access to flexible respite care in their own home and in a home from home setting for the whole family, with appropriate paediatric nursing and medical support.
11 Every family shall have access to expert, sensitive advice in procuring practical aids and financial support.
12 Every family shall have access to paediatric nursing support in the home, when required.
13 Every family shall have access to domestic help at times of stress at home.
14 Bereavement support shall be offered to the whole family and be available for as long as required.

Drugs and doses

The following section is divided into the common symptoms experienced by very ill children and outlines a management strategy for each.

- Agitation
- Anorexia
- Bleeding
- Breathlessness
- Constipation
- Convulsions
- Cough
- Gastro-oesophageal reflux
- Hiccup
- Infection
- Mouthcare
- Muscle spasm
- Nausea and vomiting
- Noisy breathing
- Pain
- Other pain syndromes
- Psychological issues
- Raised intracranial pressure
- Skin
- Sweating
- Terminal restlessness
- Emergency Drugs Summary

Introduction to drugs and doses

The approach to the care of a dying child and his/her family greatly influences the quality of their lives and the ability of the parents and siblings to cope with the child's death. Most symptoms are readily amenable to effective management. It is important, however, to adopt an individualized approach, taking into account the unique circumstances of each child and family.

Planning care

Medical assessment

* Make sure you are armed with as much information about the child and his family as possible
* Make sure you involve all the right people: this might include parents, siblings, grandparents and other carers. Whether you involve the child him/herself will depend on the child's age, understanding and state of health and the parents' wishes. It is often helpful to have another involved professional present, for example the district nurse in the community setting, so that someone else is fully aware of the discussion and can answer any questions the family might have after you have left
* Try and arrange things so that you are not in a hurry and are unlikely to be disturbed
* Be methodical: take a thorough history, and perform a full examination. Allow the child and parents time to voice their concerns as fully as possible

Explanations

* Explain symptoms and management
* Identify any misconceptions the child or family may have and address these (e.g. concerns about opioids causing addiction or hastening death)
* You may not have all the answers: if not, say so

Plans

* Identify, articulate and document the current goals of care
* Formulate a plan of action in consultation with the parents and/or child. Listen to any concerns that arise from this and be prepared to compromise on a management plan if the parents/child want something different
* Ensure there is a plan for the exacerbation of current symptoms and the development of new ones. Knowledge of the child's condition will be important here and expertise may be required from sub-specialists
* In most cases it is possible to **anticipate** either a worsening of current symptoms or the development of new symptoms, and it is vital that this is planned for so that appropriate medications and support are available
* Families need access to advice and support around the clock
* Run over the plan at the end of the consultation in language the parents and/or the child can understand
* It may be helpful to write the plan down and give a copy to the family

Review

Make a time/date when the management plan will be reviewed, and by whom.

Communication

- Make sure family members/carers know how to contact professionals, particularly out of normal working hours
- Liaise with relevant professionals and carers—leave clear written instructions in medical records or contact the community team to discuss directly—many different healthcare professionals may be involved particularly in the community, and it is important that everyone is aware of any changes in management
- It is often helpful to identify a key worker for the family

Routes for drug administration

According to the bioavailability of the drug and patient preference different routes of administration should be considered for each drug prescribed. These include:

- Oral
- Sublingual
- Buccal
- Nasal
- Intravenous
- Subcutaneous
- Transdermal
- Rectal
- Epidural

The syringe driver

A syringe driver is a small portable battery driven infusion pump used to give continuous medication parenterally, usually over a 24h period. Syringe drivers can deliver medication intravenously (e.g. via a central venous catheter) or subcutaneously. This route of delivery is particularly suitable for children who are unable to tolerate oral medication or who require immediate control of difficult symptoms, which are resistant to oral medication. Although it is a common route by which to administer medication at the end-of-life, it can also be used for short periods prior to this to gain control of difficult symptoms or when the oral route is temporarily impractical (e.g. persistent vomiting).

Indications for using a syringe driver

- Unable to absorb or refusing oral medication
- Difficulty swallowing
- Persistent vomiting
- Bowel obstruction
- Not fully conscious
- Unsatisfactory response to oral medication

Advantages of using this delivery system are:
1 Continuous blood levels of medication
2 Less requirement for needles
3 Maintenance of mobility and independence
4 The ability to deliver complex drug combinations safely

Providing they are compatible, certain common combinations of drugs can be mixed together and given in the same syringe driver. In circumstances where high concentrations of drugs are required or the agents are unstable or incompatible, separate syringe drivers may be needed. As a general rule, it is advisable not to mix more than three drugs in any one syringe—check compatibility first.

A continuous infusion delivered via a Patient Controlled Analgesia (PCA) system is an alternative to the syringe driver and has been used effectively in the postoperative setting by children as young as 7yrs. This device provides a background continuous infusion and allows the patient to administer bolus p.r.n. doses of analgesia by pressing a 'boost' button. The dose and number of p.r.n. doses available is preset and the device has a 'lock-out' facility which prevents overdose.

Setting up a syringe driver (see Chapter 6a)

Drug information

This document was written in January 2004. Whilst every effort has been made to ensure all information is accurate, it remains the responsibility of the prescriber to check this information against the most current available before administering any of the drugs in this document.

It is important to note that doses of the same medication may vary for different indications and this document should be consulted by symptom section rather than drug name.

Due to limitations of space, information regarding all side-effects and interactions for each drug are not included; further information regarding this should be sought from more detailed texts such as Royal College of Paediatrics and Child Health *Medicines for Children*[17] and the *British National Formulary*[18,19]. Many of the medications recommended in this text are not licensed for use in children or for the indications or by the routes for which they are suggested. This is a problem experienced not only by those who care for dying children but by paediatricians more generally. It is often necessary to prescribe medications 'off licence'. The recommendations that follow are based on evidence where it is available as well as the practice experience of clinicians working in paediatric palliative care and pain management. In the UK, unlicensed use is permitted at the discretion of the prescriber, and is the prescriber's responsibility.

17 Royal College of Paediatrics and Child Health (2003) *Medicines for Children*. 2nd edn. London: RCPCH.

18 Prescribing for children (2004) *British National Formulary*. **48**: 12–13.

19 Prescribing in palliative care (2004) *British National Formulary*. **48**: 15–18.

Agitation/delirium

Consider the following causes:
- Terminal restlessness
- Uncontrolled pain
- Medication (e.g. benzodiazepines, polypharmacy)
- Gastro-oesophageal reflux
- Urinary retention
- Constipation
- Dehydration
- Sepsis
- Cerebral causes: raised intracranial pressure, intracranial bleed
- Hypoxia
- Environmental irritation: too hot/cold/bright light
- Fear/anxiety
- Nausea
- Positioning

Terminal restlessness
Restlessness and agitation are not uncommon in the terminal phase of illness. Families may need reassurance that these symptoms are part of the dying process and, although difficult to witness, may not be causing distress to the child. (📖 See section on Terminal restlessness, p. 546.)

Uncontrolled pain
Take a careful history and fully examine the child before excluding pain. Children in chronic pain may not be as demonstrative as those in acute pain. Indeed, they may appear quiet and withdrawn. In children unable to communicate, ask parents and carers how their child expresses pain. Look for facial expressions such as frowning and grimacing during examination and turning/mobilizing for clues.

In the setting of uncontrolled pain, sedation does not address the underlying problem. Indeed, it may render a child in pain unable to communicate this to those caring for them.

Urinary retention
Children with neurodegenerative disease or those on opioids may have problems with retention of urine. Constipation may exacerbate this problem. Retention predisposes to urinary tract infection, which will add to the discomfort. If a urinary tract infection is suspected, consider sending an appropriate sample for analysis. Antibiotic treatment is likely to reduce any discomfort caused by infection. Retention may be relieved by gentle bladder massage or a warm bath. Bethanechol or carbechol may also be helpful. Catheterization is only occasionally necessary and need not be a permanent solution.

Constipation
Common causes include analgesia (particularly opioids), dehydration and immobility. Poor diet may be contributing but may not be rectifiable (📖 See section on Constipation, p. 492.)

Medication
Check drug chart for medications that may increase agitation.

Sepsis

Check temperature and examine for source of infection: wounds, Hickman lines and bladder are possible sites to consider. Swab/send samples as appropriate but first consider whether doing so will affect your management. Discuss whether treatment is appropriate/desirable with the child, their parents and other professionals involved. Sometimes treatment may be appropriate even in the terminal phase to control unpleasant symptoms. (See section on Infection, p. 506.)

Cerebral causes

Raised intracranial pressure, intracranial bleeds.

History and careful neurological examination may help with this diagnosis. Consider whether investigation is in the best interests of the child and whether it will influence management.

Hypoxia

Invasive tests should be avoided. Pulse oximetry may be helpful.

Environmental irritation

Too hot/cold, bright light.

Fear/Anxiety

Discuss directly with the child if possible and appropriate. Children may have concerns that adults don't consider (e.g. they might be worried about pets or who's going to look after their parents). Explanations and reassurance are helpful if the child is able to identify and talk about what is worrying them. Children are often worried about being left alone, so make sure someone they trust is with them. Placing familiar objects near the child is also useful if they are not being nursed at home. Photos of family and friends, toys and stuffed animals are examples. Many children benefit from learning simple relaxation or guided imagery techniques. Anxiolytics may be necessary if other measures fail.

Nausea

Check history and drug chart for likely causes and treat/adjust medication as appropriate.

Gastro-oesophageal reflux/indigestion

Common in very disabled children. Also a possibility in children taking steroids or undergoing chemotherapy/radiotherapy. (See section on Gastro-oesophageal reflux, p. 504.)

Positioning

The child may simply not be comfortable, and this may be frustrating for a child unable to turn himself. It may be worth adjusting the child's position if you suspect this may be a problem.

Delirium

Is characterized by:
- Disturbed consciousness and impaired attention
- Cognitive disturbances such as disorientation and memory impairment
- An acute or subacute onset and fluctuation throughout the day

Often there is a prodrome in the form of restlessness, sleep disturbance, irritability and anxiety. Early recognition and treatment are important.

Management

General measures
- Treat any reversible cause if possible and appropriate (make sure the child is not in pain)
- Nurse the child in a quiet and safe environment surrounded by familiar people and objects
- If other measures are unsuccessful, pharmacological intervention may be necessary
- Benzodiazepines are the most commonly used medication in this setting. Haloperidol may also be helpful, and is not too sedating
- Benzodiazepines are generally very effective but occasionally a paradoxical increase in irritability may be seen
- Families may need to understand that the child may not be as responsive once medication is given, but that the priority is the child's comfort

Medication

Benzodiazepines

The choice of benzodiazepine will depend on the circumstance for which it is being prescribed. Children experiencing brief periods of anxiety or panic attacks may benefit from a benzodiazepine with a very short half-life such as midazolam, given buccally or subcutaneously. Sublingual lorazepam is another option for panic attacks or anxiety related to dyspnoea. Children needing a longer duration of action may do better with diazepam or clonazepam. Levomepromazine may be an appropriate agent for children who also have nausea and pain.

Lorazepam
- Short half-life
- Form:
  - Tablets: 1mg (scored), 2.5mg
  - Oral suspension: only available as 'special'
  - Injection: 4mg in 1mL, 1mL ampoule
- Dose (sublingual, oral):all ages: 25–50 mcg/kg (max. 4mg/24h in adults)
- Injectable form can be given sublingually
- Most children will not need more than 0.5–1mg for a trial dose. Well absorbed sublingually (good for panic attacks) and parent/child has control
- Contra-indications and warnings: severe pulmonary disease, sleep apnoea, coma, CNS depression. Caution in hepatic and renal failure
- Licence: tablets are licensed as premedication in children >5yrs. Injection not licensed in children <12yrs except for treatment of status epilepticus

onazepam

Long half-life

Form:
- Drops: 2.5mg in 1mL (1 drop = 0.1mg), named patient basis
- Tablet: 0.5mg, 2mg
- Injection: 1mg in 1mL
- Oral liquid: 500 mcg in 5mL, 2mg in 5mL 'specials'

Dose (sublingual): all ages 0.01mg/kg/dose (max. 0.5mg) b.d./t.d.s.

If necessary, increase by 10–25 per cent every 2–3 days to max. 0.1–0.2mg/kg/day

Prescribe as number of drops. Count drops onto spoon before administering. Irritability and aggression not uncommon in which case drug should be withdrawn

Increased secretions may occur in infants and young children

Licence: tablets and injections licensed for use in children but not for this indication

Midazolam

Very short half-life

Form:
- Injection: 10mg in 2mL; 10mg in 5mL
- Injection may be given orally, sublingually, intranasally, or rectally
- Oral syrup 2.5mg in 1mL only available as 'special'

Single doses:
- Intravenous/subcutaneous:
  - >1month–18yrs: 100mcg/kg
- Sublingual:
  - >1month–18yrs: 500mcg/kg (max. 10mg)

Tastes bitter when given orally but can be mixed with juice or chocolate sauce

Max. effect in 30–60mins. Duration 2 h
- Intranasal:
  - >1month–18yrs: 200–300mcg/kg (max. 10mg)

Intranasal route may be unpleasant but has a fast onset of action (5–15 minutes)

Important: Drop dose into alternating nostril over 15 seconds
- Rectal:
  - >1month–18yrs: 500–750 mcg/kg
- Continuous intravenous/subcutaneous infusion:
  - >1month–18yrs: start at 2.5mg/24 h (note: this is not a per kg dose)

Titrate to effect. There is considerable inter-individual variability in the dose required and doses of up to 40mg/24 h have been used in palliative care. If high doses are needed, consider trying a different agent

Contra-indications and warnings: caution with pulmonary disease, hepatic and renal dysfunction (reduce dose), severe fluid/electrolyte imbalance and congestive cardiac failure

Avoid rapid withdrawal after prolonged treatment

Licence: injection licensed for sedation in intensive care, for induction of anaesthesia and conscious sedation in children. Other routes and indications not licensed

Diazepam
- Long half-life
- Form:
  - Tablets: 2mg, 5mg, 10mg
  - Oral solution: 2mg in 5mL and 5mg in 5mL
  - Injection (solution and emulsion): 5mg in 1mL
  - Suppositories: 10mg
  - Rectal tubes: 2mg in 1mL: 2.5mg tube, 5mg tube, 4mg in 1mL: 10mg tube
- Dose (oral):
  - 1 month–12yrs: 50–100mcg/kg/dose b.d.–q.d.s.
  - >12yrs: 2.5–5mg b.d.–q.d.s.
- Licence: rectal preparation is licensed for use in children >1yr with severe agitation. Other forms not licensed for agitation per se

Other medication
Haloperidol
- Form:
  - Tablets: 1.5mg, 5mg, 10mg, 20mg
  - Capsules: 500 mcg
  - Oral liquid: 1mg in 1mL, 2mg in 1mL. 1mg in 5 mL 'special'
  - Injection: 5mg in 1mL, 1mL ampoule; 10mg in 1mL and 2mL ampoules
- Dose (oral):
  - 2–12yrs: 10–25 mcg/kg b.d. (max. 10mg/24h)
  - >12yrs: 0.25–5mg b.d. (max. 30mg/24h)
- Dose (subcutaneous):
  - 2–12 yrs: 10–25 mcg/kg b.d. (max 10mg/24 h)
  - >12 yrs: 0.25–5mg b.d (max 30mg/24 h)
- Contra-indications and warnings: bone marrow suppression, phaeochromocytoma
- Licence: licensed for use in children

Levomepromazine
- Form:
  - Tablets: 25mg
  - Injection: 25mg in 1mL, 1mL ampoule
- Dose: (SC/i/v continuous infusion):
  - All ages: 0.5–1mg/kg/24 h then titrate to response (max. adult dose 300mg/24 h)
- Contra-indications and warnings: Parkinsonism, postural hypotension, antihypertensive medication, epilepsy, hypothyroidism, myasthenia gravis
- May reduce seizure threshold
- Sedating especially in SC doses exceeding 1mg/kg/24 h in children under 12 yrs or 25mg/24 h in children over 12 yrs
- Can be used subcutaneously but may cause inflammation at injection site
- Licence: Licensed for this indication in children

Anorexia

Poor appetite and weight loss are common in children with terminal illness, particularly towards the end-of-life. This causes a great deal of anxiety amongst many parents and carers because:

- They may consider one of their main caring roles is to keep their child well-fed
- They often perceive eating as a road to recovery
- Acceptance that their child doesn't want to eat may go hand in hand with acceptance that the terminal phase is approaching

Consider reversible causes

- Oral candidiasis
- Pain (in mouth or elsewhere)
- Nausea/vomiting
- Constipation
- Medication

Management

General measures

- Explanation and discussion with the family may be helpful. Listen to parents' concerns and reassure as appropriate. It may be helpful for families to understand that as the child becomes less mobile and as the body winds down, the child's need for fluid and food diminishes
- Provide small meals on small plates. The child may prefer to snack through the day rather than sit down to a meal
- Make food less effort to eat (e.g. by providing mashed meals or wholesome soups, ice cream and rice pudding)
- Offer 'favourite' meals
- Offer supplementary high calorie/high protein drinks
- Try not to make an issue out of meal times
- Low dose steroids will stimulate the appetite but will not change the course of the disease and may have harmful side-effects. They are almost never given for this indication

Bleeding

Management

General measures

- For children who are reasonably well but are thrombocytopenic and at risk of bleeding, regular platelet transfusions may be worthwhile
- If bleeding is likely, explain this to the parents and prepare a management plan
- If a significant bleed is a possibility benzodiazepines should be readily available (see below) and the use of red towels and blankets may be helpful. Consider a platelet transfusion if bleeding is problematic and related to low platelet count in a child with a reasonable prognosis where a transfusion would improve quality of life

Medication

Bleeding gums

Use a soft toothbrush if possible. If not, avoid brushes altogether. Consider gentle regular antibacterial mouthwash to prevent secondary infection.

Tranexamic acid
- Form:
  - Tablets: 500mg
  - Liquid: 500mg in 5mL 'special'
  - Injection: 100mg in 1mL. 5mL Amp.
- Dose (mouthwash): use undiluted preparation for injection and apply to bleeding point. Dilute preparation for injection 1:1 for oral use and use as mouthwash
- Dose (oral):
  - 1month–18yrs: 25mg/kg t.d.s.
- Caution: reduce dose in renal failure; do not use in children with haematuria because of the risk of clot retention
- Licence: licensed for use in children

Small bleeds

Tranexamic acid
See oral dose above

Topical adrenaline
- Form: 1:1000 solution
- Small external bleeds:soak gauze, apply directly to bleeding point

Sorbsan dressing
- Haemostatic dressing: apply directly to bleeding point

Catastrophic haemorrhage

An anxiolytic such as diazepam/midazolam is useful as a large haemorrhage is likely to be very frightening if the patient is conscious. If haemorrhage is likely an anxiolytic in a suitable form should be readily available, and carers/staff should be aware of how to administer it. A rapid onset of action

be desirable so provision should be made for parenteral administration.
example:

Midazolam
Form:
• Injection: 10mg in 2mL
Dose (SC/i.v. stat):
• All ages: 100–200 mcg/kg
Dose may need to be repeated
Haemorrhage is unlikely to be painful and the 'traditional' use of
Diamorphine in this instance may not be appropriate

Breathlessness

Dyspnoea, like pain, is a subjective symptom and may not correlate v
objective signs.

Consider causes and treat reversible factors as appropriate:
- Anaemia
- Anxiety
- Ascites
- Cerebral tumours
- Congenital heart disease
- Cystic fibrosis
- Infection
- Raised intracranial pressure
- Respiratory muscle dysfunction e.g. neurodegenerative disorders
- Primary or secondary tumours
- Uraemia
- Pleural effusion/pneumothorax*/haemothorax
- Pulmonary fibrosis
- Superior vena cava (SVC) obstruction*
- Increased secretions
- Pain
- Pulmonary embolism
- Pericardial effusion

* These are medical emergencies and swift treatment of these conditic
can significantly reduce symptoms; if suspected, urgent investigation a
referral to appropriate specialist should be considered.

Management

General measures

- Anxiety is likely to be an associated feature. Try reassurance, relaxati
  techniques, distraction and anxiolytics where necessary
- Provide a flow of fresh air—fan/window
- Try not to overcrowd the room
- Optimise position
- Excess secretions may respond to gentle physiotherapy +/− suction

Oxygen

May be helpful in hypoxic patients but is not without consequenc
(e.g. wearing of mask can be uncomfortable and interfere with ability
child to be close to parents and carers. Equipment can also comprom
mobility). The benefits of this intervention need to outweigh the burder

Children often refuse masks but may tolerate nasal specs. Consid
humidifying oxygen which will dry the mouth less.

Caution is needed in circumstances where chronic hypercapnia has l
the child dependent on hypoxic respiratory drive. Too much oxygen v
result in hypoventilation, so titrate carefully.

Medication

The choice of medication will depend on the underlying caus
Bronchospasm will respond to a bronchodilator. Anxiety that is unresponsi
to reassurance, distraction or relaxation techniques may require treatme

th a benzodiazepine. Excessive secretions may respond to physiotherapy d/or mucolytic agents. Opioids however, are generally very effective.

onchodilators

lbutamol

ay be helpful if bronchospasm present

Form:

- Nebulised solution 2.5mg/2.5mL. 5mg in 2.5mL
- Inhaled form: 100mcg/dose

Dose (nebulised):

- 6 months—5yrs: 2.5mg t.d.s./q.d.s.
- 5–12yrs: 2.5–5mg t.d.s./q.d.s.
- >12 yrs: 5mg t.d.s./q.d.s.

Dose (inhaled):

- All ages: 1–2 puffs 4–6 times a day (a spacer device should be used to improve delivery)

here is some evidence that small babies do not respond to salbutamol cause of receptor immaturity and it is advisable to use ipratropium first those aged <1yr.

Salbutamol may exacerbate anxiety.

Licence: licensed for use in children

ratropium

ay be helpful if bronchospasm present

Form:

- Nebulised solution: 250mcg in 1mL, 500mcg in 2mL
- Inhaled form: 20mcg/dose and 40mcg/dose

Dose (nebulised):

- <1yr: 125mcg t.d.s.–q.d.s.
- 1–5yrs: 250mcg t.d.s.–q.d.s.
- 5–12yrs: 500mcg t.d.s.–q.d.s.
- >12yrs: 500mcg t.d.s.–q.d.s.

Dose (inhaled):

- <6yrs: 20mcg/dose t.d.s.–q.d.s.
- 6–12yrs: 20–40mcg/dose t.d.s.–q.d.s.

Licence: licensed for use in children

orphine

fective in treating dyspnoea although there may be no measurable effect respiratory rate or oximetry. Morphine reduces anxiety, pain, and pul-onary artery pressure. Begin with half the paediatric analgesic dose and rate to effect (📖 See section on Pain, p. 520).

enzodiazepines

any children will be frightened by dyspnoea. Benzodiazepines may be elpful in addition to relaxation techniques and guided imagery. The choice benzodiazepine will depend on the circumstance for which it is being escribed. Children experiencing brief periods of anxiety or panic attacks association with dyspnoea may benefit from a benzodiazepine with a ry short half-life, such as midazolam, given buccally or subcutaneously. blingual lorazepam, is another option for panic attacks or anxiety related dyspnoea. Children needing a longer duration of action may do better th diazepam, clonazepam or a subcutaneous midazolam infusion.

Diazepam
- Form:
  - Tablets: 2mg, 5mg, 10mg
  - Oral solution: 2mg in 5mL and 5mg in 5mL
  - Injection (solution and emulsion): 5mg in 1mL
  - Also available as Suppositories: 10mg
  - Rectal tubes: 2mg in 1mL: 2.5mg tube, 5mg tube
- Dose (oral): 4mg in 1mL: 10mg tube
  - 1 month–12 yrs: 50–100mcg/kg 6–12 h
  - >12yrs: 2.5–5mg 6–12 h
- Contra-indications and warnings: acute porphyria. Potential for dependency. Can affect respiration if given i/v or rectally
- Licence: not licensed for this indication in children

Lorazepam
- Form:
  - Tablets: 1mg (scored), 2.5mg
  - Oral suspension only available as 'special'
  - Injection: 4mg in 1mL, 1mL ampoule
- Dose (sublingual, oral):
  - All ages: 25–50mcg/kg (max. dose in adults 4mg/24h)
- Most children will not need more than 0.5–1mg for trial dose. Well absorbed sublingually (good for panic attacks) and child has control
- Contra-indications and warnings: severe pulmonary disease, sleep apnoea, coma, CNS depression. Caution in hepatic and renal failure children >5 years
- Licence: tablets licensed as premedication in children >5 yrs. Injection not licensed in children <12yrs except for treatment of status epilepticus

Clonazepam
- Form:
  - Drops: 2.5mg in 1mL (1 drop = 0.1mg). Named patient basis
  - Tablets: 0.5mg, 2mg
  - Injection: 1mg in 1mL
  - Oral liquid: 500 mcg in 5mL, 2mg in 5mL 'specials'
- Dose (sublingual):
  - All ages: 0.01mg/kg/dose (max. 0.5mg) b.d./t.d.s.
  - If necessary, increase by 10–25 per cent every 2–3 days to max. 0.1–0.2mg/kg/day
- Long half-life
- Prescribe as number of drops. Count drops onto spoon before administering
- Irritability and aggression not uncommon in which case drug should be withdrawn. Increased secretions may occur in infants and young children
- Offers the advantage of sublingual absorption and droplet administration
- Licence: tablets and injections licensed for use in children but not for this indication

Midazolam
- Form:
  - Injection: 10mg in 2mL; 10mg in 5mL
- Injection may be given orally, sublingually, intranasally, or rectally
- Oral syrup only available as 'special': 2.5mg in 1mL

Single doses:
- Intravenous/subcutaneous:
  - >1month–18yrs: 100mcg/kg
- Sublingual:
  - >1month–18yrs: 500mcg/kg (max. 10mg)

Tastes bitter when given orally but can be mixed with juice or chocolate sauce

Max. effect in 30–60mins. Duration 2 h
- Intranasal:
  - >1month–18yrs: 200–300mcg/kg (max 10mg)

Intranasal route may be unpleasant but has a fast onset of action (5–15 minutes)

Important:Drop dose into alternating nostril over 15 seconds
- Rectal:
  - >1month–18yrs: 500–750 mcg/kg
- Continuous intravenous/subcutaneous infusion:
  - >1month–18yrs: start at 2.5mg/24 h (note: this is not a per kg dose)

Titrate to effect. There is considerable inter-individual variability in the dose required and doses of up to 40mg/24 h have been used in palliative care. If high doses are needed, consider trying a different agent

Contra-indications and warnings:caution with pulmonary disease, hepatic and renal dysfunction (reduce dose), severe fluid/electrolyte imbalance and congestive cardiac failure. Avoid rapid withdrawal after prolonged treatment

Licence: injection licensed for sedation in intensive care, induction of anaesthesia, and conscious sedation in children. Other routes and indications not licensed

Dexamethasone

May be helpful in circumstances such as bronchial obstruction, lymphangitis carcinomatosa, SVCO, and raised intracranial pressure. Administration needs to be carefully considered as steroids may produce potentially distressing side-effects in children if given for more than a few days. To avoid this, it is preferable to prescribe short courses (3–5 days) of steroids. These can be repeated if necessary.

Form:
- Tablets: 500mcg; 2mg
- Oral solution: 2mg in 5mL
- Injection: 4mg in 1mL, can be given orally

Dose (oral):
- <1yr: 0.5–1mg b.d.
- 1–5yrs: 2mg b.d.
- 6–11yrs: 4mg b.d.
- >12yrs: 8mg b.d.

Dose (SC/i/v)
- Can be given in as single doses or as continuous infusion

Higher doses may be needed in SVCO (consult paediatric oncologist)

If no effect after 3–5 days, stop steroids (no need to tail off dose)

Do not give after midday as can affect night time sleep

Co-prescribing: consider antacids and anti-thrush treatment

Contra-indications and warnings: caution in renal disease, cardiac disease or cystic fibrosis. Avoid in cardiac insufficiency

Licence: not licensed for this indication in children

Constipation

Prophylaxis and early intervention are important in managing this d.
tressing symptom. A laxative should always be prescribed when opioi
are commenced.

- What are the child's usual bowel habits?—children vary a lot; what is
  constipation for one may be a normal pattern for another
- Has there been a change in the usual pattern?

Consider cause

- Inactivity
- Metabolic: dehydration; hypercalcaemia; hypokalaemia
- Cystic fibrosis
- Reduced oral intake
- Spinal cord/cauda equina compression
- Bowel obstruction
- Fear of pain on defaecation: secondary to hard stools, rectal/anal graze
  and tears
- Drugs: opioids; anticholinergics; anticonvulsants; vincristine
  chemotherapy
- Social: shy about using toilets away from home, not knowing where th
  toilets are etc. Liaise with parents

Management

General measures

- Check for bowel obstruction, faecal impaction and rectal/anal
  grazes/tears (conduct a rectal examination only if absolutely necessary
- Consider the underlying cause and address it if appropriate/possible
- Increase fluid intake where possible and appropriate
- Increase mobility if possible
- Optimise access to the toilet
- Encourage regular toileting especially after meals
- Try oral medication first, then proceed to rectal preparations if
  necessary

Medication

It is generally helpful to use a combination of a stimulant laxativ
(e.g. senna, bisacodyl, docusate or sodium picosulphate) and a softenir
agent (e.g. magnesium hydroxide). Combined preparations are availab
(e.g. co-danthramer and co-danthrusate) for use in palliative care. Prokinet
agents such as metoclopramide and domperidone may be helpful secor
line agents (☐ See section on Nausea and vomiting, p. 512 for doses
Domperidone is less effective than metoclopramide but is less likely
cause dystonic reactions. If constipation is morphine-related and resistar
to the usual measures, it may be helpful to change to an alternative opio
such as fentanyl.

Bisacodyl

- Form:
  - Tablets: 5mg
  - Suppository: 5mg, 10mg

Dose (oral/rectal):
- Give tablets at night, suppositories in the morning
- 1month–10yrs: 5mg o.d.
- >10yrs: 10mg o.d.

Higher doses may be necessary

Acts in 12h orally, in 20–60 minutes rectally

Stimulant laxative

Senna

Form:
- Syrup: 7.5mg in 5mL
- Tablets: 7.5mg
- Granules: 15mg in 5mL

Dose (oral):
- <2yrs: Syrup 0.5mL/kg o.d.
- 2–6yrs: Syrup 2.5–5mL o.d.
- 6–12yrs: Syrup 5–10mL or 1–2 tablets o.d.
- >12yrs: Syrup 10–20mL or 2–4 tablets o.d.
- For granules use $^1/_2$ syrup dose

Stimulant laxative

Acts in 8–12h

Often used in combination with lactulose

Licence: Syrup licensed in children >2yrs, tablets not recommended in children <6yrs

Co-danthramer

Form:
- Suspension: dantron 25mg/poloxamer 200mg in 5 mL; dantron 75mg/poloxamer 1g in 5 mL (Forte)
- Capsule: dantron 25mg/poloxamer 200mg; dantron 37.5mg/poloxamer 500mg (Forte)

Dose (oral):
- Only for use in terminally ill children
- <12yrs: 2.5–5mL of the 25/200mg strength suspension or 1–2 (25/200mg strength) capsules o.d.–b.d.
- >12yrs: 5–10mL of the 25/200mg strength suspension or 1–2 (25/200mg strength) capsules o.d.–b.d., titrate as needed

Combined stimulant (dantron)/softener (poloxamer) laxative

Acts in 8–12h

Makes urine red (inform carers)

Can cause superficial burns in children who are incontinent/in nappies

Avoid in acute respiratory depression, paralytic ileus, liver disease and moderate to severe renal impairment

Licence: only licensed for use in terminally ill children

Docusate sodium

Form:
- Elixir: 12.5mg in 5mL; 50mg in 5mL. Dilute with milk or orange juice
- Capsule: 100mg
- Enemas: Fletchers' enemette: 90mg in 5mL; Norgalax microenema: 120mg in 10g

Dose (oral):
- 6 months–12yrs: 2.5mg/kg t.d.s.
- >12yrs: 100mg t.d.s.

- Dose (rectal):
  - <3yrs: 2.5mL Fletchers' enemette
  - >3yrs: 5mL Fletchers' enemette
- Softener and stimulant
- Acts in 24–48h
- Licence: capsule not licensed for children. Norgalax enema licensed for children >12yrs. Fletchers enemette licensed for children >3yrs

Lactulose

Lactulose is not very effective in opioid-induced constipation.

- Form:
  - Solution: 300mg lactose/550mg galactose in 5mL
- Dose (oral):
  - <1yrs: 2.5mL b.d.
  - 1–5yrs: 5mL b.d.
  - 5–10yrs: 10mL b.d.
  - >10yrs: 15mL b.d.
- Mild osmotic laxative, which is very sweet to taste, and can cause bloating
- Acts in 48h
- May cause colic
- Titrate dose up as required
- Can be disguised in fruit juice, milk or water

Magnesium hydroxide

Stool softener

- Form:
  - Liquid: 415mg in 5mL
- Dose (oral):
  - <3yrs not recommended
  - >3yrs 5–10mL nocte
    (adult 30–45mL nocte)

Sodium picosulfate

- Form:
  - Sachet: 10mg sachets contain sodium picosulfate 10mg + magnesium citrate powder
  - Sodium picosulfate liquid: 5mg in 5mL
- Dose (oral) sachet:
  - 1–2yrs: 1/4 sachet o.d.
  - 2–4yrs: 1/2 sachet o.d.
  - 4–9yrs: (1/2)–1sachet o.d.
  - >9yrs: 1 sachet o.d.
- Dose (oral) liquid:
  - 2–5yrs: 2.5mL nocte
  - 5–10yrs: 2.5–5mL nocte
  - >10yrs: 5–15mL nocte
- Effective within 2–3 h
- Drink plenty of water before and after administration
- Warning: can cause dehydration and electrolyte disturbance
  Caution in children with impaired renal or cardiac function

Arachis oil enema

- Form:
  - Enema 130mL arachis oil BP

Dose (rectal):
- 3–7yrs: (1/3)–(1/2) enema
- 7–12yrs: (1/2)–(3/4) enema
- >12yrs: (3/4)–1 enema

Use as required

Faecal softener

Contra-indications and warnings:hypersensitivity to arachis oil or peanuts.

Licence: licensed for children >3 yrs

odium citrate enema

Form:
- Micro-enema 450mg sodium citrate/75mg sodium laurylsulphate/5mg sorbic acid in 5mL (Relaxit). Other combinations available, but not licensed for children under 3yrs

Dose (rectal):
- 1 enema (when using in children <3yrs insert only half nozzle length)

Osmotic laxative

Licence: licensed for children >3 yrs

hosphate enema

Form:
- enema sodium acid phosphate 21.4g/sodium phosphate 9.4g in 118mL (Fleet)
- other combinations available

Dose (rectal):
- 3–7yrs: (1/3)–1/2 enema
- 7–12yrs: (1/2)–3/4 enema
- >12yrs: (3/4)–1 enema

Osmotic laxative

Licence: licensed for children >3 yrs

Convulsions

Convulsions are most commonly seen in the palliative care setting in children with neurodegenerative disorders or intracranial malignancies.

Children with neurodegenerative disorders will often already be on multiple anticonvulsant medications and their parents/carers will be knowledgeable about recognizing and treating fits. For these children fits are often variable in type and may become frequent, severe and more difficult to control towards the end-of-life.

Children with intracranial malignancy will not necessarily develop fits. However, for those who do, it is a frightening new symptom for the child and carers to learn how to manage. If fits are likely, prophylactic anticonvulsants should be considered and parents warned about what to expect. They should be given a clear plan of what to do in the event of a convulsion. The mainstay of medical treatment, diazepam, should be readily available with clear instructions as to how and when it should be administered.

Not all fits are grand mal: more subtle behaviours may also represent seizure activity. These may not require treatment if they are not troubling the child.

Investigation and treatment of persistent fitting should be tailored to the child's stage of illness and will require discussion with senior doctors and family.

Consider causes and treat as appropriate

The emergence of, or increasing frequency/severity of fits may be caused by worsening disease but other potentially reversible factors should be considered:

- Hypoglycaemia
- Electrolyte imbalance
- Sub-therapeutic anticonvulsant medication
- Infection e.g. UTI
- Raised intracranial pressure/other intracranial pathology

Management

- The choice of anticonvulsant depends on the type of fit. Advice from the paediatric unit where the child is being managed should be sought
- Single agent therapy is ideal. Where children are already on multiple medications, reducing the number of different anticonvulsants may improve seizure control
- Withdrawal or addition of anticonvulsants should be done cautiously as most agents need to be tailed off or titrated down
- Relatively higher doses of anticonvulsants are required for children <3yrs because of a higher metabolic rate and more efficient drug clearance
- Not all fits require treatment

The management of seizures will depend on the goals of care at the time. A child who is enjoying a reasonable quality of life and is in the early stages of a life-limiting illness should be treated as any other. Children in the terminal phase of illness should be kept comfortable and this will generally entail reasonable efforts to abort the seizure.

Acute management

In circumstances where the goals of care are to keep the child comfortable:
- Place the child on his/her side in a place where he/she cannot fall or be injured
- If the fit lasts longer than five minutes, prepare to give rectal diazepam (diazepam should not be given SC or i/m)

Diazepam
- Dose (rectal):
  - <1yr: 2.5–5mg
  - 1–5yrs: 7.5mg
  - 5–10yrs: 10mg
  - >10yrs: 10–15mg
- If the fit shows no signs of abating once the diazepam has been fetched and prepared, give the required dose
- Wait five minutes
- If the fit continues, the dose may be repeated
- If the fit continues after two doses of rectal diazepam, phenytoin, phenobarbital or rectal paraldehyde will be required

Alternatives

Midazolam
- Dose (buccal):
  - 500mcg/kg (max. 10mg)
- Dose (intranasal):
  - 200–300mcg/kg (dropped into alternating nostrils over 15 seconds). (Max. 10mg)

Clonazepam
- Form:
  - Drops: 2.5mg in 1mL (1 drop = 0.1mg). Only available as named patient
- Dose (sublingual):
  - All ages: 0.01mg/kg/dose (max 0.5mg)
- Prescribe as number of drops. Count drops onto spoon before administering
- Titrate up according to response
- Irritability and aggression are not uncommon in which case drug should be withdrawn. Increased secretions may occur in infants and young children.

Maintenance treatment

Medications used for emergency management of seizures do not have a prolonged effect, and if fitting is likely to be an ongoing problem, maintenance treatment is indicated. Control can usually be achieved even in the home environment but most agents will cause drowsiness. Phenytoin, phenobarbital and carbamazepine may be helpful for children able to take oral medication. For those who are unable to tolerate oral medication, phenobarbital given by subcutaneous infusion is an effective alternative. A continuous infusion of midazolam is another option. Rectal paraldehyde may also be helpful.

Provision should be made for breakthrough seizures, which may be managed with rectal diazepam, buccal intranasal or subcutaneous midazolam, or rectal paraldehyde.

Midazolam
- Form:
  - Injection: 10mg in 2mL; 10mg in 5mL
  - Injection may be used for oral, sublingual, rectal, and intranasal routes
- Dose (continuous intravenous or subcutaneous infusion):
  - Start at 5mg/24 h (note: this is not a per kg dose) and titrate to effect

Phenobarbital

Can be given orally or as a continuous subcutaneous infusion and ha anticonvulsant and anxiolytic properties.
- Form:
  - Injection 60mg in 1mL. 200mg in 1mL available as 'special'
- Dose (i/v loading dose):
  - >1 month: 15mg/kg over 5 minutes. Single dose or loading dose, no faster than 1mg/kg/min
- Maintenance dose (i/v /SC continuous infusion or as oral doses):
  - Commence 24 h after loading dose
  - 1 month–12yrs: 5–10mg/kg/24h
  - >12yrs: 600mg/24h
- Review dose after one week as drug induces its own metabolism
- Requires separate syringe driver (does not mix)

Paraldehyde
- Form:
  - Injection 100 per cent (5mL ampoule) also available as already diluted 'special'
- Dose (rectal):
  - All ages: 0.3mL/kg/dose (max 10mL) 4–8h
  - Dilute twofold with olive oil or sunflower oil or dilute 1:10 with 0.9% sodium chloride
- Incompatible with most plastics so use immediately
- Do not give intramuscularly
- Licence: not licensed for use in children

Cough

Consider causes and treat reversible factors if appropriate:

- Infection
- Bronchospasm
- Gastro-oesophageal reflux
- Aspiration
- Drug induced (e.g. ACE inhibitors)/treatment related (e.g. total body irradiation)
- Malignant bronchial obstruction/Lung metastases
- Heart failure
- Secretions
- Cystic fibrosis

Management

General measures

- Keep child as upright as possible
- Raise head of bed:Use blocks under head end of cot/bed or pillows
- Consider physiotherapy +/– suction for children with secretions. Modified physiotherapy is the mainstay of treatment for children with thick secretions
- Consider a trial of humidified air/oxygen

Medication

The choice of medication will depend upon the underlying cause. A dry throat may respond to simple linctus. Bronchospasm will respond to bronchodilator therapy. If the underlying cause cannot be reversed, a suppressant such as an opioid will be required

Simple linctus

This may be helpful if the cough is exacerbated by a dry throat.
- Form:
  - Linctus: paediatric preparation (0.625 per cent citric acid monohydrate); adult preparation (2.5 per cent citric acid monohydrate)
- Dose (oral):
  - 1 month–12yrs: paediatric preparation 5–10mL t.d.s.–q.d.s.
  - >12yrs: adult preparation 5–10mL t.d.s.–q.d.s.
- Licence: licensed for children and adults (appropriate preparation)

Codeine linctus

- Form:
  - Linctus: paediatric preparation: codeine phosphate 3mg in 5mL; adult preparation: 15mg in 5mL
- Dose (oral):
  - 1–5yrs: 5mL paediatric preparation t.d.s.–q.d.s.
  - 5–12 yrs: 2.5–5mL adult preparation t.d.s.–q.d.s.
- Licence: not licensed for use in children under 1yr
- Very constipating: laxatives should always be prescribed

Dihydrocodeine tartrate
- Form:
  - Tablet: 30mg
  - Liquid: 10mg in 5mL
- Dose (oral):
  - 1–4yrs: 500mcg/kg 4–6h
  - 4–12yrs: 500mcg–1mg/kg 4–6h
  - >12yrs: 30mg 4–6h
- Very constipating:laxatives should always be prescribed
- Contra-indications and warnings:avoid or reduce dose in moderate/ severe renal failure, chronic liver disease and hypothyroidism. Avoid in respiratory depression, cystic fibrosis, head injury and raised intracranial pressure
- Licence: licensed for moderate to severe pain in children >4yrs

Morphine linctus
- Form:
  - Solution: 10mg in 5mL
- Start with half the paediatric analgesic dose (📖 See section on Pain, p. 520) and titrate to effect

Bronchodilators

Cough can be a manifestation of hyperreactive airways and a trial of nebulised salbutamol/ipratropium may be helpful.

Salbutamol
- Form:
  - Nebuliser solution:2.5mg in 2.5mL, 5mg in 2.5mL, 5mg in 1mL. (other preparations available, see appropriate text)
  - Inhaled form:100mcg/dose
- Dose (nebulised):
  - 6months–5yrs: 2.5mg t.d.s.–q.d.s.
  - 5–12yrs: 2.5–5mg t.d.s.–q.d.s.
  - >12yrs: 5mg t.d.s.–q.d.s
- Dose (inhaled):
  - All ages: 1–2 puffs 4–6 times a day (a spacer device should be used to improve delivery)
- May induce mild tachycardia, nervousness, tremor or hypokalaemia
- Interactions: see appropriate text
- Licence: licensed for use in children

Ipratropium bromide
- Form:
  - Nebuliser solution: 250mcg/mL. 500mcg in 2mL
  - Inhaled form: 20mcg/dose and 40mcg/dose
- Dose (nebulised):
  - <1yr: 125mcg t.d.s.–q.d.s.
  - 1–5yrs: 250mcg t.d.s.–q.d.s.
  - 5–12yrs: 500mcg t.d.s.–q.d.s.
  - >12yrs: 500mcg t.d.s.–q.d.s.

- Dose (inhaled):
  - <6 yrs: 20mcg/dose t.d.s.–q.d.s.
  - 6–12yrs: 20–40mcg/dose t.d.s.–q.d.s.
  - Licence: licensed for use in children

Mucolytics

May be helpful if secretions are thick. Agents like acetylcysteine and dornase alfa may be used in patients with cystic fibrosis who have thick secretions. Their use should be discussed with the child's paediatrician.

Normal saline
- Dose (nebulised):
  - All ages: 2.5–5mL p.r.n.
- May induce cough reflex in some cases

Gastro-oesophageal reflux

Many neurologically impaired children suffer with gastro-oesophage reflux. Consider reflux if the child refuses food, vomits, has dysphagia, is irritable when supine.

Management

General measures
- Check for overfeeding
- If nasogastric/gastrostomy fed, consider changing regimen from large bolus to smaller, more frequent volumes. Continuous feeding is another option
- Thicken feeds
- Ensure optimal posture for feeds
- Adjust posture overnight to keep child more upright: use blocks unde cot/bed, or pillows
- Surgery can be considered in children with a longer prognosis. Gastrostomy and fundoplication is effective in 80 per cent but is not without complications
- Postpyloric tube feeding is also an option

Medication

Antacids

To be really effective antacids should be given four-hourly. This may lim their usefulness.

Gaviscon
- Form:
  - Tablets: alginic acid 500mg, anhydrous aluminium hydroxide 100mg magnesium trisilicate 25mg, sodium bicarbonate 170mg
  - Liquid: sodium alginate 250mg, sodium bicarbonate 133.5mg, calciu carbonate 80mg in 5mL
  - Dual Infant sachets: sodium alginate 225mg, magnesium alginate 87.5mg with colloidal silical and mannitol per dose (dose = half sachet)
- Dose (oral):
  - Birth–2yrs: 1/2–1 dual infant sachet (do not use other preparations)
  - 2–12yrs: 5–10mL liquid or 1 tablet after meals and at bedtime
  - >12yrs: 10–20mL or 1–2 tablets after meals and at bedtime
- Can cause constipation
- Licence: liquid and tablets licensed for use in children over 2yrs, for children 2–6yrs on medical advice only. Infant sachets licensed for infants and young children but, for children under 1yr, only under medical supervision

Omeprazole

Is the drug of choice for reflux oesophagitis. It is more effective than ran dine and has a good safety profile. Individuals vary in their response a doses will need titration to achieve effective acid suppression.
- Form:
  - Capsule: 10mg, 20mg, 40mg
  - MUPS dispersible tablets: 10mg, 20mg, 40mg

- Tablets: 10mg, 20mg, 40mg
- Intravenous infusion: 40mg vial
- Intravenous injection: 40mg vial

Dose (oral):
- 1 month–12yrs: 700mcg–3mg/kg o.d.—round up to nearest capsule size
- >12yrs: 20–40mg o.d. or divide dose to give b.d.

Capsules can be opened and the granules mixed in acidic drink
Tablets can be dispersed in water or mixed with fruit juice or yoghurt
Contra-indications and warnings: caution in patients with hepatic impairment
Interactions: see appropriate text
Licence: licensed for use in children >2yrs with severe ulcerating reflux oesophagitis

Ranitidine

Form:
- Injection: 50mg in 2mL
- Tablets: 50mg, 300mg. Effervescent tablets 150mg, 300mg
- Liquid: 15mg in 1mL

Dose (oral):
- 6/12 1mg/kg t.d.s.
- 6/12 2–4mg/kg b.d. (max. 150mg)

Infection

Pneumonia is often the terminal event in children with life-limiting illnesses especially those with neurodegenerative conditions. For this reason antibiotic treatment may not be appropriate. In some circumstances however, antibiotics may relieve symptoms and therefore improve the child's quality of life. Antibiotics may also be appropriate early in a life limiting illness where the child is relatively well. Wherever possible, it is helpful to discuss and record a course of action with the parents, and where appropriate the child, in advance of the terminal phase, making it clear that any decisions can be revised as time goes on. This avoids decisions being made in a crisis and may spare the child from intrusive and futile interventions.

Mouthcare

A painful mouth can cause anorexia, discomfort and difficulties eating. It can also make it difficult for the child to take oral medication. Good mouth care can significantly enhance quality of life for children in the palliative care setting.

A general examination should always include inspection of the mouth as oral problems are readily overlooked but can usually be easily managed.

Consider cause and treat as appropriate
- Oral candidiasis
- Dry mouth
- Ulcers
- Bleeding gums
- Dental caries
- Impacted teeth
- Gum hyperplasia
- Medications e.g. morphine, antidepressants, antihistamines or anticholinergics

Management

General measures
- If using oxygen, try humidifying or using nasal prongs
- Keep mouth clean and moist
- Rinse mouth after vomiting
- If possible, brush teeth, gums and tongue and other mucous membranes two to three times a day with a soft toothbrush
- Clear a coated tongue by gently brushing with a soft tooth brush, or by using effervescent vitamin C
- Sucking pineapple chunks will help maintain a clean mouth
- If the mouth is too painful to brush, regularly clean with pink sponges dipped in water or mouthwash, particularly after eating or drinking
- Avoid preparations containing alcohol
- Try water sprays or atomizers
- Ice chips may be helpful
- Artificial saliva: a number of preparations are available
- Moisten lips with petroleum jelly or lip balm
- Refer to dentist if appropriate

Medication

Oral candidiasis may present as classic white plaques or less commonly as atrophic candidiasis with a red glossy tongue. Remember that candidiasis may extend beyond the line of vision to the oesophagus.

Nystatin
- Form:
  - Pastilles: 100,000 units
  - Oral solution: 100,000 units in 1mL
- Dose (oral):
  - 1 month–18yrs: 1mL or 1 pastille 4–6h
  - For oesophageal candida in the immunocompromised: 5mL 4–6h
- The child should not eat or drink for 20 minutes after taking nystatin
- Continue 48h after clinical cure to prevent relapse
- Licence: licensed for children

Miconazole oral gel
- Form:
  - Oral gel: 24mg in 1mL
- Dose (topical to inside of mouth, then swallow)
  - Birth–1 month: 1–2mL b.d.
  - 1 month–2yrs: 2.5mL b.d.
  - 2–6yrs: 5mL b.d.
  - >6yrs: 5mL q.d.s.

Fluconazole
- Form:
  - Capsules: 50mg, 150mg, 200mg
  - Oral suspension: 50mg in 5mL; 200mg in 5mL
  - (Also available i/v)
- Dose (oral):
  - <2weeks: 3mg/kg every 72h
  - 2 weeks–1 month: 3mg/kg every 48h
  - 1 month–18yrs: 3mg/kg daily for 14 days
- Contra-indications and warnings: reduce dose in renal impairment. Co-administration with terfenadine contra-indicated, interacts with several drugs: see other texts. May cause haematological and biochemical abnormalities particularly in children with HIV or malignancies
- Licence: licensed for use in children

Ulcers/mucositis:
- Often related to neutropaenia resulting from high dose chemotherapy or radiotherapy
- Mouthwash. The type of mouthwash will depend on the severity of the mucositis. Chlorhexidine 0.2 per cent (swished for one minute or swabbed three times daily) is generally adequate for children with mild to moderate mucositis. Hydrogen peroxide mouth rinse (diluted 1 in 8 with water or saline and used two to three times daily) may need to be used in addition to chlorhexidine in children with severe mucositis
- An antifungal agent (see above) should be used. This should be given 20–30 minutes after chlorhexidine
- Mucositis can be extremely painful and analgesia appropriate to the degree of pain should be given. For children with severe mucositis, opioid analgesia may be required

Apthous ulcers
Adcortyl in orabase
- Form:
  - Oral paste
- Dose (topical):
  - All ages: Apply thin layer to affected area b.d.–q.d.s.

Choline salicylate (Bonjela)
- Form:
  - Clear gel
- Dose (topical):
  - >4 months: quarter of an inch of gel up to six times daily; may sting initially

Bleeding gums
  📖 See section on Bleeding, p. 486.

Muscle spasm

Muscle spasm may occur in the setting of an upper motor neurone lesion and can cause significant pain and distress. It can be exacerbated by factors such as pain or constipation.

Management

General measures

- Early involvement of a physiotherapist is invaluable for advice on moving, handling, positioning and seating, and is essential to prevent the problem worsening
- Discussion with a paediatric neurologist may be helpful
- Long-standing contractures in a child with a relatively long prognosis can inhibit daily caring and may be managed surgically or with botulinum toxin injection. This should be assessed by an orthopedic surgeon
- While it is generally possible to reduce muscle spasm, it may not be possible to abolish it altogether

Medication:

Analgesia (□ see section on Pain, p. 520).

Baclofen

- Form:
  - Tablet: 10mg
  - Liquid: 5mg in 5mL
  - Also available as intrathecal injection for specialist use: see below
- Starting dose (oral):
  - >1yr–12yrs: 2.5mg t.d.s.
  - >12yrs: 5mg t.d.s.
  - Increase dose every three days to maintenance dose
- Maintenance dose (oral):
  - 1yr–2yrs: 5–10mg b.d.
  - 2–6yrs: 10–15mg b.d.
  - 6–10yrs: 15–30mg b.d.
  - >12yrs: 10–20mg t.d.s.
- Baclofen can also be used intrathecally as a continuous infusion into the lumbar intrathecal space via an indwelling catheter and subcutaneous pump. The rate of infusion can be altered according to the child's clinical needs at different times of day
- Contra-indications and warnings: May cause drowsiness and increased hypotonia. Avoid rapid withdrawal. Use with caution in epilepsy. See other texts for interactions
- Doses should be reduced in renal impairment
- Licence: licensed for oral use in children >1yr

Diazepam
- Form:
  - Tablets: 2mg, 5mg, 10mg
  - Oral solution: 2mg in 5mL and 5mg in 5mL
  - Suppositories: 10mg; and rectal tubes: 2mg in 1mL: 2.5mg tube, 5mg tube, 10mg tube and 20mg tube; 4mg in 1mL; 10mg tube
- Dose (oral):
  - 1 month–5yrs: 50–100 mcg/kg b.d.–q.d.s.
  - 5–12yrs: 2.5–5mg b.d.–q.d.s.
- May cause sedation
- Licence: tablets and liquid licensed for use in cerebral spasticity and control of muscle spasm in tetany

Dantrolene
- Form:
  - Capsules: 25mg, 100mg
- Dose (oral):
  - Starting dose:
  - 1 month–12yrs: 500mcg/kg o.d.
  - >12yrs: 25mg o.d.
- Titration: Increase dose frequency to t.d.s. then q.d.s. at 7 day intervals. If response unsatisfactory continue increasing dose in increments of 500mcg/kg in children <12yrs, and 25mg in those >12yrs until maximum dose reached
- Maximum dose:
  - 1 month–12yrs: 2mg/kg (or 100mg total) q.d.s.
  - >12yrs: 100mg q.d.s.
- Contra-indications and warnings: Hepatic impairment. Caution with cardiovascular/respiratory disease. Monitor liver function tests
- Licence: not licensed for this indication in children

Nausea and vomiting

Consider cause

- Obstruction: Gastric outflow/bowel
- Constipation
- Uraemia/deranged electrolytes/hypercalcaemia
- Raised intracranial pressure
- Upper gastrointestinal tract irritation
- Anxiety
- Cough
- Pain
- Drugs: opioids, chemotherapy, carbamazepine, NSAIDS
- Intercurrent illness e.g. gastroenteritis, urinary tract infection

Management

General measures

- Treat the underlying cause if possible
- Ensure optimal pain management
- Avoid strong food smells and perfumes which may antagonize nausea
- Keep meals small and remove leftover food quickly

Medication

- Give an appropriate antiemetic according to suspected cause (see below), if this is ineffective or the cause is unclear, a phenothiazine such as levomepromazine will usually be effective. Chlorpromazine is very sedating and is used infrequently
- Levomepromazine is a very effective drug with anticholinergic, antihistaminergic, antidopaminergic and analgesic properties. It is often used in paediatric palliative care
- May need to use parenteral or rectal routes until symptoms are under control then consider oral route
- Review: if treatment is not successful, reconsider cause.

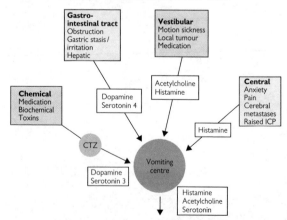

Fig. 7.2 Suspected causes of nausea and vomiting and suggested receptors/neuro-transmitters involved

Table 7.1 Receptor site affinities of antiemetics

	D₂ antagonist	H₁ antagonist	ACh antagonist	5-HT₃ antagonist
Metoclopramide	++	0	0	(+)
Ondansetron	0	0	0	+++
Cyclizine	0	++	++	0
Hyoscine hydrobromide	0	0	+++	0
Haloperidol	+++	0	0	0
Prochlorperazine	++	+	0	0
Chlorpromazine	++	++	+	0
Levomepromazine	++	+++	++	0

D_2 =dopamine, H_1 =histamine 1, Ach =muscarinic cholinergic, 5-HT$_3$ =serotonin group 3

*Adapted from Twycross R, Back I. Nausea and vomiting in advanced cancer. *European J of Pall Care* 1998; **5**: 39–45.

Opioid-induced nausea and vomiting

Opioid-induced nausea is mediated predominantly via dopaminergic pathways. Haloperidol is a dopamine antagonist which acts centrally. It is more potent in this action than metoclopramide. Metoclopramide is a dopamine antagonist and acts on both the CTZ and the gastrointestinal tract (prokinetic action). Like haloperidol, it may cause dystonic side-effects although these can be managed with benztropine. Domperidone is available for oral administration and does not cross the blood brain barrier. This means it is less effective than metoclopramide and haloperidol but is also less likely to cause extrapyramidal side-effects. Dexamethasone may be a useful adjuvant agent. Levomepromazine has antidopaminergic activity in addition to its anticholinergic and antihistamine properties.

Haloperidol
- Form:
  - Tablet: 1.5mg, 5mg, 10mg, 20mg, 500mcg
  - Capsule: 500mcg
  - Oral liquid: 1mg in 1mL, 2mg in 1mL
  - Injection: 5mg in 1mL, 1mL ampoules; 10mg in 1mL, 2mL ampoules
- Dose (oral):
  - 1 month–12yrs: 12.5–50mcg/kg b.d.
  - >12yrs: 500mcg–2mg b.d.–t.d.s.
- Dose (SC):
  - All ages: 25–50mcg/kg over 24h
- Licence: licensed for use in children

Metoclopramide
- Form:
  - Tablet: 5mg, 10mg
  - Syrup/oral solution: 5mg in 5mL
  - Paediatric liquid: 1mg in 1mL
  - Injection: 5mg in 1mL, 2mL ampoule

- Dose (oral/slow i/v /SC):
  - All ages: 100–170mcg/kg t.d.s. Max. 500mcg/kg/24h (max. 10mg) Higher doses may be needed but carry an increased risk of dystonic side-effects
- Dystonic reactions can occur with any dose although the risk increases with dose: reverse with benztropine or procyclidine
- Use with caution if intestinal obstruction suspected: if colic develops, reduce dose or stop altogether
- Caution: in moderate renal failure use 75% dose, in severe renal impairment use 25–50 per cent dose. Reduce dose in severe liver disease.
- Licence: tablets only licensed in children >15yrs.

Levomepromazine
- Form:
  - Tablet: 25mg
  - Injection: 25mg in 1mL, 1mL ampoule
- Dose (oral):
  - 2–12yrs: 0.1–1mg/kg (max 25mg) o.d.–b.d.
  - >12yrs: 6.25–25mg o.d.–b.d.
- Dose (SC/i/v continuous infusion):
  - all ages: 0.1–0.25mg/kg/24h (max. 25mg/24h)
- Highly sedative in higher doses. (SC dose >1mg/kg/24h)
- May reduce seizure threshold
- Postural hypotension especially if used with opioids
- Little experience in very small children
- Caution: Parkinsonism, postural hypotension, antihypertensive medication, epilepsy, hypothyroidism, myasthenia gravis
- Licence: not licensed for use as antiemetic in children

Domperidone
Less effective than metoclopramide but reduced risk of dystonic side effects. May be an alternative agent for a patient who has responded well to metoclopramide but experienced dystonic side-effects.
- Form:
  - Tablet: 10mg
  - Suspension: 5mg in 5mL
  - Suppositories: 30mg
- Dose (oral):
  - 1 month–12yrs: 200–400mcg/kg 4–8 h
  - >12yrs: 10–20mg 4–8 h
- Dose (rectal):
  - 2–12yrs: 15–30mg <25kg: b.d.; 25–35kg: t.d.s.; >35kg: q.d.s.
  - >12yrs: 30–60mg 4–8 h
- Use with caution if intestinal obstruction suspected: if colic develops, reduce dose or stop altogether
- Licence: only licensed for use in children in nausea and vomiting secondary to radiotherapy/chemotherapy

Chemotherapy/radiotherapy-induced nausea and vomiting
Ondansetron is very effective in relieving nausea and vomiting associated with chemotherapy. In refractory cases dexamethasone can be combined

with ondansetron. Levomepromazine is recommended as the third line agent. High dose metoclopramide is used in some centres.

Ondansetron
- Form:
  - Tablet: 4mg, 8mg
  - Tablet (melt): 4mg, 8mg
  - Oral solution: 4mg in 5mL
  - Injection: 2mg in 1mL, 2mL and 4mL ampoules
- Dose (i/v over 2–5 minutes):
  - 1 month–12yrs: 5mg/m^2(max. 8mg) b.d.–t.d.s.
  - >12yrs: 8mg b.d.–t.d.s.
- Ondansetron has been used as continuous iv/sc infusion in palliative care
- Dose (oral):
  - 1m.–12yrs: 4mg b.d.
  - >12yrs: 8mg b.d
- Consider co-prescribing laxative (ondansetron is constipating)
- Licence: licensed for post chemotherapy nausea and vomiting.

Dexamethasone
Caution is required when using steroids in children. side-effects including weight gain, and distressing behavioural and emotional changes occur if steroids are used for more than a few days. For this reason it is preferable to prescribe steroids in short courses (3–5 days) and to repeat courses if necessary.
- Form:
  - Tablet: 500mcg; 2mg
  - Oral solution: 2mg in 5mL
  - Injection: 4mg in 1mL can be given orally
- Dose (oral, i/v):
  - <1yr: 250mcg t.d.s.
  - 1–5yrs: 1–2mg t.d.s.
  - 6–12yrs: 2–4mg t.d.s.
  - >12yrs: 4mg t.d.s.
- Co-prescribing: consider antacids and anti-thrush treatment
- Caution: renal disease, cardiac disease or cystic fibrosis. Avoid in cardiac insufficiency
- Licence: not licensed for use as antiemetic in children

Levomepromazine
- Form:
  - Tablet: 25mg
  - Injection: 25mg in 1mL, 1mL ampoule
- Dose (oral):
  - 2–12yrs: 0.1–1mg/kg (max. 25mg)o.d.–b.d.
  - >12yrs: 6.25–25mg o.d.–b.d.
- Dose (SC/i/v continuous infusion):
  - all ages: 0.1–0.25mg/kg/24h (max. 25mg/24h)
- Highly sedative in higher doses. (SC dose >1mg/kg/24h)

- May reduce seizure threshold
- Postural hypotension especially if used with opioids
- No experience in very small children
- Caution: parkinsonism, postural hypotension, antihypertensive medication, epilepsy, hypothyroidism, myasthenia gravis
- Licence: not licensed for use as antiemetic in children

Raised intracranial pressure

Cyclizine

Has anticholinergic and antihistamine activity. Where raised intracranial pressure is a major factor in generating nausea and vomiting, cyclizine is often helpful. Drowsiness is a common side-effect but may be desirable in some circumstances. While it can be given subcutaneously, cyclizine has a propensity to crystallize in syringe drivers and may cause redness at the infusion site.

- Form:
  - Tablets: 50mg
  - Injection: 50mg/mL (1mL)
  - Suppositories: 25mg +12.5mg, 50mg, 100mg ('special')
- Dose (slow i/v bolus):
  - >1m.: 500 mcg–1mg/kg t.d.s. max. single dose
  - <6yrs: 25mg
  - >6yrs: 50mg
- Dose (i/v /SC continuous infusion):
  - <2yrs: 3mg/kg/24h
  - 2–5yrs: 50mg/24h
  - 6–12yrs: 75mg/24h
  - >12yrs: 150mg/24h
- Dose (oral/rectal):
  - <2yrs: 1mg/kg t.d.s.
  - 2–5yrs: 12.5mg t.d.s.
  - 6–12yrs: 25mg t.d.s.
  - >12yrs: 50mg t.d.s.
- Tablets may be crushed
- Caution: hepatic and renal failure, epilepsy, heart failure
- side-effects: dry mouth, drowsiness, blurred vision, headache, urinary retention, restlessness, insomnia, hallucinations
- Cyclizine is compatible with drugs most commonly used subcutaneously including diamorphine
- Incompatible with sodium chloride 0.9 per cent solution
- Licence: Licensed for use in adults and children aged over 6 yrs

Dexamethasone

Caution is required when using steroids in children. side-effects including weight gain, and distressing behavioural and emotional changes can occur if steroids are used for more than a few days. For this reason it is preferable to prescribe steroids in short courses (3–5 days) and to repeat courses if necessary.

- Form:
  - Tablet: 500mcg; 2mg
  - Oral solution: 2mg in 5mL
  - Injection: 4mg in 1mL can be given orally
- Dose (oral/i/v)
  - <1yr: 250–500mcg b.d.
  - 1–5yrs: 1mg b.d.
  - 6–12yrs: 2mg b.d.
  - >12yrs: 4mg b.d.
- Co-prescribing: consider antacids and anti-thrush treatment
- Caution: renal disease, cardiac disease or cystic fibrosis. Avoid in cardiac insufficiency
- Licence: not licensed for use as antiemetic in children

Noisy breathing

Excessive respiratory secretions more often cause distress to parents and carers than to the child. Reassurance may be all that is required. In circumstances where the child is distressed, pharmacological intervention may be warranted. Suction is generally not helpful.

Drug treatment is more effective if started before or immediately after the secretions are evident.

Antisecretory agents may cause drowsiness and anticholinergic side-effects: glycopyrronium has fewer CNS side-effects than hyoscine hydrobromide because it does not cross the blood brain barrier. Sometimes, however, the sedative effect may be helpful.

Management

Medication

Glycopyrronium bromide
- Form:
  - Injection: 200mcg in 1mL, 1mL ampoule
  - Tablets: 1mg, 2mg; named patient basis only
- Dose (i/v /SC):
  - 1 month–18yrs: 4–8mcg/kg (max. 200mcg) t.d.s.–q.d.s.
- Dose (continuous SC infusion):
  - 1 month–18yrs: 10–40mcg/kg/24h (max. adult dose 1200mcg/24h)
- Dose (oral):
  - 1 month–18yrs: 40–100mcg/kg t.d.s.–q.d.s.
- Contra-indications and warnings: see appropriate text
- Compatible with morphine and midazolam
- Licence: not licensed for this indication in children

Hyoscine hydrobromide
- Form:
  - Self-adhesive patch, drug released at rate of 1mg over 72h
  - Injection: 400mcg in 1mL, 1mL ampoule. 600mcg in 1mL, 1mL ampoule
- Dose (topical):
  Caution in children with intracranial malignancy: may cause agitation
  - 2–3yrs: 1/4 patch over three days
  - 3–9yrs: 1/2 patch over three days
  - >10yrs: one patch over three days
- Hyoscine patches can be cut
- Dose (SC, i/v):
  Single dose given over 2–3 minutes:
  - 1–12yrs: 10mcg/kg q.d.s.
  - >12 yrs (>40kg): 400mcg q.d.s.
- Subcutaneous continuous infusion:
  - All ages: 40–60mcg/kg/24h (max. dose 2400mcg/24h)
- Licence: transdermal preparation licensed for use in children >10yrs for motion sickness

Pain

- Adequate pain control can be achieved for the vast majority of children but requires careful attention to recognition, assessment, treatment and review
- Assessment should include a careful history and examination to elucidate the exact nature and likely cause(s) of pain so that the most effective management can be initiated
- Assessment should include discussion with parents/carers and staff as well as the child if possible
- There are a number of pain assessment tools available to aid diagnosis and monitoring of pain and analgesic effect
- Assessment of pain in children, particularly young infants and non-verbal children, may be difficult
- Pain may be under-diagnosed and therefore inadequately treated in children, particularly those unable to communicate readily
- Pain is closely associated with fear and anxiety

Recognizing pain in children with communication difficulties:
- Discuss with family/carers who know the child well
- Look for signs including: crying, becoming withdrawn, increased flexion or extension, hypersensitivity, frowning/grimacing on passive movement, poor sleep, increasing frequency of fits

Management

General measures

- Management should include reducing stress/anxiety as far as possible as well as analgesic measures
- Analgesics should be used in conjunction with non-pharmacological techniques
- Explanations and discussion often help to reduce anxiety
- A calm, quiet environment may help to reduce anxiety.
- Carefully record all information in medical records on a regular basis to enable anyone who consults the records to easily recognize changes

Medication

Choosing an analgesic:
- For mild to moderate pain, it is usual to start by using a non-opioid analgesic on a p.r.n. basis, progressing to regular use
- Some non-opioid analgesics may be used in conjunction with one another or in conjunction with opioids for added analgesic effect (🕮 see below)
- If non-opioid analgesics do not control pain effectively opioid analgesics will usually be helpful
- The oral route is preferred and adequate pain relief can be achieved using this route for most children
- In the palliative care setting where pain is constant, analgesics should be given regularly rather than p.r.n.
- Weak opioids like codeine have a dose limitation. Strong opioids do not, and the dose should be titrated until effective analgesia is achieved or side-effects prevent further escalation. If side-effects are problematic these can be treated with other medication, or the opioid can be changed to a different preparation with a different side-effect profile

- If a patient is having regular analgesia of any kind, it is important to prescribe additional p.r.n. analgesia for breakthrough pain
- Once stable, it may be possible to change to a slow release form of medication
- Discuss the management plan with the family. If opioids are to be used, a careful explanation is required so that families are prepared for drowsiness, understand that laxatives are necessary and are reassured about issues relating to addiction and dependence
- Plan for exacerbations and crises. Make sure appropriate medications and plans for their use are available to the family. This may include parenteral forms of medication for children on oral opioids
- All analgesic regimens should be regularly reviewed, particularly during titration
- Seek advice from appropriately skilled staff if you are unsure or analgesia is not quickly achieved

Non-opioid analgesics for mild/moderate pain

Paracetamol

- Form:
  - Tablet: 500mg; dispersible tablet: 500mg +120mg
  - Oral solution: 120mg in 5mL
  - Oral suspension: 120mg in 5mL; 250mg in 5mL
  - Suppositories: 60mg, 120mg, 125mg, 240mg, 250mg, 500mg, and 30mg as 'special'
- Dose (Oral):
  - Birth–3 months: 20mg/kg t.d.s. 4–6h(max. 60mg/kg/24h)
  - 3 months–1yr: 60–120mg 4–6h (max. 90mg/kg/24h)
  - 1–5yrs: 120–250mg 4–6h (max. 90mg/kg/24h)
  - 6 –12yrs: 250–500mg 4–6h (max. 90mg/kg/24h or 4g/24h)
  - >12yrs: 500mg–1g 4–6h (max. 90mg/kg/24h or 4g/24h)
- Dose (rectal):
  - Birth–1 month: 20mg/kg max. t.d.s.
  - 1 month–12yrs: 20mg/kg t.d.s.–q.d.s. (max. 90mg/kg/24h or 4g/24h)
  - >12yrs: 500mg–1g t.d.s.–q.d.s. (max. 90mg/kg/24h or 4g/24h)
- Contra-indications and warnings: dose related toxicity in hepatic failure; in moderate renal failure (creatinine clearance 10–50mL/min/1.73m^2) the minimum interval between doses is six hour. In severe renal failure (creatinine clearance <10mL/min/1.73m^2) the minimum interval is eight hours. Significantly removed by haemodialysis but not by CAPD
- May provide additional analgesia in combination with opioids
- Licence: licensed for analgesic use in children >3months, except 30mg suppository

Non-steroidal anti-inflammatory drugs

- Possess analgesic and antipyretic properties
- Are particularly useful for bone pain
- Individuals may respond better to one agent than another
- Should not be given to children with thrombocytopenia or coagulation disorders

- Can be combined with paracetamol or opioids for additive analgesia
- If gastrointestinal side-effects are likely, it may be useful to prescribe antacids and/or a proton pump inhibitor

Ibuprofen
- Form:
  - Tablet: 200mg, 400mg, 600mg
  - Tablet (slow release): 800mg
  - Capsule (modified release): 300mg
  - Liquid: 100mg/5mL
  - Granules: 600mg/sachet
- Dose (oral):
  - 1 month–12yrs: 5mg/kg t.d.s.–q.d.s. (20mg/kg/24h to a max. 2.4g/24h)
  - >12yrs: 200–600mg t.d.s.–q.d.s. (max. 2.4g/24h)
- Cautions: avoid if peptic ulcer or history of; risk of gastrointestinal bleeding if coagulation defects (ibuprofen considered safer than other NSAIDS); avoid if hypersensitivity to other NSAIDS or aspirin. Caution in renal, cardiac or hepatic impairment and asthma
- Licence: Granules and 800mg slow release tablet not licensed for children. Liquid and immediate release tablets not licensed for children <7kg/<1yr

Diclofenac
- Form:
  - Tablet: (enteric coated) 25mg, 50mg; (dispersible) 50mg; (modified release) 75mg, 100mg
  - Capsules: (modified release) 75mg, 100mg
  - Suppositories: 12.5mg, 25mg, 50mg, 100mg
  - Injection: 25mg in 1mL as 3mL ampoule
- Dose (oral/rectal):
  - 6 months–18yrs: 300mcg–1mg/kg t.d.s. (max. 3mg/kg/24h to max. 150mg/24h)
  - Dose (deep i/m* or i/v– i/v must be further diluted and given over 30–120 minutes)
  - >6 months: 300mcg–1mg/kg o.d.–b.d. (max. 3mg/kg/24h to max. 150mg/24h)
  - *Intramuscular injections not recommended in children. Consider alternative agents/routes
- Cautions and contra-indications: avoid if peptic ulcer or history of; avoid if hypersensitivity to other NSAIDS or aspirin. Caution in renal, cardiac or hepatic impairment and asthma. Avoid suppositories if ulceration of lower bowel/anus. Avoid i/v use if concurrent NSAID or anticoagulant therapy
- Licence: 25mg and 50mg tablets and 12.5mg and 25mg suppositories licensed for chronic arthritis in children >1yr. Other preparations not licensed for use in children

Opioid analgesics for moderate/severe pain
- These are usually commenced when non-opioid analgesics have been tried and have not been fully effective or if pain is severe at presentation
- Always co-prescribe a regular laxative: opioids can be expected to cause constipation and it is better to prevent this from the outset

Other side-effects which should be anticipated and promptly managed are:
- Drowsiness: usually wears off after 3–5 days. Families may need forewarning of this as they may interpret drowsiness as a severe decline in the child's condition
- Nausea and vomiting (📖 see section on Nausea and vomiting, p. 512)
- Pruritus: topical measures and antihistamines. Ondansetron may be effective
- Urinary retention: Check that constipation is not a contributory factor. Bethanechol or carbachol may be helpful. Catheterization is required infrequently
- Respiratory depression: this is very unlikely if the dose is titrated appropriately. Naloxone will reverse respiratory depression but this may be at the cost of analgesic effect if not administered carefully
- Euphoria, dysphoria
- Nightmares: a night time dose of haloperidol may be useful
- Physical dependence: opioids should be weaned and not ceased abruptly or a withdrawal reaction may occur
- Tolerance: this is the need for escalating doses to achieve the same therapeutic effect. It is managed by increasing the dose. Families may need to be reassured that tolerance is rare and does not necessarily imply disease progression

Weak opioids

Codeine phosphate
- Form:
  - Tablet: 15mg, 30mg, 60mg
  - Syrup: 25mg in 5mL
  - Linctus: 15mg in 5mL; 3mg in 5mL
  - Injection: 60mg in 1mL (for i/m use, never give i/v), 1mL Amp.
  - Suppositories (specials): 1mg, 2mg, 3mg, 6mg
- Dose (oral/rectal/i/m*):
  - Birth–12yrs: 500mcg–1mg/kg 4–6h (max. 240mg/24h)
  - >12yrs: 30–60mg 4–6h (max. 240mg/24h)
  - *Intramuscular injections not recommended in children. Consider alternative agents/routes
- Constipation common: prescribe laxatives prophylactically
- Cautions and contra-indications and warnings: little experience in young children, avoid in children <3 months. Avoid in renal impairment. Use with caution in hepatic impairment
- Licence: licensed for children >1yr

Dihydrocodeine tartrate
- Form:
  - Tablet: 30mg
  - Liquid: 10mg in 5mL
  - Injection: 50mg in 1mL
- Dose (oral/SC):
  - 1–4yrs: 500mcg/kg 4–6h
  - 4–12yrs: 500mcg–1mg/kg 4–6h
  - >12yr: 30mg 4–6h
- Constipation common: prescribe laxatives prophylactically
- Cautions and contra-indications and warnings: avoid or reduce dose in moderate/severe renal failure, chronic liver disease and

hypothyroidism. Avoid in respiratory depression, cystic fibrosis, head injury and raised intracranial pressure
- Licence: licensed for use in children >4yrs

Strong opioids

Morphine sulphate
- Form:
    - Tablets 10mg, 20mg, 50mg
    - Tablets/capsules (modified release): 5mg, 10mg, 15mg, 20mg, 30mg, 50mg, 60mg, 90mg, 100mg, 120mg, 150mg, 200mg
    - Granules for suspension (modified release): 20mg, 30mg, 60mg, 100mg, 200mg sachets
    - Oral solution: 10mg in 5mL; 100mg in 5mL
    - Injection also available but diamorphine is preferable for this purpose (see below)
    - Suppositories: 10mg, 15mg, 20mg, 30mg. 5mg available as special
- Starting dose (oral/rectal):
    - 1–12yrs: 200–400mcg/kg 4h
    - >12yrs: 10–15mg 4h
- Starting dose (SC/i/v stat):
    - 1–12yrs: 50–100mcg/kg/dose 4 h
    - >12 yrs: 2.5–10mg/dose 4 h
- Starting Dose (continuous infusion):
    - >1yr: 10–15mcg/kg/hr
- NB In children from 6 months–5 years morphine is metabolized more rapidly than in adults, in infants less rapidly
- Prescribing regimen:
    - Always prescribe breakthrough doses (total dose/24h divided by 6)
    - If pain not controlled increase dose by 25–50 per cent
    - Use 4h dosing until pain well controlled, then convert to modified release preparation and prescribe 12h (total dose/24h divided by 2)
    - Slow release preparations normally given b.d. may need to be given t.d.s. in some children
    - Keep required dose under constant review and adjust to give optimum pain control
- Contra-indications and warnings: avoid in paralytic ileus, acute respiratory depression and liver disease. Caution in raised intracranial pressure, head injury, biliary colic, hypothyroidism. Reduce dose in renal failure: use 75 per cent in moderate renal failure (creatinine clearance 10–50mL/min/1.73m^2) and 50 per cent in severe renal failure (creatinine clearance <10mL/min/1.73m^2)
- Licence: Sevredol tablets licensed in children >3yrs. Oramorph SR tablets and Morcap SR capsules are unlicensed for use in children. Oramorph is unlicensed in children <1yr: 5mg suppositories are not licensed

Diamorphine hydrochloride
- Form:
    - Injection: 5mg, 10mg, 30mg, 100mg, 500mg

- Tablets: 10mg but no advantage over morphine sulphate and only one dose available
- Diamorphine is more potent than morphine. Diamorphine is metabolized to morphine but is more water soluble and therefore considered more convenient for SC and i/v injection
- Dose (intravenous):
  - All ages: 12.5–25mcg/kg/h continuous i/v infusion
- Dose (subcutaneous):
  - All ages: 20–100mcg/kg/h continuous SC infusion
- Conversion:
  - The dose of parenteral diamorphine is one third the dose of oral morphine so if converting directly from oral dose: total dose morphine sulphate over 24h divided by three.
- Contra-indications and warnings: paralytic ileus, phaeochromocytoma. Avoid in head injury or raised intracranial pressure. Caution in acute respiratory failure and biliary colic. Reduce dose by 50 per cent in severe renal impairment
- Licence: injection form licensed for children with terminal illness

Fentanyl

Fentanyl is less sedating and less constipating than morphine but it is more difficult to adjust the dose in response to unstable pain when used transdermally. Unless contra-indicated, it is generally better to stabilize the pain using an oral or parenteral opioid before changing to fentanyl patches.

- Form:
  - Patches: for transdermal absorption over 72 h: 25mcg/h, 50mcg/h, 75mcg/h, 100mcg/h
  - Lozenge: for buccal use: 200mcg, 400mcg, 600mcg, 800mcg, 1200mcg, 1600mcg
  - Injection form available but should be used by those with specific experience in paediatric pain medicine
- Dose (transdermal):
  - All ages: To convert from total daily dose of oral morphine sulphate:

Oral morphine (total daily dose) (mg/24h)	<135mg	135–224mg	225–314mg	315–404mg	405–494mg
Fentanyl patch (mcg/hr)	25	50	75	100	125

Converting from oral morphine sulphate:

- Continue oral morphine preparation for up to 12h after first fentanyl patch applied as patch will take 6–12h to reach therapeutic levels
- Wait 24–48h after application before evaluating analgesic effect or changing dose
- Always provide p.r.n. doses of oral morphine for breakthrough pain
- Use new area of skin with each patch change
- Avoid exposure of patch to excessive heat (sun bathing; hot water bottle etc) as heat will increase absorption

- Dose (buccal):
  - Useful for incident and breakthrough pain
  - Dose not related to background analgesic dose, therefore start with 200mcg lozenge and adjust dose according to response
- Although fentanyl may be less constipating than morphine, a laxative should be co-prescribed
- Contra-indications and warnings: see diamorphine. Fentanyl is less problematic in renal failure than diamorphine
- Licence: lozenges and transdermal preparation unlicensed in children

Oxycodone
- Form:
  - Capsules: 5mg, 10mg, 20mg
  - Liquid: 5mg in 5mL; concentrate: 10mg in 1mL
  - Tablets, modified release: 5mg, 10mg, 20mg, 40mg, 80mg
- Dose (oral):
  - **For opioid naïve patients:**
  - 2–12yrs: 0.2mg/kg immediate release preparation 4 h
  - >12 yrs: 5–10mg immediate release preparation 4 h
  - **For children already on opioids:**
  - Conversion ratio from morphine to oxycodone is 2:1 (ie. total daily dose of oxycodone is half the total daily dose of morphine)
  - Alternatively: to determine dose of oxycodone, divide total morphine dose by 12 and give up to 4-h
  - Convert to long-acting preparation when stable
- Contra-indications: acute respiratory depression, paralytic ileus, liver disease, moderate to severe renal failure
- Other opioids such as hydromorphone and methadone are available but their use should be discussed with a paediatric pain or palliative care specialist.

Pain syndromes and adjuvant therapy

Bone pain

Radiotherapy

- Useful for discrete bone metastases
- May be given as a short course or single dose
- Effective treatment with minimal side-effects

Non-steroidal anti-inflammatory drugs

When used in combination with opioids, non-steroidal anti-inflammatory drugs (NSAIDS) may lower the dose of opioid required for effective analgesia. Common choices are:

Ibuprofen
- Form:
    - Tablet: 200mg, 400mg, 600mg
    - Tablet (slow release): 800mg
    - Capsule (modified release): 300mg
    - Liquid: 100mg/5mL
    - Granules: 600mg/sachet
- Dose (oral):
    - 1 month–12yrs: 5mg/kg t.d.s.–q.d.s. (max. 20mg/kg/24h to max. 2.4g/24h)
    - >12yrs: 200–600mg t.d.s.–q.d.s. (max. 2.4g/24h)
- Cautions: avoid if peptic ulcer or history of; risk of gastrointestinal bleeding if coagulation defects (ibuprofen considered safer than other NSAIDS); avoid if hypersensitivity to other NSAIDS or aspirin. Caution in renal, cardiac or hepatic impairment and asthma
- Licence: Granules and 800mg slow release tablet not licensed for children. Liquid and immediate release tablets not licensed for children <7kg/<1yr.

Diclofenac
- Form:
    - Tablet: (enteric coated) 25mg, 50mg; (dispersible) 50mg; (modified release) 75mg, 100mg
    - Capsules: (modified release) 75mg, 100mg
    - Suppositories: 12.5mg, 25mg, 50mg, 100mg
    - Injection: 25mg in 1mL as 3mL ampoule
- Dose (oral/rectal):
    - 6 months–18yrs: 300mcg–1mg/kg t.d.s. (max. 3mg/kg/24h to max. 150mg/24h)
- Dose (deep i/m* or i/v– i/v must be further diluted and given over 30–120 minutes)
    - >6 months: 300mcg–1mg/kg o.d.–b.d. (max. 3mg/kg/24h to max. 150mg/24h)
    *Intramuscular injections not recommended in children: consider alternative agent/route
- Cautions and contra-indications and warnings: avoid if peptic ulcer or history of; avoid if hypersensitivity to other NSAIDS or aspirin. Caution in renal, cardiac or hepatic impairment and asthma. Avoid suppositories if ulceration of lower bowel/anus. Avoid i/v use if concurrent NSAID or anticoagulant therapy

- Licence: 25mg and 50mg tablets and 12.5mg and 25mg suppositories licensed for chronic arthritis in children >1yr. Other preparations not licensed for use in children

Selective COX-2 inhibitors

COX-2 (cyclo-oxygenase 2) inhibitors such as celecoxib are equally analgesic when compared with non-selective NSAIDs. They offer certain advantages in that the risk of gastrointestinal bleeding is reduced, and they have no effect on platelet function.

Bisphosphonates

Bisphosphonates have been shown to reduce bone pain related to malignant and non-malignant causes in adults. They have been used in children. Seek advice before using.

'Resistant' and neuropathic pain

Most pain can be controlled with adequate doses of opioid medication and much of what is regarded as 'resistant' pain can be managed with a dose increase or an alternative route of delivery (e.g. parenteral, spinal). In some instances however, the addition of an adjuvant agent which targets a particular pain mechanism or pathway may be helpful. Neuropathic pain has particular features including a lancinating or burning quality, shock-like features or associated parasthesiae. Antidepressants or antiepileptic medications may be a useful addition to the regimen where these features are present. The choice between the two classes of drug will depend on the child's other symptoms. For example, a child with sleeping difficulties might benefit from a tricyclic antidepressant whereas a child with a coexistent seizure disorder will benefit from an anticonvulsant. If one class of drug is ineffective, a change can be made to another class.

Tricyclic antidepressants

Apart from relieving neuropathic pain, tricyclic antidepressants can enhance opioid-induced analgesia and improve sleep.

Amitriptyline

- Form:
  - Tablets: 10mg, 25mg, 50mg
  - Oral solution: 25mg in 5mL; 50mg in 5mL
- Dose (oral):
  - 1–18yrs: 0.5–1mg/kg nocte
- Starting dose should be at lower end of range, then increase dose by 25 per cent every four days until max. dose (2mg/kg/day) reached or side-effects preclude further titration. Full analgesic effect may not be seen for two weeks
- Contra-indications and warnings: see imipramine
- Licence: not licensed for treatment of neuropathic pain in children

Imipramine

- Form:
  - Tablets: 10mg, 25mg
- Dose (oral):
  - >1 month: 200–400mcg/kg nocte
  - Titrate (50 per cent increase every three days) up to 1–3mg/kg nocte

- Contra-indications and warnings: acute porphyria; hepatic impairment
- Caution with cardiac disease (monitor ECG over 150mg/day)
- Do not use for 3 weeks after discontinuing MAOIs
- Interactions and side-effects: see other texts for full information
- Causes antimuscarinic effects, sedation, cardiac arrhythmias, and lowers seizure threshold
- Licence: not licensed for neuropathic pain in children

Anticonvulsants
Carbamazepine
- Form:
  - Tablets (immediate release): 100mg, 200mg, 400mg; chewable tablets 100mg, 200mg
  - Tablets (modified release): 200mg, 400mg
  - Oral liquid: 100mg in 5mL
  - Suppositories: 125mg, 250mg
- Dose (oral):
  - 1 month–12yrs: start with 2.5mg/kg b.d.
  - Increase by 2.5mg/kg b.d. at weekly intervals to a maximum of 10mg/kg b.d.
  - >12yrs: 200–400mg b.d.–t.d.s.
- The medication should be started at the lower end of the dose range and slowly titrated until therapeutic levels are achieved, symptoms are relieved or side-effects are limiting (e.g. ataxia, drowsiness, nausea.) Titrating slowly minimizes side-effects
- The suspension is absorbed faster than tablets. This might necessitate dividing the total daily dose of suspension into 3–4 doses in order to maintain therapeutic levels
- Contra-indications and warnings: A-V conduction abnormalities, history of bone marrow depression, intermittent porphyria, MAOIs within previous two weeks, sensitivity to tricyclics. Dose reduce in advanced liver disease. Numerous drug interactions
- Licence: licensed for use in children

Gabapentin
- Form:
  - Capsules: 100mg, 300mg, 400mg
- Dose (oral):
  - All ages: start at 10mg/kg once daily for four days then b.d. for four days then t.d.s.
  - Adjust dose according to response. Max. daily dose in adults is 1.8g/24h
  - Capsules can be opened and the contents added to small volumes of fluid or food
- Contra-indications and warnings: avoid abrupt withdrawal. Caution in renal failure: reduce frequency of doses
- Licence: licensed for children >6yrs for epilepsy

Levomepromazine
May be helpful for distressed patients in severe pain unresponsive to other measures.
- Form:
  - Tablets: 25mg
  - Injection: 25mg in 1mL, 1mL ampoule

- Stat Dose (oral, SC):
  - 2–12yrs: 0.5mg/kg o.d–b.d.
  - >12yrs: 6.25–25mg o.d–b.d.
  - Titrate according to response
- Usual maximum daily dose in adults 100mg/day (can be given as a continuous SC infusion) or 200mg/day (p.o.)
- Highly sedative in higher doses. (SC dose >1mg/kg/24h)
- May reduce seizure threshold
- Postural hypotension especially if used with opioids
- Little experience in very small children
- Caution: Parkinsonism, postural hypotension, antihypertensive medication, epilepsy, hypothyroidism, myasthenia gravis
- Licence: not licensed for pain

Ketamine
Ketamine is a useful adjuvant agent for patients with neuropathic pain because of its action on NMDA receptors. It has a tendency to cause agitation and hallucinations in higher doses. Seek advice from a pain management specialist before using.

Nerve blocks/spinal administration/other neuroanaesthetic approaches
May be helpful for children who do not respond to the above measures; consult local anaesthetic team. Spinal infusions can be managed in the community by appropriately trained staff.

Pain associated with tumour-related oedema
Including pain related to intracranial tumours and nerve plexus compression.

Steroids
- Should be used with caution in children
- Short courses (up to five days) can be very effective for this type of pain
- Potential problems include mood and behaviour changes, rapid weight gain and body image changes as well as insomnia and reduced mobility caused by proximal myopathy
- Give entire dose before midday to reduce effect on sleep

Dexamethasone
- Form:
  - Tablets: 500mcg, 2mg
  - Oral solution: 2mg in 5mL
  - Injection: 4mg in 1mL can be given orally
- Dose (oral /SC/i/v):
  - <1yr: 0.25–0.5mg b.d.
  - 1–5yrs: 1mg b.d.
  - 6–11yrs: 2mg b.d.
  - >12yrs: 4mg b.d.
- Higher doses are needed for children with raised intracranial pressure or spinal cord compression
- Contra-indications and warnings: caution if renal disease, cardiac disease or cystic fibrosis. Avoid in cardiac insufficiency
- Licence: licensed for use in children for symptoms associated with brain tumours but not specifically for nerve pain

Painful procedures

- If a procedure is likely to cause discomfort take preventative action!
- Explain all procedures to parents and children as appropriate to reduce anxiety
- Undertake procedures in friendly if not familiar surroundings
- Have parents/carers or the nurse who know the child best present.
- Use anaesthetic creams and distraction techniques appropriate to the age of the child
- Benzodiazepines are often employed in small doses *in conjunction with analgesia* for more difficult procedures e.g. midazolam given buccally, i/v, or intranasally gives light sedation and some amnesia
- Oral
  - 1/12 500mcg/kg max. 15mg
- Buccal/intranasal
  - 200–300mcg/kg dropped into alternate nostrils over 15 seconds. Max. 10mg
- Inhaled nitrous oxide has analgesic and amnesic properties but is non-sedating, so is only useful for co-operative children aged five years or older. Careful supervision is required
- Ketamine is another useful agent but requires careful supervision by trained staff

Psychological issues—anxiety and depression

Management

General measures

- Provide an environment and the opportunity for the child to raise his/her concerns and fears
- Children often find relaxation techniques such as guided imagery very helpful
- Complementary therapies like music therapy may be useful particularly in non-verbal children
- Offer counselling and complementary therapies to parents if possible
- Psychotherapeutic techniques may be necessary

Anxiety

Medication

- Medication should be use in combination with non-pharmacological techniques
- Anxiety may be a manifestation of depression, in which case an antidepressant may be more appropriate
- The choice of benzodiazepine will depend on the circumstance for which it is being prescribed. Children experiencing brief periods of anxiety or panic attacks may benefit from a benzodiazepine with a short half-life, such as midazolam, given buccally or subcutaneously. Sublingual lorazepam is another option for panic attacks or anxiety related to dyspnoea. Children needing a longer duration of action may prefer diazepam

Midazolam

- Form:
  - Injection: 10mg in 2mL; 10mg in 5mL. Injection may be diluted in sodium chloride 0.9 per cent or glucose 5 per cent for buccal and intranasal routes
  - Oral syrup: only available as special
- Single doses:
  - **Intravenous/subcutaneous:**
    - >1month–18yrs: 100mcg/kg
  - **Buccal/sublingual:**
    - >1month–18yrs: 500mcg/kg (max. 10mg)
    - Tastes bitter when given orally but can be mixed with juice or chocolate sauce
  - **Intranasal:**
    - >1month–18yrs: 200–300mcg/kg (max. 10mg)
    - Intranasal route may be unpleasant but has a fast onset of action (5–15 minutes)
  - **Rectal:**
    - >1month–18yrs: 500–750 mcg/kg
    - Continuous intravenous/subcutaneous infusion:
    - >1month–18yrs: 2.5mg/24 h (note: this is not a per kg dose). Titrate to effect

Contra-indications and warnings: caution with pulmonary disease, hepatic and renal dysfunction (reduce dose), severe fluid/electrolyte imbalance and congestive cardiac failure. Avoid rapid withdrawal after prolonged treatment

Licence: licensed for sedation in intensive care and for induction of anaesthesia. Other routes and indications not licensed

Clonazepam

Form:
- Drops: 2.5mg in 1mL (1 drop = 0.1mg), named patient
- Tablets: 0.5mg, 2mg
- Injection: 1mg in 1mL (1mL ampoule)
- Oral liquid 500mcg in 5mL, 2mg in 5mL 'special'

Dose (sublingual):
- All ages: 0.01mg/kg/dose (max. 0.5mg) b.d./t.d.s
- If necessary, increase by 10–25 per cent every 2–3 days to max. 0.1–0.2mg/kg/day
- Prescribe as number of drops. Count drops onto spoon before administering

Irritability and aggression not uncommon in which case drug should be withdrawn. Increased secretions may occur in infants and young children

Lorazepam

Form:
- Tablets: 1mg (scored), 2.5mg
- Suspension: only available as special
- Injection: 4mg in 1mL, 1mL ampoule

Dose (sublingual, oral):
- All ages: 25–50mcg/kg single dose (max. 4mg in adults in 24 h)
- Most children will not need more than 0.5–1mg for trial dose

Well absorbed sublingually (good for panic attacks) and child has control

Injection can also be given sublingually

Contra-indications and warnings: severe pulmonary disease, sleep apnoea, coma, CNS depression. Caution in hepatic and renal failure

Licence: tablets licensed as pre-medication in children >5yrs. Injection not licensed in children <12yrs except for treatment of status epilepticus

Diazepam

Form:
- Tablets: 2mg, 5mg, 10mg
- Oral solution: 2mg in 5mL and 5mg in 5mL
- Injection (solution and emulsion): 5mg in 1mL
- Suppositories: 10mg
- Rectal tubes: 2mg in 1mL: 2.5mg tube, 5mg tube, 10mg tube, 20mg tube, 4mg in 1mL: 10mg tube

Dose (oral):
- 1 month–12yrs: 50–100mcg/kg b.d.–q.d.s.
- >12yrs: 2.5–5mg b.d–q.d.s.

Potential for dependency in prolonged courses

Licence: rectal preparation is licensed for use in children >1yr with severe anxiety. Tablets and liquid licensed for night terrors and sleep-walking

Levomepromazine and haloperidol are sedatives but are not effective anxiolytics.

Depression

The incidence of depression in terminally ill children (other than adolescents) is unknown, but it is likely that for many it remains unrecognized
and untreated.

The clinical picture will depend on the age and developmental stage of
the child but the usual features of depressed mood, anhedonia, social withdrawal, and disturbed sleep and appetite may be present. The diagnosis is
less dependent on somatic symptomatology because of the coexistence of
illness.

Diagnosis may be difficult: trust the instincts of parents and carers and
consult a child psychologist at an early stage.

Fluoxetine
- Form:
  - Capsules: 20mg, 60mg
  - Liquid: 20mg in 5mL
- Dose (oral):
  - 6–18yrs: 10mg o.d. increase slowly to 20mg
- Contra-indications and warnings: avoid in hepatic or renal insufficiency.
  Lowers seizure threshold. Do not use with, or within two weeks of
  taking MAOIs
- Interactions: see appropriate text
- Licence: not licensed for use in children

Amitriptyline

Although tricyclic antidepressants no longer constitute first line manage-
ment of depression in children, amitriptyline may be an appropriate choice
in circumstances where pain and disturbed sleep are also present.
- Form:
  - Tablets: 10mg, 25mg, 50mg
  - Oral solution: 25mg in 5mL; 50mg in 5mL
- Dose (oral):
  - All ages: 0.5–1mg/kg nocte
  - Start at lower end of dose range and increase by 25 per cent every
    2–3 days until maximum dose (2mg/kg/day) reached or side-effects
    preclude further dose increase. Full effect may not be seen for
    two weeks

Contra-indications and warnings: see imipramine
Licence: not licensed for treatment of neuropathic pain in children

imipramine
Form:
- Tablets: 10mg, 25mg
- Starting dose (oral):
  - 6–7yrs: 25mg nocte
  - 8–11yrs: 25–50mg nocte
  - 12–18yrs: 25mg t.d.s. or 75mg nocte
- Maintenance dose (oral):
  - 12–18yrs only:Increase stepwise to 150–200mg daily in divided doses in first seven days. Continue until definite improvement then gradually reduce dose to long-term maintenance dose of 50–100mg daily
- Contra-indications and warnings: acute porphyria; hepatic impairment. Caution in cardiac disease. Do not use with, or within two weeks of taking MAOIs. Lowers seizure threshold
- Interactions: see appropriate text
- Licence: not licensed for this indication in children

NOTE: The Committee for Safety in Medicines has advised (December 2003) that citalopram, escitalopram, paroxetine, sertraline, venlafaxine, and fluvoxamine are contra-indicated if less than 18 years old.

Sleeplessness

Disturbed sleep has a major impact upon the child and family's quality of life. Adequate sleep may be the difference between a family's ability to cope with the stresses placed upon them or not.

Management:

General measures
- Address the child's fears and concerns
- Consider the sleep pattern: the child may be sleeping a lot in the day and may be reversing the day/night pattern. It may be appropriate to keep the child awake more in the day or to provide extra stimulation during the day—this will depend on the child's stage of illness.
  The child may not be aware of when he is expected to sleep if intervention is needed around the clock
- Optimize bedtime routine: bath if possible, story, hot drink if appropriate, lights low
- Increase exposure to light in the mornings
- Consider complementary therapies to aid relaxation
- Try and disturb the child as little as possible during the night: this may mean re-scheduling medications

Medication
Temazepam
- Form:
  - Tablets: 10mg, 20mg
  - Oral solution: 10mg in 5mL
- Dose (oral):
  - 1 month–12yrs: 1mg/kg nocte
  - >12yrs: 10–20mg nocte
- Contra-indications and warnings: caution in severe liver disease. Avoid in CNS depression and acute pulmonary insufficiency
- Interactions: see appropriate text
- Licence: not licensed for use in children

Amitriptyline
This is a useful addition in circumstances where pain is also present
- Form:
  - Tablets: 10mg, 25mg, 50mg
  - Oral solution: 25mg in 5mL; 50mg in 5mL
- Dose (oral):
  - 1–18yrs: 0.5–1mg/kg nocte
  - Start at lower end of dose range and increase by 25 per cent every 2–3 days until maximum dose (2mg/kg/day) reached or side-effects preclude further dose increase. Full effect may not be seen for two weeks
- Contra-indications and warnings: see imipramine

Chloral hydrate
- Form:
  - Oral solution: chloral mixture BP: 500mg in 5mL; chloral elixir paediatric BP 200mg in 5mL, extemporaneously prepared
  - Syrup: 500mg in 5mL only available as 'special'
  - Suppositories: 25mg, 50mg, 100mg, 250mg, 750mg only available as 'specials'
  - Tablets: chloral betaine 707mg (= chloral hydrate 414mg)
- Dose (oral/rectal):
  - 1 month–12yrs: 30–50mg/kg (max. 1g) nocte
  - >12yrs: 0.5–1g nocte
- Contra-indications and warnings: avoid in liver disease and severe renal failure. Caution in cardiac disease, respiratory insufficiency, porphyria and gastritis. Avoid prolonged administration and abrupt withdrawal
- Licence: unlicensed in children

Alimemazine tartrate
- Form:
  - Tablets: 10mg
  - Mixture: 1.5mg in 1mL, 6mg in 1mL
  - Syrup: 7.5mg in 5mL
  - Syrup forte: 30mg in 5mL
- Dose (oral):
  - 1m.–12yrs: 1.5–3mg/kg nocte
  - >12yrs: 10mg t.d.s (max 90mg/day)

Promethazine hydrochloride
- Form:
  - Tablets: 10mg, 25mg
  - Elixir: 5mg in 5mL
  - Injection: 25mg in 1mL as 1mL ampoule
- Dose (oral):
  - <1yr: 5–10mg nocte
  - 1–5yrs: 10–20mg nocte
  - 6–12yrs: 20–25mg nocte
  - >12yrs: 25–50mg nocte
- May be useful in mild cases
  - Contra-indications and warnings: Porphyria; CNS depression; hypersensitivity to phenothiazines. Do not use with, or within two weeks of taking MAOIs
- Licence: licensed for use in children >2yrs

Raised intracranial pressure

Consider raised intracranial pressure if the child shows evidence of:

- Confusion
- Personality change
- Drowsiness
- Vomiting
- Headache (especially on waking)
- Focal neurology

Management

General measures

- Investigation should be considered only if it will contribute to management decisions
- Reduction of tumour bulk may improve symptoms e.g. cranial irradiation and chemotherapy. Occasionally a ventricular shunt may be appropriate
- Symptomatic management may include analgesia (see pain section), antiemetics and steroids. The antiemetic of choice is cyclizine

Medication

Dexamethasone

Caution is required when using steroids in children. side-effects including weight gain, and distressing behavioural and emotional changes occur if steroids are used for more than a few days. For this reason it is preferable to prescribe steroids in short courses (3–5 days) and to repeat courses if necessary.

- Form:
  - Tablet: 500mcg; 2mg
  - Oral solution: 2mg in 5mL
  - Injection: 4mg in 1mL can be given orally
- Dose (oral/i/v over 3–5 minutes):
  - <1yr: 0.5–1.0mg b.d.
  - 1–5yrs: 2mg b.d.
  - 6–12yrs: 4mg b.d.
  - >12yrs: 8mg b.d.
  - Do not give after midday as can affect night time sleep
- Dose (SC):
  - Can also be given in equivalent doses SC as single doses or as continuous infusion over 24h
  - If no effect after 3–5 days, stop steroids (no need to tail off)
  - Co-prescribing: consider antacids and anti-thrush treatment
- Contra-indications and warnings: caution if renal disease, cardiac disease or cystic fibrosis. Avoid in cardiac insufficiency
- Licence: licensed for use in children but not as antiemetic

Cyclizine

- Form:
  - Tablets: 50mg
  - Injection: 50mg/mL (1mL)
  - Suppositories: 25mg ('special')

Dose (i/v stat):
- 1/12 500mcg/mg/kg t.d.s. Max. single dose <6 yrs: 25mg, >6yrs: 50 mg

Dose (SC/i/v continuous infusion):
- 1m.–2yrs: 3mg/kg/24h
- 2–5yrs: 50mg/24 h
- 6–12yrs: 75mg/24 h
- > 12yrs: 150mg/24 h

Oral/rectal
- <2yr: 1mg/kg t.d.s.
- 2–5yrs: 12.5mg t.d.s.
- 6–12yrs: 25mg t.d.s.
- >12yrs: 50mg t.d.s.

Caution: hepatic and renal failure, epilepsy, heart failure

Side-effects: dry mouth, drowsiness, blurred vision, headache, urinary retention, restlessness, insomnia, hallucinations

- Tablets may be crushed
- Cyclizine is compatible with drugs most commonly used subcutaneously including diamorphine
- Incompatible with sodium chloride 0.9 per cent solution

Skin

Management

General measures

- Like adults, children with terminal illnesses have skin that is susceptible to breakdown with poor healing abilities
- Good nursing care is required to predict and prevent problems, which once established may be difficult to treat
- Frequent and appropriate turning is essential to avoid pressure areas breaking down
- The use of suitable mattresses and mobility aids should be considered
- Consult tissue viability nurse if available

Medication

- At risk areas
  - Protect with Opsite, Tegaderm or Cutifilm
- Broken areas
  - Use Duoderm, Spyrosorb
- Infection
  - Send swab for growth. Use Intrasite gel, Iodosorb paste covered with Opsite or Tegaderm +/− antibiotics
- Cavities
  - Pack with Kaltostat or Sorbsan
- Fungating tumours and odour
  - Use topical metronidazole gel, charcoal dressings or honey and sugar.
- Painful ulcers
  - Consider anaesthetic preparations e.g. lidocaine/prilocaine (EmLa cream) or a topical morphine gel

See also adult section on Skin.

Sweating

Consider cause
- Disease e.g. malignant pyrexia, lymphoma, neuroblastoma
- Drugs e.g. opioids, amitriptyline, chemotherapy
- Infection

Management

General measures
- Disease-modifying treatment may improve sweating if it is part
  of a malignant syndrome
- Fan, cotton clothing, skin care
- Encourage plenty of fluids to avoid dehydration

Medication
There is no good evidence to support the use of any of the followin
agents but they may be worth trying

Paracetamol
- Form:
  - Tablets: 500mg; dispersible tablets: 500mg
  - Oral solution: 120mg in 5mL
  - Oral suspension: 120mg in 5mL; 250mg in 5mL
  - Suppositories: 60mg, 120mg, 125mg, 240mg, 250mg, 500mg, and
    30mg as 'special'
- Dose (oral):
  - Birth–3 months: 20mg/kg t.d.s. (max. 60mg/kg/24h)
  - 3 months –1yr: 60–120mg 4–6h (max. 90mg/kg/24h)
  - 1–5yrs: 120–250mg 4–6h (max. 90mg/kg/24h)
  - 6–12yrs: 250–500mg 4–6h (max. 90mg/kg/24h or 4g/24h)
  - >12yrs: 500mg–1g 4–6h (max. 90mg/kg/24h or 4g/24h)
- Dose (rectal):
  - Birth–1 month: 20mg/kg max. t.d.s.
  - 1 month–12yrs: 20mg/kg t.d.s.– q.d.s. (max. 90mg/kg/24h or 4g/24h)
  - >12yrs: 500mg–1g t.d.s.– q.d.s. (max. 90mg/kg/24h or 4g/24h)
- Contra-indications and warnings: dose related toxicity in hepatic failure
  in moderate renal failure (creatinine clearance 10–50mL/min/1.73m^2)
  the minimum interval between doses is six h. In severe renal failure
  (creatinine clearance < 10mL/min/1.73m^2) the minimum interval is
  eight hours. Significantly removed by haemodialysis but not by CAPD
- Licence: licensed for antipyretic and analgesic use in children
  >3months, except 30mg suppository

Naproxen
- Form:
  - Tablets: 250mg, 375mg, 500mg
- Dose (oral):
  - >1 month: 5–15mg/kg b.d. (max. 1g/24h)

Contra-indications and warnings: Contra-indicated in children who have shown hypersensitivity to aspirin or other NSAIDS. Caution in asthma and cardiac, hepatic or renal failure; avoid if creatinine clearance <20mL/min/1.73m². Extreme caution if current or previous history of peptic ulceration

Licence: not licensed for use in children for this indication

ther

antrolene, steroids and H2 receptor antagonists have also been used.

Terminal restlessness

Restlessness and agitation are not uncommon during the terminal phase. Nursing the child in a calm, peaceful and preferably familiar environment is helpful as is having a parent or other trusted adult present. It is important to exclude pain or inadequate positioning as a cause of distress. Hypoxia may also be a factor.

The choice of medication will depend on the clinical circumstances. Midazolam is very effective and can be combined with morphine or diamorphine more commonly in a subcutaneous infusion. Levomepromazine is also compatible with these medications and is an appropriate choice for children who also have pain and nausea.

Medication

Midazolam

- Form:
  - Injection: 10mg in 2mL; 10mg in 5mL
  - Injection may be diluted in Sodium chloride 0.9% or glucose 5% for oral, buccal and intranasal routes
  - Oral syrup: 'special'
- Single doses:
  - Intravenous/subcutaneous:
    - >1month–18yrs: 100mcg/kg
  - Buccal/sublingual:
    - >1month–18yrs: 500mcg/kg (max. 10mg)
    - Tastes bitter when given orally but can be mixed with juice or chocolate sauce
  - Intranasal:
    - >1month–18yrs: 200–300mcg/kg (max. 10mg)
    - Intranasal route may be unpleasant but has a fast onset of action (5–15 minutes). Drop dose into alternate nostrils over 15s
  - Rectal:
    - >1month–18yrs: 500–700mcg/kg
  - Continuous intravenous/subcutaneous infusion:
    - Start at 2.5mg/24 h (note: this is not a per kg dose). Doses of up to 40mg/24 h have been necessary. If high doses required consider changing to a different agent
    - Well absorbed subcutaneously
- Midazolam is compatible in a syringe driver with morphine, diamorphine, cyclizine and other commonly used drugs
- Contra-indications and warnings: caution with pulmonary disease, hepatic and renal dysfunction (reduce dose), severe fluid /electrolyte imbalance and congestive cardiac failure. Avoid rapid withdrawal after prolonged treatment
- Midazolam raises seizure threshold making it a good choice for children likely to fit
- Licence: licensed for sedation in intensive care and for induction of anaesthesia in children >7yrs. Other routes and indications not licensed

Clonazepam

Form:
- Drops: 2.5mg/mL (1 drop = 0.1mg), named patient basis
- Tablet: 0.5mg, 2mg
- Injection: 1mg in 1mL (1mL ampoule)
- Oral liquid: 500mcg in 5mL, 2mg in 5mL 'specials'

Dose (sublingual):
- All ages: 0.01mg/kg/dose (max. 0.5mg) b.d./t.d.s.
- If necessary, increase by 10–25 per cent every 2–3 days to max. 0.1–0.2mg/kg/day
- Prescribe as number of drops. Count drops onto spoon before administering

Irritability and aggression not uncommon in which case drug should be withdrawn. Increased secretions may occur in infants and young children

Licence: not licensed for this indication

Levomepromazine

Form:
- Tablets: 25mg
- Injection: 25mg in mL, 1mL ampoule

Dose (continuous SC/i/v infusion):
- All ages: 0.5–1mg/kg/24h. Titrate to effect. (max. adult dose 300mg/24h)

Also acts as antiemetic
- May lower seizure threshold
- Can be used in conjunction with midazolam
Highly sedative in higher doses (SC dose > 1mg/kg/24h)
- Postural hypotension especially if used with opioids
- Little experience in very small children
- Caution: Parkinsonism, postural hypotension, antihypertensive medication, epilepsy, hypothyroidism, myasthenia gravis
- Licence: not licensed for use as an antiemetic in children

Emergency drugs summary

The following information is given as a rough guide for quick reference only.

Many of the following drugs, doses or indications are unlicensed in children.

Table 7.1 Analgesics

Drug	Route	1month–1yr	2–12 yrs	12–18 yrs	Notes
Morphine	p.o./PR	100mcg/kg	200–400mcg/kg	10–15mg	4-h starting doses
Diamorphine	CSCI	20–100mcg/kg/24h	20–100mcg/kg/24h	20–100mcg/kg/24h	24h starting dose
	SC/i/v stat	5–15mcg/kg	5–15mcg/kg	2.5–5mg	4-h as needed
Ibuprofen	PPO	5mg/kg	5mg/kg	200–600mg	t.d.s–q.d.s Maximum 2.4g/day

Table 7.2 Antiemetics

Drug	Route	1 month–2yr	2–12 yrs	12–18 yrs	Notes
Cyclizine	p.o./PR	1mg/kg t.d.s.	2–5yrs: 12.5mg t.d.s.	25–50mg t.d.s.	
Cyclizine	SC/i/v continuous infusion	3mg/kg/24h	2–5yrs: 50mg/24h 6–12yrs: 75mg/24h	150mg/24h (max.)	
Cyclizine	i/v stat	>1month 500mcg–1mg/kg t.d.s. (max. 25mg)	2–5yrs: 20mg (max. 25mg) 6–12yrs: 25mg (max. 50mg)	>12yrs: 50mg (max.)	Give slowly over 3–5 minutes
Haloperidol	p.o.	12.5–50mcg/kg b.d.	12.5–50mcg/kg b.d.	0.5–2mg b.d.–t.d.s.	Increased risk of extrapyramidal side-effects in children.
Ondansetron	i/v	5mg/m² b.d.–t.d.s. (max. 8mg)	5mg/m² b.d.–t.d.s. (max. 8mg)	8mg b.d.–t.d.s	Give over 3–5 minutes Can be given as continuous infusion
Ondansteron	p.o.	1mg b.d.–t.d.s	2–4yrs 2mg b.d.–t.d.s 4–12yrs 4mg b.d.–t.d.s	8mg b.d.–t.d.s	
Metoclopramide	p.o./i/m /slow i/v/SC	100–170mcg/ kg t.d.s.	100–170mcg/ kg t.d.s.	100–170mcg/ kg t.d.s.	Increased risk of extrapyramidal side-effects in children
Levomepromazine	p.o.		0.1–1mg/kg o.d.–b.d.	6.25–25mg o.d.–b.d.	Very sedating in doses over 1mg/kg/24 h
Levomepromazine	SC /i/v continuous infusion	0.1–0.25mg/kg (max. 25mg/24h)	0.1–0.25mg/kg (max. 25mg/24h)	0.1–0.25mg/kg (max. 25mg/24h)	

Table 7.3 Sedatives

Drug	Route	<1yr	1–12 yrs	12–18 yrs	Notes
Diazepam	p.o./PR	50–100mcg/kg/dose	50–100mcg/kg/dose	2.5–5mg b.d.	Repeated as needed
Lorazepam	p.o./sublingual	25–50 mcg/kg/dose	25–50mcg/kg/dose	25–50mcg/kg/dose	Max 4mg in 24 h
Midazolam	CSCI	>1 month–18yrs: 2.5mg/24h			
	SC/i/v stat	>1month–18yrs: 100mcg/kg			
	Buccal stat	1 month–18yrs: 500mcg/kg (max 10mg)			

Table 7.4 Antisialogogue (for death rattle)

Drug	Route	2–18 yrs	Notes
Hyoscine hydrobromide	SC stat	1–12yrs: 10mcg/kg <12yrs (>40kg): 400mcg	Repeat every 4h as needed Sedating
Hyoscine hydrobromide	CSCI	40–60mcg/kg/24h	Max dose 2400mcg/24h
Glycopyrronium	SC/i/v stat	1month–18yrs: 4–8mcg/kg	Repeat every 6–8h as needed Doses for drooling much lower, max. 200mcg/dose
Glycopyrronium	CSCI	1month–18yrs: 10–40mcg/kg/24h	Max adult dose 1200mcg/24h

Table 7.5 Average weights for healthy children

Age	Mean weight Kg	% Adult dose
Newborn	3.5	12.5
6 months	8	22
1 yr	10	25
3 yrs	15	33
5 yrs	20	40
7 yrs	25	50
12 yrs	40	75
Adult male	70	100
Adult female	60	100

NB Wt. in stones × 6 ≈ wt. in Kg.

The percentage adult dose should only be used as a rough guide when paediatric doses in mg/kg are not available.

Further reading

Books and articles

Bluebond-Langner M. (1978) *The Private Worlds of Dying Children*. Princeton: Princeton University Press.

Goldman A. (1994) *Care of the dying child*. Oxford: Oxford University Press.

Herbert, M. (1996) *Supporting bereaved and dying children and their parents*. Leicester: BPS Books.

Hassah SS. (2002) *Basic symptom control in paediatric palliative care: The Rainbow Children's Hospice guidelines*. 4th edn. Loughborough: Rainbow Children's Hospice.

Nikin S. (1989) A proposal concerning decisions to forgo life-sustaining treatment for young people. *J Pediatrics* **115**: 17–22.

Edstone V. et al. (2003) *Paediatric Palliative Care Guidelines*. London: The South West London and the Surrey, West Sussex and Hampshire Cancer Networks.

Orloff S., Huff S. (2004) *Homecare for Seriously Ill Children: A Manual for Parents*. Alexandria: CHI.

Royal Children's Hospital, Brisbane. (1999) *A Practical Guide to Paediatric Oncology Palliative Care*. Brisbane: Royal Children's Hospital.

Royal College of Paediatrics and Child Health (2003) *Medicines for Children*. 2nd edn. London: RCPCH.

Royal College of Paediatrics and Child Health (1997). *Withholding or Withdrawing Life-saving Treatment in Children*. London: RCPCH.

Waechter EH. (1971) Children's awareness of fatal illness. *Am J Nurs.* **7**: 1168–72.

Chapter 8

Palliative care in non-malignant disease

e majority of patients in the UK (over 90 per cent) receiving specialist lliative care services have cancer. There is increasing recognition of the met need in patients with other progressive, incurable, non-malignant agnoses which has been highlighted by recent publications. The epartment of Health in the UK is striving to redress this balance, ctating that all patients with end-stage illness should have access to the rvices offered by multidisciplinary palliative care teams.

Specialist palliative care teams have traditionally been wary about taking sponsibility for patients in whom the prognosis is uncertain, with the ar that precious resources would become overburdened by patients th longer term chronic illness. Studies in motor neurone disease (MND), owever, showed that patients did not 'block' specialist beds any more an any other patients and most hospices now accept patients with MND to their programmes. It was perhaps the emergence of AIDS in the mid 80s that made all specialist units take notice of a group of dying patients r whom they felt obliged to take some responsibility.

Patients with end-stage non-malignant disease suffer from as many stressing symptoms as those with cancer. Despite this there remains a ck of confidence in looking after patients with less familiar illnesses. This ay partly stem from the fact that the dying phase is often different from at seen in cancer. Patients dying from cancer tend to deteriorate gradu- y over time, and usually it becomes obvious when the terminal phase is itered and when treatment and interventions can be aimed more at mfort. Patients dying from chronic heart or lung disease, on the other nd, are often deteriorating over a somewhat longer period of time, terspersed by acute episodes that may be better managed within a spital environment, where acute care management is both appropriate d readily available. This may highlight educational and training issues, but es not mean that the palliative care team should take over the rôle of her specialist teams. Rather they should work alongside specialists in the her fields, ensuring that the principles of palliative care are upheld and at patients and families receive optimal treatment.

The percentage of the population over 65 years has increased and 'll continue to do so. The main causes of mortality are heart disease, rebrovascular disorder, chronic respiratory disease and cancer. Palliative re teams will need to find a way to deliver appropriate care to all tients regardless of diagnosis. To this end, there is a higher percentage of tients with non-malignant disease in the hospice movement in the USA 0–30 per cent) and there is evidence that this trend is increasing in the K, particularly within hospital specialist palliative care services.

With increasing dialogue, partnership, research and funding, the vision providing services where they are needed should be a realistic aim.

AIDS in adults

Introduction

AIDS is a cluster of clinical conditions that inevitably occur in a person infected by the Human Immuno-deficiency Virus (HIV). As this virus attacks and weakens the cellular immune system the infected person develops an increasing number of infections, often from weak but opportunistic micro-organisms. The virus also directly attacks various body tissues, resulting in chronic diarrhoea, severe weight loss, painful peripheral neuropathy, progressive dementia or profound pancytopenia. In the advanced stages of HIV infection, there is also an increasing incidence of malignancies such as Kaposi's sarcoma and cerebral lymphoma, that were previously extremely uncommon.

HIV affects principally the T-lymphocytes, resulting in impaired cell-mediated immunity. Certain lymphocytes (T4 cells) have a surface protein (CD_4) which has a high affinity for HIV. The CD_4 count declines with advancing disease and increasing immunodeficiency. Counts below 200/microlitre are associated with a high risk of developing opportunistic infection. The viral load is high following the initial infection and then declines as the immune system partially recovers after about 12 weeks. It remains at a low level for a variable period of time and then increases again with the collapse of the immune system.

Historical background

There has been much heated debate about the origins of AIDS. It was initially recognized in the gay community in the USA in the early 1980s and since then has gradually spread to the wider world community. Transmission is through contact with blood or other body fluids infected with HIV. Those most vulnerable to HIV infection are thus persons with multiple sexual partners, intravenous drug users, babies of infected mothers, persons receiving blood transfusions and health professionals who sustain needle-stick injuries.

Complexity

The course of the illness is unpredictable, the presentation is variable and, even with anti-retroviral drugs (ARVs), death from AIDS is inevitable. Added to this complex clinical picture is the emotional, social and economic impact that this pandemic is having, especially in sub-Saharan Africa. Fear, stigma, rejection, repeated bereavement and conflicting messages accompany this disease. With the rising death rate, declining life expectancy, prolonged suffering and economic disruption that is occurring as a direct result of AIDS, this condition is the single greatest health challenge to our world in the twenty-first century.

Statistics

The confusing and sometimes conflicting statistics that are presented tend to muddle rather than help, at a time when we need clear reasoning and

constructive planning for the future. What is certain is that this pandem
is very large and is growing rapidly. Despite all the recent preventi
strategies and medical advances, it is showing no signs of abating. By 200
the WHO estimated that 40 million people worldwide were infecte
The vast majority of these live in Sub-Saharan Africa where it is estimat
that 1 in 5 adults is infected.

Even in the UK, where more than 50,000 people had been infected wi
HIV by 2000, the number of infections has continued to rise despite tl
introduction of ARVs. AIDS is also spreading rapidly in Asia and Sou
America.

Clinical features

AIDS has replaced syphilis and tuberculosis as the great mimic. It ma
present in such a myriad of ways that it should be considered as a poss
bility in any patient of any age with almost any complaint anywhere in th
world. There are, however, a number of clinical presentations that ar
typical and even some that are diagnostic of AIDS. Loss of weight of mor
than 10 per cent, diarrhoea or fevers lasting more than a month, generalize
lymphadenopathy especially including the submental and epitrochlea
nodes, are very suggestive. Herpes zoster in a young adult, dry itchy sk
and small darkly pigmented itchy bumps would also raise the suspicions c
any health worker in an endemic area. Kaposi's sarcoma, cryptococc
meningitis and cerebral lymphoma are pathognomonic.

The classification devised by the WHO is a useful way of staging
the illness clinically, especially when CD$_4$ counts and viral loads are nc
available (see Table 8a.1).

Table 8a.1 WHO clinical staging of HIV/AIDS (modified)

	Clinical stage			
	Sero-conversion (1)	Early (2)	Intermediate (3)	Late (4)
Feature				
Activity	Normal	Rests occasionally	Rests for <50% of day	Rests for >50% of day
Weight loss	No	< 10%	> 10%	Wasted/ cachectic
Fever	Mild in 50%	Occasional	> 1/12	> 1/12
Diarrhoea		Occasional	> 1/12	> 1/12
Respiratory infections		URTIs Pneumonia Pleural effusion	Recurrent pneumonia Chronic otitis media	Pneumocystis carinii pneumonia (PCP)
Pulmonary TB			Miliary Lower lobes Mediastinal nodes	Extensive bilateral Resistant
Other TB				Pericardial Peritoneum Spine/bone Meningitis
Skin		Shingles H. simplex Dry Itchy papules Tinea corporis	Severe shingles Pellagra Stevens–Johnson syndrome Vaginal thrush	Persistent genital ulcers

Table 8a.1 (Continued)

| | Clinical stage | | | |
	Sero-conversion (1)	Early (2)	Intermediate (3)	Late (4)
Mouth		Aphthous ulcers Reiter's syndrome Gingivitis	Oral thrush Progressive gingivitis	Oesophageal thrush
CNS		Bell's Palsy Guillain–Barré syndrome		Painful feet Paraplegia 25% dementia Cryptococcal meningitis Toxoplasmosis
Cancer				Kaposi's sarcoma Invasive cancer of cervix Lymphoma
Lymph nodes	Generalized	Generalized	Generalized	Generalized or absent

Natural history

Following infection by HIV, the natural progression of this illness is very variable. For many there are few symptoms initially and it is only after several years of relatively normal health that the typical clinical features of AIDS become apparent. In others, the initial sero-conversion may be more pronounced with fever, body pains, headache, ulceration of the mucosa of the mouth and genitalia, a maculo-papular rash, hepatosplenomegaly and generalized lymphadenopathy. These symptoms usually resolve spontaneously over a few weeks. During this phase the person may, however, develop Bell's palsy or the Guillain–Barré syndrome, indicating early neurological involvement.

After about 12 weeks the body reaches a steady state with partial recovery of the immune system and a decline in the number of circulating viral particles. Now follows a phase of clinical latency where the only clinical signs may be generalized lymphadenopathy and occasional episodes of sweating, especially at night.

While a small proportion of infected people may progress rapidly to full-blown AIDS within one or two years, in the majority AIDS takes eight to ten years to develop. A few individuals progress very slowly and may be still alive after 20 years, even without ARVs.

As the immune system begins to become exhausted, the person becomes susceptible to a wide range of infections including recurrent upper respiratory tract infections, pneumonia, tuberculosis, a wide variety of intestinal micro-organisms, cryptococcal meningitis, herpes zoster and monilial infections of the mouth, vagina and oesophagus.

The variability of the resilience of the immune system and the potentially fatal nature of some of the infections, make it difficult to estimate the prognosis of an individual.

The effects and limitations of highly active anti-retroviral therapy (HAART)

The advent of Highly Active Anti-Retroviral Therapy (HAART) has radically changed the prospects for many people with AIDS. An emaciated person who appears to be beyond all help may start rapidly improving on ARVs. This has been nicknamed the 'Lazarus Syndrome'. In Europe and North America, numerous hospices and hospital wards dedicated to caring for dying AIDS patients have been able to empty their beds and concentrate on other forms of care.

ARVs are the best form of palliation for AIDS that is available at present. The decision of when to start ARVs and which combination to use may at first seem complex. The key to success is for the affected person and the doctor to negotiate the most suitable timing of the start of ARVs and the most suitable combination.

Good stories are a very effective way of explaining the use of ARVs and getting the right message across to less well developed educated communities e.g.

Imagine you are hiking through the bushveld and enjoying the birdlife and the game. But, in the distance, you see a lion stalking you. You aren't too worried because you have a gun. But there are only two bullets in the gun, so you need to be quite sure about the best time to shoot. If you shoot too soon there is a good chance that you will miss the lion, and that the explosion will chase away all the wildlife. If you leave it too late the lion may be on top of you before you can take aim.

The lion represents AIDS and the distance between you and the lion shows how strong your immune system is—the closer the lion the weaker your immune system. The gun with the two bullets is your anti-retroviral therapy, which you need to learn how to use properly so that you don't hurt yourself. The sound of the gun being fired represents the potential side-effects of the antiretroviral therapy—a real nuisance if the lion is far away, but the last thing you'd worry about when the lion is getting close!

The decision to start ARVs must not be hurried. Anti-retrovirals (ARVs) need to be used responsibly.[1] Time needs to be taken to help the person understand as fully as possible the various options and the need for strict adherence.

- Treatment needs to be taken for life
- It is very important to choose the first treatment regimen carefully as it is the one most likely to have the best results
- Once the virus has been exposed to ARVs, subsequent regimens are less likely to give good results
- The start of ARVs should be delayed until the CD_4 count is below 200/microlitre, or the symptoms of the infection are very troublesome
- Social and psychological problems, especially depression, need to be resolved where possible before starting ARVs as these will make adherence difficult
- The choice of drugs is growing rapidly. The inexperienced clinician should ask for advice from someone experienced with using ARVs

- In an effort to make the decision as simple as possible, the WHO is recommending fixed combinations in a similar way to the TB regimens. See www.who.int/hiv/pub/prev_care/draft/en/
- Efavirenz or nevirapine (NNRTIs) should be used in combination with zidovudine and lamivudine or stavudine and lamivudine (NRTIs from different categories) (see Table 8a.2).

Table 8a.2 Classification of anti-retroviral drugs*

Category I (NRTIs)	Category II (NRTIs)	Category III (NRTI)	Category IV (NNRTIs)	Category V (PIs)
Stavudine (d4T)	Didanosine (ddI)	Abacavir (ABC)	Nevirapine (NVP)	Nelfinavir (NFV)
Zidovudine (AZT)	Lamivudine (3TC)		Efavirenz[†] (EFV)	Indinavir/RTV (IDV)
	Zalcitabine (ddC)			Saquinavir/RTV (soft gel) (SQV)
				Lopinavir/RTV (combination)
				Ritonavir (RTV)[‡]

NRTI = nucleoside reverse transcriptase inhibitor

NNRTI = non-nucleoside reverse transcriptase inhibitor

PI = protease inhibitor

*For initiation of therapy in an ARV-naïve patient use 2 NRTIs (one from category I and one from category II) together with one NNRTI (category IV).

[†] EFV is teratogenic.

[‡] RTV is most often used in combination with another PI at a low dose of 100 mg twice daily. Here it is used as a $_p$450 inhibitor to boost the levels of the combined PI. It is not a useful anti-retroviral agent at this low dose. In adults it is rarely used as an anti-retroviral in its own right (600mg twice daily) due to increased adverse events (e.g. diarrhoea).

- The immune-compromised person who develops TB presents the clinician with an additional dilemma, as ARVs do not combine well with the standard anti-TB drugs. Where possible, the TB should be treated first
- The initial euphoria about ARVs is now abating somewhat as the problem of viral resistance to many of the drugs becomes apparent. Already 10 per cent of new infections in Europe are resistant to at least one drug. Strict adherence (>97 per cent) to complex drug regimens is needed to suppress the replication of the virus. Poor compliance leads to resistant strains developing rapidly with resultant treatment failure and disease progression. Although minor side-effects such as rashes are common, usually soon after initiating treatment, these can be managed symptomatically. Serious side-effects, such as lactic acidosis, may occur on d4T, ddI or AZT and may be fatal if not detected early

1 Brechtl JR., Breitbart W., Galietta M. et al. (2001) The use of highly active anti-retroviral therapy (HAART) in patients with advanced HIV infection: impact on medical, palliative care, and quality of life outcomes. *Journal of Pain & Symptom Management.* **21**: 41–51.

Initial small, well-controlled trials of ARVs have been shown to be very effective in some African countries. Patients adhere to their drugs as well as patients in Europe and America. The distribution of ARVs on a large scale, however, is likely to overwhelm the already over-extended primary health services in countries such as South Africa unless there is a massive injection of funds into the health system. The cost of the drugs needed to cope with this pandemic is large, but even more will be needed to build up the infrastructure and improve the capacity of the hospitals and health centres to provide the treatment and monitor patients. The vast distances and poor public transport services in rural areas will limit access to ARVs for many patients.

A number of companies, especially the large mining companies in South Africa, have made ARVs available to their staff at no cost. They have realized that it is better to keep their skilled staff healthy rather than constantly to recruit and retrain new workers.

The 'brain drain' of skilled doctors and nurses from developing countries to places such as Canada, Australia, the UK and the Middle East is compounding the difficulties. The Melbourne Manifesto on the recruitment of health professionals, adopted at the World Rural Health Conference in May 2002, needs to be taken seriously.

See http://www.globalfamilydoctor.com/aboutwonca/working-groups/rural_training/melbourne_manifesto.htm

The rôle of palliative care

As mentioned, current ARVs do not cure AIDS, but merely delay its natural progress. For many years to come the vast majority of infected people in the world will not have access to such drugs, some who are able to obtain them will not respond well or will be unable to adhere to the strict regimens required to suppress the virus. In the forseeable future we will still be faced with millions of people, dying slowly of AIDS, who will need effective palliative care. Such care should have the same focus as palliative care in other situations, namely promoting quality of life, excellent symptom control, effective communication and appropriate support for both patient and family.

Pain

Pain is common and is often undertreated. Surveys have shown that up to 98 per cent of advanced AIDs sufferers will have significant pain.

- Headache is a frequent symptom and cryptococcal meningitis (CM) and tuberculous meningitis (TBM) need to be excluded as these are treatable if diagnosed early. CM may be associated with raised intracranial pressure and the resulting severe headache can be relieved by daily serial lumbar punctures (LPs), draining off 15–20 mL of cerebrospinal fluid (CSF) with great care. Focal signs may indicate a space-occupying lesion. If possible a scan should be done to confirm the diagnosis. In Africa toxoplasmosis is the commonest cause
- Severe sensory neuropathies are present in 30 per cent of patients. Most are due to direct damage to peripheral nerves by the virus, but some may occur from the toxic effects of anti-TB treatment or ARVs (ddC, d4T and ddl)

- Herpes zoster may occur early in the course of the illness and may be severe with persisting post-herpetic neuralgia
- Persisting mouth and genital ulcerations are common and very debilitating. Once again, treatable conditions such as candida and sexually transmitted infections (STIs) should be sought. Chronic ulceration due to persisting herpes simplex can be very frustrating, but some good results are reported from resource poor areas in Africa where aciclovir tablets are crushed and applied topically
- Painful swallowing (odynophagia) may be due to oesophageal candidiasis, acid reflux and TB, which are treatable, or due to infection by cytomegalovirus (CMV) or Kaposi's sarcoma (KS), which often respond poorly to treatment
- Abdominal pain occurs in 20 per cent of patients and may be due to many different causes. Patients with abdominal pain should be approached like all other patients. Surgical emergencies should be referred appropriately, rule out lactic acidosis or pancreatitis due to ARVs (ddl, ddC, and d4T), treat infections such as salmonella, shigella or tuberculosis and provide effective analgesia for all
- Muscle and joint pains are also common. The same approach applies. Identify treatable infections and conditions and provide effective analgesia for all. Pyrazinamide used to treat TB commonly causes severe arthralgia

Follow the principles of pain management: 'By mouth', 'By the ladder', 'By the clock' with careful follow-up and review. (📖 See Chapter 6a.)

The biggest challenge in poorly resourced areas is making morphine and other effective drugs available and accessible. Great progress has been made in Uganda with the introduction of appropriate legislation allowing the distribution of morphine at clinic level. In Zimbabwe, trained palliative care nurses are able to prescribe morphine. Other developing countries need to follow their example.

Diarrhoea

Recurrent and persisting diarrhoea may be present in more than 50 per cent of patients with advanced AIDS. In places with poor sanitation, good hygiene has been shown to reduce this percentage significantly. Half of the patients with chronic diarrhoea will have an identifiable infection. The presence of fever or blood in the stool should be investigated for a treatable cause. In resource-poor areas, a short empirical trial of metronidazole and co-trimoxazole may be tried. Loperamide or morphine should be titrated up to an effective dose to reduce the frequency of diarrhoea to manageable levels. Trying to cope with profuse diarrhoea without proper sanitation or easily accessible running water is a reality for most affected families in many areas in third world countries. This places an extra burden and risk on already overwhelmed families. Chronic diarrhoea needs to be taken just as seriously as pain.

Fever

Sweating and fever are frequent throughout the course of AIDS. It may be part of the immune response or it may indicate the onset of yet another opportunistic infection. Careful assessment for possible treatable causes such as pneumonia or TB needs to be made. Extra fluids and antipyretics can be given until any possible treatable cause is identified.

Neurological

See p. 622.

Skin problems

Almost all patients with AIDS will have some kind of skin problem.

- Dry skin and itching is frequent. Discourage excessive bathing, especially in warm water, and apply aqueous cream twice a day to the whole body. The judicious use of appropriate steroid creams and oral antihistamines (especially H_1 blockers) may bring relief of itching
- Itching may also be caused by 'Itchy bump disease' (pruritic papular eruption). This is very common in Africa and is a group of conditions causing inflamed, very itchy, papules that leave small darkly pigmented bumps on the limbs and trunk
- Seborrhoeic dermatitis and psoriasis are common and should be treated appropriately
- Scabies should be considered in any patient with itching. It may present in the usual form of red itchy papules with burrows in the web spaces of the fingers and around the ano-genital area. Occasionally scabies may present in a scaly, less itchy form (hyperkeratotic scabies) on the scalp, hands and trunk. Large thick crusts on the body with cracking may also be due to scabies
- Multiple purple-brown nodules of varying size scattered all over the body especially, on the face and in the mouth, are characteristic of Kaposi's sarcoma. It may occur at any stage of the illness and although it is often slowly progressive at first, it may spread to involve internal organs and be rapidly fatal. Pain and dyspnoea are then often present and may be controlled with morphine. Palliative radiotherapy, intralesional chemotherapy and topical cryotherapy can be tried especially if the patient is still reasonably well (CD_4 < 200/microlitre)

Emotional and mental symptoms

The diagnosis of being HIV positive presents the infected person not only with the prospect of a fatal illness but also the stigma associated with AIDS. Many strong emotions crowd the mind including:

- fear of rejection by others
- fear of infecting others
- anger and sense of betrayal
- sense of shame for having contracted the disease
- sorrow in anticipation of the loss of everything
- worry about how to cope and how one's children will survive

It is little wonder that anxiety and depression are common throughout the course of illness, especially shortly after the diagnosis and again as the symptoms of advanced AIDS become apparent. Family and community support, however, can help the infected person come to terms with the tuation. Without support, the HIV positive person may lose hope. uicide then becomes a strong possibility.

Support groups for people living with AIDS have proved very effective Africa in countering the despair and hardship that so often accompanies his illness. Many HIV positive people have become involved in caring for hose that are sick at home, looking after the infants left behind and comorting the grieving. Some have been brave enough to speak out in public nd have been very effective in breaking down stigma and prejudice. This as never been easy and at times it has been dangerous, kindling the wrath f an already outraged community.

Being a neurotropic virus, over 80 per cent of people with AIDS will how some cognitive impairment while 25 per cent will go on to develop IIV-associated dementia or psychosis. Most are apathetic and withdrawn vhile a few may become delirious and agitated, requiring sedation.

Nutrition

Vhile good nutrition is essential to maintain an adequate immune system, reat care needs to be taken to ensure that the rôle of particular diets, such s the use of garlic, lemon juice and olive oil, is not seen as an alternative to ffective medical care. The sick have always been vulnerable to exploitation y quacks and 'snake oil' salesmen. While vitamins and other micronutrients ave their place, 'a round pill' should not replace 'a square meal'.

In the underprivileged areas of developing countries, vegetable gardening nd small-scale subsistence farming needs to be encouraged both as a means f survival and for the sense of well-being that it encourages.

Social issues

he young adult is the main age group affected by the AIDS pandemic. oung adults may be the main 'bread-winners' and the parents of small hildren. Their deaths have a devastating effect on the community. In eveloping countries, the loss of income, the multiple bereavements, the rowing orphan population, the child-headed households or children having o leave school to care for dying parents and siblings are all causing great conomic and emotional suffering.

Impact on Africa

In a survey of affected households in South Africa in 2002, it was found that 45% had an income of less than $150 a month, 57% had no running water inside their homes and 25% had no toilet. The plight of children is desperate. It was found that 22% of children under 15 years had lost at least one parent and 50% of children often went to bed hungry. The sick family members required care for extended periods, often as long as 12 months. Twenty per cent were too weak to wash and 16% were incontinent. The average life expectancy in South Africa has dropped by 10 years. (SA Health Review 2002)[2]

Despite some countries having child support grants and disability pensions, multiple administrative obstacles may prevent access to these funds. he capacity of the health and social welfare services to cope in most ub-Saharan countries is being stretched to the limits.

http://www.hst.org.za/publications/527

Spiritual issues

Fear, discrimination, stigma, rejection and isolation have added to the burden of those affected and infected by HIV/AIDS. While community organizations and religious groups are playing a rôle in helping those in need, the perception that AIDS sufferers have 'only themselves to blame' is still prevalent and will take much wisdom and compassion to overcome.

Health professionals need to be aware of the way different communities perceive illness and misfortune. In Africa there is a common perception that some conditions are 'natural' while others are not. Unfamiliar illnesses or conditions that are not easily cured may be attributed to evil influence of 'sorcerers' or the jealousy of neighbours. In addition to seeking help from health professionals at a hospital or clinic for the symptoms of the disease, the affected person will consult a traditional healer to discover the person responsible for the misfortune. The 'victim' will also expect to be given some means of protection from this evil.

An example of this is the common interpretation for the persistent painful feet of the peripheral neuropathy that so often accompanies AIDS. This will be interpreted as being caused by an enemy who has sprinkled 'poison' just outside the front gate of the home of the affected person. Unless the poison can be neutralized there will be no lasting cure.

Great care is needed in dealing with spiritual issues, especially if there are cultural and language differences between the ill person and the healthcare worker. A helpful approach is for the health professional to admit his/her ignorance of the beliefs and customs of the community and to ask the ill person or the family for help in understanding their needs.

Medico-legal issues

AIDS is a minefield of medico-legal issues. The right to confidentiality, the concerns of the public and the fears of the health professionals have caused many heated debates and even several court cases. The way information is entered into medical records and on death certificates has needed to be revised and improved. Disclosure even to another health worker must be on a legitimate 'need to know' basis and only after proper informed consent.

Laws relating to employment, dismissal and benefits need to be reviewed. When others are at risk, especially within a family, the infected individual needs to be helped and encouraged to disclose their HIV status.

Communities also need to deal with the issues of HIV positive children attending community schools. Proper education and the introduction of universal precautions have helped to allay the fears of parents in most cases.

Care during the dying phase

The transition from fighting against a terminal illness to preparing for death is never easy, especially when the person is young. In addition, the opportunistic infections are often treatable. Thus both doctor and patient may remain focused on cure. Families find it equally difficult to let go. However, a time comes sooner or later when despite all efforts, recovery does not take place. The same approach is needed to care for patients dying from AIDS as for those dying with cancer. The medication regime should be simplified to only those drugs needed for good sympto control. This may include stopping ARVs and even anti-TB treatment. As long as the person is no longer sputum positive for TB, there is little risk to others. It may be prudent to continue antifungals and agents for herpes simplex.

Treatment and ongoing prophylaxis for CMV retinitis may also be important, especially if retinal lesions are near the optic nerve or fovea. Fifty per cent of patients develop progressive sight deterioration within 2–3 weeks of stopping treatment.

Home-based care in developing countries has become a practical alternative to overcrowded public hospitals. With the support of established hospices, community groups have taken on the task of supporting affected families.

Bereavement and AIDS

Loss and grief are difficult to deal with at the best of times. Friends, neighbours and family members usually rally round and help to bear the burden of coping without the lost loved one. In developing countries, the multiple deaths of the AIDS epidemic are leaving the survivors with little support. It is not uncommon for an elderly widow who has been struggling to survive on her small pension, to find herself having to care for six or seven grandchildren whose parents have died one by one in a short space of time. In this state of 'distracted grief' there is little time for anything other than survival. The stigma of AIDS creates further barriers within the wider community.

Frustrations, fears and compassion fatigue

Despite the warnings and predictions of the scale and complexity of the AIDS epidemic in the late 1980s, most health services in developing countries were ill prepared for the numbers of sick and dying patients that began to crowd hospitals and clinics in the 1990s. In South Africa, this dramatic rise began in 1997. Wards in public hospitals became overcrowded with emaciated men and women with chronic diarrhoea and persisting cough. More than 50 per cent of deaths in the adult wards could be directly attributed to AIDS while in the paediatric wards the figure was closer to 85 per cent.

Advances

The identification of the causative organism, accurate diagnostic testing, HAART and the initial development of vaccines against this virus are some of the advances that have taken place. Although there is a long way to go yet before we can even begin to consider that AIDS is under control, the future looks a lot brighter than it did ten years ago.

The challenge

> AIDS is no longer just a disease, it is a human rights issue.
>
> Nelson Mandela, November 2003.

The WHO is leading the challenge with its new '3 x 5' campaign. It hopes to have three million people on ARVs by 2005. It rightly acknowledges that to achieve that will require more than the money for the drugs: the entire infrastructure of health services in developing countries will need supporting.

Resources

The following are a small selection of internet sites with information on AIDS:

Africa Alive—a forum for sharing ideas and strategies.
Web site: http://www.africalive.org
AIDS Education Global Information System—a wide range of HIV/AIDS related topics.
Web site: http://www.aegis.com
Aidsmap—The British HIV Association
Web site: http://www.aidsmap.com/
JAMA HIV/AIDS Information Centre—recent developments and treatment guidelines.
Web site http://www.ama-assn.org/special/hiv/hivhome.htm
Medscape—a web site of educational activities
Web site: http://hiv.medscape.com/

Further reading

Books

O'Neill J., Selwyn P. and Schietinger H. (eds) (2003) *A Clinical Guide to Supportive and Palliative Care for HIV/AIDS*. Washington: US Dept of Health and Human Services. (The guide is available as a free download from www.hab.hrsa.gov.)

Wilson D., Naidoo S., Bekker L.-G., Cotton M. and Maartens G. (eds) (2003) *Handbook of HIV Medicine*. Oxford: Oxford University Press.

Articles

Cameron D. (2002) Saving the history of the defeated and the lost—ethical dilemmas in the midst of the AIDS epidemic. *SA Fam Pract*, **25, 4**: 15–18.

Fassin D. and Schneider H. (2003) The politics of AIDS in South Africa: beyond the controversies. *BMJ*, **326**: 495–7.

Orrell C. and Wilson D. (2003) The art of HAART: a practical approach to antiretroviral therapy. *CME*, **21, 6**: 306–12.

Palliative care in non-malignant respiratory disease

Introduction

- The course of chronic respiratory disease is often marked by slow, inexorable decline with prolonged periods of disabling dyspnoea, reducing exercise tolerance, recurrent hospital admissions and premature death
- This is associated with loss of dignity, social isolation and psychological problems for the individual and pressure on family and carers. There is much potential gain with the application of a holistic approach to care
- Recent studies have recognized the similarity in symptoms between patients dying with malignant and non-malignant disease, and it is accepted that, regardless of diagnosis, the needs of the dying patient should be met by palliative care services

A difficulty with this is determining when chronic disease becomes terminal, as most end-stage respiratory disease progresses with periods of stability interrupted by major life-threatening exacerbations.

The potential requirement for palliative care in end-stage pulmonary disease

Respiratory disease accounted for 153,168 of 632,062 (24.2 per cent) deaths in the United Kingdom in 1999:

Condition	Deaths (%)
All respiratory disease	deaths 153,16 cases (100)
Pneumonia and TB	67,591 cases (44.1)
Cancer	35,879 cases (23.4)
Progressive non-malignant causes	39,939 cases (25.1)
COPD + asthma	(21.0)
Pulmonary circulatory disease	(4.1)
Pneumoconiosis	(0.8)
Cystic fibrosis	(0.1)
Sarcoidosis	(0.07)
Others (congenital, foreign body, etc.)	9,759 cases (6.4)

Research into symptomatology, survival, appropriate care and utilization of services is needed if the needs of this population are to be met.

Terminal symptoms, quality of life, and survival of patients with end-stage pulmonary disease

Symptoms presenting in the final weeks and months of life include dyspnoea, cough, fever, haemoptysis, stridor and chest wall pain—a similar picture to symptoms experienced by lung cancer patients.

The inability to predict disease trajectory in patients with non-malignant terminal disease makes end-of-life decisions difficult. Studies indicate that quality of life is at least as poor as those suffering from malignant lung disease.

Symptom pathophysiology and assessment

Less than 5% of patients with non-malignant disease die in hospices compared to at least 20% of lung cancer patients. More palliative care services are available to cancer patients.

Dyspnoea

Dyspnoea can be defined as difficult, uncomfortable or laboured breathing or when an individual feels the need for more air. It is the most frequently experienced symptom in those with end-stage respiratory disease and is multifactorial in origin.

Not clearly understood, the mechanism of dyspnoea has been described as a mismatch between central motor activity and incoming afferent information from chemo- and mechanoreceptors. A person's emotional state, personality and cognitive function also influence its perception.

A good history and examination is invaluable. (📖 See Chapter 6e.)

Recurrent aspiration

This is often a feature in the development of respiratory failure. There may be a bulbar cause e.g. MND, CVA or there may be repeated micro-aspiration leading to bronchiectasis.

The right main bronchus is the most direct path to the lungs leading more commonly to right lower lobe infections. Diagnosis can be made clinically, on CXR or on barium swallow.

Treatment includes:
- Nursing in semi-recumbent position
- Speech and language therapy assessment
- Thickened foods
- Nasogastric tube
- Treatment of the associated pneumonia with antibiotics and physiotherapy

Management of end-stage respiratory disease

The end-stage is not easy to recognize but usually comprises:
- Persistent dyspnoea despite maximal therapy
- Poor mobility
- Increased frequency of hospital admission
- Decreased improvements with repeated admission
- Expressions of fear, anxiety
- Panic attacks
- Concerns expressed about dying

Drugs For dyspnoea

Anxiolytics

Anxiety can exacerbate breathlessness. Clinical experience suggests that low dose anxiolytics (diazepam) can result in improvements despite a lack of evidence.

Antidepressants

TCAs and serotonin selective re-uptake inhibitors have been shown to be beneficial

Oral opioids

- Site of action may be central (brain stem) or peripheral lung receptors or help by decreasing anxiety. Opioids can cause serious side-effects such as CO_2 retention, nausea, drowsiness and respiratory depression, so care is needed
- A trial of opioid in COPD patients without CO_2 retention is appropriate with close monitoring
- Low doses and small increments should be used e.g. 2.5mg morphine elixir 4-h
- Subcutaneous diamorphine can be used in patients not able to swallow
- In the terminal phase, opioid therapy is justified for treatment of dyspnoea even in the presence of CO_2 retention

Nebulised opioids

Currently no good evidence to support use. 'As effective as nebulised saline.'

Mucolytics

N-acetylcysteine can be used, as can steam inhalers and nebulised saline.

Palliative oxygen therapy

A significant proportion of patients will have resting hypoxia, although its degree does not correlate with the level of dyspnoea. Symptoms may be improved by oxygen. Even in the absence of hypoxia, oxygen may relieve dyspnoea in COPD patients.

Non-pharmacological measures

General

- Vaccinations—influenza and pneumococcal
- General nursing care—fan, open windows, regular repositioning, relief of constipation
- Good nutrition
- Physiotherapy—forced expiratory technique, controlled coughing, chest percussion

- Psychological support—help patient cope, provide strategies to relieve symptoms, maximize quality of life etc.
- Pulmonary rehabilitation—centres around exercise conditioning by general exercise and specific muscle training
- Controlled breathing techniques—pursed lip/slow expiration etc.
- Non-invasive mechanical ventilation—shown to decrease need for intubation
- Lung reduction surgery—initial benefit in FEV_1 lasts only 3–4 years
- Lung transplantation—emphysema is most common indication

COPD

Pharmacological treatments

Bronchodilators

- beta-2 agonists, e.g. Salbutamol
- anticholinergic agents (may aggravate prostatism or glaucoma) e.g. ipratropium bromide
- Inhaled bronchodilators +/− spacers should be used where possible as nebulizers deliver medication less efficiently

Inhaled/oral steroids

These benefit 15–20 per cent of stable COPD patients and as such a trial with steroids is indicated, where at least a 20 per cent increase in FEV_1 should indicate continued use.

Theophylline

The pharmacokinetics are unstable and there is a narrow therapeutic range, but if used judiciously they have a place in COPD management.

Oxygen

- Has a definite place in the management of selected hypoxic patients
- Usually employed overnight, followed by intermittent daytime use through to continuous use
- Care needs to be taken where headaches, drowsiness or confusion appear indicating potential carbon dioxide retention

Long-term oxygen therapy (LTOT)

This can extend life expectancy if administered for 12–15 h per day, although there is a lack of evidence to support increased quality of life.

> **Indications for LTOT:**
> - $PaO_2 < 7.3$ kPa when breathing air
> - $PaCO_2$ may be normal or > 6.0 kPa
> - Two measurements separated by 4 weeks when clinically stable
> - Clinical stability = no exacerbations or peripheral oedema for four weeks
> - $FEV_1 < 1.5l$ and $FVC < 2.0l$
> - Non-smokers
> - PaO_2 between 7.3 and 8.0 kPa together with secondary poly-cythaemia, peripheral oedema or pulmonary hypertension
> - Nocturnal hypoxia (SaO_2 below 90 per cent for > 30 per cent of the night)
> - Interstitial lung disease or pulmonary hypertension where $PaO_2 < 8$ kPa
> - Palliation of terminal disease

Interstitial/fibrotic lung disease

These include:
- Idiopathic fibrotic disorders, e.g. idiopathic pulmonary fibrosis, autoimmune pulmonary fibrosis
- Connective tissue disorders, e.g. SLE, rheumatoid arthritis, scleroderma etc.
- Drug-induced diseases, e.g. nitrofurantoin, amiodarone, gold, radiation etc.
- Occupational, e.g. silicosis, asbestosis, farmer's lung etc.
- Primary unclassified, e.g. sacoidosis, amyloidosis, AIDs, adult respiratory distress syndrome (ARDS) etc.

These conditions are, however, rare.

Treatment includes immunosuppressants such as steroids, cyclophosphamide, azathioprine, and penicillamine with variable success.

Neuromuscular, restrictive and chest wall disease

These cause respiratory muscle weakness or loss of compliance in the respiratory cage. Muscular function can be affected at various sites from the spinal cord to the muscles themselves.

Features that characterize some of these conditions include:
- Increased ventilatory drive with inadequate ventilatory response
- Sleep disorders
- Unbalanced weakness of spinal and thoracic muscles leading to kyphoscoliosis
- Bulbar incoordination
- Diaphragmatic paralysis
- Pulmonary embolism

Supportive treatments:
- Oxygen
- Antibiotics
- Physiotherapy
- Techniques to clear secretions
- Inspiratory muscle training
- Beta-2 agonists

Ventilatory support can include:
- Rocking beds
- Abdominal pneumatic belts
- Negative pressure body ventilators
- Non-invasive positive pressure ventilation
- Nasal continuous positive airways pressure
- There have been many advances in this field, but many patients still choose to refuse such invasive treatments

Bronchiectasis

Survival of patients has improved markedly with the advent of antibiotic therapy. Conditions associated with bronchiectasis include:
- Cystic fibrosis
- HIV infection
- Rheumatoid arthritis
- Infection, inflammation
- Bronchopulmonary sequestration

- Allergic bronchopulmonary aspergillosis
- Alpha1-antitrypsin deficiency
- Congenital cartilage deficiency
- Immunodeficiency
- Yellow nail syndrome
- Bronchial obstruction
- Unilateral hyperlucent lung

Diagnosis is usually made by high resolution CT scanning.
Treatment involves:
- Antimicrobial drugs—directed by sputum microbiology, usually treated for longer periods
- Bronchodilator therapy
- Chest physiotherapy
- Nebulised recombinant human deoxyribonuclease
- Anti-inflammatory treatment
- Supplemental oxygen
- Immunoglobulin administration/enzyme replacement
- Surgery
- Management of haemoptysis
- Management of halitosise—e.g. broad-spectrum antibiotics, mouth and gum care

Cystic fibrosis
- Affects 1 in 2,500 newborns
- Marked by alteration in ion and water transport across epithelial cells resulting in recurrent pulmonary infection, bronchiectasis, lung fibrosis and pancreatic insufficiency
- Most care takes place in specialized units with home support teams trained in the principles of palliative care

HIV-associated
Pulmonary complications:
- bacterial e.g. Strep. pneumoniae, Pseudomonas aeruginosa
- mycobacterium e.g. M. tuberculosis, M. avian complex
- fungi e.g. Pneumocystis carinii, Cryptococcus neoformans
- viruses e.g. Cytomegalovirus
- parasites e.g. Toxoplasma gondii
- Malignancies e.g. Kaposi's sarcoma, non-Hodgkin's lymphoma
- Interstitial pneumonitis e.g. lymphocytic pneumonitis
- Other e.g. COPD, pulmonary hypertension

Tuberculosis
Recurrent reactivation results in severe pulmonary scarring, cavitation and secondary aspergillosis infection and, if left unchecked, respiratory failure, recurrent bacterial infection and massive haemoptysis.

Chronic bronchitis and emphysema

These conditions cause 80 per cent of pulmonary hypertension. Treatment usually involves:

- Oxygen
- Non-invasive ventilation
- Beta-2 agonists
- Diuretics in the management of fluid retention in acute phase of cor pulmonale
- The use of pulmonary vasodilators is of doubtful significance

Obstructive pulmonary hypertension

- This is often caused by repetitive, silent pulmonary embolism. Other causes include vasculitis, sickle cell anaemia and infective endocarditis
- Treatment can involve anticoagulation, and occasionally pulmonary thromboendarterectomy or the insertion of inferior vena caval filter

Primary pulmonary hypertension

- Of unknown aetiology
- Symptoms can include progressive dyspnoea, decreased exercise tolerance, central chest pain and syncope
- Occasionally it is associated with haemoptysis, fluid accumulation and sudden death
- Treatment involves oxygen, anticoagulation and vasodilators such as hydralazine and nifedipine

Pulmonary embolism (📖 see Chapter 6l)

There is an increased incidence of thromboembolism in dependent, hospitalized patients.

- The triad of venous stasis, alteration in coagulation and vascular injury are fundamental in the pathogenesis
- A clinical suspicion is possible with dyspnoea, pleuritic pain and haemoptysis being classical symptoms
- Forty per cent of high-risk patients with proximal DVT's are asymptomatic when pulmonary embolism occurs

Investigation includes:

- Arterial blood gas (Not commonly available in in-patient palliative care units.)
- ECG
- CXR
- Doppler ultrasonography/contrast venography
- V/Q scan
- Angiography
- Enhanced spiral CT scan

Prevention involves adequate hydration, promotion of mobility, the avoidance of venous obstruction, compression stockings and low molecular weight heparin (LMWH).

Treatment usually involves heparinization with LMWH and consideration of warfarinization, or vena-caval filters.

For patients with metastatic malignancy there is increasing evidence that warfarin is not as effective as LMWH. (See Chapter 6l.)

Pneumothorax and pleural disease

Pathogenesis includes spontaneous and iatrogenic causes. Treatment usually involves intercostal tube drainage if appropriate, or oxygen, analgesia and opiates in the terminally ill.

- Causes of pleural effusion are multiple but include infection, cardiac failure, hypoalbuminaemia and renal impairment
- Treatment may consist of intermittent aspiration +/− chemical pleurodesis
- Localized pleural pain may be secondary to rib fracture, infection or pneumothorax and may respond to normal analgesia, or may require a local anaesthetic intercostal nerve block

Respiratory terminal care and palliative sedation

In terminal phase, simple measures are important:
- constant draught from fan or open window
- regular sips of water
- sitting upright

In the terminal stages, the emphasis changes from active interventions to supportive and symptomatic measures.
- Non-invasive ventilatory support and active physiotherapy may be withdrawn
- Drugs for palliating symptoms are often unavoidable
- The oral route should be used where possible, but failing this, drugs may be given by the subcutaneous route

The 'rattle' associated with loose respiratory secretions, although probably not distressing to the patient, may be addressed by re-positioning, or by the use of hyoscine hydrobromide or glycopyrronium bromide.

- As many patients approaching death with end-stage respiratory disease will have uncontrolled dyspnoea, sedation and opioid use should not be withheld because of an inappropriate fear of respiratory depression
- Options include benzodiazepines or opioids. The risks and benefits must be carefully considered and the justification for sedation clearly defined. Such decisions are often made by teams rather than individuals and it is appropriate that patients and families are fully involved in the decision making process

Further reading

Books

Ahmedzai S. (1998) Palliation of Respiratory Symptoms. In D. Doyle, G. Hanks, N. MacDonald: *Oxford Textbook of Palliative Medicine*. 2nd edn. Oxford: Oxford University Press.

Back, I. (2001) *Palliative Medicine Handbook*. 3rd edn. Cardiff: BPM Books.

Davis C. L. (1998) Breathlessness, Cough and Other Respiratory Problems. In M. Fallon, B. O'Neill (eds.) *ABC of palliative care*. London: BMJ Books.

Doyle D., Hanks G., Cherny N. and Calman K. (2004) *Oxford Textbook of Palliative Medicine.* 3rd edn. Oxford: Oxford University Press.

Fallon M. (ed.) *ABC of Palliative Care.* London: BMJ Books.

Watson M. and Lucas, C. (2003) *Adult Palliative Care Guidelines.* London: The South West London and the Surrey, West Sussex and Hampshire Cancer Networks.

Wilcock A. (1997) *Dyspnoea.* In P. Kaye (ed.) *Tutorials in palliative medicine*, pp. 227–49. Northampton: EPL Publications.

Palliative care in heart failure

Definition

Chronic heart failure is a progressive, fatal disease and is the final common pathway of many cardiovascular diseases. Heart failure is defined by the European Society of Cardiology as the presence of symptoms of heart failure at rest or during exercise, and objective evidence of cardiac dysfunction (usually on echocardiography).

Incidence

Heart failure is the only major cardiovascular disease with increasing incidence. It is predominantly a disease of old age (mean 75 years). There are 63,000 new cases per annum in the UK.[1] A diagnosis of heart failure has huge cost implications: patients with heart failure occupy up to 2 per cent of all inpatient bed days and account for up to 2 per cent of NHS costs (most of which are hospital not community).

Prognosis

An estimated 5 per cent of all deaths in the UK (24,000 per annum) are from heart failure. (Death certification explicitly discourages doctors from recording heart failure as a cause of death—the true number is probably much higher). Forty per cent of patients die within one year of diagnosis. Fifty per cent of patients with heart failure die suddenly and 25 per cent without worsening of their heart failure symptoms. This can occur at any stage of the disease. There are no reliable prognostic models either for poor overall prognosis or sudden death.

Relevant pathology and physiology

Coronary artery disease and hypertension are the commonest causes of heart failure. The direct insult is of mechanical pump failure, but this initiates an ongoing, complex cascade of haemodynamic, metabolic, neuroendocrine and renal dysfunction that is the syndrome of chronic heart failure.

Clinical features

Breathlessness and fatigue are the classic symptoms of heart failure. Orthopnoea is a sensitive 'measure' of fluid overload.

Fluid retention causes not only breathlessness, cough and dependent oedema, but also anorexia, nausea, abdominal bloating and pain.

Other common symptoms which are poorly recognized and therefore frequently not treated include:

- Pain (common, severe, prolonged and distressing). Probably due to a combination of angina, liver capsule distension, lower limb swelling and co-morbid disease, e.g. arthritis

Petersen S., Rayner M., Wolstenholme J. (2002) Coronary heart disease statistics: heart failure supplement 2002 edition.

- Anxiety and depression (severe in a third of hospitalized patients). Depression adversely affects mortality and hospital readmission[2]
- Disordered sleep
- Memory loss and confusion
- Anorexia, nausea, vomiting and constipation
- Weight loss (usually mild, but severe cachexia is a poor prognostic sign)
- Loss of libido

Poor information, communication and understanding for patients are widespread and contribute to psychological morbidity.

Significant functional impairment in activities of daily living and social isolation are common, long before the end-of-life. Despite this there is poor access to social and therapy services. The pattern of functional decline is slow, compared to the classic patient with cancer who exhibits precipitous decline approximately five months before death.[3]

Disease burden

The burden of chronic heart failure has physical, psychological and social dimensions. These needs have been demonstrated to be prevalent, severe, prolonged and usually unrecognized and unrelieved.

The disparity in symptom control and support offered to those dying from heart failure compared to cancer is described tellingly by those who have lost a parent to each disease.

Table 8c.1 New York Heart Association (NYHA) functional classification (summary)

Class	Symptoms
I	Heart disease present, but no undue dyspnoea.
II	Comfortable at rest; dyspnoea on ordinary activities.
III	Less than ordinary activity causes dyspnoea, which is limiting.
IV	Dyspnoea present at rest; all activity causes discomfort.

Management

Disease-specific management

Education of patients and carers including diet (salt intake, alcohol, weight), smoking and exercise advice.

The cornerstones of drug treatment are angiotensin-converting enzyme (ACE) inhibitors and beta blockers. They both improve symptoms and slow disease progression. Diuretics are used to control fluid overload. Angiotensin-II antagonists, spironolactone and digoxin are used where appropriate.

Symptom management

1 Ensure specific heart failure treatments are optimal. This is the first step in achieving good symptom control. Diuretics may need quite frequent dose changes to control fluid overload. Avoid over-diuresis which may cause dizziness, nausea, poor sleep and fatigue.

Avoid where possible drugs which may worsen cardiac function. These include some drugs commonly prescribed in cancer palliative care practice. (See Table 8c.2).

Actively seek out and manage other likely symptoms. Bear in mind the likely causes of symptoms in a patient with heart failure and the renal function.

- Pain: follow the WHO ladder. Avoid NSAIDs and alter opioid dosing schedules as per renal function
- Nausea: try haloperidol for a biochemical cause and metoclopramide for gastric stasis
- Anxiety and depression: treat conventionally (with or without drugs). Newer classes of antidepressant such as sertraline (a selective serotonin re-uptake inhibitor) and mirtazepine are safer than tricyclics. They are less likely to affect cardiac conduction, cause postural hypotension or interact with other drugs
- Breathlessness management: this may include correction of anaemia, low dose opioids and the non-pharmacological approaches used in respiratory rehabilitation and lung cancer management
- Adopt a palliative approach to psychological, social, spiritual, information and communication needs, actively pursuing and managing identified needs. Patients and carers may need help to manage the uncertainty of a future with a high chance of sudden death

End-of-life care

Diagnosing dying in heart failure is extremely difficult. The disease trajectory is of a steady decline punctuated by unexpected sudden death.

Features suggested as characterizing a subgroup of patients with a poor prognosis are:[4]

- Previous admissions with worsening heart failure
- No identifiable reversible precipitant
- Optimum tolerated conventional drugs
- Deteriorating renal function
- Failure to respond soon after admission to changes in vasodilators or diuretics

In these patients, invasive treatments and monitoring should be reviewed and emphasis on palliation should predominate. Discontinuation of cardiac drugs may be appropriate. When a patient is clearly dying, use of a guideline such as the Liverpool care pathway for the dying patient[5] is recommended.

Models of care

Although chronic heart failure is increasingly being managed across the community/hospital interface by multiprofessional heart failure teams, most

2 Jiang W., Alexander J., Christopher E., Kuchibhatla M., Gaulden L. H., Cuffe M. S. et al. (2001) Relationship of depression to increased risk of mortality and rehospitalization in patients with congestive heart failure. *Arch Intern Med*, **161, 15**: 1849–56.

3 Teno J. M., Weitzen S., Fennell M. L., Mor V. (2001) Dying trajectory in the last year of life: does cancer trajectory fit other diseases? *J Palliat Med*, **4, 4**: 457–464.

4 Ellershaw J. and Ward C. (2003) Care of the dying patients: the last hours or days of life. *BMJ*, **326**: 30–4.

5 http://www.lcp-mariecurie.org.uk

patients currently never see a heart failure specialist. These teams should aim to address the disease management and supportive and palliative care needs of the majority of patients with heart failure. The minority of patients with extraordinary palliative needs may need direct involvement from specialist palliative care services, often in concert with active heart failure team management. Mutual support and education, plus joint management by heart failure and specialist palliative care teams should be objectives for the future.

Table 8c.2 Key drugs to avoid in heart failure patients

Drugs	Reason for avoidance
Non-steroidal anti-inflammatory (NSAID)	Salt and water retention and worsen renal function
Tricyclic antidepressants	Cardiotoxic
Lithium	Salt and water retention
Cyclizine	Probably cardiotoxic
Steroids	Water retention
Progestogens	Water retention
Flecainide/mexiletine	Depress myocardial function

Diuretics

Furosemide is less effective when given orally rather than parenterally in heart failure, cirrhosis and probably any hypoalbuminaemic state. It is more affected by food intake than bumetanide which may be better absorbed orally than furosemide. Continuous infusion of furosemide may be given i/v and has been given by CSCI. Spironolactone is used for ascites particularly if associated with liver metastases, steroid-induced fluid retention and possibly heart failure. Metolazone is a weak thiazide diuretic which can be used alone but is also synergistic with furosemide.

Further reading

Articles

Gibbs J. S. R., McCoy A. S., Gibbs L. M., Rogers A. E., Addington-Hall J. M. (2002) Living with and dying from heart failure: the rôle of palliative care. *Heart*, **88** (Suppl. 2): ii36–ii39.

Remme W., Swedberg K. (2001) Task Force for the Diagnosis and Treatment of Chronic Heart Failure. *European Heart Journal*, **22**, **17**: 1527–60.

Ward C. (2002) The need for palliative care in the management of heart failure. *Heart*, **87**, **3**: 294–8.

Palliative care in non-malignant neurological disease

Multiple sclerosis (MS)

There are an estimated 80,000 to 90,000 people with multiple sclerosis in the UK. In the majority (70–80 per cent), the course of the disease is relapsing and remitting in nature at the onset. Half of these patients will enter a progressive phase within 10 years (secondary progressive MS). In a smaller group of patients the disease is progressive from the onset (~15 per cent). In a population of patients with MS approximately 20–30 per cent have marked paraparesis, hemiparesis or paraplegia, 15 per cent are wheelchair-bound and 5 per cent have severe cognitive impairment. It is estimated that only about 25 per cent of patients who are severely disabled are alive at 10 years.

Death is commonly due to secondary complications of MS (e.g. aspiration pneumonia, pulmonary embolus). If sudden neurological deterioration occurs, precipitating factors such as infection should be looked for. If there is no resolution of symptoms, a course of steroids is usually given which has a high chance of improving symptoms for a further year or so.

Symptom management

Immobility
Walking is usually affected if the disease is progressive, through a combination of weakness, spasticity, fatigue, disuse, pain, cerebellar ataxia and sensory loss particularly proprioception. Immobility inevitably becomes difficult towards the end-of-life, leading to many problems, which need to be addressed by the majority of members of the multidisciplinary team.

Pain
Chronic pain may be present in 60 per cent and some studies have shown inadequate control in 40 per cent of patients, with significant adverse effects on quality of life. Neuropathic pain, which may present as a persistent burning discomfort often affecting the lower limbs, is usually treated with standard agents for neuropathic pain such as the tricyclic antidepressants.

Trigeminal neuralgia is a common paroxysmal pain and is classically treated with carbamazepine. Gabapentin has also been used. Neurosurgical procedures such as percutaneous denervation may be considered, although this may leave the patient with paraesthesiae.

Lhermitte's sign is a syndrome of intermittent burning sensations or 'electric shocks' occurring on neck flexion. It is probably due to demyelination in the posterior columns of the spinal cord and can occur in up to two-thirds of patients at some time during the course of the disease. It is often self-limiting but, if persistent, a cervical collar and carbamazepine may be needed.

Musculoskeletal pain is common, particularly back pain, and results from prolonged immobility, poor posture and gait abnormalities. It is probably caused by a combination of spasticity leading to muscular pain and abnormal stresses resulting in mechanical pain. Osteoporosis should also be considered and treated as appropriate. Simple analgesics or NSAIDs can be prescribed. Physiotherapy is needed to improve poor posture and to ensure that correct seating and wheelchair adaptations are provided. Passive and active exercises, TENS, massage and acupuncture may also be helpful.

Spasticity

Increased muscle tone occurs in the majority of patients with MS. It may cause difficulty with function of the affected limb, painful muscle spasms and, when severe, difficulty in nursing care. Neurophysiotherapists teach patients and their carers stretching techniques for shortened spastic muscles and passive joint exercises to maintain movement which should be carried out regularly. Splints may be used and TENS may alleviate the frequency of painful muscle spasms and improve sleep. Aggravating factors such as urinary tract infections, pressure sores and constipation should be avoided and/or treated.

Baclofen can be built up slowly by 5mg every few days starting from 5mg t.d.s. up to a maximum of 80mg daily. Transient neuropsychiatric and gastrointestinal symptoms may occur. Reduction of baclofen should be gradual to avoid fits or hallucinations. Intrathecal baclofen can be used for severe spasticity and muscle spasms if they are affecting quality of life and have proved unresponsive to other therapies.

Benzodiazepines such as diazepam can be given at night if painful spasms disturb sleep.

Dantrolene is less sedating than other muscle relaxants but can further weaken muscles and is therefore often reserved for those patients who are wheelchair-bound. Liver function should be monitored.

Tizanidine, an alternative to baclofen, is associated with less muscle weakness than baclofen or diazepam. The starting dose is 2mg increased every 3–4 days in 2mg increments up to 24mg daily in divided doses. It can cause sedation and dry mouth and liver function should be monitored for the first four months. Gabapentin is an alternative.

Intramuscular botulinum toxin can be effective for focal spasticity that interferes with hygiene or nursing care. It is generally only used when maintenance of function is less important. It should always be accompanied by a physiotherapy regime of passive stretching.

Tenotomies (surgical release of tendons) or other nerve blocks most commonly obturator, perineal, adductor, or pudendal may be needed.

Ataxia and tremor

Feeding, correct seating and head control can be very difficult. The rôle of the occupational therapist is crucial. There is some evidence, although minimal, for the benefits of propranolol and clonazepam. Severe tremor can be treated with stereotactic thalamotomy but with initial benefit only. Other techniques of deep brain stimulation may be promising.

Urinary system

Assessment and treatment is important in order to improve symptoms and to minimize complications such as pressure atrophy of the kidneys, urinary tract infections and skin breakdown secondary to incontinence. Incontinence can lead to profound embarrassment and social breakdown. Adequate fluid intake, bladder emptying (particularly if residual volume is more than 100ml) and treatment of infection are the principle priorities.

Hyperreflexia of the bladder is associated with a low volume capacity bladder and possible symptoms of mild urgency, frequency and incontinence. Treatment is usually with anticholinergic drugs such as oxybutinin or tolterodine. Incomplete bladder emptying, induced by these drugs, may require intermittent self-catheterization. Nocturnal incontinence may be relieved with desmopressin nasal spray 10–40 mcg at night. If the overactive bladder is resistant to conventional management, transvesical phenol capsaicin may provide some benefit.

Bladder hypotonia and sphincter dyssynergia (sphincter contracts when voiding) results in incomplete emptying, of which the patient may be unaware. Catheterization will be needed. Intermittent catheterization is associated with less risk of UTI than a permanent indwelling catheter. However, the latter may be needed if all other methods fail to fully empty the bladder frequently enough to avoid problems. Even with a permanent catheter, an anticholinergic may still be needed for bladder spasm and urinary bypassing. If all else fails a urinary diversion may be the only viable option.

Constipation

Constipation is common due in large degree to delayed gut transit time, immobility and anticholinergic medication. Adequate dietary fibre and fluid intake are important and regular oral laxatives or suppositories/enemas are frequently needed.

Fatigue

Fatigue is severe and disabling in the majority of patients, reflecting muscle weakness and sleep interruption (e.g. from nocturia or spasms). It presents as overwhelming tiredness which is not relieved by exercise or rest. It does not necessarily directly correlate with mood disturbance or the severity of the MS.

Precipitants such as exposure to hot baths and hot weather should be avoided. Amantadine and modafinil offer modest benefit. Explanation, reassurance, and advice on modification in lifestyle such as pacing activities, taking rest periods and gentle exercise are essential.

Mood/cognitive disturbance

Clinical depression is common in MS. The estimated lifetime risk of developing depression is 50 per cent and the risk of suicide is 7.5 times that of the healthy population. Depression is contributed to by many factors including the breakdown in family relationships, public embarrassment, social isolation and other losses of work, money, sexual abilities and confidence. Antidepressants should be selected according to their side-effect profile; for example, a tricyclic antidepressant might be used if an overactive bladder and additional neuropathic pain are a problem. Conversely, an SSRI which is less sedating than a tricyclic would be preferable if the patient feels fatigued.

There is some degree of cognitive impairment in 50–60 per cent of patients. The most common deficits relate to short-term memory, attention and speed of processing information and impaired learning. Personality and behaviour may change. Moderate to severe dementia is seen in 10 per cent of patients with long-standing MS. Pathological laughing and crying is a problem in 10 per cent, for which amitriptyline may be tried.

Multiple sclerosis is usually only managed in late advanced-stage disease by specialist palliative care teams, although they may have an earlier rôle in providing respite. The principles of palliative care apply through the illness trajectory and should aim to provide the best and most acceptable quality of life for the individual. Good symptom control and support for families are paramount.

Further reading

Articles

Cornish C. J. et al. (2000) Symptom management in advanced multiple sclerosis. *CME Bulletin Palliative Medicine*, **2, 1**: 11–16.

Gibson J., Frank A.O. (2003) Supporting individuals with disabling multiple sclerosis. *Journal of the Royal Society of Medicine*, **96, 5**: 256–7.

Parkinson's disease

Parkinson's Disease (PD) is the commonest neurodegenerative disease, after Alzheimer's disease, with an estimated incidence of 2/1000. It affects just under 1 per cent of people over the age of 65 years. PD is probably not one disease but several with common clinical features.

Criteria for the diagnosis of Parkinson's Disease

Bradykinesia (slowness and progressive decrease of amplitude of movement) plus at least one of the following:

- Tremor (frequently 'pill rolling')
- Rigidity (often cogwheeling in nature) or
- Disorders of posture (flexion of neck and trunk)
- Disorders of balance (loss of righting reflexes)
- Disorders of gait (short steps, shuffling, festination and freezing)

Classical pathological lesions seen in PD include loss of dopaminergic neurones in the substantia nigra and locus coerulus with formation of Lewy bodies in the cytoplasm. Degeneration of the nigrostriatal pathway leads to depletion of the neurotransmitter dopamine.

The aetiology is unknown, although neurotoxins such as 1-methyl-4-phenyl-1,2,3,6-tetrahydropyridine (MPTP), pesticides and herbicides have been linked to causation. There is a two- to threefold risk of developing PD in first-degree relatives.

Management

Research is underway into transplantation of human and animal foetal cells or allogenic stem cells, and therapy with nerve growth factors.

Surgical options such as subthalamic nucleus (STN) lesions may be effective for disabling dyskinesias (abnormal, involuntary movements), relieving rigidity and tremor. Alternatively, deep brain stimulation using implantable electrodes and a pacemaker-like generator may be used, allowing flexibility to modify the response and reduce side-effects.

The mainstay of management is the control of symptoms with medication with the aim of achieving optimal quality of life. Patients with PD should be monitored by doctors and teams specializing in PD, who should be alerted if there are any changes to the basic clinical pattern; reversible factors adversely affecting the PD should be pursued and subtle changes in medication advised, where appropriate.

Motor symptoms

Levodopa preparations

Dopamine does not cross the blood–brain barrier (BBB). To circumvent this problem, levodopa, which is able to cross the BBB, is used. Levodopa is converted to dopamine by the enzyme aromatic-L-amino-acid decarboxylase. The striatum is thus provided with the essential dopamine. However, the presence of too much dopamine outside the blood–brain barrier causes side-effects such as nausea. To circumvent this problem, inhibitors of the converting enzyme, which do not cross the BBB, are given to reduce peripheral dopamine. Carbidopa and benserazide are used in this way and combined with levodopa as the preparations sinemet and madopar respectively.

These compounds are available as modified release and immediate release preparations. They are also available in the dispersible form to aid administration with an oral syringe or through a nasogastric or gastrostomy tube where necessary. The timing of medication and dose are individualized, some patients benefitting from a 'kick start' dose in the mornings and others by avoiding late night medication which may interfere with sleep. Others benefit from long-acting medication at night to reduce painful stiffness. Any changes in dose should be undertaken slowly, allowing several weeks for the change in regimen to stabilize. The drugs should never be withdrawn unless severe side-effects develop, since patients may become unable to move, swallow and adequately protect the airway.

Unfortunately, the efficacy of levodopa is marred by unwanted actions that become progressively more prominent with advancing disease. These patients may develop severe drug-induced dyskinesia, often alternating with sudden unpredictable loss of mobility (freezing and hesitancy).

Dopamine agonists

These act directly on dopamine receptors and include bromocriptine, pergolide, ropinerole, pramipexole and cabergoline. Lisuride is rarely used in the UK. They are more likely than levodopa to cause dopaminergic side-effects such as nausea, vomiting, drowsiness, hallucinations and confusion and should be titrated up slowly; domperidone cover may be needed to treat the nausea.

Apomorphine is usually administered subcutaneously either as boluses or as a continuous infusion using a portable minipump. Its rapid onset of action can 'rescue' patients from sudden 'off' periods. It is most commonly reserved for patients experiencing severe and frequent motor fluctuations despite adequate trials with other oral medications. Domperidone is needed for three days prior to starting treatment to prevent nausea. Painful nodules which ulcerate may develop and sites of injection should be changed daily. Apomorphine treatment should be guided by a specialist in PD.

Drugs that delay the breakdown of levodopa

Entacapone achieves this by inhibiting the enzyme catechol-0-methyl transferase (COMT). It usually relieves motor fluctuations and allows dose reduction of levodopa-containing drugs.

Anticholinergics

These are sometimes effective for tremor but not bradykinesia and rigidity. Dry mouth, urinary retention, drowsiness and confusion often limit their usefulness.

Glutamate inhibitors (e.g. amantadine)

Amantadine may help rigidity and bradykinesia. It can be useful as adjunctive therapy and may be beneficial in reducing levodopa-induced dyskinesias. Common side-effects include peripheral oedema, livedo reticularis and hallucinations.

Monoamine oxidase type B selective inhibitor (e.g. selegeline)

This boosts the dopamine available in the brain by reducing the metabolism, and may be useful symptomatically. It is controversial as to whether or not selegeline has a neuroprotective rôle. Selegeline is now available as both an oral and a buccal melt preparation.

Other general measures for management of motor symptoms include input from members of the multidisciplinary team, particularly the physiotherapist, occupational therapist, speech therapist and dietician.

Nausea and vomiting

This may be due to drug treatment for PD or for another unrelated reason. Neuroleptics should not be used, in particular haloperidol, metoclopramide and prochlorperazine. (Most phenothiazines should be avoided since they may aggravate PD, except for clozapine and quetiapine which do not have extrapyramidal side-effects.) The safest drug to use is domperidone which can be given orally or rectally. A 5-HT$_3$ inhibitor such as ondansetron may also be tolerated.

Depression

This may occur in 40 per cent of patients with PD. It is not known whether it is an inherent feature of PD or secondary to a reaction to the disability caused by PD. Drugs such as the tricyclic antidepressants may aggravate postural hypotension and cause dry mouth. The selective serotonin reuptake inhibitors (SSRIs) may be helpful although they may worsen symptoms of PD and can cause postural hypotension. Mirtazepine has proved helpful in relieving depression and anxiety and reducing tremor.

Constipation

This may be caused by a lack of adequate neurotransmitter in the myenteric plexus. Advice on diet, adequate fluids and exercise should be given. Aperients are usually needed.

Swallowing difficulties

The ability to take food, chew and swallow may vary during the day, especially in more advanced disease. The speech and language therapist may be able to analyse the cause of the difficulty and to provide useful advice. Also the dietician may be required to advise on diet. The occupational therapist can help by providing appropriate feeding implements. Special seating and head and neck supports may be required.

Patients often lose a significant amount of weight in late stage PD, since the severe dyskinesias use up a significant amount of calorific energy. Feeding difficulties are often associated with periods of motor disability. Patients may choose to use their good functional moments to attend to activities of daily living or to pursue what they want to do, rather than wasting these precious moments on eating. They should be advised to eat little and often to make efficient use of time and energy intake. A deterioration of PD can be triggered by minimal dehydration and patients should be encouraged to drink adequately, especially during hot weather. High calorific drinks and other nutritional additives are useful to supplement an often inadequate diet.

Urinary urgency and nocturia

Urinary urgency may be helped with drugs such as tolterodine, oxybutynin and trospium. Severe distressing nocturia may be helped by a nocturnal dose of desmopressin, but care should be given to ensure that hyponatraemia and congestive cardiac failure are not induced by this treatment.

Postural hypotension

Patients should be given general advice on rising carefully from a lying or sitting position. It may be helpful to raise the head of the bed and some patients may tolerate compression stockings. If symptoms are severe, fludrocortisone may be needed. If dizziness is experienced, encourage the patient to take a full glass of water with medication, especially with the first dose of the day.

Sleep

Sleep disorders occur in 70–80 per cent of patients with PD and are distressing for patients and carers alike. The patient may be awoken by motor fluctuations; they may wake up and be unable to move and any effort to turn may cause painful muscle spasms; painful neck extension and leg cramp may occur. Attempts should be made to maintain nocturnal levels of levodopa, including avoiding high protein meals in the late evening (amino acids compete with dopamine for receptor sites) and by giving domperidone in the evenings (if needed) to avoid a delay in gastric emptying. Restless leg syndrome (RLS), characterized by an urge to move the legs, with painful cramps, paraesthesiae and a burning sensation in the calves may be relieved by standard levodopa therapy and dopamine agonists.

Amantidine and selegeline are stimulant and should be avoided if possible in the evenings. If PD is associated with dementia a reversal of the sleep-wake cycle may occur. Short-acting hypnotics can be used if necessary. Hallucinations and panic attacks may also keep patients awake at night and may be due to dopamine agonists and other antiparkinsonian medication therapy. (📖 See the section on confusion/hallucinations below).

Communication

Difficulties in communication can be very distressing, especially if the patient is cognitively intact but has unpredictable episodes of being unable to communicate adequately. As with other symptoms in PD, it may worsen in stressful situations. Impaired emotional expression (mask-like facies), so characteristic of PD, impairs the very important non-verbal aspects of communication and should be recognized. Speech therapists can be helpful in improving symptoms.

Dementia

May occur in up to 40 per cent of patients.

Confusion/hallucinations

This may occur as part of the PD itself or as a result of medication. Nocturnal hallucinations are a particular problem and may improve if medication is avoided just prior to sleep. Patients will sometimes tolerate a degree of hallucinosis provided that the other features of the disease, such as motor disability, are reasonably well controlled. The newer antipsychotic agents such as clozapine (beware agranulocytosis), risperidone or olanzepine may help, although should be avoided if there is cerebrovascular disease. Quetiapine is also a very useful medication in this regard but for some is too sedating. Antimuscarinics should be avoided if possible. All medication may have to be reduced if symptoms persist. The anti-dementia drugs such as donepezil, rivastigmine, galantamine and memantine are proving very effective in suppressing drug-induced hallucinations and confusion.

Pain

Pain is a feature of PD and may be relieved by treating the stiffness with levodopa or dopamine agonists. Pain of a sensory nature often occurs in PD and should be treated appropriately. It is important to remember that patients, if demented, may not be able to communicate the presence of pain.

Anxiety

This occurs in 40 per cent of patients but in over 90 per cent of depressed patients with PD. Symptoms of PD such as tremor and dyskinesia often worsen in situations induced by anxiety or emotional excitement (even watching a television programme). A benzodiazepine may help, although it may result in muscle weakness and falls due to loss of muscle tone. Very small doses such as diazepam 1mg b.d. can be effective, therefore this dosage should be carefully titrated from this low start dose.

The terminal phase

PD may worsen with infection, dehydration or other illnesses. Any reversible factors should be corrected where appropriate alongside the management of the PD itself, preferably in a specialist centre. Care and consideration needs to be given to continuing on the antiparkinsonian drugs for as long as possible in order to keep patients as comfortable as possible and able to communicate and swallow. However, if the patient is developing distressing side-effects from the medication, withdrawal of therapy may be in the patient's best interests.

All patients should be encouraged, with help from the family and professionals, to discuss their attitudes and wishes for the management of acute life-threatening medical problems that may occur, such as pneumonia. An Advanced Directive may be helpful in ascertaining patients' wishes for interventions.

Multiple system atrophy (MSA)

MSA is a progressive neuro-degenerative disorder that results in autonomic dysfunction in addition to parkinsonian and at times cerebellar features. It is not hereditary and affects adults usually in the fourth or fifth decade. Post-mortem studies of patients diagnosed with PD indicate that between 10–25 per cent had MSA. It is poorly responsive to levodopa. The mean survival is nine years. As with PD, a multidisciplinary approach is essential.

Progressive supranuclear palsy (PSP)

PSP is the most common cause of an atypical Parkinsonian syndrome with dementia. It occurs more commonly in men than women, with a peak incidence in the early 60s. It comprises postural instability associated with parkinsonism, vertical opthalmoplegia and progressive subcortical dementia. Patients are limited in their ability to move their eyes downwards on request, although the eyes are able to move downwards reflexly, such as when a patient is asked to stare at a stationary object and the head is gently rotated backwards.

Limited upwards eye movement is also common in PSP, but is not diagnostic. Within one year of diagnosis the majority of patients have frequent falls, are slow in performing activities of daily living and have speech difficulties. Twenty-five per cent are confined to a wheelchair by one year following diagnosis increasing to 70 per cent by four years. The mean duration of the illness is four–six years, though this is often shorter in older patients.

Further reading

Bhatia K. et al. (2001) Updated guidelines for the management of Parkinson's disease. *Hospital Medicine* (London) 62, **8**: 456–70.

Global Parkinson's Disease Survey (GPDS) Steering Committee (2002) Factors impacting on quality of life in Parkinson's disease: results from an international survey. *Movement Disorders*, 17, **1**: 60–7.

O'Sullivan J. (2000) What PD therapies to use and when. *Health and Ageing*, January: 16–18.

Olanow CW. (2001) An algorithm (decision tree) for the management of Parkinson's Disease: treatment guidelines. *Neurology*, **56** (11 Suppl 5): S1–S88.

Rascol O. et al. (2002) Treatment interventions for Parkinson's Disease: an evidence-based assessment. *Lancet*, **359**: **9317**: 1589–98.

Schapira AHV (1999) Science, medicine and the future: Parkinson's disease. *British Medical Journal*, **318**: 311–314

Scott S. (2002) *Swallowing Problems and Parkinson's*. PDS Information Sheet 52. London: PDS.

Motor neurone disease

When I wake each morning I decide ...
This can be a good day or a bad day—my choice.
I can be happy or sad—my choice.
I can complain or I can cope—my choice.
Life can be a chore or a challenge—my choice.
I can take from life or give to life—my choice.
If all things are possible,
How I deal with those possibilities is—my choice.

Steve Shackel, diagnosed with MND, (alternatively referred to as amyotrophic lateral sclerosis (ALS))[1]

Motor neurone disease (MND) is a disease of unknown aetiology in which there is progressive degeneration of both upper and lower motor neurones, leading to wasting of muscles and weakness. The average survival is 40 per cent at five years although older patients presenting predominantly with bulbar signs may have a worse prognosis and conversely, younger patients with largely lower motor neurone involvement may have a better than average prognosis. The mean age of onset is 56 years.

UPPER MOTOR NEURONE involvement leads to generalised spasticity, hyper-reflexia and often emotional lability.

LOWER MOTOR NEURONE involvement leads to flaccidity, muscle wasting and fasciculation.

Involvement of BULBAR innervated muscles leads to dysarthria and dysphagia. Interestingly the third, fourth and sixth cranial nerves and those of the lower segments of the spinal cord are usually spared such that eye movements, bladder, bowel and sexual function are generally unaffected. Furthermore intellect, memory, sight and hearing are also usually preserved.

Symptoms in MND are often similar to patients with cancer and include:
- weakness (100 per cent)
- constipation (65 per cent)
- pain (50–60 per cent)
- cough (50–60 per cent)
- insomnia (40–50 per cent)
- breathlessness (40–50 per cent)
- dribbling (30–40 per cent)
- anxiety and depression

In addition problems related to mobility, communication and psychosocial issues, both for the patient and their families, must be addressed necessitating a fully multidisciplinary approach.

1 http://home.goulburn.net.au/~shack

Symptoms

Weakness

Attention to individual needs for maximum comfort is crucial in order to prevent pain and other problems such as skin trauma, contractures and joint dislocation. The rôle of the physiotherapist is important, not only for the patient but also to educate and advise relatives. Although it is important to maintain muscle function and to keep joints mobile, over-enthusiastic physiotherapy may tire the patient and be counterproductive.

Insomnia

It is important to ascertain as far as possible the cause of insomnia, which may range from pain and depression to the overwhelming anxieties of choking and the fear of dying. There is a general reluctance to prescribe night sedatives to patients with MND for fear of respiratory depression. In practice this rarely happens and is insignificant in relation to the morbidity associated with chronic fatigue.

Pain

Management of cause of pain
- Stiff joints—careful positioning/physiotherapy
- Inflammation—NSAID
- Joint pains—Intra-articular steroid injections
- Muscle cramp—quinine sulphate
- Muscle spasm diazepam/baclofen
- Skin pressure—regular turning/turning beds, analgesic ladder

Neuropathic pain is not a feature of MND per se, however patients may complain of pain associated with sensory disturbance and tricyclic antidepressants may help.

The use of opioids in MND

There has been a reluctance to prescribe opioids for fear of respiratory depression in patients whose lung function may already be compromised. However, one study showed that over 80 per cent of patients had been treated with morphine without detriment.

Dysphagia

The speech therapist will help in analysing the exact cause of dysphagia in order to recommend specific techniques to aid swallowing. A common cause is spasticity of the tongue causing difficulty in propelling a food bolus to the pharynx.

Ice packs applied to the neck or chips of ice placed in the mouth may result in relaxation of the tongue and ease swallowing.

The subject of artificial feeding via a gastrostomy tube should be discussed with the patient and the advantages and disadvantages outlined. In the end-stages of the disease, tube feeding may not necessarily prolong life. However, earlier in the disease, particularly if the patient is ambulant, gastrostomy feeding may slow the inevitable weight loss and its associated weakness and depression.

The dietician will advise on food consistency and general nutritional requirements, and the speech therapist on the timing of endoscopic percutaneous gastrostomy tube insertion.

Dysarthria

The speech therapist should be involved early to teach the patient various techniques relevant to his/her own special needs. Various aids are available and include Lightwriters with or without synthesized voice function. Other computerized systems are available from specialized centres including electronic equipment, telephone devices and communication boards which may be adapted to the physical abilities of the individual patient. It is essential to plan ahead since motor function may deteriorate rapidly.

Breathlessness

This is due to diaphragmatic and respiratory muscle weakness. The physiotherapist may suggest breathing techniques and help with chest drainage if appropriate. Antibiotics may be useful in controlling symptoms but if the patient is in a terminal stage they may be inappropriate, serving only to prolong dying.

Nocturnal hypoventilation is characterized by poor sleep and nightmares, early morning headaches and daytime tiredness with subsequent impaired concentration. At an early stage in the disease, it may be appropriate to consider some form of limited ventilatory assistance, such as non-invasive positive pressure ventilation to aid respiration at night time. As breathing becomes weaker, this form of ventilation may continue during the day time.

Patients must be fully informed of the pros and cons of assisted ventilation. More invasive ventilation through a tracheostomy is generally not used in the UK. The wishes of patients for respiratory support should be discussed well in advance of acute problems arising. Patients with MND may die suddenly and unexpectedly with respiratory failure.

Choking

The normal reflexes which protect the airway are impaired so that swallowing food or saliva may result in choking. Although it is a common fear, patients rarely, if ever, die as a result of choking. Speech therapists may help by advising different techniques for protecting the airway such as chewing carefully and slowly, breathing in, swallowing and then deliberately coughing. This technique serves to clear the larynx and to minimize the possibility of choking.

Some patients find suction to the upper airways useful. For others it is avoided since it not only causes trauma, fright and discomfort but may also be very distressing for the relatives to witness.

The Motor Neurone Disease Association (MNDA) supplies a box known as a Breathing Space Kit which provides support for patients and carers. It is a small box with two drawers which contain drugs prescribed by the GP. One side may contain rectal diazepam for the family to administer in an emergency and the other side, drugs such as diamorphine, hyoscine and diazepam, for the doctor or nurse to give.

The multidisciplinary team

All members of the team will have been involved in the care of a patient with MND at some time. These include the neurologist, physiotherapist, occupational therapist, speech therapist, dietician, case manager, GP, district nurse, palliative physician and palliative home care team.

The MNDA provides an invaluable service not only in terms of liaising, supporting and educating patients and carers but also in facilitating the loan of equipment and helping financially.

Further reading

Borasio G., Voltz R. (1997) Palliative care in amyotrophic lateral sclerosis. *Journal of Neurology*, **244**(Suppl. 4): S11–S17.

Borasio G. D. *et al.* (2001) Clinical characteristics and management of ALS. *Seminars in Neurology*, **21**: 155–66.

Carter H. *et al.* (1998) Health professionals' responses to multiple sclerosis and motor neurone disease. *Palliative Medicine*, **12, 5**: 383–94.

Dawson S., Kristjanson L. (2003) Mapping the journey: family carer's perceptions of issues related to end stage care of individuals with Muscular Dystrophy or Motor Neurone Disease. *Journal of Palliative Care*, **19, 1**: 36–42.

Leigh N. *et al.* (2001) Motor neurone disease. *European Journal of Palliative Care*, **8**, 1: 10–12.

Oliver D. (1998) Opioid medication in the palliative care of motor neurone disease. *Palliative Medicine*, **12, 2**: 113–15.

Oliver D. *et al.* (eds) (2000) *Palliative Care in Amyotrophic Lateral Sclerosis (Motor neurone disease)*. Oxford: Oxford University Press.

Polkey M. I. *et al.* (1999) Ethical and clinical issues in the use of home non-invasive mechanical ventilation for the palliation of breathlessness in motor neurone disease. *Thorax*, **54, 4**: 367–71.

Neurological complications of AIDS

Prevalence: up to 65 per cent.

AIDS dementia complex

- A syndrome of progressive cognitive loss with motor and behavioural dysfunction in HIV- infected patients
- Clinical features: apathy, social withdrawal, impaired concentration, slowing of speech and movement, unsteady gait, can progress to being bedridden with paraparesis, urinary incontinence and faecal incontinence
- Investigations:
  - Need to exclude opportunistic infection with toxoplasmosis or CMV
  - CT scan—cerebral atrophy and ventricular enlargement
  - MRI scan—white matter abnormality
- Management: anti-retroviral drugs may improve symptoms and prolong survival

Vacuolar myelopathy

- Aetiology: unclear but vacuolization of the white matter in spinal cord is seen at post-mortem
- Clinical features: progressive weakness, spasticity and ataxia, urinary incontinence, faecal incontinence
- Management: no current treatment

Peripheral neuropathy

- Distal symmetrical polyneuropathy is the most common feature and may occur in 10–30 per cent. It is characterized by a symmetrical distal painful sensory loss which is associated with weight loss and dementia
- Management: trial of amitriptyline
- Inflammatory demyelinating neuropathy is characterized by progressive weakness and loss of tendon reflexes. It is usually mild
- Inflammatory polyradiculopathy can be due to CMV infection and is characterized by a progressive distal weakness, sensory problems and incontinence
- Management: no treatment available
- Cranial nerve neuropathy, can involve the facial nerve

HIV-associated myopathy

Symptoms are progressive with symmetrical painless weakness of the proximal limbs and facial muscles.

- Investigations: electromyography (EMG), muscle biopsy
- Management: consider corticosteroids and plasmapheresis

Opportunistic infections of the CNS

- Common organisms: Toxoplasmosis gondii, cryptococcus neoformans, JC virus, CMV
- Clinical features: headache, confusion, fever, seizures, focal signs
- Investigations: CT scan, MRI scan, lumbar puncture—CSF analysis
- Management:
  - Cerebral toxoplasmosis—pyrimethamine and sulphadiazine
  - Cryptococcal meningitis—amphotericin B

- Progressive multifocal leucoencephalopathy (JC virus)—no effective treatment
- CMV infection—ganciclovir

Further reading

Article

Janssen R. S. *et al.* (1989) Human immunodeficiency virus (HIV) infection and the nervous system: report from the American Academy of Neurology AIDS Task Force. *Neurology*, **39, 1**: 119–22.

Creutzfeldt-Jakob disease (CJD)

CJD is a rare degenerative disorder of the central nervous system. Prion proteins occur naturally but it is the abnormal development and accumulation of rogue prion proteins in brain cells that leads to the development of CJD.

The most common form of the disease, accounting for 80 per cent of all cases, is '**sporadic**', presenting as a rapidly progressive multi-focal dementia with poor memory and cognition, impaired balance and mobility, myoclonic jerks, slurred speech and visual problems. The incidence of sporadic CJD 0.5–1 new case/million population per year.

'**Inherited**' prion disease, accounting for around 10 per cent of cases, due to autosomal dominant inheritance of a genetically-mutated prion protein. The clinical course of inherited forms is usually more protracted than other forms.

'**Acquired**' prion disease occurs when rogue proteins have inadvertently been introduced into the individual (e.g. secondary to treatment with human derived growth hormone, following transplant of infected organs such as corneas, or the inadvertent use of contaminated neurosurgical instruments).

'**Variant**' (vCJD) was first described in 1996 and has been linked to the UK Bovine Spongiform Encephalopathy (BSE) epidemic of the 1980s. The median age at onset is younger than for patients with sporadic disease, at 26 years. Common early features are dysphoria, withdrawal, anxiety and hallucinations, with subsequent neurological decline. The time course is longer than for sporadic disease (14.5 months mean duration compared with four months).

Unpublished research into the palliative care of patients with CJD has shown that many patients are being cared for by specialist palliative care services, and that the key issues in their care include managing agitation and movement disorders, impaired communication and the dilemma associated with end-of-life decisions. There is frequently a high level of distress amongst those emotionally close to the patient, in keeping with the younger age of patients, the distressing nature of the illness and its high media profile.

Following the death of a patient, the case should be discussed with the coroner, who may require a *post-mortem*. As with any coroner's case, a *post-mortem* can be carried out without permission from the next of kin, which may cause great distress, particularly with some cultural/religious groups who will need a great deal of support at this time. All *post-mortems* for CJD are usually carried out in designated neuropathology institutions. Following removal of the brain and spinal cord, families are able to view the body again if they wish. There is usually no visual evidence that the body has been tampered with. The brain and spinal tissue are then sent to the CJD Surveillance Unit where a formal tissue diagnosis may take months. The Unit has information for relatives and handles the situation sensitively, organizing the return of body parts to the family's funeral director for cremation or burial when the tests are completed.

Further reading

Articles

Carter H., McKenna C. *et al.* (1998). Health professionals' responses to multiple sclerosis and motor neurone disease. *Palliat Med*, **12, 5**: 383–94.

Oliver D. (1998) Opioid medication in the palliative care of motor neurone disease. *Palliat Med*, **12, 2**: 113–5.

Bailey B., Aranda S., Quinn K., Kean, H. (2000) Creuzfeldt-Jakob disease: extending palliative care nursing knowledge. *Int J Palliat Nurs*, **6**: 131–9.

Brown P. (2001) Bovine Spongiform Ecephalopathy and variant CJD. *British Medical Journal*, **322**: 841–4.

Spencer M., Knight R., Will R. (2002) First hundred cases of variant CJD: retrospective case note review of early psychiatric and neurological features. *BMJ*, **324**: 1479–82.

Meek J. (1998) A case study: team support for a patient with CJD. *Community Nurse*, **4**: 27–28.

Useful contacts

Multiple Sclerosis Resource Centre
7 Peartree Business Centre
Peartree Road
Stanway
Colchester
Essex CO3 5JN
Tel: 01206 505444
Freephone: 0800 783 0518
E-mail: themsrc@yahoo.com
Web Site: http://www.msrc.co.uk
Also provide a 24 hour MS telephone counselling service on 0800 783 0518

Multiple Sclerosis Society
MS National Centre
372 Edgware Road
London NW2 6ND
Tel: 020 8438 0700
MS Helpline: Freephone 0808 800 8000, 9am–9pm
E-mail: info@mssociety.org.uk
Web Site: http://www.mssociety.org.uk
Provides information, support and practical help to anyone affected by MS
and to those working with them. Also provide respite care centres and
holiday homes.

Motor Neurone Disease Association
PO Box 246
Northampton NN1 2PR
Tel: 01604 250505
Fax: 01604 638289/624726
Helpline: 08457 626262
E-mail: enquiries@mndassociation.org
Web Site: http://www.mndassociation.org
Links to other sites and documents can be accessed through this site.
Telephone: 0131 537 2128
National Prion Clinic: www.st-marys.nhs.uk/specialist/prion/clinicinfo.htm

The National C-JD Surveillance Unit
Western General Hospital
Crewe Road
Edinburgh EH4 2XU
Web Site: http://www.cjd.ed.ac.uk

NHS National Prion Clinic
Box 98
National Hospital for Neurology and Neurosurgery
Queen Square
London WCIN 3BG
Tel: 020 7405 0755
E-mail: help.prion@st-marys.nhs.uk
Web Site: http://www.st-marys.nhs.uk/specialist/prion/clinicinfo.htm

Palliation in the care of the elderly[1]

Old age is associated with disease, it does not cause it.

The large majority of the population over the age of 85 years live at home; 20 per cent live in nursing homes. Elderly patients with palliative care needs often have a constellation of complex and chronic requirements including:

- Appropriate therapeutic interventions that can preserve function and independence and help patients maintain quality of life
- Clear communication on the usual course of illness so that they and their family members can make appropriate arrangements
- Recognition and management of caregiver stress
- Management of physical and psychological symptoms of both acute and chronic illnesses

Elderly people in the UK may receive palliative care in a number of settings, including;

- At home with the care of a GP and community nursing team
- In a residential or nursing home with the care of a GP and local nursing staff
- In a Community Hospital
- On a care of the elderly unit/facility
- In an acute hospital following an acute admission

Background

- While a child born in 1900 could expect to live fewer than 50 years, life expectancy for a child born in 2010 is expected to increase to 86 years for a girl and 79 years for a boy.[2] The implication for increasing input from supportive and palliative care is clear
- In developed nations, the overwhelming majority of deaths occur in elderly patients suffering from multiple coexisting and progressive chronic illnesses
- Some studies suggest that elderly patients are excluded from life-prolonging interventions even if they might be appropriate. This difference may be due to *de facto* rationing based on age rather than emphasis on individualizing the goals of care. Specialists in care of the elderly are skilled at devising goals of care which are appropriate for the individual's particular needs
- Data suggests that elderly patients receive less pain medication than younger persons for both chronic and acute pain. Chronic pain syndromes such as arthritis, and other musculoskeletal problems affect 25–50 per cent of the community-dwelling elderly and are also typically undertreated

1 Meier D. and Monias A. (2004) In D. Doyle, G. Hanks, N. Cherny and K. C. Calman *Oxford Textbook of Palliative Medicine.* 3rd edn. pp. 935–44. Oxford: Oxford University Press.

2 Field M. J. and Cassel C. K. (1997) Approaching death: Improving care at the end of life. In Institute of Medicine, ed. Washington, DC: National Academies Press.

Caregiver burden

- The tremendous growth in numbers of people over 65 years with chronic health problems has challenged both national and personal resources
- In the UK, the duration of caring for an elderly relative may exceed ten years
- Fifty per cent of caregivers have financial difficulties
- Caregiving in general is not valued in western societies, where sometimes those involved in full time caring can be made to feel that life is passing them by

Risks to the carer include:
- Physical risks
  - Development of musculoskeletal diseases through lifting and handling
  - Increased mortality—Many of the carers are themselves elderly and vulnerable
- Emotional risks
  - Major depression, and associated comorbidities
- Social risks
  - Isolation and loss of contact with friends and social circle. Close to 90 per cent of caregivers say they need more help in caring for their loved ones in one or more categories including
  - Personal care
  - Nursing
  - Transportation
  - Loss of income
  - Loss of status within society

How can we address the needs of an elderly, frail and depressed woman who is shortly to be bereaved, and who through the course of caring for her demented husband over many years has lost contact with any support network of friends or family?

Medical goal-setting in care of the elderly with chronic illness

Table 8e.1 A checklist for palliative care throughout the course of chronic illness in the elderly

Early	Middle	Late
Discuss diagnosis, prognosis, and course of disease	Assess efficacy of disease-modifying therapy	Discuss goals of care with patient and family
Discuss disease-modifying therapies	Review course of disease	Confirm previous advance directives
Discuss goals of care, hopes, and expectations	Reassess goals of care and expectations	Actively manage symptoms
Discuss advance care planning	Confirm advance directives and ensure a health care proxy is appointed	Review financial resources and needs

Table 8e.1 (Continued)

Early	Middle	Late
Manage comorbidities Advise financial planning/consultation with a social worker for future needs including long-term care	Recommend physio/ occupational therapies to preserve function and promote socialization Behavioural and pharmacological symptom control	Review long-term care needs and discuss options
Inform patient and family about support groups Inquire about desire for spiritual support	Treat mood disorders Suggest support groups for patient and caregiver	Consider if palliative care needs are being well met in current care setting
Behavioural and pharmacological symptom control	Offer social and emotional support to caregivers	Referral/planning to ensure peaceful death
Treat mood disorders	Review long-term care options and resource needs	Assess spiritual needs Offer respite care

Reproduced from *Oxford Textbook of Palliative Medicine*.[3]

Early in illness

Health care professionals should discuss goals of care with their patients. These goals may change as the disease progresses but may include:
- Prolonging life
- Preserving autonomy and independence
- Maintaining social activities
- Forming a plan for advanced stages of disease
- Staying at home.

Mid-disease

The middle disease period is characterized by:
- Increased medical needs
- Declining function
- Loss of independence, and increased dependence on caregivers for assistance in basic activities of daily living, e.g. patients with dementia require increased supervision while patients with Parkinson's disease, heart failure, or rheumatological diseases may need more assistance with ambulation.

Needs during mid-disease period include:

Patient needs
- Treating physical symptoms of chronic disease such as pain, dyspnoea, anorexia, nausea, vomiting, changes in bowel habit and insomnia which may become prominent during this phase of disease. These symptoms should be effectively treated as outlined in other chapters

3 Meier D. and Monias A. (2004) In D. Doyle, G. Hanks, N. Cherny and K. C. Calman *Oxford Textbook of Palliative Medicine*. 3rd edn. pp. 935–44. Oxford: Oxford University Press.

Caregiver needs
- Help in supervision of the patient, the lack of which results in great caregiver stress, leading to unnecessary consideration of nursing home placement
- Information for carers about local resources for adult day care, respite care, home care services, and support groups
- Helping the caregiver to maintain physical, financial, and emotional strength for the multi-year tasks ahead by providing opportunities to discuss and address their particular difficulties
- Where appropriate encourage a regular rotating schedule of respite support from family and friends

Ageism and the care of the Elderly

Ageist attitudes can inhibit the quality of palliative care available to elderly patients. Such attitudes may be displayed overtly or covertly by:
- Society at large— 'a disproportionate percentage of patients who are left waiting on trolleys for hospital admission in the UK are elderly'
- Doctors and Nurses—'He is too old to benefit from a hip replacement'
- Relatives—'Granny wouldn't want to be told about her disease'
- The elderly themselves—'Why should anyone bother with me? I've had my day'

Home needs
- Home evaluation for adaptive devices such as raised toilet seats, shower seats, and grab bars

Late in disease of chronic illness

In later stages of disease, goals may shift to providing maximum comfort and security.

Patient needs
- Careful attention to symptom control as, particularly in the last few months of life, patients may lose the ability to complain of pain and other symptoms. (e.g. Pain is often undertreated in end-stage dementia.)
- To be treated as an individual, and as a person with particular characteristics and needs
- Ensuring that patients' wishes, fears, and concerns as far as possible are discussed and addressed
- Enjoyment in the modalities of life where joy is possible, e.g. food which the patient enjoys
- At this stage of disease, mortality is 50 per cent at six months, and the goals of care shift to minimise suffering and maximize quality of life, according to the values and expressed wishes of the patient
- Physicians should discuss the merits, or otherwise, of continuing painful routine procedures with the patient and carers

Carer needs
- Patients in the end-stage of a chronic disease may be bed or chair-bound. They can become completely dependent on caregivers for feeding,

toileting, bathing, and dressing and are often incontinent, which can be extremely distressing both for the patient and the carer
- As patients deteriorate carers can enter a chronic state of loss as they witness their relative's physical and mental deterioration. Recognition of the loneliness and pain of such a state can bring important comfort and help
- Due to increased care demands and exhaustion of family caregivers, patients' families may benefit from respite admissions in order to allow the patient's choice to stay at home long term to be achieved

Placement needs
- It is important that efforts are made to find out where a patient would prefer to die, and where possible to ensure that this decision is respected
- Patients who reside in a nursing home and want to remain in the comfort and security of familiar surroundings may not want to be transferred routinely to the hospital for intercurrent illness or for symptoms that can be managed in the nursing home. 'Do not transfer' instructions should be discussed with patient, family, and staff where possible, and if appropriate, to prevent an emergency move to an acute setting when the patient's condition deteriorates
- No one place is the ideal setting for terminal care for every person, as physical, emotional and social resources will all need to be balanced in the selection of place of care

Common issues in palliative care of the elderly

Physical issues

Infection

- The late stages of many terminal illnesses are commonly complicated by life-threatening infections
- Immobility, malnutrition, incontinence, lung aspiration, and decreased immunity increase the risk of pneumonia, cellulitis, decubitus ulcers, urinary tract infections, and sepsis
- Decreased ability to express oneself and atypical presentation may lead to delayed recognition of infections
- Palliative care should focus on reducing risk factors for infection in providing patients with good skin care, ambulation training, and aspiration precautions
- As with all other treatments, the risks and benefits of antibiotic therapy need to be weighed

Pressure ulcers

- Many patients who are bedbound, incontinent, and poorly nourished do not develop decubitus ulcers in large measure due to the excellence of care provided
- Importantly those who do develop ulcers often do so in spite of excellent care—the appearance of the ulcer being a marker of deteriorating physical condition rather than deteriorating medical or nursing care
- Use of pressure relieving mattresses and cushions prior to the development of skin problems, and quality nursing care are the mainstays in preventing ulcers developing
- In the terminal phase, care should focus on relieving pain and limiting odour, not on aiming for ulcer cure
  - Analgesia should be provided prior to all dressing changes
  - Odour can be controlled with topical metronidazole gel, silver sulfadiazine, or charcoal dressings
- Although the development of decubitus ulcers is not an independent risk factor for death, the presence of a pressure wound is a marker of advanced stage of disease and poor prognosis

Pain

Treatment of pain in the elderly generally follows the same guidelines as in younger adults. Studies on clinical pain perception indicate that pain from headache and visceral pain decrease in the elderly, but musculoskeletal, leg, and foot pain increase with aging. Pain is undertreated in the elderly.

Concomitant diseases likely to cause chronic pain have a higher prevalence in the elderly and often exist alongside the prime pain causing problem, i.e. the development of bowel cancer will not prevent a patient from continuing to suffer the pain of rheumatoid arthritis.

Such chronic illnesses include:

- Arthritis
- Polymyalgia rheumatica

Atherosclerotic disease
Cancer
Herpes zoster

Such diseases cannot be ignored if holistic quality symptom control is to take place.

Nausea and vomiting

Common causes of nausea and vomiting in the elderly include:
Drug reactions, including opioids
Gastroparesis due to autonomic system dysfunction (especially caused by diabetes)
Constipation

Management for nausea and vomiting in the elderly is the same as for younger patients, with particular attention being paid to possible side-effects from antiemetic medication. ('Start low, go slow.')

Constipation

Constipation is a nearly universal complaint of elderly patients. Over half of the community-dwelling elderly report constipation.
Risk factors include:
female gender
medication
depression
immobility
chronic diseases—Parkinson's disease, hypothyroidism, diabetes mellitus, diverticular disease, irritable bowel syndrome, and haemorrhoids
Common medication includes opioids, calcium, iron, calcium channel blockers, antihistamines, tricyclic antidepressants, and diuretics

Management

A patient who presents with a history of constipation should always be examined rectally to exclude faecal impaction. If impaction is present, the patient should be manually disimpacted, with some sedation to minimise distress, and treated with suppositories and/or enemas prior to receiving oral laxatives. (□ See Chapter 6b.)

Diarrhoea

If patients are bedbound this symptom can be particularly exhausting and demeaning to patients and caregivers.
Common causes of diarrhoea in the elderly include:
Overflow incontinence
Antibiotics
Clostridium difficile enterocolitis
Malabsorption
Enterocolitis
Stress

Note: The onset of diarrhoea can also herald the onset of a gastro-intestinal haemorrhage.

Management

Exclude reversible causes
Consider bulking agents if patient mobile and able to drink enough fluid

- Loperamide, co-phenotrope or codeine may help
- Octreotide is effective to reduce intestinal secretions and leaking fistulae in special circumstances

Cough

Non-malignant causes of chronic cough in the elderly include oesophage reflux disease, COPD, heart failure, and post-nasal drip. Cough can also b a result of medications such as ACE inhibitors.

Dizziness

- Dizziness is a common symptom in elderly patients with chronic disease. Prevalence ranges from 13–38 per cent
- It is multifactorial in origin and can be due to decreased proprioceptior secondary to diabetic neuropathy, vascular disease, vestibular disorders, and cardiac arrhythmias. Postural hypotension may also result in dizziness, as can certain medications
- Dizziness has been identified as a syndrome of the elderly because of its prevalence and the frequency with which no single cause is isolated

Drug management includes treating any obviously reversible pathology an appropriate consideration of antihistamines, such as betahistine, or occa sionally anxiolytics. Secondary prevention is also important, reducing th risks of falls through education, and risk assessment of the patient's home.

Oral symptoms

Elderly patients can present with mouth pain, dryness, and halitosis.
- The differential diagnosis of mouth pain includes aphthous ulcers, mucositis from chemotherapy, fungal infection secondary to decreased immunity or antibiotics, dental caries, periodontal disease, and poorly fitting dentures
- Infection should be treated appropriately and patients and caregivers instructed on oral hygiene
- Medications are the most common cause of dry mouth in elderly patients and should be kept under constant review
- When symptoms are not relieved with sips of water or ice, artificial saliva or commercial preparations containing mucin may provide relief
- Some patients experience mouth pain despite a normal oropharyngeal examination. These patients often benefit from viscous lidocaine

Ethical issues

Artificial nutrition and hydration (📖 See Chapter 1)

General issues
- Patients suffering from end-stage dementia and other chronic neurological illnesses may develop dysphagia, which predisposes them to aspiration pneumonia
- In the late stages of dementia, patients frequently refuse food, clamp their mouths shut, or hold food without swallowing
- Feeding may become a frustrating battle between the patient and caregiver, who may feel that the patient is deliberately being difficult. Carers will need support and information to understand that this may be involuntary and due to the dementia

Possible management options

- Changing the texture of the diet to purée, or liquids thickened with cornstarch or potato starch, may support safe swallowing
- Improving the taste of food may provide increased enjoyment of the process of eating
- Caregivers should be trained to feed the patient in an upright position, with the head forward, using small spoonfuls

Artificial nutrition and hydration is an emotionally charged issue for many caregivers.

They may believe that their loved one would suffer hunger without artificial nutrition and hydration.

Family members should understand that loss of appetite is an integral part of the dying process

📖 For a fuller discussion of these issues see Chapter 1.

Prescribing in the elderly

This is a huge issue, and many patients are admitted to hospital each year due to the effects of injudicious prescribing, particularly in the elderly population.

Particular concerns include the following:

- Decreased renal function and liver metabolism places elderly patients at higher risk of drugs accumulating to toxic levels
- Multiple complex physical and psychological conditions can lead to a wide range of medication being prescribed for different complaints, with increasing likelihood of drug interactions causing dangerous side-effects
- Complexity of prescribing schedules and lack of support networks can lead to irregular medicine ingestion with higher risks in a population where memory, eyesight and dexterity may not be as good
- It is easier to increase medication than it is to reduce or stop drugs which have been started by another specialist team
- Elderly patients may be particularly sensitive to the confusional side-effects of medication, and in situations where patients suddenly develop confusion it is important to exclude iatrogenic cause
- Medication which a patient has taken faithfully for many years to help with a symptom due to e.g. high blood pressure may no longer be strictly necessary, but the patient or family may have a belief in that particular tablet, which makes stopping it even in the last days of illness very difficult
- Routes of administration can become an important issue in prescribing if an elderly patient loses the ability to swallow

General rules

- As few medications as possible
- Start medication at low doses and slowly increase
- Regular review of medication and reduce any unnecessary tablets
- Use of pre-filled drug administration boxes or other devices may help with compliance
- Age should not exclude patients from either effective, expensive, or innovative drug therapy where it is appropriate and prescribed with care and consultation

Emotional issues

Dementia: 'a syndrome consisting of progressive impairment in two or more areas of cognition sufficient to interfere with work, social function or relationships in the absence of delirium or major non-organic psychiatric disorders.'

Some 5–8% of all people over the age of 65 suffer from moderate to severe dementia, with the prevalence doubling every 5 years reaching over 20% in 80 year olds

Agitation in the chronically confused
- Seventy per cent of patients with dementia may have insomnia or 'sun-downing', a syndrome of increasing confusion during the evening
- Daytime exercises, a consistent bedtime routine, and minimizing daytime napping can help improve sleep patterns
- Encouraging patients to participate in their own grooming and bathing may decrease agitation
- Sponge baths and adjusting water temperature may make bathing less threatening
- Familiar music and frequent social activities may also exert a calming influence
- Early in the disease, behavioural abnormalities in patients with dementia can be helped by disease-specific cholinesterase inhibition with drugs such as donepezil, galantamine, or rivastigmine. (Often such improvement does not last more than a few months.)
- Low doses of neuroleptics can ameliorate confusion, hallucinations, and delusions
- Second-generation antipsychotic medication (risperidone, and olanzapine) causes less extrapyramidal toxicity than first-generation antipsychotics; however, patients still need to be monitored for parkinsonism, and doses should always be started as low as possible to minimise side-effects
- Successful management of agitation can prevent hospital admissions and nursing home placement

Anxiety
Being elderly and ill can often provoke considerable anxiety. Such anxieties may relate to:
- Concern about the process of dying. Such patients may have had experiences of illness and dying which lead them to believe it will inevitably be pain-filled and difficult
- Concerns about leaving dependent relatives, or family, particularly if there are unresolved conflicts or issues within the family
- Concerns about financial or housing matters

Such anxieties will usually be helped by open discussion and isolation of the particular points of concern. General, non-specific, 'don't worry' advice tends to increase rather than decrease anxiety levels, as patients need a plan as to what they can do to address their concerns.

Common sources of suffering and discomfort in the elderly

- Patients may suffer even when they are free of pain or other symptoms
- Health care professionals need to ask about suffering as well as pain
- Questions should be open-ended in order to help make the patient comfortable with discussing fear, anxiety, and other non-physical symptoms. 'How are you feeling inside yourself?'
- A sample question to family members is, 'are you concerned that your family member may be suffering or uncomfortable?'

As in younger patients, relief of pain goes hand in hand with treatment of the emotional and spiritual components that contribute to it.

Care of the caregiver

Caregivers of elderly patients in the end-stage of chronic disease often need as much or more attention from the medical team as the patient. While family caregivers may take enormous satisfaction from their ability to provide safe and loving care for their loved one, most also feel varying degrees of exhaustion, guilt, and frustration.

- Listening to and trying to help address the concerns of caregivers, the medical team conveys the fact that the caregiver is not alone and that the concerns are legitimate and important
- Caregiver stress does not end after placement of the patient in a nursing home
- Caregivers continue to worry about the patient as well as suffer guilt over the necessity of nursing home placement
- Caregivers universally face difficult medical (and goals of care) decisions when the question of tube feeding, hospitalization for predictable infection, and use of antibiotics arise

Hospice Care and the Elderly Population

Concern exists within the palliative services of being overwhelmed by elderly patients with chronic long term care needs

- Although hospice care may be appropriate for certain patients with end-stage dementia and other chronic illnesses, hospice is accessed less frequently for these patients than for those with cancer
  This may be because: It is more difficult to accurately identify a limited prognosis among such patients
- The needs of elderly patents suffering from long term illnesses in the last year of life may far exceed the needs of patients with malignancy, yet the services available to meet those needs are often much less
- Quality palliative care does not require admission to a hospice but does require access to a healthcare team committed to providing holistic, individualised, planned and communicated care in whatever setting is appropriate for the particular patient

Conclusions

Growing old is a natural process which often changes our bodies, mind and what we regard as being important. A life which has been well live can provide an elderly person with great comfort and satisfaction as the contemplate their pending death.

Having the opportunity to 'sort things out' and to 'tidy up loose ends can provide ease of mind to someone who is coming to the end of thei life, and is a process that should be facilitated and not regarded a 'morbid'.

The essence of palliative care is providing holistic care tailored to th particular needs of individual patients. The same can be said of care of the elderly.

Remaining open to all the possibilities of old age and the dying journe will prevent our care of the elderly in this very important part of their live becoming stereotyped or sentimental and help carers face the realities o their own mortality.

Further reading

Books

Meier D. and Monias A. (2004) *Oxford Textbook of Palliative Medicine*. 3rd edn. pp. 935–44. D. Doyle, G. Hanks, N. Cherny and K. C. Calman. Oxford: Oxford University Press.

Articles

Bernabei R., Gambassi G. *et al.* (1998) Management of pain in elderly patients with cancer. SAGE Study Group. Systematic Assessment of Geriatric Drug Use via Epidemiology. *JAMA*, **279, 23**: 1877–82.

Feldt, K. S. and Gunderson J. (2002) Treatment of pain for older hip fracture patients across settings. *Orthop Nurs*, **21, 5**: 63–4, 66–71.

Krulewitch H., London M. R. *et al.* (2000) Assessment of pain in cognitively impaired older adults: a comparison of pain assessment tools and their use by nonprofessional caregivers. *J Am Geriatr Soc*, **48, 12**: 1607–11.

Lawlor P. G., Fainsinger R. L. *et al.* (2000) Delirium at the end of life: critical issues in clinical practice and research. *JAMA*, **284, 19**: 2427–9.

Chapter 9

Spiritual care

The awareness and appreciation of a patient's individual spiritual orientation (spiritual issues, spiritual needs, spiritual pain, spiritual care, spiritual practices and nurturing) is essential to holistic care.

Holistic care in human life is governed by social, psychological, physical and spiritual influences. A dying person is more than a failing physiological system.

The doctor most often credited with founding the modern hospice movement, Dame Cicely Saunders, approached palliative care from the rather unique perspective of multiprofessional training. Her insights into the dying journey were enhanced by her social work background—listening and recording the experiences and feelings of patients, her nursing experience—dealing in practical terms with the physical needs of patients and her medical training—scientifically and systematically diagnosing and treating the cause of distressing symptoms.

The concept of holistic care was not discovered in St Christopher's Hospice, but the search to improve care for patients who appeared to have been sidelined by modernist over-confidence in scientific and medical advances resonated with a deeply felt need throughout the world.

Spiritual care is inseparable from holistic care, despite the difficulties which it brings with it in secular, multi-faith societies and to communities divided by religious and ethnic conflicts. Spirituality remains a challenging and vital presence at the heart of palliative care provision.

- The concept of spiritual care is inherent in the practice of holistic palliative care
- Spiritual matters are often referred to as those things that give life meaning and value
- In order to carry out holistic care, we must attend to the three indivisible facets of the human condition—the mind, body and spirit of humankind.[1]

In one study, 93 per cent of patients with cancer said that religion helped sustain their hopes.[2]

1 Hopper A. (2000) Meeting the spiritual needs of patients through holistic practice. *European Journal of Palliative Care*, **7, 2**: 60–3.

2 Roberts J. A. et al. (1997) Factors influencing views of patients with gynecologic cancer about end-of-life decisions. *American Journal of Obstetrics and Gynecology*, **176**: 166–72.

Definitions

Central to the problematic nature of 'spiritual care' is how 'spirituality' is defined.

- A definition which *includes* religious elements may cause a sense of exclusion among those who hold to a different belief system
- A definition which *excludes* all religious elements may exclude those within society who subscribe to a particular belief

The term 'spirituality' has strong religious connotations in the monotheistic religions of Christianity, Judaism and Islam, and it has been used in the religious context for hundreds of years to refer to particular practices and theological meanings.

In the context of eastern religions, with growing influences in the West both directly and through new age movements, spirituality has a less defined but no less central significance.

To disentangle completely 'spirituality' from such religious associations which have interpreted and developed understandings and insights into 'spirituality' over hundreds of years in the context of faith communities seems disingenuous.

However, paradoxically 'spirituality' is also used, in the context of patient care, as a term to refer to a particular characteristic of an individual which can exist without reference to any particular body of beliefs.[3]

Thus no single definition of 'spirituality' can capture its full meaning.

O'Brien defines spirituality very broadly as: That which inspires one to transcend the realm of the material.[4]

> Spirituality can be defined as what we do with our pain. We can either transform it or transmit it.
>
> R. Roar

. . . the word 'spiritual' has become a portmanteau into which we tend to stuff what is left over when we have removed what we can identify with and describe in terms of the body or the mind. Theologically, this runs the risk of leaving only the gaps in our understanding to God. Philosophically, it is perhaps an extension of Descartes' reductionist emphasis on the division of mind and body, adding a third dimension—the spirit.[5]

Spirituality is therefore not simply an intellectual proposition but consists of cognitive, emotional, and behavioural components that contribute to defining a person and to the way life is experienced.[6]

> The essence of what it means to be human, spiritual issues are the issues of the soul and concern our deepest values and meaning.
>
> M. Kearney

> And almost everyone when age,
> Disease, or sorrows strike him,
> Inclines to think there is a God,
> Or something very like him
>
> From 'There is no God', Arthur Hugh Clough 1819–61

- The concept of spirituality, which may seem abstract and ethereal to a scientifically trained doctor or nurse, is ignored at the peril of providing substandard care

- Spirituality forms the context in which patients respond to care, choose their treatment options, deal with relationship matters and face death
- The type of care shown to the patient will inevitably impact on the patient's own sense of meaning, worth and hence 'spirituality'
- The expression of spirituality is shaped by the accepted practices and beliefs of a particular culture, as well as by other influences such as institutionalized religion, or reaction to institutionalized religion
- How people live and understand their life can provide a framework for helping them face their own mortality and death
- Being forced to face imminent mortality can challenge belief systems profoundly, and sometimes beliefs cannot withstand such challenge without changing. A disintegration of beliefs evidenced by doubts, conflict and confusion can cause severe distress to the individual and family involved
- Conversely, spiritual beliefs which have long lain dormant can sometimes become central when a person experiences the suffering associated with a serious life-threatening illness
- It is important to realize just how dynamic the concept of spirituality is, especially in the palliative care setting
- Those involved in looking after patients need to be aware of the spiritual impact that their interaction with the patients can have
- Spiritual beliefs have been shown to affect the ways in which a patient deals with illness. Holland studied patients with malignant melanoma and discovered that those who rated religious and spiritual beliefs as highly important often used successfully active—cognitive means of successful coping. She felt that such coping strategies provided a sense of connection, involvement and meaning which helped patients accept their illness.[8]
- Others have claimed that those with strong religious beliefs, including atheistic convictions, are better able to deal with mortality issues, than those who have lukewarm beliefs which can contribute to increased anxiety and fear as death approaches

Spirituality and religion

'Religious practices have been developed to impose sense and order on the inherent mysteries of spiritual things, and sacraments have evolved to express the seemingly inexpressible.'[5]

The tension between the religious elements of 'spirituality' and the non-religious elements cannot be ignored. To ignore one aspect will lead to a distorted concept of spirituality that is either so culturally rooted to a particular set of beliefs as to manifest itself as tribalism, or to be so unrelated

3 Cobb M. (2003) Spiritual care. In M Lloyd-Williams (ed.) *Psychosocial Issues in Palliative Care*, pp. 135–47. Oxford: Oxford University Press.

4 O'Brien M. E. (1978) The need for spiritual integrity. In H. Yura and M. B. Walsh (eds) *Human Needs and the Nursing Process*. Norwalk, Connecticut: Appleton-Century-Crofts.

5 Hopper A. (2000) Meeting the spiritual needs of patients through holistic practice. *European Journal of Palliative Care*, **7, 2**: 60–3.

6 Argyle M. (2000) *Psychology and Religion*. London: Routledge.

7 Murray R. B., Zentner J. P. (1989) *Nursing Concepts for Health Promotion*. London: Prentice Hall.

8 Holland J. (1999) The rôle of religious and spiritual beliefs in coping with malignant melanoma. *Psycho-oncology*, **8, 1**: 14–26.

to human existence, as experienced by the vast majority of the population in their day-to-day existence, as to be irrelevant.

Experiencing the tension of such a paradox can be uncomfortable for those unused to paradoxical thinking, though less so for those whose philosophical or religious upbringing has provided insight into paradox.

Various understandings in the nature of the relationship between spirituality and religion have been explored.

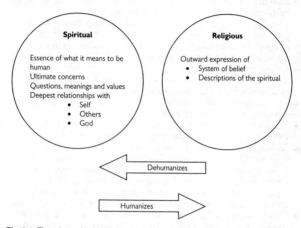

Fig. 9.1 The relationship between spirituality and religion. Leonard Lunn/ Margaret, 1990.

When Rajendra was admitted to the Hospice it was clear that his prognosis was very limited. His district nurse had asked that he be admitted to a side room because his family, who were devoutly Hindu, wanted to be able to fulfil their familial and spiritual responsibilities to him without upsetting other patients. The family were extremely attentive to his personal physical care and also to his religious requests.

Through the reading of the Hindu scriptures and the burning of incense Rajendra seemed to derive great comfort.

The Hospice was a Christian foundation, with strong links to the local churches and an active chaplaincy department who visited Rajendra regularly at his request.

Several members of staff found the overt Hindu practices very distressing as they were concerned about demonic influences. A decision was taken that such members of staff would be assigned to different patients.

Several weeks after his death the family returned to say how much they had valued their last days together with Rajendra in the Hospice. They had been nervous when admission had been suggested because they had been aware of the Christian ethos of the Hospice.

They also shared how Rajendra's greatest spiritual comfort and solace in his last days had come from the sense of love, care, and acceptance he had received from hospice staff, particularly because in his business life as a shop owner, he had had to put up with a great deal of racial and religious harassment.

Faith practices

Compare spirituality with nutrition; neither is a subject that healthcare providers can take for granted. Inadequate nutrition is costly. If people are not fed properly, resistance weakens and wounds do not heal. Evidence is growing in volume and quality that this holds for spiritual sustenance too. [9]

For many people spirituality is not just an idea but has daily practical, social and material meaning. In short 'spirituality' has form as well as content.
  These forms may include:
- **Rituals:** such as prayer, meditation, pilgrimage, and sacraments
- **Social group values**: beliefs, dietary restrictions, and morals
- **Material manifestations**: buildings, icons, prayer beads, symbols etc
- Patients may have practices and rituals which they would wish to maintain because of their beliefs
- These practices may be disrupted because of illness
- Illness and treatment may affect energy levels and therefore interfere with the routines of normal life and the opportunities for contact from other members of the faith community
- Those from minority faith traditions may find particular difficulty in accessing religious support

Faith practices can be very helpful particularly in times of stress and change. In the context of illness and the inevitable medicalisation inherent in modern treatment pathways, faith practices can help to maintain an identity separate from that of 'patient'.

For the carers of such patients it is *dangerous to make assumptions* about faith practices.
- Those with no identifiable religious affiliation may wish to be involved with, and derive obvious comfort from, faith rituals or prayer and meditation
- Conversely those with identifiable religious affiliations may find the expected practice of their faith rituals unhelpful and burdensome

Faith practices have a particular importance around the period of death which underscore the transition from life to death and help patients and relatives make sense of their loss, to be supported through hurt and to provide a framework for dealing with the process of letting go.

9 Koening H. K. et al. (2001) *Handbook of Religion and Health*. Oxford: Oxford University Press; Quoted by Culliford L. (2002) Spirituality and clinical care. *BMJ*, **325**: 1434–5.

Suffering

> The realization that life is likely to end soon may well give rise to feelings of the unfairness of what is happening, and at much of what has gone before, and, above all, a desolate feeling of meaninglessness. Here lies, I believe, the essence of spiritual pain.[10]
>
> Dame Cicely Saunders

This is echoed by Frankl's dictum that: 'Man is not destroyed by suffering, he is destroyed by suffering without meaning.'[11]

Suffering involves more than the activation of nerve pathways and the experience of physical pain. Suffering involves the experience which a person undergoes when their personhood is threatened or damaged.

In the palliative care context this threat often relates to that posed by a serious illness which not only threatens the individual's physical health, but also their emotional well-being, social standing and identity.

Suffering affects people in very personal ways which are particular to the individual involved. How people respond to such suffering will vary greatly. Some will find a resilience to transcending their suffering, others may feel completely overwhelmed by it. In part, the different responses are nurtured by previous encounters with suffering and what methods people have used in the past to deal with it.

Some will focus on accepting their suffering, others will talk in terms of 'fighting it'. Some will try to play their suffering within a larger landscape, in which all of their life experience can be incorporated and in which they seek to find wholeness through incorporating the many differing experiences of being human.

The religious traditions of the world have different interpretations of suffering and have practices and theologies which help people to transcend their immediate suffering through prayer, meditation or other religious ritual.

For others, suffering may so completely overwhelm them that they may describe themselves as 'living in hell'—isolated, hopeless and abandoned. Such patients may need psychiatric assessment to exclude a major depressive episode. For those providing spiritual care, such suffering provides a severe challenge in which words offered in an attempt to bring comfort can sound platitudinous and trite.

Remaining in contact with such patients can be exhausting, as their alienation and aloneness can quickly drain those carers who feel they have a responsibility to find an answer to the suffering.

Maintaining a regular presence and offering the chance of connectedness is more sustainable if carers recognize that not all suffering can be 'cured'.

Less suffering	More suffering
• Identified cause of pain	• Life threatening cause of pain
• Pain can be dealt with	• Intractable
• Short lived	• Reflects hopeless prognosis

Twycross 1994

When I was diagnosed with lung cancer, in the space of a few days everything changed. I had to stop working. I went onto chemotherapy which made me tired, and at home suddenly instead of being the person who provided for my wife and children, they were having to look after me. I felt myself to be nothing more than a burden, no longer fit to be a husband, or father. I just felt that I might as well be dead'

Spiritual pain

Spiritual pain can be defined as an individual's perception of hurt or suffering associated with seeking to transcend the realm of the material It is manifested by a deep sense of hurt stemming from feelings of loss or separation from one's God or deity, a sense of personal inadequacy before God and man, or a lasting condition of loneliness of spirit Spiritual pain has been defined as: 'a disruption in the life principle that pervades a person's entire being and that integrates and transcends one's biological and psychosocial nature'

Given that spirit is experienced, not proven, it may be suggested that the spirit manifests itself through the expression of its needs (Mount 1993)
- Need to find meaning, purpose in life, suffering, death. 'The person who has a 'why' to life can bear with it almost any how,' (Victor Frankl 1971)
- Need for hope and creativity
- Need for a belief and love in self, others and a power beyond the self
- Need to find forgiveness and acceptance
- Need to be listened to with respect
- Need for a source of hope and strength
- Need for trust
- Need for expression of personal beliefs and values
- Need for spiritual practices

Some Elements of Spiritual Pain
Experience of:-
- Disconnection
- Disharmony

- Lack of meaning (why me?)
- Hopelessness
- Feeling of emptiness
- Despair
- Feelings of injustice
- Pointlessness
- Powerlessness
- Feelings of being abandoned
- Spiritual guilt
- Anxiety/fear of God (What will happen after death? Heaven, hell, annihilation)

0 Saunders C. (1998) Spiritual pain. *Journal of Palliative Care*, **4**: 29–32.

1 Frankl V. (c. 1962) *Man's Search for Meaning*. London: Hodder & Stoughton.

Assessment

Spiritual needs can be broadly categorized as the need for meaning and purpose in life, the need for love and harmonious relationships with humans, living entities and God, the need for forgiveness, the need for a source of hope and strength, the need for trust, the need for expression of personal beliefs and values, and the need for spiritual practices.[12] The point of assessing a patient's spirituality is so that an appropriate response can be initiated to meet such needs.

An assessment provides information for the whole palliative care team which allows decisions to be made in the context of the patient's beliefs and spirituality. Conversely the assessment process can illustrate clearly to the patient how important the individual's beliefs are to the professional caring for them. Assessment continues beyond the initial interview, as a patient's spirituality may change during the course of an admission.

Information gained from the initial and the subsequent assessment must be recorded in the patient's notes along with other physical and psychosocial assessment information.

- Spiritual assessment for its own sake, without any potential benefit to the patient, is of dubious ethical status
- Spiritual assessment needs to be carried out using a methodology which acknowledges each person's 'right to their own values and beliefs and to respect their right to remain silent about them'.[13]
- The initial assessment needs to address the importance of spirituality to the patient
- If the patient has indicated that spirituality is a meaningful aspect of their life and that they are willing to talk about it, then questions clarifying the nature of the patient's spirituality are appropriate
- Finally the patient should be offered the opportunity to speak further about their spirituality

Examples of helpful questions in an initial assessment
(Cobb, M. Spiritual care. In: Lloyd-Williams M, editor. (2003). *Psychosocial Issues in Palliative Care*. Oxford: Oxford University Press: 135–147.)

'I see from your notes that you describe your religion as Jewish, can you tell me about this?'
Or
'Do you have any spiritual or religious beliefs?'/'Can you tell me about them?'
'Is your faith/spirituality/religion helpful to you?'
'Are there ways in which we can support you in your faith/spirituality/religion?'
'Are there things we need to know about your faith/spirituality/religion that would help us in caring for you?'
'Would you like to talk to someone about these matters?'
'We have a chaplain who is part of our team, would you like to see him/her?'
'Would you like us to arrange a member of your faith community to come and see you?'

Providing spiritual care

'Having no solution is not the same as having no response'.

Leonard Lunn

Before initiating effective spiritual care, professionals must know and understand their own level of spiritual awareness, which involves an examination of personal beliefs and values, combined with a positive attitude towards spiritual health.

An awareness of one's own prejudices and biases will ensure that clients are dealt with sensitively, and that one's own values and beliefs are not imposed on others, especially spiritual doctrines. Self-awareness helps to prevent forming judgements or attempting to convert another to one's own beliefs or cultural understanding.[12]

In a much-quoted paper about spiritual pain, Cicely Saunders wrote that although work is pressing, patients are very ill and there may be no available opportunity to talk about matters of the spirit, but 'we can always persevere with the practical'. She seems to suggest that while spiritual care on one level is related explicitly to what we say, it is in practice implicit in the detail of care. It rests not just in what is said, but rather in what is to be done. The very word 'palliative' conveys some sense of this. That which is palliative is not 'what one can do when nothing else can be done', but rather 'what there is to do'.[14]

It is instructive to distinguish cure of symptoms from healing of people.[15,16] The words 'heal' and 'whole' have common roots. Healing entails restoration of psychobiological integrity, with the implication of personal growth and a sense of renewal.[17]

12 Dom H. (1999) Spiritual care, need and pain—recognition and response. *European Journal of Palliative Care*, **6, 3**: 87–90.

13 Stoll R. (1979) Guidelines for spiritual assessment. *American Journal of Nursing*, **79**: 1574–7.

14 Leone S. (1997) Pain as an ethical and religious problem. *European Journal of Palliative Care*, **4, 2**: 54–7.

Some Principles of Spiritual Care

Presence: To be maximally useful to patients and their experiences, we must be fully aware of our own biases and distortions

Listening: Listening attentively with genuineness and acceptance.

Facilitate exploration: Meaning cannot be given by another, it must be found by the person him/herself.

Allow for mystery: Some issues will always defy explanation.

Allow for paradox: Conflicting priorities in the care of patients may mean that some questions are difficult to answer. The emotional pain of this needs to be recognised and supported.

Foster *realistic* hope: To give unrealistic hope that life will be prolonged is unethical but there is always something more that can be done to bolster hope in a realistic way.

Create 'space' for patients: Patients need to feel that they still have some choice and control.

Combination: Professionalism with compassion.

Remain in touch with your own spiritual needs: To maintain spiritual equilibrium.

Skills needed to provide spiritual care

The spirituality of those who care for the dying must be the spirituality of the companion, of the friend who walks alongside, helping, sharing and sometimes just sitting, empty handed, when one would rather run away. It is a spirituality of presence, of being alongside, watchful, available, of being there.[18]

- Spiritual care is relevant in all aspects of a patient's care and may include giving good support during treatment such as radiotherapy, providing tasty food and privacy and the opportunity for prayer, or laughter etc. according to wishes. Spiritual need is best addressed by offering practical care in a way that responds to the patient as a unified individual experiencing life and dying in every facet of their being
- Excellent communication skills
- Empathetic and active listening, where the patient is unconditionally accepted
- Being able to detach from your own orthodoxies and concentrate on your orthopraxies (from beliefs to practices)
- Helping a patient to deal with:
  - Past issues
  - Present issues
  - Future issues

15 Swinton J. (2001) *Spirituality and Mental Healthcare: Rediscovering a Forgotten Dimension.* London: Jessica Kingsley.

16 Culliford L. D. (2002) Spiritual care and psychiatric treatment—an introduction. *Advances in Psychiatric Treatment*, **8**: 249–58.

17 Culliford L. (2002) Editorial: Spirituality and clinical care. *BMJ*, **325**: 1434–5.

18 Cassidy S. (1998) *Sharing the Darkness.* London: Darton, Longman & Todd.

- Ability to foster hope and provide strategies to support or restore hope in some way
- A broad perspective

'Compassion is about being with others in their suffering. It is about entering into that pain in such a way that one is no longer an observer but an integral participant.

Compassion does not mean 'feeling sorry for someone'. Rather, compassion is to 'get inside the skin' of the one who hurts, to experience with him or her the pain that is there; to sense a kinship with the one who is suffering.

Before we can be compassionate with others we must first enter our own suffering and extend loving kindness to ourselves.

True compassion insists that we enter into the sufferings of others. Yet we cannot become so absorbed by someone else's pain that we cease to have a life of our own. There is a delicate balance between these two dimensions, and sometimes life is such that this delicate balance is shattered. The intensity of someone's painful situation can be so demanding that it swallows our emotional life for a time.'

Your sorrow is my sorrow, Joyce Rubb.

Further reading

Books

Doyle D., Hanks G., Cherny N., Calman K. (2004) *Oxford Textbook of Palliative Medicine*, 3rd edn. Oxford: Oxford University Press.

Green, J. (1991) *Death with dignity*. London: Macmillan Magazines.

Green, J. (1993) *Death with dignity, volume II*. London: Emap Healthcare.

Lloyd-Williams M. (ed.) (2003) *Psychosocial Issues in Palliative Care*. Oxford: Oxford University Press.

Neuburger J. (2004) *Caring for Dying People of Different Faiths*, 3rd edn. Oxford: Radcliffe Medical Press.

Speck P. (1988) *Being There*. London: SPCK.

Stanworth R. *Recognizing Spiritual Needs in People who are Dying*. Oxford: Oxford University Press.

Wilcock P. (1996) *Spiritual Care of Dying and Bereaved People*. London SPCK.

Chapter 10

The contribution to palliative care of allied health professions

Palliative care has been very successful at taking ideas, values, and techniques from other disciplines in health care. Such borrowing of ideas has nearly always included considerable adaptation from the parent discipline. However, the notion of cross-boundary, interdisciplinary working is now highly developed in palliative care. Some disciplines such as medicine and nursing have become core parts of the specialist team, whereas others such as speech and language therapy and dietetics have been accessed on an as-required basis. Increasingly, individual allied health professions (AHPs) have seen the need to evolve palliative care specialism within the generic discipline. Example of such AHPs include occupational therapy, physiotherapy, social work, and chaplaincy.

Rehabilitation

Palliative rehabilitation improves the quality of survival, so that patients' lives will be as comfortable and productive as possible with a minimum level of dependency, regardless of life expectancy.

The length of survival for most patients with cancer and other chronic progressive cardiac, respiratory and neurological illnesses has increased over the past 25 years. In some patients this is associated with prolonged disability due to the disease itself and/or the side-effects of treatment.

In general medicine, rehabilitative techniques are generally associated with chronic benign disease and disability and aim to *restore* a person's ability to live and work as normally as possible. In palliative medicine, rehabilitation shares the same principles of maximizing a person's potential but aims to help patients to *adapt* to their clinical situation.

Most patients are fearful of being dependent on others. Regardless of life expectancy, patients can be helped to be as independent as possible and to live a fulfilled life within the constraints of their illness. This not only helps patients but also relieves the stress of caregivers. Patients within palliative care settings are deteriorating and techniques need to be individually tailored to the rate of clinical deterioration. Techniques include setting realistic and achievable goals which are determined in conjunction with the multidisciplinary team. These goals must be reassessed continually in parallel with exacerbations and remissions of disease and symptoms. At different stages of the illness goals may vary. It may be appropriate for a patient with a prognosis of weeks/months to set goals for mobilizing with comfort in order to get away for a holiday or to attend an important family event. For patients with days/weeks prognosis, goals may include providing physical, emotional, social and spiritual support to both patient and carers to manage a home death with confidence.

Palliative rehabilitation helps patients to gain opportunity, control, independence, and dignity.

Assessment of potential for successful palliative rehabilitation

Biological/medical status

A careful medical assessment of the underlying disease, and other disease pathologies which may be contributing to morbidity, needs to be undertaken in order to direct treatment to optimize the control of symptoms (e.g. correction of anaemia or congestive heart failure). In the absence of reversible pathology the empirical control of symptoms is paramount. Consideration should also be given to prognosis. In this way, patients will be in the best position to be able to achieve their own realistic goals.

Psychological status

Patients experience many losses as their illness progresses. These include loss of mobility, self-esteem, position or role in the family and expectation for the future. These factors, together with loss of control over their lives, may intensify their feelings of anger, apathy, depression and hopelessness, which will have a negative impact on rehabilitation.

A lack of motivation may need to be explored, to ensure that there are no reversible factors such as clinical depression which may impede their ability to think in any positive way about the future. A competent unwillingness to participate in rehabilitation, on the other hand, should be respected. Palliative rehabilitation offers positive psychological support to overcome lack of confidence, providing goals to stimulate motivation to maintain activity.

- **Decreased cognition:** patients must be able to follow instructions and retain information in order to benefit maximally from palliative rehabilitation. However, limited functional goals can still be met despite limited cognition
- **Social factors** such as family and social support, both emotional (and sometimes financial), impact on a patient's confidence in goal-setting and achievement

Successful palliative rehabilitation depends on:-

- Speed of team response
- Setting of realistic goals
- Adapting constantly to changing circumstances
- Supporting patients and carers through change

Rehabilitation team
- The patient, family and carers
- Medical staff
- Nursing staff
- Occupational therapist
- Physiotherapist
- Social worker
- Chaplain
- Psychologist
- Complementary therapists
- Nutritionists
- Other specialists, according to need

Further reading

Eva G., Lord S. (2003) Rehabilitation in malignant spinal cord compression. *European Journal of Palliative Care*, **10, 4**: 148–50.

Fialka-Moser V., Crevenna R., Korpan M., Quittan M. (2003) Cancer rehabilitation: particularly with aspects on physical impairments. *Journal of Rehabilitation Medicine*, **35, 4**: 153–62.

Hopkins K. F., Tookman A. J. (2000) Rehabilitation and specialist palliative care. *International Journal of Palliative Nursing*, **6, 3**: 123–30.

Montagnini M., Lodhi M., Born W. (2003) The utilization of physical therapy in a palliative care unit. *Journal of Palliative Medicine*, **6, 1**: 11–17.

Watson P. G. (1990) Cancer rehabilitation: the evolution of a concept. *Cancer Nursing*, **13, 1**: 2–12.

Wells R. J. (1990) Rehabilitation: making the most of time. *Oncology Nursing Forum*, **17, 4**: 503–7.

Occupational therapy

Occupational therapy is the treatment of people with physical and psychiatric illness or disability, through specific selected activities, for the purpose of enabling individuals to reach their maximum level of function and independence in all aspects of life (World Federation of Occupational Therapists).

The occupational therapist (OT) uses a symptom-led rather than a disease- or diagnosis-led approach to treatment, concentrating on dysfunction as it presents while anticipating and preparing for further problems that may arise. The occupational therapist assesses various factors prior to advising on a useful strategy.

Occupational history

A profile of the patient is built up based on family history, past self-care abilities, work experience and leisure and recreational patterns. A functional assessment is then made which includes:

- **Self-maintenance** (looking after oneself)
- **Productivity** (productive to life, either in the form of domestic activities or earning a living)
- **Leisure**

Self-esteem

A degree of social equilibrium and homeostasis is needed for a peaceful life, in harmony with all that life brings. When patients are diagnosed with a life-threatening illness and are changing from being totally independent to becoming dependent, chaotic feelings emerge. The natural protective reactions to this assault on self-esteem include anger, resentment, bitterness and hostility.

These feelings are energy wasting, serve no useful purpose and can lead to withdrawal, apathy and depression. Furthermore, carers are inevitably entrenched in this vicious circle of trying to cope not only with their own feelings but those of the patient, who may be continuing to verbalize that their present life is unacceptable. This extra burden and stress can trigger feelings of helplessness, hopelessness, and uselessness in both patients and carers.

People are only able to feel self-worth if they are in a position to contribute, as a result of which they can engender respect in others. The rôle of the OT is to help identify and analyse the cause of these feelings and reactions and to redirect them towards an attitude of positivism and control.

Physical systems

An analysis of the patient's physical capabilities will depend on the diagnosis and the course of the illness. The OT will need to have an understanding of the likely prognosis in order to advise realistically, sensitively and appropriately.

The OT assesses physical dysfunction as it relates to muscle strength and endurance, assessing the degree to which disuse may have affected this and to what extent some rehabilitative potential might exist. The OT will need to be aware of muscle spasms and other pain and what factors trigger them. They will also assess ambulation and balance. The impact of cognitive abilities will also be relevant and techniques will be found to compensate for these.

Locus of control

An OT will need to gain insight into the personal effectiveness of the individual and how they normally respond and adapt in everyday life situations.

The internal profile is characterized by the person who seeks out environmental opportunities and pays attention to feedback as a way of correcting performance. These individuals take a moderate amount of risk, have a basic belief in their skills and a measure of expectancy of success or failure.

The external profile is characterized by the person who does not seek out opportunities and pays no attention to feedback to correct performance. These individuals do not engage in moderate risk taking and do not believe they have skills or ability to control what happens to them.

Quality of life

Quality of life is defined by the individual. As professionals, we can see potential and give advice that we believe might improve satisfaction (subjectively) in the patient and carer and from which achievement can be measured (objectively). However, it is ultimately the choice of the individual, which must be valued and respected, to take or reject advice. A patient may, for example, feel that they gain more by not fighting physically or mentally to retain any vestige of their independence.

Goals

With the full cooperative involvement of the patient, the OT can help to set realistic goals. The goals must be feasible, and structured in such a way that they can be achieved dependently and ultimately independently according to the goal in question. If a patient has always been very independent and is 'internally motivated', it may be very difficult for them to accept having to adapt to different methods of performance and what they perceive as unacceptably low goals yet still maintain their pride and dignity.

Carers may find pursuing goals a burden. They may worry about hurting the patient or themselves. They should not be asked or be required to do more than they are physically or emotionally capable of doing. They are often reassured by being told that they will be taught what to do. They need support from health professionals and other support groups, and advice for the often unspoken, unrecognized and unrewarded burden of care.

Treatment planning

Patients and families are vulnerable and often fearful of the uncertain future. They may vacillate chaotically between objective, logical thought and subjective, emotional despair. The aim is to work alongside these feelings and to raise the level of functioning by helping independence. A semblance of order, structure, purpose and control can hopefully be regained.

Examples of occupational therapy interventions

- Home assessments and modification to enable independence.
  Retraining in personal activities which include toileting, feeding,
  bathing and dressing. Retraining in domestic activities with the
  use of appropriate equipment, e.g. kitchen activities
- Ensuring a safe environment: this relates particularly to hoists and other
  equipment adapted for use by the individual
- Liaison with appropriate organizations in the community for packages
  of care
- Encouraging increasing engagement in purposeful activity. Teaching
  time management and the usefulness of daily routines. Redeveloping
  a sense of purpose and accomplishment to increase self-esteem
- Facilitating lifestyle management with continued engagement in hobbies
  and leisure pursuits. Promoting therapeutic activity programmes, such
  as involvement in creative activities and socialization, while achieving
  individual treatment goals is encouraged
- Relaxation training and stress management. Training in energy
  conservation and work simplification techniques to cope with
  fatigue
- Supporting and educating carers
- Facilitating psychological adjustment to loss of function. Retraining in
  cognitive and perceptual dysfunction, e.g. learning compensatory
  techniques to improve procedural memory during domestic tasks
- Assessment for and prescription of wheelchairs, pressure relief posture
  management and seating. Assessment of muscle flexibility and
  positioning. Splints made where necessary and transfers aided.
  Both indoor and outdoor needs are incorporated

Occupational Therapists define a clear, structured plan of action with the
patient and carers to provide strength of purpose and dignity. Life is a
delicate balance: a matter of coping and adapting to a situation in which
being productive and feeling valued are paramount. The OT is critical to
facilitating a person's sense of mastery and competence and re-instilling
substance and control into the quality of living.

Further reading

Armitage K., Crowther L. (1999) The rôle of the occupational therapist in palliative care.
European Journal of Palliative Care, **6, 5**: 154–7.

Bye R. (1998) When clients are dying: occupational therapists' perspectives. *Occupational
Therapy Journal of Research*, **18, 1**: 3–24.

Cooper J. (ed.) (1997) *Occupational Therapy in Oncology and Palliative Care*. London: Whurr.

Ewer-Smith C., Patterson S. (2002) The use of an occupational therapy programme within
a palliative care setting. *European Journal of Palliative Care*, **9**: 30–3.

Dietetics and nutrition

'Laughter is brightest where food is best.'

Nutrition is not solely concerned with refuelling the body, but has profound emotional and cultural significance. Food preparation symbolizes tangible care and affection and, as far as possible, should continue to be part of daily social interaction. For carers, a good intake is often thought of as a hopeful sign whereas a decreasing intake, particularly as the patient deteriorates, often causes much conflict and distress. The patient may feel guilty for not eating and often forces him/herself to eat in order to please the family.

You must eat up if you want to get better.

Good assessment of factors affecting nutritional status is important. Nutritional intervention focuses on ensuring that symptoms of disease or side-effects of treatment are managed well and initiating appropriate dietary advice and strategies to prevent further morbidity. The aims of nutritional support in palliative care will change as disease progresses. In the earlier stages of illness *aggressive nutritional intervention* is needed, allowing the patient to cope with:
- Metabolic demands of illness and treatment
- Repair of tissue and prevention of infection
- Maintaining well-being and quality of life

Palliative nutritional care, on the other hand, concentrates on symptom control and targetted nutritional intervention later in the disease process, in order to enhance quality of life.

Anorexia (□ see Chapter 6c)
Anorexia is the absence or loss of appetite despite obvious nutritional needs. Reversible causes of anorexia must be addressed.

Cachexia
Cachexia is the metabolic inability to use nutrients effectively resulting in weight loss, lipolysis, loss of muscle and visceral protein, anorexia, chronic nausea and weakness.

Role of the dietitian in palliative care
State registered dietitians are experts in nutrition and are able to translate scientific theory into practical advice for patients, carers and other health professionals depending on the patient's needs. They can be accessed within the hospital or the community setting and work closely with other members of the multidisciplinary team. Their role is to enhance quality of life.

Tasks for the professional advising on nutrition:
- Assess a patient's nutritional status
- Elicit the patient's goals regarding nutrition
- Provide specialized nutritional advice at diagnosis, during treatment and in the palliative phase

- Advise on food preparation/fortification/supplementation as appropriate
- Relax dietary restrictions if possible i.e. for diabetics, hypercholesterol states
- Recommend and calculate feeding regimens to suit an individual patient's requirements, using enteral or parenteral access
- Provide psychological and emotional support
- Listen to patients' fears

Dietitians don't just give out nice little boxes of milky supplements!

Dietary management of common symptoms affecting nutritional status

The common symptoms experienced require a multidisciplinary team approach.

Loss of appetite

- Eat small frequent meals or snacks
- Eat slowly and relax after meals
- If unable to manage full meals use nutritious snacks e.g. baked beans, scrambled egg, cheese on toast, or tinned, frozen or convenience meals i.e. macaroni, ravioli, cottage pie
- 'Take-aways' and pre-cooked, delivered meals do not need to be prepared so can be useful to stimulate appetite
- Simple exercise or a glass of alcohol, if permitted, can be useful stimulants
- Consider avoiding soups pre-meals since the volume may prevent further appetite for more nutritious foods

Sore mouth

- Choose foods with plenty of sauce or gravy e.g. casseroles, fish in parsley sauce
- Moisten food with milk, butter, cream
- Choose soft foods e.g. pasta dishes with sauces, creamy soups, egg dishes, milk puddings and mousses
- Avoid irritants such as citrus fruits (or juice), spicy or salty foods and rough, coarse, dry foods such as raw vegetables, toast, crackers
- Cook foods until they are soft and tender and cut into small pieces
- Use a blender or food processor to puree foods
- Sipping fluids is more refreshing than gulping
- Keep the mouth clean—brush teeth, gums and tongue at least three times a day with a soft toothbrush
- Use mouth washes regularly
- Sucking ice before being treated with 5-fluouracil, other than in head and neck cancer, is helpful in preventing mucositis

Nausea and vomiting

- Cold foods may be more acceptable than hot
- Eat small amounts slowly
- For morning sickness, eat prior to getting out of bed e.g. plain biscuits, dry toast, or cracker

- Keep meals dry, do not add gravy or sauces
- Sip fluids after meals
- Keep upright whilst eating and for two h afterwards
- Fizzy drinks—especially ginger ale and soda water—can help with nausea
- Use a fan to direct away odours, especially in hospital
- Fatty foods may make nausea worse, so grill foods instead
- Check for other reversible causes such as opioid medication, constipation, patient anxiety

Taste changes

- If red meat tastes unpleasant, try chicken, fish, milk, cheese, beans or nuts. These foods are bland in taste and may be more acceptable
- Marinate meat in lemon juice or vinegar to improve flavour
- Use herbs and spices to mask the taste of meat
- Oranges, grapefruit, pineapple and lemon fruits or juices will freshen the mouth
- Cold food may taste better than hot food. It may suit the patient to have frequent cold snacks throughout the day rather than a more traditional three meal pattern
- Food may have a bitter taste—avoid food and drink which contains saccharin or other artificial sweeteners
- It is important to keep the mouth clean—brush teeth three times a day and use a recommended mouth wash
- Use plastic utensils if the patient experiences a metallic taste

Diarrhoea

- High fibre intake should be discouraged i.e. reduce bran, fruit, vegetable, pulses
- Avoid strong tea and coffee which are gut stimulants
- Avoid spicy foods
- Consider malabsorption
- Certain fats may make diarrhoea worse—reduce greasy, fatty foods
- Check inappropriate laxative use

The above includes only some of the advice available and is a guideline only to the merits of a formal dietetic assessment.

Nutritional supplements

In UK see the *British National Formulary* for a full range and nutritional composition of prescribable products.

Oral supplementation is available to assist rather than replace food, but it will not increase weight or prolong the life of patients with cancer. There are many products on the market which range in nutritional support and can be expensive. They should be ideally recommended after assessment by a state-registered dietitian who will select the most appropriate for the individual, according to preferred taste and perceived need.

The challenge for dietitians working with patients in the palliative care setting is to use their expertise to cater for the particular needs of the individual patient whose requirements and goals may change rapidly.

Oral nutritional supplements can be divided into the following categories:

Oral sip feeds
- Some are nutritionally complete and provide a full range of vitamins and minerals
- Milk, juice or yoghurt options are available
- Good source of protein and energy

Fortified puddings
- Provide protein and calories in small volumes
- Useful for dysphagic patients

Modular supplements
- Concentrated source of carbohydrate/protein fat
- Beneficial only if used in conjunction with a diet plan to ensure a range of nutrients is provided
- Carbohydrate drinks are not suitable for diabetics without supervision
- In powder form they can be incorporated into foods without increasing volumes
- Need to be calculated to patient requirements to maximize use and reduce risk of volume overload

Tube feeding
Tube feeding is generally nasogastric or gastric through a percutaneous endoscopic gastrostomy (PEG) or radiologically inserted gastrostomy (RIG) but rarely may be duodenal or jejunal. The aim of feeding may be to replace normal food intake or to supplement it.

There is some evidence that artificial feeding prior to definitive oncological treatment, including surgery, may assist in stabilizing weight, improving quality of life and contributing to better treatment results. There is no evidence that artificial feeding prolongs life in patients with advanced cancer.

The decision to feed artificially requires clinical judgement within the multidisciplinary team and good understanding of the patient's needs and feelings. If used appropriately (e.g. some neurological conditions where proper counselling and discussion have taken place and occasionally in head and neck cancer), it can be useful and take the pressure off patients and carers when eating has become a burden and food can no longer be tolerated or enjoyed.

Ethical issues
Healthcare professionals working within the palliative care setting are faced with ethical dilemmas daily. Decisions should be made with the support of the team and consideration of the patient and carers. In order to make a justifiable, considered decision, the following questions should be considered prior to commencing artificial feeding:
- What are the patient's wishes?
- What benefit will it bring to the patient?
- How much discomfort is caused by eating and drinking normally?
- How keen is the patient to continue eating and drinking?
- What are the risks and discomforts associated with artificial feeding?

Documents are available to offer guidance on nutrition and hydration to health professionals and some are listed below.

Further reading

British Medical Association (2001) *Withholding and Withdrawing Life-Prolonging Treatment.* 2nd edn. London: BMA.

Lennard-Jones, J. E. (ed.) (1998) *Ethical and Legal Aspects of Clinical Hydration and Nutritional Support.* The British Association for Parenteral and Enteral Nutrition.

National Council for Hospice and Specialist Care Services (1995) *Ethical Decision-Making in Palliative Care: Artificial hydration for people who are terminally ill.* London: NCHSPCS.

Physiotherapy

A physiotherapist is 'a healthcare professional who emphasises the use of physical approaches in the promotion, maintenance and restoration of an individual's physical, psychological and social wellbeing, encompassing variations in health states'.

In palliative care, the rôle of the physiotherapist is to reduce the degree to which disabilities, caused by the disease or the treatment, interfere in everyday life. This is particularly pertinent when the disease trajectory may be short and the patient is deteriorating rapidly.

Physiotherapists are important members of the multidisciplinary palliative care team. They may be involved in all healthcare settings in the treatment of patients with any actively progressive condition which most commonly includes cancer, chronic end-stage respiratory, neurological and cardiac disease.

As part of rehabilitation, the specialist physiotherapist is in a good position to identify the needs and coordinate the responses of colleagues working in a wide variety of complementary fields.

The physiotherapist, with a knowledge of the underlying pathological condition, adopts a problem-solving approach in which goals of treatment are planned jointly with the patient. This gives the patient, who may feel helpless because of a loss of independence, a measure of control. These goals must be realistic and achievable for the phase of the disease and continually reassessed. Goals may be simple (to be able to sit comfortably in bed) or more complex (to attend and enjoy a wedding). This is known as 'active readaptation'.

A physiotherapist has a detailed knowledge of functional anatomy and ergonomics, and is able to analyse movement and posture in its relationship to the environment. For instance, weakness and immobility may lead to poor posture, which places a strain on muscles and ligaments and can cause pain, particularly around joints. These stresses may be relieved by strategic physical positioning.

The physiotherapist may be the first professional to be alerted to the signs and symptoms of spinal cord compression due to malignant disease. Alongside immediate medical treatment, the aim initially will be an attempt to minimize loss of function. Should a more complete picture of motor, sensory and autonomic impairment develop, the physiotherapist will be instrumental in helping the patient cope with adapting to a drastic reduction in functional ability by helping the patient to develop a strategy for the future. This may involve balance training, development of upper body strength, instruction in transfers and the use of a wheelchair. Relatives and carers will also require instruction in passive movement, the positioning of paralysed limbs, the use of wheelchairs, and in moving and handling techniques.

Physiotherapy techniques used

Touch

Massage and exercise therapy are core skills of all physiotherapists. Touch is probably the oldest method of relieving pain and discomfort. Therapeutic massage using stroking and gentle kneading may be used to reduce muscle spasm, relieve pain and aid relaxation. Joints become painful and stiff if not moved regularly, leading to the rapid development of shortening of some muscle groups and contractures. Maintenance of joint range is important in the management of neurodegenerative diseases, and passive movements and active assisted exercises need to be implemented and taught to relatives and carers.

Electrotherapy

Physiotherapists are trained in the safe use of electrotherapy. Bone pain and neuropathic pain due to cancer are notoriously difficult to manage. Relief may be obtained by the use of transcutaneous electrical nerve stimulation (TENS) which they may also use for the control of nausea. Physiotherapists use therapeutic ultrasound, interferential or pulsed shortwave diathermy for the relief of pain and muscle spasm. Local applications of heat and ice are also used for pain relief. Physiotherapists provide and fit splints, collars and various supports for weakened muscles, to correct or reduce deformity and to facilitate improved function.

Symptom management

Breathlessness

Breathlessness is very frightening and distressing for patients and carers, making them feel out of control. All physiotherapists are trained in respiratory care and can teach patients and their carers techniques to reduce the work of breathing, to encourage relaxation, to aid expectoration of secretions and coping strategies to improve breathing control. Physiotherapists often help in the management of patients, using noninvasive ventilation for respiratory failure secondary to neuromuscular disability such as motor neurone disease.

Some physiotherapists are trained in various complementary therapies that can be used to help the control of breathlessness such as acupuncture, reflexology, and aromatherapy.

Lymphoedema

Chronic oedema, which may develop in an arm following treatment for breast cancer or as a manifestation of recurrent axillary lymph node disease, or in the legs secondary to impedance of lymphatic drainage from disease in the pelvis, is often managed by physiotherapists. A swollen limb is heavy and affects posture and mobility, placing stresses on weakened muscles and joints.

Gravitational oedema may develop in an immobile, dependent limb, causing discomfort, functional disability, and nursing management problems.

Management of lymphoedema includes using exercise, correct positioning, hosiery, bandaging and manual lymph drainage techniques and skin care. See page 309.

Psychological issues

The physiotherapist works on a one to one basis with patients. Patients often discuss their hopes and fears with a sensitive listener. They feel safe to ask searching questions in these situations, and the physiotherapist needs to be adequately prepared and informed to deal with these issues and to communicate relevant issues with the team, within the bounds of confidentiality.

Walking aids

A physiotherapist can give advice on the use of walking sticks. However, many patients will start using a walking stick without guidance, and the following simple advice can help ensure appropriate use:

- A walking stick should usually be used on the *opposite* side from the affected leg if painful on weight bearing (to halve the weight carried through the affected leg)
- Use on the *same* side if neurological or muscle leg weakness, for extra support
- To check the correct height, the handle of the walking stick should be level with the wrist joint when the arm is resting beside the body
- A rubber cap on the end of the stick will help prevent it slipping

Further reading

Doyle D., Hanks G., Cherny N. and Calman K. (2004) *Oxford Textbook of Palliative Medicine.* 3rd edn. Oxford: Oxford University Press.

Robinson D. (2000) The contribution of physiotherapy to palliative care. *European Journal of Palliative Care,* **7, 3**: 95–8.

Speech and language therapy

Speech and language therapy (SALT) should be available to palliative care teams as patients often have difficulties in communication (particularly verbal) and swallowing. These factors are integral to the patient's feeling of worth, their contribution to and place in society and are a significant contributing factor to their quality of life. SALT plays a pivotal rôle not only in palliative rehabilitation but also in the terminal stages of illness. The aim of therapy is to help the patient compensate for deficits rather than to restore original function.

Communication difficulties

Expressive dysphasia (difficulty in finding and expressing words) interferes with communication. It is seen frequently in palliative care as a result of cerebrovascular accident or intracerebral disease commonly due to primary or secondary cerebral tumours.

The patient should be able to cooperate fully with and benefit from the SALT, if there are no receptive difficulties in understanding what is being said or significant cognitive impairment.

Dysarthria (difficulty in articulating) commonly occurs in chronic neurological conditions such as motor neurone disease, in which cognition is usually preserved, and in multiple sclerosis. It is also a problem for those with cancers in the region of the throat and mouth.

Impairment in comprehension and expressive language skills is not uncommon in the terminally ill, for a variety of different reasons. Patients may have difficulty in understanding long or complex sentences, and may have poor memory retention, poor recall of new information and word finding difficulties. Furthermore, poor breath support and motor control of speech because of general weakness may lead to dysarthria or weakened voice projection, which may contribute further to impairing their communication skills.

However mild, these communication difficulties cause stress not only for the patients themselves but also for the carers. It is frustrating for the patient to be unable to express what would normally be considered as trivial such as 'I am hungry', and emotionally draining if they wish to convey more complex thoughts and wishes such as 'I need to write a will'.

As speech deteriorates, it is not uncommon for patients to insist on trying to continue to try to speak 'normally', delaying having to resort to other means. Understanding what is said may be relatively easy and efficient for the main carer who has become attuned, but difficult for friends who are unaccustomed to the deteriorating speech.

Friends may have to concentrate very hard to pick up a mixture of words, non-verbal clues and nuances only to have to admit finally, when the patient has become exhausted, that they have not understood what is being said. The embarrassment may result in friends visiting less frequently to avoid their own feelings of guilt and inadequacy, leaving the patient feeling ever more embittered, isolated, withdrawn and a burden on others. Communication in these situations often takes a considerable amount of time and perseverance.

In general, patients prefer carers to be honest and to admit that they have not understood, with a willingness to try again, rather than to mislead them by encouraging the 'conversation' to continue when there has been little understanding.

The speech and language therapist can offer advice to carers on facilitating communication. This can include giving patients extra time to understand what is being said to them and allowing the patient time to formulate a response.

- Patients who feel under time pressure to communicate will feel anxious and even less able to make themselves understood
- If it is difficult for the patient to understand complex sentences, these can be separated into simpler sentences
- Reduction of background noise and distractions is essential to aid communication

The therapist may teach compensatory techniques. It may be important to establish a consistent 'yes/no' response before communication can successfully take place. Strategies for 'word finding' difficulties include talking around the subject (circumlocution), the use of gesture, focussing on the initial sound of a target word and writing this down or thinking of a substitute word.

Patients with severe breathing difficulties can be trained to make optimal use of the available breath support by speaking at a slower pace and in manageable segments.

If speech is unclear, picture charts can be used for efficient communication of general needs. These are available from the speech and language therapist, or a simple chart can be devised until a more formally robust one is available. An alphabet chart to which the patient can point may also be useful to spell the first letter of the word or spell out the word.

The therapist assesses the patient for the most suitable communication aid for his unique difficulties. Communication aids such as voice amplifiers, lightwriters with visual displays or electronic speech and other computerized equipment may be appropriate.

Speech problems in head and neck cancer (☐ see Chapter 6h)

Swallowing difficulties

There are numerous causes of swallowing difficulties in palliative care. A speech and language therapist is necessary in the situation in which the reflex mechanism of swallowing has become impaired to such a degree that the larynx and airways are no longer adequately protected from oral contents.

In palliative care, the majority of patients who need specialist input from SALT are those with bulbar symptoms in motor neurone disease and late Parkinson's disease, benign or malignant cerebral disease, head and neck tumours or malignant invasion of the base of the skull directly involving the cranial nerves.

The ability to swallow is inherent in maintaining life naturally. It is very frightening to lose the ability to swallow with ease. Mealtimes may become an anxious time when attempts to eat result in episodes of, or fear of, choking. The SALT, through analysing the unique difficulties of the patient, may be able to recommend a strategy to improve the situation.

- The act of ingesting food begins as the food enters the mouth. The patient may be unable to hold food in the mouth because of a difficulty in lip closure. This can be helped by teaching the patient to carry out exercises to strengthen the lips
- The food, once in the mouth, is chewed and an assessment of any correctible features to improve chewing are analysed
- A food bolus is then formed by the action of the tongue, which may not be functioning adequately
- The bolus is then propelled over the posterior aspect of the tongue, which may be difficult if the tongue is spastic: this may occur in motor neurone disease
- The tongue may be encouraged to relax by placing ice chips in the mouth or applying a cold object around the front of the neck
- If there is a chance of aspiration of contents into the larynx, patients may be advised to cough before and after swallowing

In some cases, if one side of the palate is paralysed, the patient will be advised to turn the neck to the paralysed side, effectively 'blocking' the non-functioning side of the pharynx to make maximum use of the fully functioning side.

The SALT might also suggest other helpful postural tips for patients, and will advise on consistency of food in conjunction with a nutritionist.

The SALT will also advise on meticulous mouthcare, in particular the routine of mouth cleaning after eating, to ensure that no debris collects which could result in an unpredictable and frightening episode of choking.

There may come a point at which the patient is at severe risk of aspirating through inadequate swallowing technique. This needs to be discussed fully with the patient and family and, if strategies to improve swallowing fail, the patient may want to opt for another method of receiving nutritional intake, such as a percutaneous endoscopic gastrostomy (PEG).

The speech and language therapist, conversant in the philosophy of palliative care and the clinical situation and prognosis of the patient, may be very helpful in discussing the merits and burdens of these methods of feeding.

Further reading

Logemann J. (1998) *Evaluation and Treatment of Swallowing Disorders*, 2nd edn. Austin, Texas: PRO-ED.

Salt N. et al. (1999) The contribution of speech and language therapy to palliative care. *European Journal of Palliative Care*, **6**, **4**: 126–9.

Clinical psychology

Clinical psychologists are concerned with the psychological well-being of the patient and family and others in the provision of general emotional care and support. They are not the only professionals able to provide this care, but they are specifically trained to work with all individuals 'across the lifespan' with problems from mild to severe.

Experiencing loss through the death of close family members may be the most stressful event in a person's life. Dealing with patients and their families facing the end of life and the loss of important relationships is a central part of the work of psychologists working in palliative care.

Palliative care has traditionally been associated with cancer, but this remit is changing to encompass patients with chronic diseases. These patients, who are often elderly, may be dying over longer periods of time. This is interspersed with acute episodes of care and partial recovery, requiring physical and psychological rehabilitation, as the illness progresses. This gradual change in emphasis will challenge the Multidisciplinary Team (MDT) to help patients and their families adjust to progressively limited functional—and sometimes cognitive—abilities. The specialist palliative care psychologist is becoming a core component of the MDT, facilitating the understanding of the psychological effects of chronic progressive disease.

Theoretical models and understanding of human behaviour

A wide range of theories are used to explain how people respond cognitively, emotionally and behaviourally to issues related to illness. These are based on the assumption that there are normal patterns in human life cycles which inescapably include life and death. One theory is that changes or transitions may be considered as *normal*, permitting psychosocial development and growth as people learn how to cope successfully with change and loss or, alternatively, to consider bereavement and loss as *stressors*, to which individuals are required to adapt.

Another theoretical model, known as restoration-focused coping, suggests that people oscillate in their styles of coping between focusing on the emotional expression of grief and the need to continue with everyday living; the dying and bereaved can be helped to achieve the balance between being overwhelmed by loss and being able to function on a daily basis.

Direct psychological interventions

Sadness and depression are relatively common in palliative care. It may not be clear whether a patient or family member is displaying an appropriate adjustment reaction to loss or change, or whether they have become clinically anxious or depressed. Furthermore, professionals may be reluctant to refer to other specialists for assessment and management of these problems, fearing that their patients will be labelled with the stigma of mental illness. Psychologists are trained in understanding human behaviour and in recognizing psychopathology; whereas professionals, other than psychologists, are relatively poor at detecting psychological morbidity, particularly in palliative care. They have the skills to encourage expression of thought and emotion in a safe, supportive and reassuring environment and, through counselling and skilled communication, to provide resources for coping. They are trained in the objective measurement of psychological functioning and morbidity, which could form part of routine palliative care assessment (forming baseline and change measures). This would be in line with holistic palliative care and good clinical governance in addition to recent[1] National Institute for Clinical Excellence (NICE) guidance.

Psychologists address a variety of clinical issues including:

- Complex grief reactions, such as prolonged grieving
- Adjustment disorders, such as fear of leaving the hospice/hospital
- Psychological morbidity, such as anxiety and depression
- Relationship and communication problems, such as excessive dependency
- Symptom management, such as control of anticipatory nausea or pain by means of relaxation and other techniques (eg cognitive behavioural interventions)
- Anxiety-reducing techniques such as relaxation training, guided imagery and systematic desensitization
- Psychological distress detection and appropriate management

Working with teams and organizations

Palliative care professionals work in MDTs, believing this to be the best model for the holistic management of patients. However, MDT working is not always straightforward. Psychologists are trained in understanding complex interpersonal and interdisciplinary relationships and the difficulties encountered. They can, therefore, facilitate the process of working as a team. Their understanding of group dynamics can help support and further improve patient-focused care.

Psychologists have a rôle in helping staff to support and contain their distress when a clinical issue has been challenging. They may work constructively in groups, reflecting on the difficult issues in an interactive, confidential, non-judgemental manner. This form of support is commonly used following a difficult death, which may have strained the team to its limits. Critical incident learning and learning from the patient, their family and others are aspects of good clinical governance which can both improve care and staff learning.

Psychologists have an important rôle in clinical supervision, because the psychological elements of care are essential to the protection, maintenance and development of the skills of the caregivers. A forum for teaching psychological skills and providing some quality control over these skills can avoid staff 'burn out', which is high in this area of care delivery.

All professionals should have a basic understanding of good psychological care in order to practise in a way that is not damaging to patients, relatives and colleagues. This is particularly pertinent in palliative care. Psychologists provide high-level communication skills supported by their theoretical knowledge and experience of complex human interactions. The basic counselling skills of the MDT may enable patients and families to find their own solutions to concerns, but a minority may lack the necessary insight or psychological coping resources to resolve their difficulties. Families overwhelmed by loss will be helped by the specialist skills and unique perspective of the psychologist.

Research

Psychologists have research skills, often using tools to measure attitude, mood, personality, cognitive and neurological functioning and change generally. Psychometric tools and other techniques are used to assess the usefulness of interventions.

Psychologists may help to bridge the gap between biomedical research and social science research. Substantial practical and ethical problems surround research with the frail and vulnerable. Qualitative research techniques which circumvent some of these problems are becoming increasingly popular, but can also usefully be combined with quantitative techniques. When the taboos of research in the dying lessen, the prospect of action research in which patients and carers lead the research show promise for gaining future palliative care knowledge.

Further reading

Books

Lloyd-Williams M. (2003) *Psychosocial Issues in Palliative Care*. Oxford: Oxford University Press.

Whitaker D. S. (2001) *Using Groups to Help People*, 2nd edn. London: Routledge.

Articles

Brennan et al. (2001) Adjustment to cancer-coping of personal transition? *Psycho-oncology*, **10**: 1–18.

Payne S., Haines R. (2002) Doing our bit to ease the pain. *Psychologist*, **15, 11**: 564–7.

Payne S., Haines R. (2002) The contribution of psychologists to specialist palliative care. *International Journal of Palliative Nursing*, **8, 8**: 401–6.

NICE (2004) *Improving supportive and palliative care for adults with cancer*. London: NICE.

Social work

Social workers are an integral component of the palliative care team, and address many of the non-physical issues so crucial to the holistic care of patients and their families. It is relatively easy to recognize physical problems such as shortness of breath, but healthcare professionals often make assumptions about what they think is important to the patient. Social workers usually approach clinical problems from a different angle, being guided first and foremost by the patient and family, empowering them to identify and express what they feel are their most important needs.

Patients with terminal illness have emotional, spiritual and practical needs which may not always be revealed until distressing physical symptoms are managed. All members of the multidisciplinary team broadly address some of these needs, but patients may not want to talk about their emotional feelings to the professionals who are giving them physical care. The social worker's focus is on the effects of life-threatening illness on the family system: he or she is therefore often in the best position to allow patients to express emotional issues, helping them to reduce fear and anguish and to re-enable them to feel in touch with friends and family.

Friends, family and partners also need help to cope with their fear and anger at the situation. They need to feel involved in care and decision-making, which is essential in order to avoid a complicated bereavement. Patients, families, partners and friends can be helped to say their goodbyes, to be given the opportunity to heal rifts and to complete unfinished business. At-risk families will be recognized by the social work team following full assessment and offered appropriate support.

A full assessment is often aided by constructing the family genogram, finding out who is important to the patient and highlighting relationship issues. The social network may include ethnic and cultural issues that need understanding in order to facilitate family communication. Strong, unfamiliar and often conflicting feelings can be a barrier to open communication. Rifts within families may emerge and will need managing sensitively, often allowing reconciliation and rebonding of relationships. Barriers to communication can also occur when families want to protect each other from the pain of bad news and the limited future. Families may need help so that they feel more confident about knowing how to tell and involve their children.

Spiritual pain can also be addressed, helping to relieve isolation and giving comfort, knowing that concerns, even if unanswered, are taken seriously and recognized as being important and valid. Difficulties such as body image, sexuality and intimacy may need discussion. Patients rarely volunteer these problems and may need prompting to see if they want to talk about them. Appropriate guidance is needed to help patients and families cope with the changing circumstances.

Practical help involves enabling patients to make decisions and exercise choice, both for practical reasons and also to promote a sense of worth and dignity. They may need basic assistance in paying bills or getting a telephone in the house, or to execute more complicated tasks such as preparing a will and thinking about the future of dependants. It is important to ensure that patients receive benefits to which they are entitled, such as Attendance Allowance and Disability Living Allowance. Similarly carers may be entitled to Carers Allowance. Carers themselves may need support at such a distressing time and can have their own needs assessed to ensure they receive appropriate help. The patient and family may want to know about the law and other social institutions, family and mental health legislation and community services according to their particular situation. Ensuring that patients receive packages of care and help with decisions around placement, if required, are part of the social work rôle.

Social workers seek to enable patients and families retain or regain control and promote empowerment and choice, to help people find inner strength and confidence. Realistic goal plans can be set, to stop families feeling so powerless and enable them to plan for and enjoy the important time that is left.

After death, bereavement support is fundamental to the rôle of palliative care social workers, who commonly work with bereavement counsellors within the team. Families are offered one to one, family or group counselling. Special bereavement sessions for children may also be available.

Financial and practical help in the UK

Attendance Allowance

This provides financial help with personal care for people over 65 years. It is paid at variable rates according to dependency. People with a terminal illness (prognosis of six months or less) can receive the benefit faster and the formalities are simpler.

Disability Living Allowance

This provides financial help for personal care and/or mobility for people under the age of 65 years. The same rules apply for dependency and terminal illness (see above).

Other possible benefits

- Council Tax benefit
- Housing benefit
- Statutory Sick Pay
- Disability working allowance
- Funeral payments (social fund)
- Bereavement payment
- Bereavement allowance
- Widowed parents allowance
- Severe disablement allowance
- Income support
- Invalid care allowance
- Incapacity benefit

Social Services may be able to provide:

- Home care for personal care
- Help with housework
- Occupational therapy aids
- Meals on wheels or frozen meals
- Residential/nursing care
- Dial a ride access to community transport

The chaplain

Training levels
There is no current universally required palliative care chaplaincy qualification, though there are masters degrees in healthcare chaplaincy, training courses for new chaplains, and recommendations from the Association of Hospice and Palliative Care Chaplains. Most chaplains will be trained for ordination or other ministry in the church or other religious body. In-service training is expected.

Denominations and faiths
The religious affiliations of chaplains are intended to reflect proportionally the affiliations of the patient group. A chaplain will know how to access minority religious groups not represented on the chaplaincy staff, and will be able to provide information about the usual needs of religious minorities.

Ethos
Respect for religious positions of first, patients and second, relatives is paramount. Chaplains should cater for spiritual needs and must not create them.

Multidisciplinary working
The chaplain expects to be treated as part of the multidisciplinary team. Communication should occur both ways, and chaplains should be involved as far as possible in multidisciplinary meetings.

Availability
Chaplaincy staffing levels depend upon the healthcare setting in the unit, though provision is a requirement. Most units have 24-hour cover from chaplains, and possibly from local clergy; chaplaincy time with patients will be variable. Some units have teams of chaplains.

Bereavement caseloads
Some chaplains are centrally involved in bereavement.

Chapel space
There may be a dedicated chapel, or a multipurpose space. However it is constituted, as far as possible provision that respects both the sensibilities and needs of all religious groups must be made.

Assessment
Patients' spiritual needs must be assessed initially and then on a continuing basis. Spiritual assessment may be undertaken by any member of the multidisciplinary team. There are a number of assessment models available.

Patient and family care
This includes listening, life review, prayer and sacraments. There may be some hostility from patients towards organized religion, which chaplains should accept. The chaplain's rôle must be non-judgemental.

Families may have technical questions about funerals, access to services and beliefs.

Healing

A ministry of healing is now normative in all mainline Christian churches, with new formal services being both devised and adopted. Healing in these terms is not usually presented as a full physical cure, but as the divine having an effect upon both the human spirit and the human body, and may describe death as healing.

Some 'charismatic' believers will encourage belief in the possibility of miracles up to the point of death. Spiritual healers may or may not be aligned to any religious faith; most have been involved in training by one of the professional associations in this country. Healing and prayer for healing are central to most religious traditions. 📖 See Spiritual healing, p. 693.

Marriage

Institutional chapels may be used for marriages of those who cannot be moved elsewhere, and registrars normally come at very short notice *in extremis*. Those who have been divorced have to take special care to present all necessary documents to the registrar. Church of England clergy may not marry the divorced except in a church to which one of the couple marrying belongs by residence or attendance, and therefore cannot do this in hospitals etc.

Funerals

Hospital or hospice chaplains may be requested to take funerals for those patients with whom they have developed a special relationship. Practice varies between always, sometimes or never acceding to requests. Reasons why the chaplain might conduct a funeral are to continue an established pastoral relationship, to personalize the funeral, and to encourage a more open attitude to funeral liturgy. Reasons for not doing so include avoiding the subversion of community-based provision of bereavement and pastoral aftercare.

Remembrance services

These may be included in the bereavement service events, or be free-standing. In many hospice units there is an annual remembrance event at Christmas-time.

Staff support

Chaplains invariably have a rôle in staff support in the organization.

Education

Chaplains teach, but subjects will vary according to the interests and experience of the individual.

Awareness of different faiths

When caring for a terminally ill patient, it is important to obtain a general outline and understanding of their philosophy of life, religious beliefs and expectations of the continuity of life after death. Such knowledge is valuable if a dying patient is to be sensitively and efficiently cared for. The best way of obtaining this information is by talking tactfully to the patient and family.

Spiritual beliefs, even without a particular religious discipline, vary enormously, and a religious label noted down on a hospital form may have little to do with the patient's past or current ways of thinking. Moreover the behaviour and beliefs of an individual enjoying full health may change dramatically when they become terminally ill and reach the threshold of a previously unconsidered period of life.

Most religions provide both ritual procedures and pastoral (or existential) care. Although a Christian priest will administer both, this may not be the case in other religions. Existential care and comfort may well be provided by lay groups.

In this chapter brief guidelines are set out regarding the care of dying patients of the most commonly encountered faiths.

Denominationalism

Buddhism, Christianity, Islam, Judaism and Hinduism all have a wide range of denominations or variations. They all contain fundamentalist groups for whom the correct procedures are most important and liberal groups who are unlikely to take offence provided sensitivity and openness are displayed.

Religious demands and taboos are frequently found with relation to the following subjects:

1 Food
2 Alcohol
3 Privacy
4 Washing
5 Cross-gender care
6 Touching/preparing the body after death
7 Religious objects.

There are two rules:-
 1 **Always check** with the patient (and/or family) as to their beliefs and affiliations even if these are many years past.
 2 **When in doubt**, follow the more orthodox procedures.

Faiths, preferences and demands

Buddhism
Preferences
- Buddhists may want a Buddhist (or even a Christian!) priest to help with prayer and meditation. With regard to food, Buddhists are commonly vegetarian. It is also usual that Buddhists may prefer cremation to burial
- Buddhists may wish to avoid palliative treatments that lessen either the experience of pain, mental control, or awareness of the moment of death

Demands
- None, except to inform a Buddhist priest of his/her persuasion after death

Christianity
Preferences
- Christians may want a priest/minister of their persuasion for confession (formal or informal), prayers, communion or annointing. In many denominations, lay people fulfil these functions adequately

Demands
- None.

Islam
Preferences
- Muslims may have special dietary requests and strict Muslims will not accept even medicines if they contain alcohol
- There are special fasting times during the year but an ill patient is allowed to eat as necessary. During festivals, routine medical examinations and tests should be avoided
- Women may want to be seen by a female doctor

Demands
- Muslims require plenty of facilities for washing, which is an essential part of worship. The family should be consulted to ensure that the body is specially prepared for burial. Disposable gloves must be used if a body is to be touched. The eyes should be closed and the limbs straightened; the head should be turned towards Mecca and the body wrapped in a plain sheet. The family may wish to wash the body themselves. Muslims are always buried and this should/must be arranged as soon as possible. Post-mortem examinations or any operation on the body is forbidden unless ordered by the coroner, in which case it must be carried out as soon as possible
- Traditional demands for burial within 24 h of death and in the deceased's native country need sensitive handling and explanation

Judaism
Preferences
- Jewish people may want 'Kosher' meals or vegetarian food
- They will probably want a Rabbi and women may want to remain fully clothed and have their hair covered. The religious emphasis on life may mean that the family or patient will question any treatment that could be seen to weaken the fight for life

Demands
- Orthodox Jews have strict dietary laws, and the family or Rabbi should be consulted for advice. At death the body must be handled as little as possible and even then only by his/her children and then covered
- The family, or in their absence a Jewish undertaker, should be informed immediately and a funeral held within 24 h. The exception is during the Sabbath (Friday dusk to Saturday dusk)

Further reading

Cassidy, S. (1988) *Sharing the Darkness. The spirituality of caring*. London: DLT.

Chapter 11

Complementary therapies in palliative care

Complementary therapies are based on the belief that mind, body and spirit are interconnected and that health depends on wholeness and balance between them. This is often called the 'holistic' approach.

Definitions
- **Alternative** cancer treatments claim to reduce tumour burden, or to prolong the life of a patient and generally replace conventional treatments.
- **Complementary** treatments, in contrast, can be used alongside mainstream (orthodox, conventional) medicine; this is the *integrated* approach. However, there is no absolute distinction between what is a 'complementary' therapy and what is a 'conventional' one.

The primary aim of complementary therapies is to provide comfort and to increase quality of life by promoting relaxation, improving sleep, reducing stress and anxiety, relieving pain and other symptoms and by reducing the adverse effects of conventional treatments. Some complementary therapies also claim a direct anti-cancer effect.

Types of therapy
A comprehensive list of all the complementary therapies is not appropriate here, but the following are among the most widely practised, particularly within oncology and palliative care: homeopathy, acupuncture, herbalism, spiritual healing, relaxation, aromatherapy, reflexology and hypnotherapy.

For convenience, the individual therapies to be described in this chapter will be considered under four headings: therapies involving direct bodily contact, therapies involving ingestion of substances, mind–body therapies and creative therapies.

Principles and philosophy
A central tenet of complementary and alternative medicine (CAM) is the strong belief in the uniqueness of the individual and the power of the body to heal itself. The body will always strive to establish homeostasis, thereby maintaining good health: hence the logic that the whole person should be treated and not just the area of the body affected. Individuals are encouraged to adopt a way of life that is in harmony with nature, a view supported by Hippocrates who advocated eating simple, good quality nutritious food, exercise, rest, and fresh air, as well as clean water and sunlight.

People who consult complementary practitioners usually have long-standing conditions or illnesses that are difficult to manage such as HIV infection, multiple sclerosis, psoriasis, rheumatological conditions and, in particular, cancer. The interest in complementary therapies in the palliative care setting is perhaps not surprising given the inherent need for the terminally ill to feel supported holistically, with regard to physical, psychosocial, emotional and spiritual domains, in achieving an acceptable quality of their remaining life.

Prevalence

Prevalence studies in the USA show that 30–50 per cent of the general population use complementary therapies either in health maintenance or for illness or symptoms.[1] United Kingdom (UK) surveys, although fraught with methodological inconsistencies, have produced similar results.[2]

A systematic review revealed that a third of all patients with cancer consult complementary therapists.[3] Seventy per cent of all departments of oncology in Britain employ at least one type of complementary therapy practitioner in the palliative care setting. Most hospices now offer a range of complementary therapies for their patients. Therapists are largely volunteers, although some units are beginning to recognize complementary therapies as part of basic and expected care, and salaried posts are emerging.

There are estimated to be 50,000 complementary and alternative practitioners in the UK.

Reasons for seeking complementary therapies

Many years ago, having a paucity of effective treatments, doctors concentrated on the relief of physical and spiritual suffering. The last 50 years have seen unprecedented technical advances, which have encouraged a paternalistic approach to patients and a perceived decrease in respect for them as individuals. The disillusioned patient body is now recognizing that longer survival from cancer is often obtained at the expense of suffering due to orthodox treatments. Patients now demand more involvement in their care and open, honest, empathic communication with their healthcare advisers. The complementary therapies provide some of these needs, making patients feel better recognized as entire individuals and not just as scientific statistics.

There are multiple reasons why patients with terminal illnesses might seek complementary therapies. It is natural for patients to hope for cure or prolongation of life which, even if unrealistic, may be a motivational factor. Patients hope that complementary therapy will improve control of their symptoms, including stress and anxiety, and facilitate their emotional adjustment to the advancing illness.

In addition, complementary therapies provide patients with a greater sense of choice and control than they might achieve with conventional medicine alone.

Motivation for using CAM

Positive
- Perceived effectiveness
- Perceived safety
- Philosophical/spiritual/holistic/natural concepts
- Control over treatment
- High touch/low tech
- Good patient/therapist relationship with time and empathy
- Non-invasive
- Accessibility
- Pleasant therapeutic experience
- Affluence

Negative
- Dissatisfaction with conventional healthcare and its adverse effects
- Rejection of science and technology
- Rejection of the establishment
- Desperation
- False hopes of cure

Evaluation

Relatively little good research into complementary therapies has been conducted, largely because they have developed without a research tradition, organized infrastructure or financial backing. Furthermore, there are those who argue that scientific measurement or clinical validation is not needed since patients feel better after therapy (even if it is not proven significantly better than placebo in a formal research study).

The negative attitudes towards research in the palliative care setting, which encompass ethical and methodological issues, particularly when patients are reaching their last few weeks of life, are pertinent in this regard. However, this attitude, and the lack of research evidence, has been a barrier to collaboration between conventional and complementary practitioners.

The view that we do have a responsibility to investigate the cost-effectiveness, potential future value and adverse effects of complementary therapies is gaining ground. The provision of complementary therapies in mainstream medicine can only be justified with research backing.

From the available literature, there is no compelling evidence to support 'alternative' medicine (which includes diets, herbal medicines and supplements), as an effective treatment for reducing tumour burden or prolonging the life of patients with cancer. Some patients, however, choose to start or continue with this approach in preference to orthodox treatment. This is their choice. The place of complementary medicine, on the other hand, working alongside orthodox medicine is less controversial. It can be very difficult to design studies appropriate for a population of terminally ill patients and many studies are flawed. However, some well-conducted studies using different therapies in palliative care show statistical improvement in various parameters. For instance, a randomized trial of aromatherapy massage using essential oils showed significant benefits in psychological, physical and global quality of life.

Relaxation techniques, used to manage breathlessness in lung cancer patients, demonstrated a reduction in physical and emotional distress combined with improved coping strategies, despite a deteriorating performance status.[4] A retrospective survey of patients receiving hypnotherapy suggested improved coping as a positive outcome.

1 Astin J.A. et al. (1998) A review of the incorporation of complementary and alternative medicine by mainstream physicians. *Archives of Internal Medicine*, **158, 21**: 2303–10.

2 Zollman C., Vickers A. (1999). ABC of complementary medicine: users and practitioners of complementary medicine. *BMJ*, **319, 7213**: 836–38.

3 Ernst E., Cassileth B. R. (1998) The prevalence of complementary/alternative medicine in cancer: a systematic review. *Cancer*, **83, 4**: 777–82.

4 Bredin M. et al. (1998) Multicentre randomised controlled trial of a nursing intervention for breathlessness in patients with lung cancer. *Palliative Medicine*, **12, 6**: 470 (research abstract).

However, patients diagnosed with a terminal illness are vulnerable and can be exploited easily, and every effort should be made to ensure that they are making a fully informed decision about CAM. They should be made aware of the lack of evidence of efficacy compared with conventional treatment, the possibility that their hopes might be unrealistically raised and the chance that treatment may be a financial burden and a source of stress for the family.

Adverse effects

There is no formal register for monitoring adverse events associated with alternative and complementary therapies. However, reports in the literature confirm that they are not without risk. A report on acupuncture citing 30,000 needle insertions described minor local reactions, tiredness, drowsiness, infection and several cases of pneumothorax. Hypnosis may be associated with negative physiological and psychological effects. Some herbal or dietary additives are known to have side-effects and to interact with conventional medication.

Emotional turmoil in already distressed families can be compounded by patients who either adhere too rigidly or too haphazardly to a therapy or regime that is thought to be beneficial. This is particularly relevant if a patient becomes too unwell to continue with the treatment. Either situation can leading to feelings of anger, blame and guilt for both patient and family which may interfere adversely with family life and relationships.

Practitioner accountability

There is no legislation that restricts the practice of complementary and alternative therapies in the UK. Concerns over this lack of regulation of standards and training together with a paucity of research data prompted the establishment of the Foundation for Integrated Medicine in 1993. This organization is pivotal in the encouragement of research, development, education, regulation and delivery in the UK.

Conclusion

The use of complementary therapies alongside conventional medicine may have advantages in terms of improved symptom control, well-being, satisfaction and cost-effectiveness. This is now seen as an essential component of best practice in cancer care and is supported by the National Cancer Strategy, and the NICE Guidance on Support and Palliative Care for Adults with Cancer[5].

Foundation for Integrated Medicine
13 Sherwood Street
London W1F 7DR
Tel: 020 7439 7332

British Holistic Medical Association
59 Lansdowne Place
Hove
East Sussex BN3 1FL
Tel: 01273 725951

5 NICE (2004) Improving Supportive and Palliative Care for Adults with Cancer. London: NICE.

Bristol Cancer Help Centre
Grove House
Cornwallis Grove
Bristol BS8 4PG
Confidential helpline: 0845 123 2310
Switchboard: 0117 980 9500

Further reading

Books

Mitchell A., Cormack M. (1998) *The Therapeutic Relationship in Complementary Health Care.*
Edinburgh: Churchill Livingstone.

Novey D. (2000) *Clinicians Complete Reference to Complementary and Alternative Medicine.* St Louis:
Mosby.

Articles

Astin J. A. *et al.* (1998) A review of the incorporation of complementary and alternative
medicine by mainstream physicians. *Archives of Internal Medicine*, **158**, 21: 2303–10.

Biley F. C. (2002) Primum non nocere: thoughts on the need to develop an 'adverse
events' register for complementary and alternative therapies. *Complementary Therapies
in Nursing and Midwifery*, **8**, **2**: 57–61.

Bredin M. *et al.* (1998) Multicentre randomised controlled trial of a nursing intervention for
breathlessness in patients with lung cancer. *Palliative Medicine*, **12**,6: 470 (research abstract).

Clover C., Kassab S. (1998) Complementary medicine for patients with cancer. *European
Journal of Palliative Care*, **5**, **3**: 73–6.

Ernst E. (2000) The rôle of complementary and alternative medicine in cancer. *Lancet
Oncology*, **1**, 3: 176–80.

Ernst E. (2001) Complementary therapies in palliative cancer care (review).
Cancer, **91**, **11**: 2181–5.

Ernst E., Cassileth B. R. (1998) The prevalence of complementary/alternative medicine in
cancer: a systematic review. *Cancer*, **83**, 4: 777–82.

Finlay I. G., Jones O. L. (1996) Hypnotherapy in palliative care. *Journal of the Royal Society of
Medicine*, **89**, **9**: 493–6.

Jacobson J. S. *et al.* (2000) Research on complementary/alternative medicine for patients with
breast cancer: a review of the biomedical literature. *Journal of Clinical Oncology*, **18**, **3**: 668–83.

Kainz K. (2003) Avoiding patient self-blame. *Complementary Therapies in Medicine*, **11**,1: 46–8.

Lewith G., Holgate S. (2000) CAM research and development. *Complementary Therapies in
Nursing and Midwifery*, **6**, **1**: 19–24.

Mason S. *et al.* (2002) Evaluating complementary medicine: methodological challenges of
randomised controlled trials. *BMJ*, **325**, **7368**: 832–4.

NICE (2004) Improving Supportive and Palliative Care for Adults with Cancer. London: NICE.

Pan C. X. *et al.* (2000) Complementary and alternative medicine in the management of pain,
dyspnea, and nausea and vomiting near the end-of-life: a systematic review. *Journal of Pain
and Symptom Management*, **20**, **5**: 374–87.

Penson J. (1998) Complementary therapies: making a difference in palliative care. *Complementary
Therapies in Nursing and Midwifery*, **4**, **3**: 77–81.

Vickers A. (1996) Complementary therapies in palliative care. *European Journal of Palliative
Care*, **3**, **4**: 150–3.

Vickers A. (2000) Recent advances: complementary medicine. *BMJ*, **321, 7262**: 683–6.

Vincent C., Furnham A. (1999) Complementary medicine: state of the evidence. *Journal of the Royal Society of Medicine*, **92**: 170–7.

Walker L. A., Budd S. (2002) UK: the current state of regulation of complementary and alternative medicine. *Complementary Therapies in Medicine*, **10, 1**: 8–13.

White P. (1998) Complementary medicine treatment of cancer: a survey of provision. *Complementary Therapies in Medicine*, **6, 1**: 10–13.

Wilkinson S. (1995) Aromatherapy and massage in palliative care. *International Journal of Palliative Nursing*, **1, 1**: 21–30.

Wilkinson I. (2002) The House of Lords Select Committee for Science and Technology. Their report on complementary and alternative medicine and its implications for reflexology. *Complementary Therapies in Nursing and Midwifery*, **8, 2**: 91–100.

Zollman C. Vickers A. (1999) ABC of complementary medicine: users and practitioners of complementary medicine. *BMJ*, **319, 7213**: 836–8.

Group 1: Therapies involving direct body contact

Acupuncture
Background and theory
The history of acupuncture dates back 2000 years and it is an integral part of and based on the principles of traditional Chinese medicine (TCM). *Acupuncture* involves the stimulation of certain points in the body by the insertion of fine needles, whereas *acupressure* involves firm manual pressure on these selected points.

The workings of the human body are thought to be controlled by a vital force or energy called Qi (pronounced *shee*) which circulates between organs along channels called meridians. There are 12 main meridians, corresponding loosely to 12 major functions or organs of the body. On these meridians, more than 350 acupuncture points have been defined. Qi energy must flow in the correct strength and quality through each of the meridians and organs for health to be maintained. The acupuncture points are situated along the meridians and through these the flow of Qi can be altered. Traditional acupuncture theory is based on the concept of yin and yang, which should be in balance: any imbalance (particularly blockage or deficiency) in the continuous flow of energy causes illness. Acupuncture redresses this balance, allowing the healthy unimpeded flow of Qi.

There are many different schools of acupuncture. Conventional Western health professionals relate acupuncture points to physiological and anatomical features such as peripheral nerve junctions. The concept of 'trigger points', whereby areas of increased sensitivity within a muscle cause referred pain in relation to a segment of the body, has also been recognized.

There is no evidence to confirm the physical existence of Qi or the meridians. A possible explanation for the points is that they are sites at which nerves can be stimulated. There have been attempts to explain the effects of acupuncture within a conventional physiological framework. It is known that acupuncture stimulates A delta nerve fibres which enter the dorsal horn of the spinal cord and mediate segmental inhibition of pain impulses carried in the slower unmyelinated C fibres. Through connections with the midbrain, descending inhibition of C fibre pain impulses is also enhanced at other levels of the spinal cord. Acupuncture is also known to stimulate the release of endogenous opioids and other neurotransmitters such as serotonin, which are involved in the modulation of pain. It has also been noted that the electrical conductivity of organ-related acupuncture points is altered when the corresponding organ is diseased.

All organs of the body are represented on the helix of the ear in an inverted foetal position. Tender points in the ear have been shown to match sites of chronic pain in corresponding distant parts of the body. Acupuncture needles or studs can be used in these sites (auriculoacupuncture).

Uses
Acupuncture is used, for example, in the management of pain, anxiety, fatigue, breathlessness, dry mouth and digestive disorders.

Practical application

Acupuncture may be delivered in a number of different ways. In the UK, typically between 4 and 10 needlepoints are selected. These points are often located in areas where they represent the relevant local, regional and distant meridians. Needlepoints may also be centred around the area of pain to boost the local 'dose' to the area. This is often referred to as 'surrounding the dragon'.

In the UK, the practice in palliative care is to use sterile disposable needles which are usually inserted to a depth of about 5 millimetres (or more deeply into muscle). Needles are left *in situ* for approximately 15 minutes. Needle sizes differ but typically measure up to about 30 mm long and 0.25 mm in diameter. It is possible that the sensation of 'de Qi' (pronounced *deshee*) which causes feelings of heaviness, soreness or numbness at the point of needling is necessary both to indicate that the anatomically correct site has been needled and that the treatment will work well. However, this is by no means universal, the treatment often being successful even in the absence of de Qi or any sensation at the point of skin puncture.

It is not common in palliative care in the UK to increase the stimulation of the acupuncture point other than by gentle turning/manipulation of the needles, although an increase in dose may be achieved using a small electric current, laser beams or ultrasound. Acupuncture studs remain *in situ* and may be pressed by the patient as necessary to give more sustained stimulation. In moxibustion, points are heated by smouldering a substance called moxa over the points.

Acupuncture treatments are often given once a week for a few weeks and thereafter as necessary.

Safety

Acupuncture is generally considered to be a relatively safe form of treatment with a low incidence of serious side-effects. There is no official reporting mechanism for adverse events. One prospective study of 65,000 treatments from Japan recorded only 94 minor adverse events, the most common being forgotten needles and faintness. No serious events were recorded (Yamashita 1999). The conclusion was that acupuncture is probably safe in skilled hands. However, there have been reports of pneumothorax, infection, spinal injuries and hepatitis B transmission. Acupuncture studs in the ear may result in perichondritis of the underlying cartilage.

Acupuncture should be used with care in any patient in whom there is a risk of infection or bleeding. It should be avoided in patients with valvular heart disease. Deep needling should be avoided in patients with bleeding disorders or taking anticoagulants. Acupuncture to spinal muscles should be safe unless there is an unstable spine, in which case it is contraindicated. Extra care should be exercised in patients receiving their first acupuncture treatment as they may react strongly, with dizziness and drowsiness. The initial treatment should be given supine and patients should be advised not to drive or to operate machinery for a few hours.

Further reading

Books

Filshie J., White A. (eds) (1998) *Medical Acupuncture*. Edinburgh: Churchill Livingstone.

Articles

Dibble S. L. *et al.* (2000) Acupressure for nausea: results of a pilot study. *Oncology Nursing Forum*, **27, 1**: 41–7.

Dillon M., Lucas C. (1999) Auricular stud acupuncture in palliative care patients. *Palliative Medicine*, **13, 3**: 253–4.

Ezzo J. *et al.* (2000) Is acupuncture effective for the treatment of chronic pain? A systematic review. *Pain*, **86, 3**: 217–25.

Rampes H., James R. (1995) Complications of acupuncture. *Acupuncture in Medicine*, **13, 1**: 26–33.

Vickers A. (2001) Acupuncture. *Effective Health Care* **7**: 2.

Yamashita H. *et al.* (1999) Adverse events in acupuncture and moxibustion treatment: a six year survey at a national clinic in Japan. *Journal of Alternative and Complementary Medicine*, **5, 3**: 229–36.

Massage

Background and theory

Massage is one of the oldest healthcare practices in existence. It is documented in Chinese texts more than 4000 years ago and has been used in Western healthcare since Hippocrates in the fourth century BC. Massage therapy is the scientific manipulation of the soft tissues of the body for the purpose of normalizing these tissues. It consists of manual techniques that include applying moving or fixed pressure, and movement of the body. These techniques affect all body systems, in particular the musculoskeletal, circulatory, lymphatic and nervous systems. The basic philosophy is to help the body to heal itself, in order to achieve or increase well-being. Touch is the fundamental medium of massage therapy. Touch may involve a degree of pressure which is sensitively defined for each individual and concentrated on areas of muscle tension and soft tissue. Touch is also a form of communication, sensitive touch conveying a sense of caring, an essential element in the therapeutic relationship.

Uses

Massage is widely used in a variety of conditions including lymphoedema, stress, anxiety, back and other pain and insomnia. Through the relaxation of muscle tension and relief of anxiety, massage therapy may reduce blood pressure and heart rate. Massage may also enhance the immune system and increase the capacity of cytotoxic agents to work better. Abdominal massage may be useful for constipation.

Practical application

Either the whole body or relevant specific parts may be treated. Practitioners ensure warmth and modesty and may play background music depending on patient preference. Patients may be encouraged to breath steadily and to communicate with the therapist. Oils, including aromatherapy oils, may also be used, depending on the individual patient and the aims of treatment. Massage usually lasts one hour.

Safety

Massage is comparatively safe and there is no evidence that it encourages the spread of cancer, although it would also be contraindicated in any situation where it might damage tumour or frail tissue, particularly in treatment-related areas.

It is generally contraindicated for advanced heart disease, phlebitis, thrombosis and embolism, kidney failure, infectious diseases, contagious skin conditions, acute inflammation, infected injuries, unhealed fractures, conditions prone to haemorrhage and psychosis. It is also contraindicated in the acute flare up of rheumatoid arthritis, eczema, goitre and open skin lesions.

📖 For aromatherapy massage see the Aromatherapy section, p. 684.

Further reading

Books

Rich G. J. (2002) *Massage Therapy: the Evidence for Practice.* Edinburgh: Mosby.

Articles

Vickers A., Zollman C. (1999) ABC of complementary medicine: massage therapy *BMJ*, **319**: 1254–7.

Reflexology

Background and theory

The therapeutic use of hand and foot pressure for the treatment of pain and various illnesses existed in China and India over 5000 years ago.

It is suggested that there are ten longitudinal, bilateral reflexes or zones running along the body which terminate in the hands and feet. All systems and organs are reflected onto the skin surface, particularly that of the palms and soles. By applying gentle pressure to these areas it is possible to relieve the congestion or imbalance along the zone. Specific organs and the interrelationship between organs and bodily systems can be influenced to regain and maintain emotional, physical and spiritual homeostasis. This results in the relief of symptoms and facilitates the prevention of illness and healing, with the aim of promoting good health and well-being.

Malfunction of any organ or part of the body is thought to cause the deposition of tiny crystals of calcium and uric acid in the nerve endings, particularly in the feet. These deposits are then broken down and eliminated by gentle pressure. This is referred to as 'detoxification' which may lead to a 'healing crisis' including 'flu-like symptoms, a feeling of being light headed and lethargic, feeling cold 3–4 days post-treatment, reduction in blood pressure, increase in excretory functions and alteration in sleep pattern. Following this, healing can then begin.

Uses

Treatment may be used for a variety of clinical problems. Of particular relevance to palliative care are control of pain and anxiety (Stephenson et al. 2000), induction of deep relaxation and improvement in sleep.

Practical application

There are different schools of teaching in the application of reflexology, although the underlying principles are consistent.

The foot is treated by applying gentle pressure along each zone systematically until the dorsum, sides and sole have been covered. The practitioner then repeats the treatment on the other foot. Initially gentle massage and stroking movements are used followed by deep thumb and finger pressure. The reflex areas on the foot may feel tender or painful if 'blocked', but this is relieved as the treatment works and the 'blockage' is removed. Treatment may take up to an hour and be repeated weekly as necessary, effects being apparent within a few sessions depending on the individual.

Safety

Contraindications to reflexology include the first trimester of pregnancy. Care should be taken in depressive and manic states, epilepsy and acute conditions. Reflexology practitioners should work closely with medical colleagues, particularly where they are integrally involved in a patient's ongoing medical management.

Patients receiving reflexology may notice an increase in urination and body discharges, leading to fears that medicinal drugs such as chemotherapy agents might be eliminated more quickly from the body and thus be less effective. There is no evidence for this.

Further reading

Article

Stephenson N. L. N. *et al.* (2000) The effects of foot reflexology on anxiety and pain in patients with breast and lung cancer. *Oncology Nursing Forum*, **27, 1**: 67–72.

Group 2: Therapies involving ingestion of substances

Aromatherapy

Background and theory

Aromatic plants, and infusions prepared from them, have been employed in medicines and cosmetics for thousands of years. Aromatherapy uses oils extracted from plants, which are usually referred to as 'essential oils'. These are the pure, concentrated essences of plants, flowers (e.g. rose) leaves (e.g. peppermint), barks (e.g. cinnamon), fruits (e.g. lemon) and seeds (e.g. fennel), grasses (e.g. lemongrass) and bulbs (e.g. garlic) and other plant substances. Fresh plant material usually yields 1–2 per cent by weight of essential oil on distillation. A typical essential oil is a complex mixture of over 100 different chemical compounds which give the oil its smell, therapeutic properties and in some cases its toxicity.

Essential oils are considered to act not only on the body, by stimulating physiological processes, but also on the emotions and the mind. Odour stimulates the olfactory senses and these relay to the limbic system, which is central to the emotions and memory. The limbic system in turn is associated with the hypophyseal–pituitary axis which regulates the endocrine system, affecting reactions to fear, anger, metabolism and sexual stimulus. Pure essential oils exert a positive influence on these reactions. Some oils have an affinity for a particular organ whilst others have a more general effect, promoting homeostasis and well-being. The body uses what it needs and excretes the remainder via the lungs and excretory organs.

Practical application

Aromatherapy oils can be used in the bath and can also be inhaled once vaporized. Essential oils for use on the skin are always diluted by mixing them in an inert unperfumed vegetable carrier such as almond oil, or in lotion or cream. A typical dilution would be two drops of essential oil to 10ml of carrier oil (i.e. 1–5 per cent dilution) for external use and 0.5–2.5ml (10–50 drops) daily for oral use, although this may be diluted further as necessary.

Oils may be light, stimulating, energizing and uplifting e.g. eucalyptus, or try: levelling, balancing and calming e.g. lavender, or calming, sedative and relaxing e.g. benzoin. These three broad types of oil are often mixed, the exact oil depending on the symptoms. For instance:

- Treatment for influenza might include a mixture of eucalyptus (for sore throat/blocked sinuses), lavender (for headache/insomnia) and benzoin (for aching joints)
- Aching muscles and back pain might benefit from a mixture of juniper, rosemary and lavender
- Constipation may usefully be managed with lemon, rosemary and mandarin
- An irritable bowel may benefit from a mixture of peppermint, chamomile and lavender
- Nausea may respond to peppermint and ginger

Safety

The total quantity of oil absorbed into the body from an aromatherapy massage varies according to the percentage dilution of the oil, the total quantity applied and the total area of skin to which the oil is applied. Warmth, massage and applying the oil to hydrated skin increases the amount absorbed. The amount absorbed orally may be 8–10 times greater than that received in a massage. It is possible for small regular amounts to lead to unrecognized chronic toxicity.

Skin reactions can include irritation, sensitisation and phototoxicity. It is potentially dangerous to apply undiluted essential oils to damaged, diseased or inflamed skin and patch testing should therefore always be carried out prior to treatment.

The oils used in clinical aromatherapy are not considered to be carcinogenic or toxic. Potentially carcinogenic oils found in camphor oil, tarragon oil, sassafras oil and methyluegent are not usually found in the range of oils used by aromatherapists.

Patients with cancer are often highly sensitive to the sense of smell, which may have altered due to chemotherapy. Certain smells can be very nauseating, and this should be assessed with the patient before therapy.

Certain oils should be avoided in specific situations. For example, Cade, Ravensara anisata, basil, sassafras, camphor and tarragon shoud be avoided in patients with cancer and anise and fennel should be avoided in those with oestrogen-dependent tumours such as carcinoma of the breast.

Further reading

Books

Tisserand R., Balacs T. (1995) *Essential Oil Safety: A Guide for Health Care Professionals*. Edinburgh: Churchill Livingstone.

Vickers A. (1996) *Massage and Aromatherapy: A Guide for Health Professionals*. London: Chapman & Hall.

Articles

Corner J. *et al.* (1995) An evaluation of the use of massage and essential oils on the well-being of cancer patients. *International Journal of Palliative Nursing*, **1, 2**: 67–73.

Kite S. M. *et al.* (1998) Development of an aromatherapy service at a Cancer Centre. *Palliative Medicine*, **12, 3**: 171–80.

Soden K. (2004) A randomised controlled trial of aromatherapy massage in a hospice setting. *Palliative Medicine*, **18**: 87–92.

Wilkinson S. (1995) Aromatherapy and massage in palliative care. *International Journal of Palliative Nursing*, **1, 1**: 21–30.

Wilkinson S. (1999) An evaluation of aromatherapy massage in palliative care. *Palliative Medicine*, **13, 5**: 409–17.

Dietary therapies and supplements

Background

The rôle of diet in health is of great interest to patients, but has generally been neglected in orthodox medicine. Dietary manipulation, such as decreased consumption of calories, fat, alcohol and smoked or pickled food, has been shown to reduce the incidence of specific adult cancers, while increased dietary fibre appears to have a protective rôle. There are few quality research studies, however, that show that dietary manipulation is influential in altering the prognosis in established cancer.

Theory

The transformation from normal cells to cancer cells is thought to result from successive and cumulative genetic defects. Cancer cells themselves are genetically unstable, defective aspects of malignant DNA metabolism contributing to tumour growth and progression. This genetic instability can be increased through metabolic mechanisms associated with diets high in fat and low in antioxidants (e.g. vitamin E and C).

Radical diets

There are anecdotal reports, although not controlled trials, of dramatic remissions in cancer associated with radical diets, which naturally captures the imagination of patients desperate to find a cure. The Gerson diet is one such example.

Gerson (1996) believes that cancer cells have been pathologically transformed in their ability to digest and exchange proteins and fats, with the result that enzyme metabolism is altered. Proponents believe that most metabolic processes are concentrated in the liver and that treatment therefore needs to detoxify and stimulate the liver.

Detoxification refers to the elimination of any potentially accumulated chemicals including pesticides, hydrocarbons and heavy metals, in addition to the unwelcome products of packaged, processed foods including refined sugars and flours, sweets, caffeinated beverages, dairy products, meats, preservatives and other food additives. It relies on the body's inherent ability to cleanse itself if given the opportunity. Detoxification involves avoiding the intake of toxins, facilitating elimination of waste products and promoting a healthier diet and lifestyle while building the body's nutrition. Gerson proposes intensive detoxification, which is the basis of coffee enemas which are believed to stimulate the enzyme systems of the liver, thereby effectively eliminating the toxins.

Many diets, including the Gerson diet, encourage the drinking of quantities of fresh raw juice, including carrot and celery. Strict diets may include organically grown fruit, vegetables and whole grains with supplements which include potassium, thyroid hormone, vitamins and pancreatic enzymes from organic materials. Salt, fat, coffee, berries, nuts and all bottled, canned, refined, preserved and frozen foods are not permitted.

Dietary burden

Strict adherence to diets may become a burden to the patient and family and for this reason only a minority of patients choose this option. Great effort and determination is needed to adhere to a strict diet, especially if it is not enjoyed. Patients may take the diet willingly or may be under pressure to start or continue, feeling that they will let the family down if they do not do everything in their power to try to fight the cancer.

The family may feel uncomfortably committed to supporting the patient's belief that the diet is imperative to control the cancer. The organization and preparation of the food and associated practices may involve a considerable part of each day and become a burden for families who see that, despite their efforts, the patient is continuing to deteriorate.

Shared family meals may no longer take place, leading to breaks in family cohesion. The diet may begin to dominate family life, altering family dynamics unhealthily at a time when all members need to support each other. Conflict may develop at a time when attention should be turned to quality of life and allowing patients to eat and drink what they feel like. Furthermore, special diets and supplements are often very expensive and may also lead to side-effects from high dose supplements and nutritional deficiencies, adding to further burden.

Since the 1980s, The Bristol Cancer Help Centre have moved away from an emphasis on strict diet and metabolic therapies to a more gentle, caring approach empowering patients to concentrate on self healing and to live with cancer. Greater importance is now afforded to psychological care and integration of transpersonal psychology supporting the holistic complementary approach to patient care. Relaxation and the permission for free expression of emotion and feelings enhances the healing experience and promotes the enjoyment of life by reducing negative influences and increasing positive inputs, while still recognizing the importance of diet.

Guidelines for healthy eating

The tumour host environment depends on a number of factors, including diet. It seems sensible therefore to recognize the influence that diet can have and to base it on ingredients that are thought to promote health. Healthy diets are characterized by low fat, moderate protein (chiefly from vegetarian sources), high vegetable/fruit and whole grain cereals, bread and pasta and other essential nutrients. Other influences may include phytochemicals (e.g. soy products) with known anticancer and detoxification properties and biologically active agents including, among others, vitamin E, A and eicosapentaenoic acid (EPA), all of which demonstrate antitumour effects.

Further reading

Articles

Bloch A. (1999) Alternative nutritional regimens targeted to persons with cancer. *Cancer Practice*, **7, 3**: 151–3.

Weir M. W. (1993) Bristol Cancer Help Centre: success and setbacks but the journey continues. *Complementary Therapies in Medicine*, **1, 1**: 42–5.

Weitzman S. (1998) Alternative nutritional cancer therapies. *International Journal of Cancer Supplement*, **11**: 69–72.

Herbal medicine

Background and theory

Plants have been used for their medicinal properties for many years. With the advent of the purification of plant extracts of morphine from the opium poppy in 1805, the use of penicillin in the 1940s and the increasingly sophisticated scientific domination of more clinically specific compounds, the practice of using plants fell into disfavour. However, the use of herbal remedies is becoming increasingly popular again. Over £40 million a year is spent on herbal products in the UK, mainly on over-the-counter products for self-medication.

Herbalists treat disease and also promote health awareness and enhance quality of life, physically and spiritually. Herbalists use the entire plant kingdom, not just what botanists would define as a herb.

Ancient Chinese herbalism is based on the concepts of yin ('cooling') and yang ('stimulating') and of Qi energy. Herbs are used according to the deficiencies or excesses of these qualities in the patient. Modern Western herbalism matches the effects of herbs to the individual body systems, diseases or symptoms.

There are three important differences between herbal and conventional medicine.

1 Herbalists often use several different herbs together, whereas conventional medicine aims to minimize polypharmacy. The claim for using a mixture is that the different constituents work synergistically and additively, and toxicity is minimized.

2 Herbalists use unpurified plant extracts. Conventional medicine, on the other hand, aims to use more purified substances.

3 Diagnostic principles differ from those of conventional medicine. For instance, arthritis is considered to be caused by a defect in elimination of waste products resulting in their accumulation. A medication resulting in elimination such as a diuretic or laxative may then be used alongside a herb with anti-inflammatory properties.

Uses

The aim is to improve and maintain well-being by correcting patterns of dysfunction which are thought to be causing the underlying disease. In laboratory settings, plant extracts have been shown to have a variety of pharmacological effects, including anti-inflammatory, vasodilatory (or haemostatic), antimicrobial, anticonvulsant, sedative and antipyretic effects. In humans, randomized controlled trials support the use of ginger for treating nausea and vomiting, feverfew for migraine prophylaxis, gingko for cerebral insufficiency and dementia and St John's Wort for mild to moderate depression. St John'sWort could be a useful remedy for mild depression in palliative care.

Practical application

Medication is usually given in the form of tinctures (alcoholic extracts) or teas which can smell and taste unpleasant. Syrups, pills, capsules, ointments and compresses may also be used.

Safety

Many plants are highly toxic due to their direct pharmacological effects, contamination, adulteration or misidentification. In general, patients taking herbal medication on a regular basis should receive regular follow-up and appropriate biochemical monitoring.

A system is being set up to record adverse events and interactions. Some well-known interactions exist which should be less likely to occur with qualified practitioners who take a detailed drug history.

Table 11.1 Chart of potential toxicity with conventional medication

Herb	Conventional drug	Potential problem
Echinacea (> 8 weeks)	Anabolic steroids, methotrexate, amiodarone, ketoconazole	Hepatotoxicity
Feverfew, garlic, ginseng, gingko, ginger	Warfarin	Altered INR
Ginseng	Oestrogens, corticosteroids	Additive effects??
St John's Wort	MAOIs and SSRIs Iron	Insufficient evidence of safety. May limit iron absorption
Valerian	Barbiturates	Sedation
Kyushin, liquorice, plantain, uzara root, hawthorn, ginseng	Digoxin	Monitor drug levels
Evening Primrose oil	Anticonvulsants	Lowered seizure threshold
Kava	Benzodiazepines	Sedative effects
Kelp	Thyroxine	Interference
Liquorice	Spironolactone	Antagonism
Karela, ginseng	Insulin, sulphonylureas, biguanides	Interfere with glucose control

Further reading

Books

Mills S. (1991) *Out of the Earth: the essential book of herbal medicine*. London: Viking.

Newall C. A. et al. (1996) *Herbal Medicines: A Guide for Health-care Professionals*. London: Pharmaceutical Press.

Reviews

Linde K., Mulrow C. D. (1998) St John's wort for depression. *The Cochrane Database of Systematic Reviews*. Issue 4.

Articles

Vickers A., Zollman C. (1999) ABC of complementary medicine: Herbal medicine *BMJ*, **319**: 1050–3.

Homeopathy

Background and theory

Practitioners of homeopathy treat disease using highly diluted preparations of a variety of different substances. The principle of homeopathy is that 'like should be cured with like'. Patients are given preparations that will produce the symptom that the patient is presenting with. For instance, hayfever which presents with lacrimation, stinging and irritation around the eyes and nose might be treated with the remedy Allium cepa, derived from the common onion.

Remedies are prepared by a process of serial dilution and succussion (vigorous shaking). The greater the number of times this process of dilution and succussion is performed, the greater the potency of the remedy.

Prescribing strategies vary considerably. In 'classical' homeopathy, practitioners aim to identify a single medicine that is needed to treat a patient holistically, taking into account current illness, medical history, personality and behaviour. 'Complex' homeopathy involves the prescription of combinations of medicine.

Common homeopathic medicines include those made from plants (such as belladonna, arnica and chamomile), minerals (such as mercury and sulphur), animal products (such as sepia (squid ink) and lachesis (snake venom), and more rarely, biochemical substances (such as histamine or human growth factor).

About 10–20 per cent of the UK population have bought homeopathic medication over the counter and it is even more popular in Europe.

Homeopathic medicines are diluted to such a degree that not even a single molecule of the original solute is likely to be present. Conventional scientists remain sceptical about its efficacy although it is possible that some, as yet undefined, biophysical mechanism may exist. One possible explanation, currently being investigated, is that during serial dilution the complex interactions between the solvent (water) molecules are altered to retain a 'memory' of the original solute material. Some laboratory studies have reported biological effects on animals, plants and cells at ultramolecular dilutions.

Uses

Many different, often chronic and recurring conditions are treated with homeopathic medication. Self prescription for various conditions such as the common cold, bruising, hayfever and joint sprains is common.

Practical application

A detailed history is taken paying attention to the 'modalities' of presenting symptoms such as whether they change according to the weather, time of day, season and so on.

Information is also gathered about mood and behaviour, likes and dislikes, responses to stress, personality and reactions to food. A 'symptom' picture is thus built up and matched to a 'drug picture' described in the homeopathic Materia medica. One or more homeopathic medicines are then prescribed, usually in pill form, either as one or two doses or on a more regular basis.

A patient's initial symptom picture commonly matches more than one drug picture. Follow-up allows the practitioner to define the best medication for a particular patient.

Safety

Serious, unexpected adverse effects of homeopathic medicines are rare. Symptoms may become acutely and transiently worse (aggravation reactions) after starting treatment and patients should be warned of this possibility. The occurrence of an aggravation reaction may be a sign that the treatment will be beneficial.

The more serious issue is the view of some practitioners who adamantly believe that conventional medication reduces the efficacy of homeopathic remedies. Serious adverse effects have occurred when patients have failed to comply with conventional medication. For instance, some practitioners feel that vaccination can do more harm than good.

Further reading

Book

Swayne J. (1998) *The Homeopathic Method: Implications for Clinical Practice and Medical Science*. Edinburgh: Churchill Livingstone.

Articles

Kleijnen J. *et al.* (1991) Trials of homeopathy. *BMJ*, **302, 6782**: 960.

Linde K. *et al.* (1997) Are the clinical effects of homeopathy placebo effects? A meta-analysis of placebo-controlled trials. *Lancet*, **350, 9081**: 834–43.

O'Meara S. *et al.* (2002) Homeopathy. *Effective Health Care*, **7, 3**: 1–12.

Ramakrishnan A. U. (1997) The treatment of cancer with homeopathic medicine part 2: case studies. *Journal of the American Institute of Homeopathy*, **90, 3**: 126–31.

Thompson E. A. (1999) Using homeopathy to offer supportive cancer care in a National Health Service outpatient setting. *Complementary Therapies in Nursing and Midwifery*, **5, 2**: 37–41.

Thompson E. A., Reilly D. (2002) The homeopathic approach to symptom control in the cancer patient: a prospective observational study. *Palliative Medicine*, **16, 3**: 227–33.

Vickers A., Zollman C. (1999) Homeopathy. *BMJ*, **319**: 1115–18.

Group 3: Mind–body therapies

Relaxation

Relaxation aims to release tension from both body and mind. There are many different methods of relaxation, one of the most used being the progressive clenching followed by conscious relaxation of all the muscles in the body in parallel with concentration on the control of breathing. It can be quickly learnt in groups or classes or by listening to tapes or reading guides. One study used relaxation techniques to manage breathlessness in patients with lung cancer, demonstrating significant reduction in physical and emotional distress combined with improved coping strategies, despite deteriorating performance status.

Hypnotherapy

Background and theory

Hypnotherapy involves the induction of deep physical and mental relaxation, leading to an altered state of consciousness. In simple terms, the individual becomes able to concentrate more and more on less and less, which leads to a greatly increased susceptibility to suggestion. We store much more memory than we can consciously remember. Once guided into a hypnotic trance, patients may recall data not easily accessed by the conscious mind. The dissociation between the conscious and unconscious mind can be used to give therapeutic suggestions, thereby encouraging changes in behaviour and the relief of symptoms. Hypnotherapy can be a powerful, non-invasive tool which can be used for relaxation and also for psychotherapeutic purposes.

Hypnotherapy induces a unique behavioural state with a demonstrable neurophysiological basis. Electroencephalogram (EEG) studies reveal that hypnosis induces an altered state of consciousness in which the subject is in a state of relaxation but not sleep.

Uses

Hypnotherapy is more commonly used for anxiety, for disorders with a strong psychological component (such as asthma and irritable bowel syndrome) and for conditions that are modulated by levels of arousal, such as pain. There is good evidence that hypnotherapy reduces anxiety related to stressful situations such as chemotherapy. It also helps in panic disorder and insomnia. There is evidence that it is effective in reducing cancer-related anxiety, pain, nausea and vomiting in adults and in children.

Practical application

Patients often see a practitioner on a one to one basis for a course of treatments which may last up to an hour or so, although hypnotherapy may also be carried out in groups of up to 12 patients. It is possible to teach patients self-hypnosis. Ninety per cent of the population can be hypnotized to varying degrees, the depth of trance determining the potential success of treatment.

Safety

Hypnosis can sometimes exacerbate psychological problems. Patients with post-traumatic stress disorder who are re-traumatized through revival of memories may be particularly affected. False memories may be induced in the psychologically vulnerable. Hypnosis may be implicated in bringing on latent psychosis, and is therefore best avoided in established or borderline psychosis and personality disorders.

Guided imagery and visualization

This makes use of the imagination in order to focus the mind and induce relaxation through pleasant thoughts. Words create a picture for the mind of some pleasant scene, special to the patient, which is revisitable at any time. All the senses are called upon to make the mind-picture come alive with descriptions of pleasant warmth, smells, sounds, taste and associated feelings. Relaxation tapes may contain music or sounds such as the sea or birdsong. Relaxation training combined with imagery may help reduce side-effects from cancer treatments, and enhance patients' well-being and sense of control.

The underlying hypothesis is that physical processes in the body are affected by what the imagination creates and that, with training, an individual can learn to develop powers of imagination and use them to combat cancer. People with cancer who are interested in these techniques are helped to visualize their cancer being attacked by their immune system. The actual images are chosen by the patient, the cancer being represented by a weak and feeble opponent and the immune system by a strong powerful force. Patients are encouraged to see themselves as healthy and active in the future. The image is used for a short period once or twice a day and is combined with techniques of relaxation. Feelings of regaining control are experienced and this is seen as a positive step to counteracting the negativity of the disease.

Meditation

Meditation aims to quieten the body and the mind. This can be achieved by learning to concentrate, perhaps on an object such as a candle or a word that is special to the individual, their own mantra. Concentration on breathing helps achieve this peaceful state. Patients can then let go of the incessant busyness of life and relentless speed of thoughts, letting them come and go until they reach a state of inner quiet, a silent space. The skill of meditation takes time to learn but books, tapes and classes are available.

Spiritual healing

Background

Spiritual healing is one of the oldest known therapies and is used in every culture around the world. It has been largely rejected by Western medicine because it is alien to conventional ways of relating to health and illness. However, since the 1950s, its benefits have become more recognized. Healers work to a standard code of conduct and medical practitioners now accept this form of treatment within conventional healthcare settings.

Uses

Healing can alleviate symptoms and recovery in a variety of clinical situations such as headache, backache, arthritis, wound healing, anxiety and bereavement. It is often used when other treatments have failed, which probably masks the extent of its potential usefulness.

Practical application

Spiritual healing is generally given in two ways, *laying-on of hands* or *distant healing*. In the former, healers hold their hands near to but not touching, or only lightly touching, the body. They focus their minds on being able to help and heal the patient by transfer of energies. Most healers report that patients flush, sigh and relax within minutes of starting the treatment. In the latter, healers send signals mentally as meditation, prayer or healing wishes from a location that can be many miles away from the patient.

Several treatments are given weekly over several months, during which time healing occurs gradually.

Many varieties of healing are available. Therapeutic touch is the most familiar. *Reiki*, derived from Japanese traditions, is also popular. *Shamanism* may include chanting and dancing.

Safety

Healing is a safe treatment with no known deleterious effects, although in situations where pain is being treated, temporary increases in pain may be seen, which may however indicate a positive response to treatment.

Further reading

Books

Edmonds C., Phillips C., Cunningham A. (2001) The focused mind: hypnosis, relaxation, guided imagery, and meditation. In J. Barraclough (ed.) *Integrated Cancer Care: Holistic, Complementary and Creative Approaches.* Oxford: Oxford University Press.

Vachon M., Benor R. (2003) Staff stress, suffering, and compassion in palliative care. In M. Lloyd-Williams (ed.) *Psychosocial Issues in Palliative Care*, pp. 165–82. Oxford: Oxford University Press.

Articles

Benor D. J. (1995) Spiritual healing a unifying influence in complementary therapies. *Complementary Therapies in Medicine*, **3, 4**: 234–8.

Bredin M. *et al.* (1998) Multicentre randomised controlled trial of a nursing intervention for breathlessness in patients with lung cancer. *Palliative Medicine*, **12, 6**: 470 (research abstract).

Buckley J. (2002) Holism and a health-promoting approach to palliative care. *International Journal of Palliative Nursing*, **8, 10**: 505–8.

Burkhard P. (1997) Hypnosis in the treatment of cancer pain. *Australian Journal of Clinical and Experimental Hypnosis*, **25, 1**: 40–52.

Gauthier D. M. (2002) The meaning of healing near the end-of-life. *Journal of Hospice and Palliative Nursing*, **4, 4**: 220–7.

Mason R. (2003) Spiritual healing: the quantum medicine of Dan J. Benor, MD. *Alternative and Complementary Therapies*, **9, 3**: 130–5.

Kanji N. (2000) Management of pain through autogenic training. *Complementary Therapies in Nursing and Midwifery*, **6, 3**: 143–8.

Peter B. (1996) Hypnotherapy with cancer patients: on speaking about death and dying. *Australian Journal of Clinical and Experimental Hypnosis*, **24, 1**: 29–35.

Spiegel D., Moore R. (1997) Imagery and hypnosis in the treatment of cancer patients. *Oncology* (Huntington) **11, 8**: 1179–89.

Reviews

Anderson R. (1999) Psychoneuroimmunoendocrinology: review and commentary.
Townsend Letter for doctors and patients, **164**: 48–9.

Carroll D., Seers K. (1998) Relaxation for the relief of chronic pain: a systematic review.
Journal of Advanced Nursing, **27, 3**: 476–87.

Fife A., Beasley P., Fertig D. (1996) Psychoneuroimmunology and cancer: historical perspectives
and current research. *Advances in Neuroimmunology*, **6, 2**: 179–90.

Kirsch I. *et al.* (1995) Hypnosis as an adjunct to cognitive-behavioural psychotherapy:
a meta-analysis. *Journal of Consulting and Clinical Psychology*. **63, 2**: 214–20.

Curtis C. (2001) Hypnotherapy in a specialist palliative care unit: evaluation of a pilot service.
International Journal of Palliative Nursing, **7, 12**: 604–9.

Group 4: Creative therapies

Introduction

The attitude to and acceptance of terminal illness is influenced by different cultures worldwide. In the West, with advances in medicine, there is the expectation that we will enjoy long and healthy lives. When this aspiration is shattered, it often leads to feelings of loss of control and desperation. Families may be fragmented, and busy pursuing material wealth and ambitions, leaving little time to support their sick and dying members.

The suffering that cancer brings can be frightening, and lead to a questioning of life values which can be emotionally destructive but also enriching. Thoughts may be overwhelming and confusing, leading inexorably to fears of isolation, dependence, becoming a burden and loss of identity.

In recent times medicine has been led largely by scientific thought, but there is a growing acceptance of the art of medicine encaptured by the humanities and concepts of holism. The concept of healing through marrying body and soul is no longer anathema to medical thought. The recognition that creativity can help in bridging this divide has led to the burgeoning of the creative therapy movement.

The creative therapies such as art, music, prose and poetry can be used to explore meaning by symbolic communication. They are used as vehicles to address suffering and to explore inner feelings. Patients and families do not need to have any talent in these areas in order to benefit, although the unexpected unveiling of hidden talent may result in a sense of achievement and personal fulfilment. The therapies act as powerful media for self-expression when communication by word alone is too difficult.

Therapy may release suppressed deep fears and feelings and evoke memories that, with careful and sensitive guiding by the therapist, may be used in trying to help the patient make sense of the situation. Desperation and hopelessness may be challenged to allow a maturation towards coping and adjusting to the illness. These powerful feelings are explored in a secure, trusting and impartial relationship with the therapist.

Art therapy

Modern art therapy began in the 1940s within psychiatric hospitals. The British Association for Art Therapy was founded in 1964. More recently it has been recognized as having a useful rôle in palliative care, helping with feelings of loss, fear, anger, guilt, anxiety and depression for patients either individually or in groups. Disturbed images of macabre, chaotic scenes are not uncommon at the start of therapy. Images such as trees, rainbows, bridges, and other symbols with which hope can be explored, may then develop.

Music therapy

Patients are encouraged to listen actively to music and to the sounds of nature and natural vibration. Therapists may induce a state of relaxation prior to the session to enhance its effect. Therapeutic suggestion through the medium of the music is then used to induce further relaxation and feelings of comfort. Rhythmical, melodious and harmonious music aids the alleviation of discomfort and provides a calm space. Alternatively other types of music can be used to represent patients' destructive feelings such as anger and pain, and to resolve the inevitable emotional stresses. Patients can be encouraged to verbalize or express their feelings in some form so that they can work through them constructively and positively. Therapists may use recorded music, play an instrument themselves or encourage the patient (regardless of their musical talent) to play the instrument, sing or to compose music. This may encourage the expression of conflict of emotions and provide a pathway to some inner peace.

Listening to music can be combined with other complementary modalities such as therapeutic touch.

Further reading

Books

Aldridge D. (1999) *Music Therapy in Palliative Care: New Voices.* London: Jessica Kingsley.

Connell C. (1998) *Something Understood: Art Therapy in Cancer Care.* London: Wrexham Publications.

Pratt M., Wood M. (1998) *Art Therapy in Palliative Care: the Creative Response.* London: Routledge.

Articles

Hardy D. (2001) Creating through loss: an examination of how art therapists sustain their practice in palliative care. *Inscape*, **6, 1**: 23–31.

Hilliard R. E. (2001) The use of music therapy in meeting the multidimensional needs of hospice patients and families. *Journal of Palliative Care*, **17, 3**: 161–6.

Mandel S. E. (1993) Music therapy: variations on a theme: the rôle of the music therapist on the hospice palliative care team. *Journal of Palliative Care*, **9, 4**: 37–55.

Nicholson K. (2001) Weaving a circle:a relaxation program using imagery and music. *Journal of Palliative Care*, **17, 3**: 173–6.

O'Callaghan C. C. (1996) Complementary therapies in terminal cancer: pain, music creativity and music therapy in palliative care. *The American Journal of Hospice and Palliative Care*, **13, 2**: 43–9.

Tyler J. (1998) Nonverbal communication and the use of art in the care of the dying. *Palliative Medicine*, **12, 2**: 123–6.

Chapter 12

Palliative care in the home

The significance of community palliative care—Why is it important?

> The major part of continuing care for palliative patients is provided by the primary healthcare team, whether with malignant or non-malignant diagnoses: such continuing care cannot realistically be the responsibility of specialist palliative care. The reality is that primary care and the generic hospital services currently provide, and will continue to provide the great majority of palliative care.[1]

Palliative care in the community is important. Primary care contributes a vital rôle, which is greatly appreciated by patients and carers, and has a significant impact on other services. Many general practitioners (GPs) and district nurses feel that palliative care represents the best of all medical care, bringing together the clinical, holistic and human dimensions of primary care. They know their patients well, and are in a key position to provide best support for them and their families at this most crucial stage, with the backing of specialist palliative care and hospice expertise, advice and resources. GPs and district nurses often prioritize care of the dying, some claiming that it reconnects them with their reasons for entering healthcare and affects their standing in a community. However, care at home can break down or become suboptimal, for a variety of reasons: poor communication, limited round-the-clock coordination, difficulties in symptom control, inadequate support for carers, etc.

> Good palliative care is appreciated by our patients and their families, and is at the core of good primary care, and in many ways is probably the best thing we do.
> (Northern Ireland GP)

First paradox of community palliative care[2]
Most dying people would prefer to remain at home, but most of them die in institutions.

Second paradox of community palliative care
Most of the final year of life is spent at home, but most people are admitted to hospital to die.

Despite most patients expressing a preference to remain at home and to die there if adequately supported, most patients die in institutions. Disturbingly, most are not even formally consulted as to their wishes. 'Home is the place that reminds us of living as well as dying and is where we feel more fully ourselves.'

1 Barclay S. (2001) Palliative care for non-cancer patients: a UK perspective from primary care. In J. Addington-Hall, I. Higginson (eds) *Palliative Care for Non-cancer Patients.* Oxford: Oxford University Press.

2 Thorpe G. (1993) Enabling more dying people to remain at home. *BMJ*, **307**: 915–8.

Community provision of palliative care services is therefore a vital part of the jigsaw, and affects hospital and hospice admission rates and capacity, particularly for non-cancer patients. As many cancer patients die in care homes as in hospices, so good palliative care here is also essential. Many hospice-based hospice-at-home services successfully supplement generic services. The original principles espoused and modelled by Dame Cicely Saunders, the founder of the modern hospice movement, and others, are being mainstreamed into standard healthcare across the world. From the early days of the movement there was discouragement for the proliferation of hospices, in favour of broad dissemination of 'terminal care' principles throughout the health service, including acute hospital and community services.

Ideally, there should be a means to optimize generalist palliative care at home, so that regardless of the setting, the diagnosis and the possible disease timescale, patients should receive the highest standard of palliative care at all times, i.e. the '... care of the dying should be raised to the level of the best' (NHS Cancer Plan England 2000). 'Palliative care at home embraces what is most noble in medicine: sometimes curing, always relieving, supporting right to the end.'[3]

> I think that terminal care is probably if not the most important then certainly one of the most important things that GPs can become involved in. I feel it's that personal involvement that is often the most important thing.[4]

Community palliative care key facts

- Ninety per cent of the final year of life for most patients is spent at home
- People are now living longer with serious illnesses, and mainly in the community
- GPs have always been, and will continue to be the main providers of palliative care for the majority of patients

Patients especially appreciate:

- continuity of relationship
- being listened to
- an opportunity to ventilate feelings
- being accessible
- effective symptom control
- GPs' palliative care rôle can be optimized by specialist support, especially if there is some formalized engagement.[5] 'It is better to help a colleague with a difficult case than to tell him he is wrong, and that he should make way for the expert' (Pugsley and Pardoe 1986).[6]
- On average, each GP will look after 30–40 patients with cancer at any one time, or about 200 patients per practice team of 10,000 patients, or 3,500 for every Primary Care Trust (PCT)
- On average there will be 8 patients newly diagnosed with cancer/GP/year, 50 per practice and 750 per PCT
- The 'average' UK GP will have about 20 patient deaths/year, of which about five will be from cancer, five from organ failure e.g. heart failure or COPD, 7–8 from multiple pathology, dementia and decline, and 2–3 from sudden death e.g. myocardial infarction, road traffic accident etc

- Palliative care occupies a greater proportion of a district nurse's time, including out-of-hours care, than patient numbers would indicate
- There is less support available for patients and carers with non-malignant end-stage illness, and limited support for GPs managing such patients
- There is a steady shift in the place of care for many patients with palliative care needs, away from the hospital setting into the community, for the majority of the last year of life
- Hospital death is more likely if patients are poor, elderly, have no carers, are far from other services or have a long illness trajectory
- The home death rate in England is low (23 per cent for cancer patients and 19 per cent for all deaths)
- The hospital death rate in England is high (55 per cent cancer patients and 66 per cent of all deaths)
- There is a clear preference from most patients and carers for a home death and an increasing choice of hospice death
- For hospitals, improving community palliative care services will help reduce patients with palliative care needs occupying acute beds, improve capacity and waiting lists, and reduce the standard hospital mortality ratio
- It is estimated that 4000 patients a day could be discharged from hospital if there were adequate community places for them according to the National Audit Office
- Gaps are apparent in community care e.g. symptom control management, 24h nursing care, night sitters, access to equipment, out-of-hours support, and there are concerns that this picture may worsen in future with changes in out-of-hours provision
- Specialist palliative care has raised standards of care and symptom control
- Hospice care is changing: with the average length of stay now reduced to two weeks
- Fifty per cent of patients admitted to hospices will be discharged back to the community
- Improved palliative care services can have a very positive effect on a family's bereavement journey
- GPs and district nurses repeatedly demonstrate they are keen to improve the quality of the palliative service they provide, and they regard palliative care as important and intrinsic to primary care
- In England national directives emphasize the vital rôle of community palliative care

'The care of the dying is a test of a successful NHS' (NHS Chief Executive Sir Nigel Crisp March 2003).

3 Gomas J.-M. (1993) Palliative care at home: a reality or 'mission impossible'? *Palliative Medicine*, **7 (Suppl. 1)**: 45–59.

4 Jeffrey D. (2000) *Cancer from Cure to Care*. Hochland and Hochland.

5 Mitchell G. (2002) How well do general practitioners deliver palliative care? A systematic review. *Palliative Medicine*, **16**: 457–64.

6 Pugsley R., Pardoe J. (1986) The specialist contribution to the care of the terminally ill patient. *Journal of Royal College of General Practitioners*, **36**: 347–8.

Patients' needs

The user viewpoint

You matter because you are you. You matter to the last moment of your life and we will do all we can not only to help you die peacefully but to live until you die.

Dame Cicely Saunders

John had wanted to stay at home as he became weaker. But suddenly one weekend it all went badly wrong and he went into hospital in the middle of the night. He never came home. I will never forgive myself for this. I will have to live with this feeling of guilt all my life, wishing I could have done more.

Mary, wife of John, a cancer patient

Listening to patients

The care provided both in the provision of day to day clinical care at the bedside and strategically in the planning of services must be based on the needs of patients. Listening to the 'user view' is obvious, increasingly important in both scenarios, yet sometimes still avoided. The importance of the views of the patient and their carers is becoming recognized more formally with the emergence of 'User groups' in cancer networks and elsewhere.

How much do we listen to patients' needs and respond accordingly? Unfortunately the pressure of workload and the daunting task of facing sensitive situations that require good communication skills, can easily deflect from taking time to acquire the patient's view. Some assessment tools have been developed to help facilitate this important task, such as the Problems and Concerns Assessment Tools or Patient/Carer Feedback sheets.

'I think that the most important thing is that we must listen to what the question is and try to hear what is behind the actual words used.'[7]

Truth telling, communication skills and retaining control

Patients and carers cannot be full contributors in decision-making without clear information, and if left uninformed, there will be less sense of retaining autonomy and control. There is a common, well-intentioned but misguided assumption, present at all stages of cancer care, that what people do not know does not harm them.

'Truth may hurt but deceit hurts more.'[8] Healthcare professionals often censor the information they give to patients in an attempt to protect them from potentially hurtful, sad or bad news. However, less than honest disclosure and the desire to shield patients from the reality of the situation often create even greater difficulties for patients, carers and other members of the healthcare team. Although well meant, such a conspiracy of silence often results in a heightened state of fear, anxiety and confusion for patient's who may even feel betrayed by such a process which actually does little to promote patient calm and equanimity. Ambiguous or deliberately misleading information may afford short-term benefits, but denies individuals and their families opportunities to reorganize and adapt their lives towards the attainment of achievable goals, realistic hopes and previously planned-for aspirations. Having said this, breaking bad news is always difficult. Skills in discussing sensitive information can be learned and practised, and most areas run communication skills learning, now an integral part of the Supportive and Palliative Care Guidance in England.

As the Age Concern 12 Principles of a Good Death confirms in 8 out of 12 assertions, retaining control is a vital element for patients, and our rôle should be more to enable than to instruct, ever respectful of the boundaries set by our patients.

Age Concern 12 principles of good death[9]

1 To be able to retain **control** of what happens
2 To have **control** over pain relief and other symptom control
3 To have **choice and control** over where death occurs (at home or elsewhere)
4 To have **access** to hospice care in any location, not only in hospital
5 To have **control** over who is present and who shares the end
6 To be able to issue **Advance Directives** which ensure wishes are respected
7 To know when death is coming, and to understand what can be expected
8 To be afforded dignity and privacy
9 To have **access** to information and expertise of whatever kind is necessary
10 To have **access** to any spiritual or emotional support required
11 To have time to say goodbye, and **control** over other aspects of timing
12 To be able to leave when it is time to go, and not to have life prolonged pointlessly.

Preferred place of death

Asking and noting where patients would like to be cared for in their dying phase is a very significant step towards the tailoring of services to meet patient preferences and needs. This is a key issue in developing a real sense of choice, maintaining some control and self-determination in a world seemingly turned upside down for patients and their carers. The literature confirms that where someone has been asked about preference for place of care it is more likely to be attained, and choice of place of death is increasingly seen now as a patient's right. However, many may express a preference for home or hospice care, but are currently unable to achieve this. Carers are our patients in primary care and also have their own needs, as the toll of caring for the dying patient may be considerable.[10]

Patient needs

We all have needs, whether acknowledged or not. In 1943[11] Maslow proposed that we are all motivated by our wish continually to satisfy our needs. He commented that there were at least five sets of goals which he called basic needs. Briefly, these are:

1 Physiological (food, sleep, warmth, health)
2 Safety (security, protection from threats)

7 Clark D. (2002) *Cicely Saunders, Founder of the Hospice Movement—selected letters 1959–1999.* Oxford: Oxford University Press.

8 Fallowfield L. J., Jenkins V. A., Beveridge H. A. (2002) Truth may hurt but deceit hurts more: communication in palliative care. *Palliative Medicine.* **16**: 297–303.

9 Henwood M. (1999) *The Future of Health and Care of Older People.* London: Age Concern.

10 Simon C. (2001) Informal carers and the primary care team. *British Journal of General Practice,* **51**: 920–3.

11 Maslow A. H. (1943) A theory of human motivation. *Psychological Review,* **50**: 370–96.

3 Social (belonging, association, acceptance, friendship, love)
4 Esteem (self-respect, reputation, status, recognition)
5 Self-actualization (personal growth, accomplishment, creativity, achievement of potential).

Maslow described a hierarchy of needs to show that at any moment we concentrate almost exclusively on one of our unmet needs. We do not bother much about our social status if we are starving. Once the most immediate need is fairly well satisfied we are impelled to move on to the next most pressing need. Patients recently diagnosed with cancer find themselves returned starkly to the bottom of Maslow's hierarchy, to the level of the need to survive.

Dying is not just a physical or medical journey, it is essentially a human one, common to us all: something of metaphysical or spiritual significance set within a cultural context. If we as healthcare professionals can fully support our patients in the first two stages of the hierarchy above, i.e. as far as possible maintain comfort, freedom from symptoms and provide a sense of security and support, then patients are more likely to be able to proceed with other stages of the journey towards greater depths of relationships, self-acceptance and spiritual peace. By alleviating symptoms and reducing fear we create the space for people to travel. Our prime business is to play our rôle within the medical context; hence maintaining patients symptom free, secure, supported and enabled to die in the place of choice. These are three of the goals of the Gold Standards Framework.

> The essential concept is that the doctor, or at least the practice, will stay firmly with the patient and relative at their time of need and not desert them … When a patient is dying at home, it makes a big difference if the doctor continues to call regularly … otherwise patient and family are likely to feel abandoned and deserted when they least expect it … The promise of a regular visit gives a special kind of support unlike any other.[12]

What do patients and carers want from the services?

1 *Being treated as a human being.* People want to be treated as individuals, and with dignity and respect
2 *Empowerment.* The ability to have their voice heard, to be valued for their knowledge and skills, and to exercise real choice about treatments and services are central to patients' and carers' wishes
3 *Information.* Patients and carers should receive all the information they want about their condition and possible treatment. It should be given in an honest, timely and sensitive manner
4 *Having choice.* Patients and carers want to know what options are available to them from the NHS, voluntary and private sectors, including access to self-help and support groups and complementary therapy services
5 *Continuity of care.* Good communication and coordination of services between health and social care professionals working across the NHS and social sectors is essential
6 *Equal access.* People want access to services of similar quality wherever they are delivered

7 *Meeting physical needs.* Physical symptoms must be managed to a degree acceptable to patients

8 *Meeting psychological needs.* Patients and carers need emotional support from professionals who are prepared to listen to them and are capable of understanding their concerns

9 *Meeting social needs.* Support for the family, advice on financial and employment issues and provision of transport are necessary

10 *Meeting spiritual needs.* Patients and carers should have support to help them explore the spiritual issues important to them.

(From *Cancerlink* survey)

Examples of needs-based predicting and fulfilling needs

Two examples of refocusing and structuring care around patients' needs are:

- **The Seven Promises**, produced in the USA by Joanne Lynn, President of ABCD (Americans for Better Care of the Dying) and co-director of the Institute of Healthcare Improvements Breakthrough Series
- **Summary of suggested needs-based care**, which was the basis of the development of the Gold Standards Framework in the UK

Lynn, writing about the current position of end-of-life care in the USA, asks why do we feel 'lucky' if things go well in the final stages of life, in an age when we are surrounded by highly complex and sophisticated innovations that we take for granted at any other stage?

Ask any American about the death of a family member or friend and you will usually hear a sad tale of pain, fear, confusion, along with a mismatch of services offered and services needed. Less often, you will hear about a decent close of life, one that included appropriate and respectful healthcare, time with family and friends and support from the community. Even so, that good story will have a strange conclusion: 'Weren't we lucky!' How odd! We don't attribute good conclusions from other important events to luck—we know that airplanes land safely and patients wake up after surgery because lots of people do their jobs well, in systems designed to help people do their jobs well. Yet, we accept almost without question that the last few months or years of life—when we are most often chronically ill, dependent and frail—will be miserable. Should our final days be comfortable only with good luck?

How did we come to do so poorly on care at the end-of-life? A fundamental reason is we have simply never been here before. We face problems our grandparents would envy—the problems that come from growing quite old and dying rather slowly ... So what will we need when we have to live with eventually fatal chronic disease? More than anything else we need reliability. We need a care system we can count on. To make excellent care routine we must learn to do routinely what we already know must be done ... All it takes is innovation, learning, reorganisation and commitment. People should not expect end-of-life care to be miserable and meaningless... we should get good care for our expense without having to hope for good luck.[13]

---

12 Brewin T. (2001) Personal view: deserted. *BMJ*, **322**: 117.

13 Accelerating Change Today (2000) *Promises to keep.* Boston: The National Coalition on Health Care and the Institute for Healthcare Improvement.

The Seven Promises—a vision of a better system

For patients with advanced stages of serious illnesses, it is not possible to promise cure or restoration of health. However, here are seven promises that really seem to make a difference to such patients. In each case, we define the promise, its core statement, and list a few examples of what it might mean to put practices in place to deliver on that promise.

1 Good medical treatment
   - You will have the best of medical treatment, aiming to prevent exacerbation, improve function and survival, and ensure comfort
   - Patients will be offered proven diagnosis and treatment strategies to prevent exacerbations and enhance quality of life, as well as to delay disease progression and death
   - Medical intervention will be in accord with best available standards of medical practice and evidence-based when possible

2 Never overwhelmed by symptoms
   - You will never have to endure overwhelming pain, shortness of breath or other symptoms
   - Symptoms will be anticipated and prevented when possible, evaluated and addressed promptly and controlled effectively
   - Severe symptoms, such as shortness of breath, will be treated as emergencies
   - Sedation will be used when necessary to relieve intractable symptoms near the end-of-life

3 Continuity, coordination and comprehensiveness
   - Your care will be continuous, comprehensive and coordinated
   - Patients and families can count on having certain professionals to rely upon at all times
   - Patients and families can count on an appropriate and timely response to their needs
   - Transitions between services, settings and personnel will be minimized in number and made to work smoothly

4 Well-prepared—no surprises
   - You and your family will be prepared for everything that is likely to happen in the course of your illness
   - Patients and families come to know what to expect as the illness worsens, and what is expected of them
   - Patients and families receive supplies and training needed to handle predictable events

5 Customized care, reflecting your preference
   - Your wishes will be sought and respected, and followed wherever possible
   - Patients and families come to know the alternatives for services and expect to make choices that matter
   - Patients never receive treatments they refuse
   - Patients who want to live out the end of their life at home, usually can

6 Use of patient and family resources—financial, emotional and practical
   - We will help you and your family to consider your personal and financial resources, and we will respect your choices about the use of your resources
   - Patients and families will be aware of services available in their community and the costs of those services

- Family caregivers' concerns will be discussed and addressed
- Respite, volunteer and home aid care will be part of the care plan when appropriate

7 Make the best of every day
- We will do all we can to see that you and your family will have the opportunity to make the best of every day
- The patient is treated as a person, not a disease, and what is important to the patient is important to the care team
- The care team responds to the physical, psychological, social and spiritual needs of the patient and family. Families are supported before, during and after the patient's death

Table 12.1 Summary of suggested needs-based care—for the Gold Standards Framework

Need	Outcome	Process		Structure
Hierarchy of need of patient (after Maslow)	Patient feeling—'inner' dimension	Provision—'outer' determinant		Practical measure—examples of suggested means or intervention
1 Physiological	Comfort Health Functioning body	Symptom relief—free of physical symptoms		Assessment-physical Specialist advice out-of-hours palliative care and access to 24h DNs SC Register—identification
2 Safety	Security and support Lack of fear + anxiety Protected from threats	Emotional support Information Continuity of care Practical support Anticipatory care Financial help		Assessment—psychosocial/holistic Information out-of-hours Protocol access to key person Equal access to resources+equipment SC Register—identification PHCT planning and co-ordination Financial + benefits advice

3 Social	Love Belonging Acceptance Harmonious relationships	Supportive, loving relationships Dealing with emotions	Active listening Communication skills Information Family dynamics and carer support
4 Esteem	Dignity Self respect Feeling good about themselves	Control, choice, confidentiality Respect Humane treatment Empowerment Being valued Truth and honesty	Consultation Information e.g. Home pack Agenda-sharing Patient Review sheets in Home Pack
5 Self-actualization	Spiritual peace Personal growth Inner calm	Acceptance Finding meaning Hope, wisdom Dealing with inner fears and all of the above	Time, prayer Supportive relationship Spiritual needs addressed, religious support and all of the above

SC = Supportive Care
PHCT = Primary Healthcare Team

Barriers to community palliative care

The care of all dying patients must improve to the level of the best.
The NHS Cancer Plan, DOH, September 2000

Palliative care is a barometer for all our other care... and we only have one chance to get it right.

DN Liverpool

Several studies confirm that GPs, district nurses and other community professionals prioritize care of the dying. Yet, despite this high priority, service provision can be less than optimal. This may be due to lack of communication, poor team working, out-of-hours factors, limited carer support or difficulties with symptom control. But commonly the major problem is that the different instruments in the orchestra are not playing together.

The challenge is to orchestrate the service so that the patient and carers feel enveloped in professional, seamless, supportive care allowing them 'a good death' in the place of their choice.

Current gaps in community palliative care provision include (key factors in **bold**):
1 Clinical competence
   • Assessment of symptoms and diagnostic skills
   • **Symptom control** and drug usage
   • When to refer or seek help
2 Organizational
   • Communication and information transfer
   • Access to other support—social care and **carer support**
   • Continuity including **out-of-hours**
   • Primary care issues—workforce, time and workload
   • **Teamwork** and co-working with specialists
3 Human dimension
   • Patient **control**, autonomy and choice
   • **Supportive care**
   • Listening to deeper underlying needs and spiritual reflections

Specific issues

• **Rôle of the primary healthcare teams.** Primary care teams play a pivotal rôle in the delivery and coordination of care. Using a framework to increase consistency of standards and formalize good practice ensures fewer patients 'slip through the net'. District nurses play a crucial rôle in needs assessment, the development of a therapeutic relationship and are well placed to liaise across the boundaries of care between community and inpatient services
• The main barriers to effective community palliative care however, are lack of an organized system or plan of care, communication and team working issues, out-of-hours care, carer support, good symptom control and effective involvement of specialists

- **Out-of-hours palliative care and 24h district nurses.** The out-of-hours gap in provision can cause significant breakdown in home care and inappropriate crisis admissions to hospitals. Anticipatory planning along with better access to information (e.g. via a handover form), drugs left in the home or carried by the on-call provider (as in palliative care bags held by GP cooperatives) and better access to support at home and specialist advise, can prevent many crises. Lack of out-of-hours district nursing is an important issue and is a first step to improving community palliative care. More terminally ill patients are kept at home where there is 24h district nursing availability
- **The social care of patient and carer at home** is seen consistently as one of the key factors that will prevent institutionalization of care, as confirmed in the literature and the experience of professionals. So the availability and coordination of night sitters, Marie Curie nurses, social services input, rapid response teams etc. play a vital rôle in maintaining home care. This is sometimes overlooked in the strategic planning of services. Well functioning co-operation between healthcare and social services is crucial, with continuing care funds or their equivalent, carer assessments, non-medical support, respite care, carer support groups, grants and financial advice being of vital importance
- **Preferred place of care.** Care customized to patient need is another crucial factor, and one vital element of this is choice over where a person wishes to be in their final days. Most people would chose to remain at home to die but this is less likely to occur with some groups of patients, particularly the poor, the elderly, women etc. *Asking and recording the patient's preferred place of death/care has been shown to makes this more likely to be fulfilled. This requires time, good communication skills and a trusting relationship with the patient and carers.* Good use of assessment tools, discussion with the patient and family of their management plans (a 'death plan' in a similar manner to a 'birth plan' in obstetrics), Advance Directives, discussion of 'Do Not Resuscitate' (DNR) decisions (and informing of ambulance staff), route-maps of likely options. These all help to involve patients and families in decisions, enabling some retention of control and self-determination. With better planning and communication, this may also prevent some disasters e.g. emergency calls, failed attempted resuscitations in the ambulance or inappropriate coroner's cases
- **Specialist palliative care and effective symptom control.** There is a need for specialists to work effectively with generalists and there are many good examples of this working well in the UK. Clear referral criteria and regular formalized contact at primary care team meetings, plus availability of telephone advice, can enable more effective working relationships. Symptom control in the community can be difficult, so supportive relationships with specialists helps, along with targeted education programmes, better assessment tools, and agreed guidelines
- **Communication and transfer of information.** Poor organization in this area can create an unbridgeable chasm for all involved, reducing patients' confidence in their professional carers and adding stress to staff. Several factors have been shown to improve information transfer:
  - Using practice registers
  - Handover forms for out-of-hours providers

- Patient held records or medication cards, electronic transfer of information
- Ensuring patients and carers have written information at home to consult when problems arise
- Home packs (potentially needed medication and equipment)
- **Non-cancer patients.** There is less access to services for patents with non-malignant disease than that for cancer patients. GPs will have as many patients dying from organ failure, e.g. heart failure or COPD, as from cancer and yet the disease trajectory is less predictable and the end-stages harder to recognize. Crisis hospital admissions are more frequent, yet there is less specialist involvement or access to supportive cancer-related services such as Marie Curie or Macmillan nurses. Those dying from chronic 'multiple pathology' illnesses causing general decline or dementia may be disadvantaged further. The learning gained from cancer patients may be transferred to care for other end-stage illnesses (as in the Gold Standards Framework) and there is increasing recognition that patients with other end-stage illnesses should be able to benefit from palliative care symptom control, advice, and services
- **Other care settings.** Some patients dying in other settings may be significantly disadvantaged, as they currently do not benefit from specialist palliative care services or even from the generic skills of generalists within the primary care teams. Provision for good palliative care in other settings therefore needs to be included in the area-wide strategic plan, e.g. in care homes, private hospitals, prisons and community hospitals

Improving community palliative care—the Gold Standards Framework

Increasingly within primary care there are agreed protocols of care, just as in the management of patients with other conditions such as diabetes or hypertension. Often however there are no such systems for the effective organization of care for the most seriously ill patients nearing the end-of-life. Not every patient has diabetes or hypertension, yet every one of our patients eventually dies. There is a need to formalize a model of good care to ensure that every dying patient receives top quality care. Hospices and palliative care specialists have largely led the way in this, but this needs also to be mainstreamed into generalist care, to encompass all dying patients. In primary care, the use of a framework such as the Gold Standards Framework in community palliative care can bridge this gap, but can also enable local ownership and release the creativity of the staff to respond to the needs of patients relevant to their area.

In our team, we didn't have a system of care before for dying patients so sometimes patients would slip through the net—now we do, and we all feel better for it, patients and their families, as well as doctors and nurses.

District nurse

Developing a system-best care for every patient every time

It is said that care should be:

- Knowledge-based—best science, best practice, best evidence
- Systems minded—*co-operation across boundaries, working at systems delivery*
- Patient centred—*put patients in control of care, ACTIVELY customize care to patients' needs*[14,15]

In other words:

1 **Clinical competence**—*knowledge-based* e.g. assessment and diagnostic skills, knowledge of what to do, which treatments to use, when to refer, symptom control etc. the 'what to do'—the head.
   Response: Education and training, audit etc

2 **Good organization**—*systems minded* protocols/processes /systems, e.g. communication and information transfer, accessing other support, coordination and continuity out-of-hours, workload issues and managed systems of care—the 'how to do it'—the hands
   Response: improve system—e.g. Gold Standards Framework

3 Affirmation of **the human dimension of care**, including the commitment to improve the patient experience of care, compassion, preserving patient dignity, patient and carer autonomy/choice, 'loving medicine' the 'why' we do it—the heart
   Response: e.g. patient/carer involvement, needs focussed, preferred place of care etc.

We need all three elements—focusing purely on education will miss the importance of developing practical systems or protocols leading to continuous quality improvements.

We know what we'd like to do—but it doesn't always seem to happen.

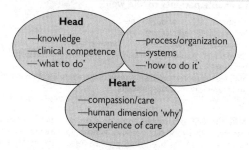

Fig. 12.1 The head, hands and heart of palliative care

It is most often the systems organization or 'hands' that let us down.

The Gold Standards Framework in community palliative care[16]

The Gold Standards Framework (GSF)

The aim of the Gold Standards Framework is to develop a practice based system to improve and optimise the organisation and quality of supportive/palliative care for patients in their last 6–12 months of life.

GSF is cited as an example of a generalist community framework in the Improving Supportive and Palliative Care for Adults with Cancer guidance[17] and is currently being used extensively across the UK to improve primary palliative care.

There are three central processes of GSF, all of which involve improved communication.

1 **Identify** the key group of patients i.e. using a register
2 **Assess** their main needs, both physical and psychosocial, and that of the carers
3 **Plan** ahead for problems, including out-of-hours—move from *reactive* to *proactive* care by anticipation and prevention

14 Berwick D. (2002) A Users Manual for the IOM's Quality Chasm Report. *Health Affairs*, **21**: 30: 80.

15 Berwick D., Nolan T. (1998) Understanding medical systems. *Ann Intern Med*, **128**: 293–8.

16 Thomas K. (2003) *Caring for the Dying at home: Companions on the journey.* Oxford: Radcliffe Medical Press. Or contact gsf@macmillan.org.uk

17 NICE (2004) *Improving supportive and palliative care for adults with cancer.* London: NICE.

The five goals of the Gold Standards Framework are to enable patients to 'die well'

G1 Symptom-free as far as possible
G2 In their preferred place of choice
G3 Feeling safe and supported with fewer crises
G4 Carers feeling supported, involved, empowered and satisfied with care
G5 Staff feeling more confident, satisfied, with better communication and teamworking with specialists.

Essentially the GSF is a simple common-sense approach to formalizing best practice, so that good care becomes standard for *all* patients *every* time. GSF users find it affirms their good practice, regularizes quality palliative care activities and improves consistency of care.

We are doing much of it 'piecemeal' already, but it formalizes and coordinates what we do, so under pressure it's more likely to happen.

GP, Halifax

The GSF is the one thing in palliative care over recent years that has really made a difference.

District nurse, Glasgow

It is in the attention to such details, in the context of an overall management plan, that transforms the quality of palliative care provision in the community.

3. Plan

Communicate

2. Assess

Communicate

1. Identify

Communicate

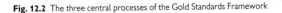

Fig. 12.2 The three central processes of the Gold Standards Framework

Key elements of the Gold Standards Framework[18]

The seven 'gold standards' of community palliative care—The Seven C's

- **C1** Communication
- **C2** Co-ordination
- **C3** Control of symptoms
- **C4** Continuity including out-of-hours
- **C5** Continued learning
- **C6** Carer support
- **C7** Care in the dying phase

The seven C's

C1: Communication

Practices maintain a supportive care register (paper or electronic) to record, plan and monitor patient care, and act as a focus for regular monthly PHCT meetings. The aims of these meetings are:

- To improve the flow of information
- Advanced planning/proactive care
- Measurement and audit, to clarify areas for future improvement at patient, practice, Primary Care Trust and network level

C2: Co-ordination

Each PHCT has a nominated coordinator for palliative care (e.g. District nurse) to ensure good organization and coordination of care in a practice by overseeing the process, i.e.:

- Maintaining the register of problems/concerns, summary care plans, symptom sheets, handover forms, audit data, etc
- Organizing PHCT meetings for discussion, planning, case analysis, education, etc
- Using tools such as a checklist of potential symptoms that need to be assessed

Coordinators meet regularly together with the local facilitator to share experience and discuss ways to overcome local barriers to good care.

C3: Control of symptoms

Each patient has their symptoms, problems and concerns (physical, psychological, social, practical and spiritual) assessed, recorded, discussed and acted upon, according to an agreed process. The focus is on actively assessing and responding to the patient's agenda.

C4: Continuity

Transfer information to the out-of-hours service for palliative care patients, for example, using a handover form, ensuring appropriate drugs are available in the home, and use of an out-of-hours protocol.

This builds in anticipatory care to reduce crises and inappropriate admissions. Information should also be passed on to other relevant services, such as hospice/oncology departments. Record and minimize the number of professionals involved, i.e. note lead GP, lead district nurse, etc.

C5: Continued learning

The PHCT will be committed to continued learning of skills and information relevant to patients seen: 'learn as you go'.

- Practice-based or external teaching, lectures/videos
- Use of Significant Event Analysis (SEA)
- Practice and personal development plans
- Audits/appraisal
- Assemble a practice reference resource
- Learning involves clinical, organizational/strategic and attitude domains
- Involvement and co-working of specialists is crucial
- Protected time for a review meeting e.g. after six months allows audit, assessment of current practice, planning for improvement and development of a practice protocol

C6: Carer support

Carers are supported, listened to, kept fully informed, encouraged and educated to play as full a rôle in the patient's care as they wish. They are regarded as an integral part of the team.

- Practical support:
  - Practical hands-on support is supplied where possible, for example, night sitter, respite, commode
- Bereavement:
  - Practices plan support, target 'high risk bereavement' visits, notes tagged, others informed, etc
- Staff support
  - Inbuilt, leading to better teamwork and job satisfaction
  - A shift to no-blame culture (eg SEA) enables 'systems thinking' and improving care

C7: Care of the dying

Patients in the last days of life (terminal phase) are cared for appropriately, for example by following the Liverpool Integrated Care Pathway. (☐ See Chapter 13.)

This includes:

- stopping non-essential interventions and drugs,
- considering comfort measures,
- psychological and religious/spiritual support,
- bereavement planning,
- communication and care after death being assessed, recorded and acted upon.

18 Thomas K (2003) Caring for the Dying at home: Companions on the Journey. Radcliffe Medical Press.

Table 12.2 Minimum protocol for the dying—C7 of GSF

1 Diagnosis of dying—awareness of signs of the terminal phase
2 Current medication assessed, non-essentials discontinued, essential treatment converted to subcutaneous route via syringe driver
3 As required drugs written up as per protocol including pain, agitation, respiratory secretions and nausea and vomiting
4 Ensure the carers know the patient is dying
5 Spiritual, religious needs assessed and met regarding patient and carers
6 There is an agreed plan of ongoing assessment and care including symptom control (pain, agitation, respiratory tract secretions, mouth care, pressure areas, psychosocial support)
7 Relatives are aware of what to do when the patient dies at home
8 Communication with others—handover form for out-of-hours providers updated, secondary/specialist services informed and hospital appointments cancelled after a death etc

Adapted from the Liverpool Care Pathway. (📖 See also Chapter 13)

Once the above minimum protocol is established, consider developing this further as an area/PCT, by adopting an integrated care pathway for the dying e.g. the Liverpool Care Pathway, used in the last few days of life to ensure standardising and benchmarking of best care. Contact lcp@mariecurie.org.uk or see Ellershaw and Wilkinson (2003).[19]

Doing both?

Suggested plan for introduction of GSF and Liverpool Care Pathway (LCP)
● in the community—GSF first then add LCP
● in care homes—LCP then add GSF
● in hospitals and hospices—LCP and then link with GSF practices

The Gold Standards Framework has transformed our practice's approach to the care of the dying. The whole team no longer perceives palliative care as all doom and gloom and is more confident that we can make a positive contribution. The teamworking, care coordination and anticipation of problems mean that our patients experience fewer crises and have a much better outcome. We are so pleased that we have decided to start applying the principles of the Gold Standards Framework to all of our cancer patients from the point of referral onwards.

GP, Runcorn GSF Phase 2

How to do it
Gold Standards Framework—how to implement in your primary healthcare team

1 **Pick out and identify** palliative care patients within the practice population—using a register to centralize information. Discuss these patients as a team regularly—encouraging better proactive planning, communication. Give someone in the practice the task of coordinating the care and ensuring things come together e.g. Handover form sent, drugs left in home, patients choice of place of death noted etc. (C1 and C2)

19 Ellershaw J., Wilkinson S. (2003) *Care of the Dying: A pathway to excellence.* Oxford: Oxford University Press.

2 Use tools to **assess** patient and carer choices, needs, symptoms and problems and **respond or refer**; as appropriate. (C3)
   • Reflect on your practice, linking in learning with palliative care specialists, e.g. local Macmillan hospice community nurse;
   • Audit your care to target changes and commission better local resources;
   • Link with practice clinical governance and set your own standards;
   • Measure improvement and celebrate teamwork and success. (C5)
3 Proactive **planning** and improved **communication.**
   • Send a handover form to the out-of-hours team and leave appropriate drugs and equipment in the home (C4)
   • Link with social services. Consider carers' needs and provide information and contact details, especially for a crisis (C6)
   • Build in bereavement care and be aware of other local services for the bereaved
   • Plan for good care in the last days of life (C7 checklist).
   • Review and reflect on achievements and learning after six months. Agree a practice protocol for all dying patients, so that the best of care becomes normal practice—'this is what we do for our palliative care patients'

Gold Standards Framework—a 6–12 month plan of how to implement in an area (such as a UK Primary Care Trust)
For more details and resources see the web sites—www.gsf.org.uk and www.macmillan.org.uk
1 Each area funds a **GSF facilitator** e.g. one day a week with administrative back-up.
2 Facilitator **introduces GSF** to a few interested practices e.g. 4–10 at a time.
3 Each practice team agrees to use GSF for at least 6–12 months, nominates a practice **GSF coordinator** (DN or manager) (C2) backed by supportive GP and DN, and undertakes a baseline questionnaire.
4 GSF Facilitator **links** with larger group e.g. Cancer Network, Macmillan, project team etc. and receives training in GSF and ongoing support plus resources, to be distributed to each practice team via coordinator.
5 GSF Facilitator organizes regular **coordinators meetings** (e.g. monthly at lunchtime) to teach principles of GSF, share experiences, audit, develop local commissioning, develop new ideas etc. This group is an important backbone of the work as it nurtures relevant local ownership and momentum, commissions local changes and develops sustainability. It raises awareness of palliative/supportive care and builds better relationships between teams and with specialists. Specific teaching can be tailored to learning needs.
6 Practice coordinator sets up Supportive care **registers** using suggested templates provided (amended if needed) (C1). Criteria for inclusion are initially cancer patients with a prognosis of 6–12 months i.e. those eligible for attendance allowance via form DS1500—later extended to patients with other end-stage illnesses, but recommended to begin with cancer patients who have a more predictable illness trajectory.

If preferred, this can be prioritized into those with most need, moderate need and future need e.g. colour coded, star rated, 'poorlies and pending' etc.
  • Pre-printed forms for identification, planning, and handover are available
7 Practice coordinator organizes a regular primary healthcare team **meeting** to discuss relevant patients on the register, patient and carer needs, management plan, preferences for place of care and anticipated requirements—this builds in better communication and proactive care. Palliative care specialists can be invited and teaching integrated.
8 Practice coordinator develops **system of tasks** i.e. sends information/handover form to out-of-hours provider (C4), agrees assessment tools in line with local arrangements (C3), provides information to carers e.g. Home pack (C6), uses a minimal protocol for the last days of life or Care Pathway (C7) etc.
9 Practice coordinator plans a team **review meeting** e.g. six monthly, to review and audit care, reflect on positive and negative issues (e.g. use of significant event analysis), develop and refine an agreed practice protocol which then embeds changes into mainstream care.
10 **Extend** application of GSF to patients with other end-stage illnesses, to other settings e.g. in care homes or community hospitals and to supportive care at an earlier stage e.g. from diagnosis. Improve carer support and patient information and empowerment. Introduce e.g. Liverpool Care Pathway for the Dying if agreed locally and continually improve generalist palliative care in the community with education and strategic planning of services.

The results in practice

One of the big shifts in practice using such a framework is the move from reactive to proactive care. Here are two examples of typical patient journeys, as described by two District nurses, Rosie Norbury and Anne Fearnley of West Yorkshire. NB The first may not be considered to be a 'bad death' by many, but one that may be suboptimal but not untypical, especially after team reflection or discussion with the carer. Much worse situations can occur, occasionally leading to complaints, media exposure or litigation.

Reactive patient journey before GSF

Mr B in the last months of his life

GPs and District nurse ad hoc visiting arrangements—no agreed care plan and no preferred place of death discussed or communicated among the team

Problems with symptom control—high anxiety-carer uninformed

Crisis call out-of-hours e.g. no information, plan or drugs available

Admitted to hospital (Inappropriate use of an 'acute' bed.)

Dies in hospital—(over intervention/medicalisation of natural process)

Carer given minimal support in grief

No reflection or improvements by primary care team

GSF Proactive patient journey using GSF

Mrs W in last months of life

On Supportive Care Register—needs and care plan discussed at team meeting

Social benefits administration such as the UK DS1500 form and information given to patient + carer (e.g. Home pack)

Regular support, visits phone calls—anticipatory not reactive visits

Assessment of symptoms—referral to specialist palliative care services considered—customized care to patient and carer needs

Carer assessed including psychosocial needs—information given for crises

Preferred place of care noted and provision organized

Handover form sent to out-of-hours service—drugs issued for home

Minimal protocol for terminal care/Liverpool Care Pathway used

Patient dies in preferred place—bereavement support

Staff reflect—significant event analysis, audit gaps, learn, improve care.

---

20 measurable outcomes in GSF Seven C's GSF goal
📖 **see pp. 738, 740**

 1 Identification of palliative care patient using a register* C1 G2
 2 Team meeting to discuss advanced care planning* C1 G2
 3 Co-working with specialists C1 G1, G3
 4 Team Coordinator named—cross-boundary communication C2 G2
 5 Management plans including advanced care planning noted C2 G2
 6 Preference for place of care/death noted* C2 G2
 7 Preferred place of death attained* C2 G2
 8 Staff teamwork satisfaction and confidence* C5 G5
 9 Symptom control better—assessment tools used C3 G1
 10 Confidence in assessment of symptoms and management* C3 G1
 11 Out-of-hours information/handover form sent* C4 G3
 12 Required drugs left in home* C4 G3
 13 Crises reduced e.g. fewer acute admissions in last days* C4 G3
 14 Review meeting (e.g. six monthly), audit and reflection C5 G5
 15 Targeted learning, use of SEA and protocol developed C5 G5
 16 Information given specifically to carer* C6 G4
 17 Carer separately assessed and supported* C6 G4
 18 Staff support, communication and teamwork improved* C6 G5
 19 Use of protocol for last days of life* C7 G1
 20 Application to non-cancer patients, other settings etc.
      (* most important)

Specific issues in community palliative care

Out-of-hours palliative care

'It was awfull—just panicked! My husband was in agony. It was three o'clock in the morning. We were at home all alone. It was dark and frightening and we didn't know what to do or who to turn to. Things all came together to make his pain seem much worse than it really was.'

Reducing the burden of symptoms suffered by patients and their carers at home remains a challenging round-the-clock priority. For this to be addressed we need to plan for out-of-hours palliative care services in the community, dovetailing generalist palliative care from GPs, district nurses and their out-of-hours providers with the available specialist palliative care skills and resources.[20] Several protocols have been developed[21]—one such four point plan has been shown to improve care as judged by practitioners' experience.[22]

Suggestions to improve out-of-hours palliative care in the UK

1 **Develop a local protocol**—coordinate a meeting of all out-of-hours health professionals involved in care of the seriously or terminally ill. This would include the GP cooperative, the deputizing service, PCT or health authority, district nurses and specialist doctors. Improve anticipatory care and proactive planning by the PHCT.
2 Look at **communication** and efficient transfer of information between those working in hours and out-of-hours. Use a paper or electronic handover form which is kept by the patient/the district nurse and out-of-hours service. Make sure the patient and the carer know what to do in an emergency.
3 Ensure 24h **carer support**, including 24h access to nursing care. Night sitters and respite care should also be easily available. Preventing a breakdown in the carer system is key to avoiding inappropriate crisis admissions.
4 Make best use of the **specialist advice** out-of-hours and expertise available through the local hospice/SPC service.
5 Keep in the patient's home an adequate supply of **drugs** (including a range for dose increases) and p.r.n. drugs for predictable symptoms, such as hyoscine, midazolam, diamorphine and cyclizine/haloperidol. Coordinate equipment access. On-call cars or out-of-hours centres could hold special palliative care bags.

See the five recommendations of the Macmillan Out of hours Palliative Care report—www.macmillan.org.uk or gsf@macmillan.org.uk

Improving access to palliative care drugs

1 Suggested list of drugs to be left in the home of every palliative care patient Diamorphine, cyclizine, midazolam, hyoscine butylbromide
2 Suggested drug list in palliative care bags carried by out-of-hours provider to be locally agreed
   • Midazolam, haloperidol, cyclizine, hyoscine butylbromide, levomepromazine, rectal diazepam, dexamethasone, metoclopramide, ?glycopyrronium, ?diclofenac, controlled drugs used with special CD measures—diamorphine, oral morphine solution

Summary of four point plan for out-of-hours palliative care
From Calderdale and Kirklees Health Authority West Yorkshire

1 Communication:
   • use handover form—GP/DN to write and fax to on-call service, keep in DN notes
   • inform others e.g. hospice
   • does the carer know what to do in a crisis?
2 Carer support:
   • coordinate pre-emptive care e.g. nightsitters, 24h district nursing service
   • give written information to carers
   • emergency support e.g. Rapid Response Team
3 Medical support:
   • anticipated management in handover form
   • crisis pack, guidelines etc and ongoing teaching
   • 24h specialist advice available from hospice
4 Drugs/equipment:
   • leave anticipated drugs in home
   • Special palliative care bag with drugs and information available on-call
   • on-call stocked pharmacists

Communication—handover form
The handover form has two important functions:
1 To improve information transfer
2 To build in anticipatory care.

The process of completing such a form is part of the benefit—if you think that a patient might become agitated or develop a 'rattly chest' over a weekend, leave some midazolam or hyoscine in the home, for administration either by the on-call doctor or district nurse. If the on-call doctor presented with the handover form notes that the patient has stated a preference to remain at home, there is more chance that they will be enabled to do so. Many are developed electronically and being used by central

20 Thomas K. (2000) Out-of-hours palliative care—bridging the gap. *Eur J Pall Care*, **7**: 22–5.

21 Munday D. (2002) Out-of-hours and emergency palliative care. In R. Charlton (ed.) *Primary Palliative Care*. Oxford: Radcliffe Medical Press.

22 King N., Bell D., Thomas K. (2003) An out-of-hours protocol for community palliative care. *International Journal of Palliative Nursing*, **9, 7**: 277–82

coordinating agencies e.g. NHS Direct. Once discussed with the family (and if possible the patient), some have added 'not for CPR' or 'Do Not Resuscitate' statements, to inform emergency staff, and prevent the tragic indignity of inappropriate resuscitation. Confirming written details with the carers of what to do in an emergency and informing other agencies such as hospice staff is also important.

Carer support

Round the clock access to nursing care is a basic pre requisite for good palliative care in the community. Some areas have Rapid Response Teams, a crisis-only service for patients who would otherwise be admitted to hospital. There are examples of good coordination of care with a centralized number for all services (NHS Direct may increasingly be involved in this in England).

Medical support

Handover forms inform the visiting on-call doctor of the GP's care plan and the current medication. When faced with a difficult medical symptom, crisis symptom sheets (often kept in the palliative care bags in the on-call cars) or local guidelines are invaluable, backed by teaching. Most specialist palliative care services provide some on-call advice.

Drugs and equipment

For drug access, there are three suggestions:
1 Leaving anticipated drugs in the home, prompted by the handover form
2 Keeping a stock of drugs with the out-of-hours service
3 Stocking the on-call pharmacist with an approved list of drugs.

Carer support

It is worth reminding ourselves that the principal providers of care are actually the relatives. We are still not doing nearly enough to empower, strengthen, educate and support carers and to use imaginative means to help and support them through this ghastly time.[23]

> When my wife, Joy, was diagnosed with cancer of the liver, our excellent GP said three things: first, we can do a great deal to control pain these days; second, we must see that the quality of life will be as good as it can be; third, we must see that she dies at home. With the help of our Macmillan nurse all these points were met. At every stage of the next 14 months our GP, district nurse and Macmillan nurse were on hand to suggest, reassure and predict, helping not only Joy but me and our children. Their assistance in dark days was priceless.
>
> M. C., widower and carer

If the needs of carers cannot be addressed, an almost inevitable result will be the breakdown of home care, with the majority of patients dying in institutions.

Carer support is one of the most important aspects of the care provided by primary healthcare teams. The experience of most healthcare professionals, reflected clearly in the literature, is that carer breakdown is often **the** key factor in prompting institutionalized care for dying patients. Some suggest that the impact of cancer (or other serious illness) on the carer can be even greater than that of the patient. Certainly, there is resounding evidence that without support from family and friends it would be impossible for many patients to remain at home. Those without carers are less likely to be able to remain at home to die—they present particular difficulties for primary care.

Carers' anxiety is rated alongside patients' symptoms as the most severe problems by both patients and families.[24]

> The reason my husband had to go into a nursing home in the end was quite simply that I couldn't lift him to the commode. It all came to a head after a fall and I felt I couldn't cope on my own any more. We were both heartbroken.
>
> Elderly carer of cancer patient

For the carer, despite their natural feelings of trepidation beforehand, there can be a great sense of consolation in bereavement if they have been able to fulfill the patient's wishes to remain at home during their final days. However this places a great strain on carers, both emotionally and physically.

The NHS Executive White Paper *Caring about Carers: a National strategy for Carers*[25] describes the difficulties that carers face, and emphasizes that carers should be treated as partners in the team but with specific and sometimes unmet needs of their own.

> We intend to make progress so that more carers—and eventually all carers feel adequately prepared and equipped to care if that is what they choose to do, feel cared for themselves, and feel their needs are understood.

A primary care team response to carer needs[26,27]

- Acknowledge carers, what they do, and the problems they have.
- Flag the notes of informal carers so that in any consultation you are aware of their circumstances
- Treat carers as you would other team members and listen to their opinions
- Include them in discussions about the person they care for
- Give carers a choice about which tasks they are prepared to take upon themselves
- Ask after the health and welfare of the carer as well as the patient
- Provide information about the condition the person the carer is looking after suffers from
- Provide information about being a carer and support available
- Provide information about benefits available
- Provide information about local services available for both the person being cared for and the carer
- Be an advocate for the carer to ensure services and equipment appropriate to the circumstances are provided
- Liaise with other services

23 Doyle D. (1998) The way forward. In National Council for Hospice and Specialist Palliative Care Services: *Promoting Partnership: Planning and Managing Community Palliative Care*, pp. 44–50. London: NCHSPCS.

24 Ramirez A., Addington-Hall J., Richards M. (1998) ABC of Palliative care; the carers. *BMJ*, **316**: 208–11.

25 Department of Health (1999) *Caring about Carers*. London: DoH.

26 Piercy J. (2002) The plight of the informal carer. In R. Charlton (ed.) *Primary Palliative Care*. Oxford: Radcliffe Medical Press.

27 Simon C. (2001) Informal carers and the primary care team. *Br J Gen Pract*, **51**: 920–3.

- Ensure staff are informed about the needs and problems of informal carers
- Respond quickly and sympathetically to crisis situations
- Training—e.g. in lifting, giving medication etc
- Confiding in and being listened to, needs expressed and supported, often outside the home
- Coping strategies, both internal (faith, positive attitude etc) and external (social networks)
- Development of a bereavement protocol and raising awareness of bereaved patients in practice teams. Assemble a list of local contacts for bereavement support

> I was terrified at first when they said they would discharge him home—I didn't think I could cope. But in looking after Peter dying at home, I felt I was fulfilling his wishes and we were a real family—this really helps me now. Our GPs and district nurses were really caring and professional and kept pace with us at every stage—we felt very grateful to them. Although it was so sad, it was also in some ways a very good and satisfying experience, etched forever on our minds. The children and I are glad that we were able to look after him at home, where he wanted to be, with the help of our marvellous team.
>
> Maureen, wife of Peter, a cancer patient

The vast majority of care in the last year of life is not provided by professionals, but by relatives and friends, especially wives and daughters. The support provided by a family caregiver may make all the difference for the dying person in their place of death: some have reported that up to 90 per cent of terminal admissions to hospice are due to the stress of caring on the relatives, or lack of resources available to support the patient at home. The relationship between carers and professionals is often an ambiguous one. For over half the carers, the only supportive service that they are in touch with is their GP.[28]

Bereavement (📖 see Chapter 14)
The loss of a loved person is one of the most intensely painful experiences any human being can suffer, not only is it painful to experience, but it is also painful to witness.[29]

There is a significant increase in morbidity and mortality in grief, making dying of a broken heart a reality for some. The main causes of bereavement associated death are heart disease, alcohol-induced cirrhosis, suicide, road accidents or other violent death. Bereavement is the greatest psychological trauma people can go through, and yet in some cases the carers are not given the 'preventative care' that could ameliorate future problems. The immediate bereavement visit straight after a death is much appreciated but will not in itself constitute the kind of help that heals. Initiating regular support and contact, actively listening, planning even brief follow-up care, tagging notes, awareness of risk factors etc. as well as referral to specialist groups are all proactive means of caring for carers and preventing the feeling of desertion at this most vulnerable time. Recognizing the sense of loss that staff may feel is also important and is where the development of a team approach through shared meetings can be of benefit, especially when there is a sense of guilt of less than perfect care. Care of dying patients, though very rewarding, is also an area of care that many professionals find stressful and challenging, so support for staff is essential.

Other providers of community palliative care

Specialist palliative care services
Clinical nurse specialists, Macmillan and Marie Curie nurses, hospice general staff and home care teams and Hospice at Home initiatives have long been involved in bringing quality palliative care services into patients' homes.

This can only be successfully achieved *in partnership* with generalists from the patient's usual primary care team.

Care homes
Care homes provide important nursing and residential care especially for the frail and alone, although numbers of beds are limited. More people die in care homes than in hospices and, although the palliative care provided in such homes can vary in quality, there is great interest in palliative care education and use of protocols to improve standards of care.

Community hospitals
Particularly in rural areas, community hospitals are a valuable and greatly appreciated resource, allowing continuity of care from GPs and nurses in a more localized environment. Guidelines and protocols exist to maintain high standards.

The 'key worker' rôle
User and patient groups consistently emphasize the value of having one person, a key worker, to relate to, as advocate, advisor and supporter. Some primary care teams have developed this rôle within the practice team, allowing continuity of support from diagnosis, through treatment to bereavement care. For others, a hospital clinical nurse specialist, hospice staff member or other professional may take on this rôle for part of the time and a trusting relationship may develop. Support at the life-changing time of diagnosis and also for the carer are crucial, and may otherwise be overlooked. This person may also be able to reduce inappropriate hospital admissions, unwanted interventions or appointments, thus improving hospital capacity.

Marie Curie staff
Marie Curie community nurses and sitters in the UK work usually through the night to enable patients to remain at home in the final days of illness *and support* carers. Their rôle is acknowledged and appreciated at this critical time.

Allied health professionals and others in the community
There are many others who contribute considerably—pharmacists, physiotherapists, occupational therapists, chaplains, clergy and other religious leaders, voluntary groups, bereavement services and mobilizers of local resources can all play crucial roles in providing quality holistic care.

28 Barclay S. (2001) Palliative care for non-cancer patients: a UK perspective from primary care. In J. Addington-Hall, I. Higginson (eds) *Palliative Care for Non-cancer Patients*. Oxford: Oxford University Press.

29 Bowlby J. (1969) *Attachment and Loss, Vol. 1*. Harmondsworth: Penguin.

Different GPs—GP facilitators, primary care cancer leads and GPs with a special onterest (GPwSIs)

Macmillan GP facilitators have the rôle of:

- educating their colleagues within primary care
- enhancing local service provision for patients in the community

Primary Care Organization (PCO) cancer leads in England focus on improving the strategic planning of services for cancer patients.

GPs with a special interest (GPwSIs) include some with extra clinical training in palliative care and are a new initiative, especially useful in areas short of palliative medicine specialists.

Supportive care guidance

Supportive care is defined as care designed to help patients and families cope. The Supportive and Palliative Care Guidance,[30] commissioned in England as part of the NHS Cancer Plan, makes recommendations to improve the vital areas of care not directly related to curative treatment, i.e. that of palliative care (generalist and specialist), psychological, social and family care, rehabilitation, coordination, communication, information, spiritual support etc. underpinned throughout by user involvement. This guidance is likely to be used in the future planning and commissioning of services, including those in the community, for patients throughout their cancer journey.

---

30 National Institute for Clinical Excellence (2004) *Guidance on Cancer Services: improving supportive and palliative care for adults with cancer: the manual.* London: NICE.

Working partnerships with palliative care specialists

Good effective partnerships with palliative care specialists will ensure best care for patients and their families. Involvement of specialists in primary palliative care can be very fruitful e.g. in local education and training programmes, targeted teaching on individual patient case histories, invitations to team meetings, agreed use of assessment tools and templates, out-of-hours protocols and advice, strategic planning of services and hospice outreach etc. With good relationships and lines of communication, and with roles and responsibilities clarified, there can be excellent dovetailing of generalist and specialist skills, for the benefit of all.

Referral to specialist palliative care services

Eligibility criteria for specialist palliative care help clarify what is expected of both generalist and specialist palliative care providers.[31] By attempting to crystallize and improve 'generalist' palliative care, and better integration with the 'specialist' services available a more comprehensive, and equitable service for those in the last stages of life could be provided.

Eligibility criteria for referrals to specialist palliative care services[32]

Eligible patients have:

1 Any active progressive and potentially *life-threatening* disease.
2 *Anticipated or actual unresolved*, complex needs that cannot be met by the caring team ie physical, psychological, social, spiritual needs e.g. complicated symptoms, specialist nursing needs, difficult family situations, ethical issues regarding treatment decisions.
3 Been recently *assessed* by a member of one of the specialist palliative care teams.

---

31 Ellershaw J. E., Boyes L.M Peat S. (1995) Assessing the effectiveness of a hospital palliative care team. *Pall Med*, **9**: 145–52.

32 Bennett M., Adam J., Alison D., Hicks F., Stockton M. (2000) Leeds Eligibility Criteria for specialist palliative care services. *Pall Med*, **14, 2**: 157–8.

Further reading

Addington-Hall J., Higginson I. (2001) *Palliative Care for Non-cancer Patients.* Oxford: Oxford University Press.

Charlton R. (ed.) (2003) *Primary Palliative Care.* Oxford: Radcliffe Medical Press.

Cooper J. (ed.) (2000) *Stepping into Palliative Care: a handbook for community professionals.* Oxford: Radcliffe Medical Press.

Doyle D., Jeffrey D. (2000) *Palliative Care in the Home.* Oxford: Oxford University Press.

Ellershaw J., Wilkinson S. (2003) *Care of the Dying: A pathway to excellence.* Oxford: Oxford University Press.

Lee E. (2002) *In Your Own Time: A guide for patients and their carers facing a last illness at home.* Oxford: Oxford University Press.

Lynn J. (2000) *Improving Care for End of Life: A sourcebook for health managers and clinicians.* New York: Oxford University Press.

Thomas K. (2003) *Caring for the Dying at Home: Companions on the journey.* Oxford: Radcliffe Medical Press.

Useful web sites are:
www.goldstandardswframework.nhs.uk/gsf
www.hospice-spc-council.org.uk
www.macmillan.org.uk
www.modern.nhs.uk/cancer
www.palliativedrugs.com
www.palliative-medicine.org

Chapter 13

The terminal phase

The terminal phase is defined as the period when day to day deterioration, particularly of strength, appetite and awareness, are occurring.

Prognosis

Patients frequently ask, 'How long have I got?' It is notoriously difficult to predict when death will occur, and it is wise to avoid the trap of predicting or making an incorrect guess. If pushed to do so, it should be made clear that any predictions are only a guide. It is best to talk in terms of 'days', or 'weeks' or 'months', as appropriate.

For example:

'When we see someone deteriorating from week to week we are often talking in terms of weeks, when that deterioration is from day to day then we are usually talking in terms of days, but everyone is different.'

Research has shown that nurses, relatives and domestic assistants in hospices are often better at predicting the approach of death than medical staff.

Signs and symptoms of death approaching[1]

The clearest signs of approaching death are picked up by the day by day assessment of deterioration.

Profound weakness	Bed-bound
	Needs assistance with all care
Diminished intake of food and fluids	
Drowsy or reduced cognition	May be disorientated in time and place
	Difficulty concentrating
	Scarcely able to co-operate with carers
Gaunt appearance	
Difficulty swallowing medicine	

Should such symptoms develop suddenly over a matter of days instead of the usual weeks, it is important to exclude a reversible cause of deterioration such as infection, hypercalcaemia, or medication changes.

Goals for the last 24 h
- Ensure the patient's comfort physically, emotionally and spiritually
- Make the end-of-life peaceful and dignified
- By care and support given to the dying patient and their carers make the memory of the dying process as positive as possible

1 National Council for Hospice and Specialist Palliative Care Services (1997) *Changing Gear— Guidelines for Managing the Last Days of Life in Adults.* London: NCHSPCS 7.

It is very important to continually seek the patient's views on, and feeling about treatment while they remain conscious, even when the weakening state makes communication difficult. Relatives also need to be given time to have their questions, concerns, and requests for information listened to and answered as clearly as possible. As the patient deteriorates, the family's advocate rôle becomes more important, though their wishes need to be balanced with the palliative care team's understanding of the patient's needs.

Where possible, families and carers should be offered the opportunity to participate in the physical care of patients. Carers should be invited to stay, if they want to, while nursing and medical procedures are carried out. Very occasionally relatives would like to participate in laying out the body after death, and this can be a very important part of their last 'duty' or behalf of their dead loved one.

The events and the atmosphere which are present at the time of a patient's death can great influence the grieving process of those left behind

Cardiopulmonary resuscitation

The issue of cardiopulmonary resuscitation (CPR) has again come to the fore with stories of patients learning that doctors had written 'Not for Resuscitation' in a patient's notes without them being consulted. The response from the medical profession has been to advise that 'Not for Resuscitation' should only be written into the notes after a full discussion with the patient and family has taken place. Nurses can face very difficult situations if they are unsure what their response should be if a particular patient suddenly deteriorates.

1 Many hospices have a policy that they do not carry out CPR and patients have to 'opt in' rather than 'opt out' of resuscitation.
2 Ultimately it is the doctor's decision whether it is in the patient's best interest for a resuscitation attempt to be made.
3 Frank and open discussion with the patient and the family, before admission, about the hospice's resuscitation policy can be a great help, provided that the information is recorded clearly in the medical records.

Different cultures

Different religious and cultural groupings have divergent approaches to the dying process. It is important to be sensitive to their possible beliefs. If in doubt, ask a family member. Offence is more likely to be caused by not asking than by asking.

The patient's wishes

Dying is a very special event for each individual. Helping to explore patients' wishes about death and dying should, if possible, take place before they reach the final 24 h. Important discussions can still, however, take place even at this late phase and professionals should encourage this dialogue. The family gain great comfort in knowing that they have made the most of precious moments and that they have the answers to issues that are important to both of them. Some of these questions can include preferred place of death or burial/cremation and financial or 'unfinished' business issues. Time to say last goodbyes to close family members, children and dependents and time to forgive and bury guilt can be crucial to enable a normal bereavement.

Collaborative multidisciplinary approach
Effective terminal care needs a team approach. No single member of the palliative care team, no matter how committed or gifted, can meet all the palliative care needs of a patient and their family.

Effective multidisciplinary working depends on:
- Recognising the centrality of patient and family needs
- Good communication
- Clear understanding and respect for the value, importance and rôle of other professionals
- Early referral to specialist palliative services if needed

Referral to Specialist Palliative Care services is appropriate when:
- One or more distressing symptoms prove difficult to control
- There is severe emotional distress associated with the patient's condition
- There are dependent children and or elderly vulnerable relatives

Assessment of patients' needs
The focus in assessment in the last 48 h is to discover what, apart from dying itself, the patient is most concerned about and which concerns need to be addressed. Patients may under-report their symptoms which distresses families. Families may be very helpful in interpreting non-verbal clues but, in their own distress, may also misperceive and exaggerate the patient's symptoms which needs careful handling.

Physical needs
Common problems that need to be addressed are nausea, pain, oral problems, sleep disturbance, weakness, feeling confused (and sometimes hallucinating), pressure sores and the burden of having to take medication. Patients rarely worry about nutritional and fluid intake, but this may be a major concern for the family.

Psychological needs
The key to psychological assessment is finding out what the patient wants to know. Gently assessing how the patient feels about their disease and situation can shed light on their needs and distress. How the patient interprets their disease and its symptoms may be a cause of suffering itself. Deep probing at this stage, however, is inappropriate as the goal is psychological comfort and peace, NOW.

Anxiety and agitation may need to be managed with medication. Patients are more often concerned about the family at this stage than about themselves.

Fears associated with symptoms	e.g. the pain will escalate to agony, breathing will stop if I fall asleep.
Other emotional distress	e.g. dependence on family, ('I am a burden and it would be better if I was out of the way').
Past experience	e.g. past contact with patients who died in unpleasant circumstances.
Preferences about treatment or withholding treatment	e.g. 'What if nobody listens to me or takes my wishes seriously?'
Fears about morphine	e.g. 'If I use morphine now, it will not work when I really need it.'
Death and dying	e.g. Patients frequently adapt to the fact that they will die, but are fearful of the process leading up to death.

Dignity

The palliative care team need to have as a goal the maintenance of the patient's dignity in a manner which is appropriate to that particular patient. What is dignified for one patient may not be for another, which is one of the reasons why many hospices have both single rooms and small wards.

Spiritual needs

There may be particular religious tasks to be accomplished such as absolution, confession, or other forms of religious preparation. Spiritual disquiet or pain may be relieved by allowing expression of feelings and thoughts, particularly fear and loss of control. Patients are more often concerned about the family at this stage than about themselves and may need to address unresolved conflict or guilt.

Families often want to know that the patient is comfortable and not suffering. If appropriate, it may be helpful for them to be aware of the experiences of people who have had near death experiences which are described as tranquil and peaceful. Many mechanisms have been used to explain this phenomenon including the release of endorphins (natural analgesics), retinal hypoxia with resultant neuronal discharge (particularly in the fovea where there are many neurones) so that a bright spot looks like the end of an inviting tunnel. Temporal lobe seizures may also provide an explanation. Whatever the mechanism, nature seems to have a way of allowing dying humans to feel comforted and at peace at the end.

Talking about death and dying

As a taboo subject, few people feel comfortable about discussing death, even though it is natural, certain, and is happening all around us all the time.

Opening up discussion can be very liberating to patients who can feel they have not been given permission to talk about dying as this would be admitting defeat.

Sometimes the direct question 'Are you worried about dying?' is most appropriate.

Often a patient's biggest fears are groundless and reassurances can be given. Where reassurance cannot be given it is helpful to break the fear down into constituent parts and try to deal with the aspects of the fear which can be dealt with.

Physical examination

Examination at this stage is kept to the minimum to avoid unnecessary distress. Examine:
- Any site of potential pain. Patients may be comfortable at rest but in pain on being turned, which they may not readily admit
- Any relevant area of the body that might be causing discomfort as suggested by history or non-verbal signs
- Mouth

Investigations

Any investigation at the end-of-life should have a clear and justifiable purpose, such as excluding reversible conditions, where treatment would make the patient more comfortable. There is little need for investigations in the terminal stages.

Review of medication

At this stage comfort is the priority. Unnecessary medication should be stopped but analgesics, anti-emetics, anxiolytics/antipsychotics and anticon-vulsants will need to be continued. Diabetes can be managed with a short-acting insulin as needed. If the patient is unable to swallow essential medicines, an alternative route of administration is necessary. These changes needs to be explained to relatives, who may become anxious that tablets which the patient has had to take for years have now suddenly stopped.

Treatment of symptoms

Dying patients tolerate symptoms very poorly because of their weakness. Important factors:
- Excellence in nursing care
- Prevention of new problems developing by e.g. using appropriate mattresses, thereby preventing bed sores
- Treating specific symptoms such as a dry mouth
- Anticipating the probable needs of the patients so that immediate response can be made when the time comes

Routes for Medicine in the Terminal Phase
The **intramuscular** route for injections should be avoided as it is too painful.

If **buccal** medicines are given it is important that the mouth is kept moist.

The **rectal** route can be very useful for certain patients though is more or less accepted in different cultures.

Topical Fentanyl patches should be avoided in the terminal stage unless they have been used before this time, since it takes too long to titrate against a patient's pain.

In many instances a **syringe driver** containing diamorphine is used so that adjustments can be made more finely in accord with the patient's changing state.

Even when patients are dying, it is often possible to communicate with them and to get their consent for certain treatment, such as subcutaneous medication. As the patient becomes less aware, however, it is the relatives and the nursing staff who become the patient's advocate. At this point a clear plan of goals needs to be agreed between the doctors, nurses and family members.

- The potentially sedative side-effects of analgesia needs to be explained
- The use of alternative routes of medication need to be discussed, as the oral route may be more difficult
- The treatment plan should define clearly what should be done in the event of a symptom breakthrough

Common problems in last 48 h
- Noisy, moist breathing
- Pain
- Restlessness/agitation
- Breathlessness
- Nausea/vomiting
- Myoclonic twitching

Noisy, moist breathing (death rattle)

This is very distressing to relatives, and should be treated prophylactically as it is easier to prevent secretions forming than removing secretions that have gathered in the upper airways or oropharynx.

Management

General measures include re-positioning the patient and giving reassurance to the relatives. It should be explained that the noise is due to secretions collecting which are no longer being coughed or cleared as normal. They should also know that the secretions are not causing suffocation, choking or distress.

Specific measures

These specific guidelines are for patients who are imminently dying and develop 'rattling' or 'bubbly' breathing (the death rattle). The following guidelines should be used with caution, particularly if the patient is still aware enough to be distressed by the dry mouth that will result from treatment.

Acute pulmonary oedema should be excluded, or treated with furosemide.

- Give hyoscine hydrobromide 400mcg stat subcutaneously, and start hyoscine hydrobromide 1.2–1.6mg/24h CSCI
- Wait for half an hour and reassess the patient. If there is still an unacceptable rattle, and there has not been a marked improvement:
- Give a further dose of hyoscine hydrobromide 400mcg stat SC
- Wait for half an hour and reassess
- If the noise has been relieved, but recurs later, give repeat doses of hyoscine hydrobromide 400mcg to a maximum of 800mcg in any 4h
- Increase CSCI to 2.4mg/24h
  NB Hyoscine hydrobromide can cause sedation and confusion

If the patient is conscious, and respiratory secretions are not too distressing, it may be adequate to use a transdermal patch (Scopaderm 1.5mg over three days or sublingual tablets (Kwells).

If the noise of secretions is not relieved:

1 Try an alternative, e.g:
   - Glycopyrronium bromide 0.2mg stat. or CSCI 0.6–1.2mg/24h
   - Glycopyrronium does not cause sedation or confusion. It is useful for the patient who is still conscious and wishes to remain as alert as possible
   - Hyoscine butylbromide (buscopan) 20mg SC stat. and 60–90mg CSCI. Since it does not cross the blood—brain barrier, buscopan is less sedating than hyoscine hydrobromide
2 If the respiratory rate is >20 breaths per minute, the noise may be reduced by slowing the respiratory rate: give diamorphine 2.5–5mg SC (or a sixth of the 24h dose if already on CSCI) and repeat after 30 minutes if respiratory rate still above 20 per minute.
3 If the noise appears to be coming from the back of the pharynx, try tipping the bed 30 degrees 'head-up', allowing the secretions to drain back into the lungs from the throat or trachea.
4 If the patient is deeply unconscious, try using gentle suction.
5 Ensure that the patient is not distressed, using sedative drugs such as midazolam if necessary.

Terminal agitation

All potentially reversible causes of agitation (see the Think list below) in the terminal phase should be excluded. A diagnosis of terminal agitation can only be made if reversible conditions are excluded or are failing to respond to treatment. Since the patient is clearly distressed, some degree of sedation will probably be warranted. This decision should be discussed with the patient if at all possible. It is helpful for the family if they are also involved in the discussions.

Think list for some common reversible causes of terminal agitation:

- Pain
- Urinary retention
- Full rectum
- Nausea
- Cerebral irritability
- Anxiety and fear
- Side-effects of medication

Cerebral Oedema: Rising intracranial pressure due to cerebral oedema, in the terminal stages of cerebral tumours, can cause a rapid and severe escalation of headache (which can be made worse by opioids) and terminal agitation. Generous doses of opioids, however, may be effective in addition to a NSAID and midazolam. Avoid drugs that will lower the seizure threshold such as levomepromazine unless given with adequate doses of benzodiazepine. In a dying unconscious or semiconscious patient, it should not be necessary to replace oral steroids with subcutaneous steroids provided that adequate pain control and sedation is given. Usually by this stage the oedema is not well controlled by steroids and at best may only serve to prolong the dying phase.

Management

Examination and explanation

Once treatable causes for agitation have been excluded it is important to inform family in attendance of your clinical findings, and of the management options, emphasizing clearly that the goals in this situation are primarily comfort and dignity, and ensuring that treatments will aim to achieve these goals.

Medication

Midazolam 5–10mg SC stat. and 30–60mg/24h given by CSCI. If the patient remains distressed, other medication (e.g. levomepromazine) should be added. Clonazepam (1–4mg CSCI/24h) is sometimes used instead of midazolam, particularly if the patient has neuropathic pain and can no longer take effective medication by mouth.

Levomepromazine 25mg SC stat. and 50–100mg/24h by CSCI. It is unusual for patients to require larger doses but, if necessary, up to 200mg/24h can be given. Haloperidol 5mg SC stat. and 10–20mg/24h **CSCI** may be used but extrapyramidal symptoms can occur, particularly at higher doses.

Phenobarbital 100mg SC stat and 300–600mg/24h by CSCI should be effective but higher doses may be needed; a second syringe driver is needed as phenobarbital in incompatible with most other drugs.

If a syringe driver is not available, alternative phenothiazines +/– benzodiazepines may be used by sublingual or rectal routes e.g. chlorpromazine 25mg PR 4–6 h with escalation to response (up to 100–200mg 4-h) and/or diazepam rectally 10mg p.r.n. or clonazepam sublingually 0.5mg and titrate upwards.

Propofol, an anaesthetic agent, has been used intravenously in intractable cases, under specialist supervision.

The Liverpool Care Pathway for the dying patient

The preceeding section detailing the last 48 h of life, practical issues and bereavement in this handbook clearly outline good practice for care of the dying. The Liverpool Integrated Care Pathway for the Dying Patient (LCP) aims to translate such best practice into a template of care to guide healthcare professionals with limited or infrequent experience of caring for dying patients. The next section will explain how this best practice can be incorporated into a care pathway which can be used both as an educational tool and to provide a template of care within practice.

There are three sections of the Liverpool Care Pathway for the dying patient:

1 Initial assessment and care of the dying patient
2 Ongoing care of the dying patient
3 Care of the family and carers after death of the patient.

Initiating the Liverpool Care Pathway for the dying patient (LCP)—diagnosing dying

Before a patient is commenced on the Liverpool Care Pathway it is important that the multidisciplinary team have agreed that the patient is in the dying phase. This decision in itself can sometimes lead to conflict within the team, but it is important to make a clear diagnosis if appropriate care and communication is to be achieved.

In cancer patients, if the patient's condition has been deteriorating over a period of time, i.e. the last weeks/days, and two of the following four criteria apply:

- The patient is bed bound
- Semi-comatose
- Only able to take sips of fluid
- Unable to take tablets

it is likely that the patient is entering the dying phase. *These criteria may not be appropriate in a non-cancer population.* It is important to highlight that a patient who is clinically in the dying phase may occasionally recover and stabilize for a period of time. However, this should not prevent the clinical team from using the LCP to provide the appropriate physical, psychological, social and spiritual care.

The three sections of the Liverpool Care Pathway for the dying patient

Section 1—Initial assessment and care of the dying patient

This section identifies the key goals that should be achieved when a patient enters the dying phase. These goals are directly related to and support the guidance given in the chapter on the last 48 h of life regarding the terminal phase. A key component of the LCP is the supporting guidelines for the symptoms of pain, agitation and respiratory tract secretions. These are shown in Figure 13.1. These guidelines ensure that appropriate oral medication is converted to a subcutaneous regimen and that patients have p.r.n. (as required) medication available should they develop

COMFORT MEASURES	**Goal 1: Current medication assessed and non essentials discontinued**
	  Yes ☐ No ☐
	  Appropriate oral drugs converted to subcutaneous route and syringe
	  driver commenced if appropriate
	  Inappropriate medication discontinued

	Goal 2: PRN subcutaneous medication written up for list below as per protocol
	  (see blue sheets at back of ICP for guidance)
	  Pain Analgesia **Yes ☐ No ☐**
	  Nausea and vomiting Antiemetic **Yes ☐ No ☐**
	  Agitation Sedative **Yes ☐ No ☐**
	  Respiratory tract secretions Anticholinergic **Yes ☐ No ☐**

	Goal 3: Discontinue inappropriate interventions
	  Blood test **Yes ☐ No ☐ N/A ☐**
	  Antibiotics **Yes ☐ No ☐ N/A ☐**
	  i V's (fluids/medications) **Yes ☐ No ☐ N/A ☐**
	  Not for cardiopulmonary resuscitation **Yes ☐ No ☐**
	  (Please record below & complete appropriate associated documentation–policy/procedure)

	Goal 3a: Decisions to discontinue inappropriate nursing interventions taken
	                  Yes ☐ No ☐
	  Routine turning regime – reposition for comfort only – consider pressure
	  relieving mattress–and appropriate assessments re skin integrity–Taking Vital Signs

	Goal 3b: Syringe driver set up within 4 h of Doctor's order **Yes ☐ No ☐ N/A ☐**

PSYCHOLOGICAL/ INSIGHT	**Goal 4: Ability to communicate in English assessed as adequate**
	  a) Patient **Yes ☐ No ☐ Comatosed ☐**
	  b) Family/other **Yes ☐ No ☐**

	Goal 5: Insight into condition assessed
	  Aware of diagnosis a) Patient **Yes ☐ No ☐ Comatosed ☐**
	         b) Family/other **Yes ☐ No ☐**
	  Recognition of dying c) Patient **Yes ☐ No ☐ Comatosed ☐**
	         d) Family/other **Yes ☐ No ☐**

RELIGIOUS/ SPIRITUAL SUPPORT	**Goal 6: a) Religious/spiritual needs assessed with patient**
	             Yes ☐ No ☐ Comatosed ☐
	  b) Religious/spiritual needs assessed with family/other
	             Yes ☐ No ☐
	  Patient/other may be anxious for self/others
	  Consider support of chaplaincy team
	  Religious tradition identified, if yes specify:............... **Yes ☐ No ☐ N/A☐**
	  Support of chaplaincy-team offered **Yes ☐ No ☐**
	  In-house support Tel/Bleep No: .... Name .... Date/Time ....
	  External support Tel/Bleep No: .... Name .... Date/Time ....
	  Special needs now, at time of impending death, at death and after death identified:-
	  ....

COMMUNICATION WITH FAMILY/OTHER	**Goal 7: Identify how family/other are to be informed of patient's impending death** **Yes ☐ No ☐**
	  At any time ☐ Not at night-time ☐ Stay overnight at hospital ☐
	  Primary contact name ....
	  Relationship to patient .... Tel no: ....
	  Secondary contact ....
	  Tel no:........

	Goal 8: Family/other given hospital information on:-
	             Yes ☐ No ☐
	  Concession car parking; accommodation; dining
	  room facilities; payphones; washrooms and toilet facilities
	  on the ward; visiting times. Any other relevant information

COMMUNICATION WITH PRIMARY HEALTHCARE TEAM	**Goal 9: GP Practice is aware of patient's condition**
	             Yes ☐ No ☐
	  GP Practice to be contacted if unaware patient is dying

SUMMARY	**Goal 10: Plan of care explained & discussed with:-**
	  a) Patient **Yes ☐ No ☐ Comatosed ☐**
	  b) Family/other **Yes ☐ No ☐**

	Goal 11: Family/other express understanding of plan care.
	          Yes ☐ No ☐
	  Family/other aware that LCP commenced and their concerns identified and documented

Fig. 13.1 Initial Assessment and care of the dying patient

2 Ellershaw J. E., Wilkinson S. (eds) (2003) *Care of the Dying: A pathway to excellence.* Oxford: Oxford University Press. (2003).

symptoms in the dying phase. In care settings where the LCP is not in common usage, healthcare professionals can use the goals of care in Figure 13.1 to guide and inform their practice.

Section 2—Ongoing care of the dying patient
The LCP promotes multidisciplinary working and a joint approach to the care of the patient and their family. In caring for a dying patient, at least four-hourly observations of symptom control, and appropriate action if there are problems identified, should occur. Particular attention is given to pain, agitation, respiratory tract secretions, nausea and vomiting, mouthcare and micturition problems. Support regarding the psychological, social and spiritual aspects of care for the family and patient need to be continued in the dying phase.

Section 3—Care of the family and carers after the death of the patient
The LCP incorporates the certification of death within the document, identifies any special needs for the patient who has died and support for the family and carers immediately after death. It particularly focuses on the information needs of the family at this distressing time and includes a leaflet on bereavement care.

How does using the Liverpool Care Pathway benefit patients?
In providing a template of care for the dying phase, the LCP promotes discussion within the clinical team with regard to the diagnosis of dying, and facilitates the initiation of care which is appropriate for the dying phase. The LCP integrates local and national guidelines into clinical practice. It is a powerful educational tool which can be used to facilitate the rôle of specialist palliative care teams and to empower generic health workers to deliver a model of excellence for care of the dying. The LCP should ensure that patients die a dignified death and that their carers receive appropriate support. Healthcare professionals also benefit by knowing that they have delivered a good standard of care to the patient. In the words of the National Cancer Plan 'The care of all dying patients must be improved to the level of the best.'

Further reading

Books
de Luc K. (2000) *Developing Care Pathways*. Oxford: Radcliffe Medical Press.

Department of Health (2000) *The NHS Cancer Plan—A plan for investment, A plan for reform*. London: DoH.

Ellershaw J. E., Wilkinson S. (eds) (2003) *Care of the Dying: A pathway to excellence*. Oxford: Oxford University Press.

Articles
Campbell H., Hotchkiss R., Bradshaw N., Porteous M. (1998) Integrated care pathways. *BMJ*, **316**: 133–7.

Ellershaw J. E., Smith, C., Overill S., *et al.* (2001) Care of the dying. *Journal of pain & symptom management*, **21**: 12–17.

Elllershaw J. E., Ward C. (2003) Care of the dying patient: the last hours or days of life. *BMJ*, **326**: 30–4.

Chapter 14

Bereavement

> How small and selfish is sorrow. But it bangs one about until one is quite senseless.
>
> Queen Elizabeth the Queen Mother, in a letter to Edith Sitwell
> shortly after the death of King George VI

Grief is a normal reaction to a bereavement or other major loss. Its manifestations will vary from person to person but will often include physical, cognitive, behavioural and emotional elements. For a close personal bereavement, grief is likely to continue for a long time and may recur in a modified form, stimulated by anniversaries, future losses or other reminders. People are likely to be changed by the experience of grieving but most, in time, find that they are able to function well and enjoy life again.

Normal manifestations of grief

Physical manifestations

Symptoms experienced by a bereaved person may include hollowness in the stomach, tightness in the chest or throat, oversensitivity to noise, feeling short of breath, muscle weakness, lack of energy, dry mouth and a sense of depersonalization.

Emotional manifestations

For many, a sense of shock and numbness is the initial emotional response to bereavement. Feelings of anger (directed at family, friends, medical staff, God, the deceased or no one in particular) and feelings of guilt (relating to real or imagined failings) are common, as is a yearning or desire for the return of the deceased. Anxiety and a sense of helplessness and disorganization are also normal responses. Sadness is the most commonly recognized manifestation of grief, but the greatest depth of sadness, something akin to depression, is often not reached until many months after the death. Feelings of relief and freedom may also be present, although people may then feel guilty for having these feelings.

Cognitive manifestations

Disbelief and a sense of unreality are frequently present early in a bereavement. For a while elements of denial may also be present. The bereaved may be preoccupied with thoughts about the deceased. It is also not uncommon for the bereaved to have a sense (visual, auditory etc.) of the presence of the deceased. Short-term memory, the ability to concentrate and sense of purpose are frequently detrimentally affected.

Behavioural manifestations

Appetite and sleep may be disturbed and dreams involving the deceased, with their attendant emotional impact for the bereaved, are not infrequent. The bereaved person may withdraw socially, avoid reminders of the deceased or act in an absent-minded way. They may also engage in restless overactivity, behaviour which suggests that they are at some level searching for the deceased or visit places or carry objects which remind them of the deceased. Some people contemplate rapid and radical changes in their lifestyle (e.g. new relationship or move of house), which may represent a way of avoiding the pain of bereavement. Such rapid changes soon after a bereavement are not normally advisable.

Psychological/psychiatric models

He was my North, my South, my East and West,
My working week and my Sunday rest,
My noon, my midnight, my talk, my song;
I thought that love would last forever: I was wrong.

W.H.Auden 1907–73: *Funeral Blues* (1936)

Grief and bereavement have been analysed over many years, and it is generally agreed that there are no single 'correct' or 'true' theories that explain the experience of loss or account for the emotions, experiences and cultural practices which characterize grief and mourning. Within broad cultural constraints, individuals manage bereavement in different ways, reflecting the diverse range of human responses. There are no strict rules in the UK about how people should behave, but the importance of ensuring that the bereaved are encouraged to express their emotions, to acknowledge the reality of the loss and to share thoughts and feelings with appropriate others, is recognized.

Theories of grief

Most cultures are aware of what happens after death and have ideas about how the bereaved should feel and behave. The range of beliefs, practices and rituals associated with death is large, particularly in multicultural societies, although many adapt to the customs of the host culture. Most religions support certain behaviours and practices both before and after death, but in an increasingly secular society this may now have less influence.

Psychological models

These are based on developmental notions of change and growth. It is assumed that bereavement is a process in which there is an outcome: individuals need to progress through phases or stages and tasks need to be accomplished. The theory is based on the fact that people have some control over their feelings and thoughts and that these can be accessed through talk. Individuals need to accept the reality of the loss so that the emotional energy can be released and redirected.

The effortful, mental process of withdrawing energy from the lost object is referred to as 'grief work'. It is essential to break relationships with the deceased, and to allow reinvestment of emotional energy and the formation of new relationships with others.

The most influential and earliest theories emerged from psychoanalysts such as Freud (1917), who also described normal and pathological grief. Bowlby (1969) proposed a complex theory of close human relationships in which separation triggers intense distress and behavioural responses.

Parkes (1996) proposed that people progress through phases in coming to terms with their loss and that they have to adapt to changes in relationships, social status and economic circumstances. Kubler Ross (1969) also proposed a staged model of emotional expression of loss described in terms of shock/denial, anger, bargaining, depression and ultimately acceptance.

Worden (1991) based his therapeutic model on phases of grief and tasks of mourning. He suggested that grief was a process, not a state, and that people needed to work through their reactions to loss to achieve a complete adjustment. Tasks that need to be accomplished in order to allow recovery from mourning included:

Task 1—To accept the reality of the loss

Task 2—To experience the pain of grief

Task 3—To adjust to an environment in which the deceased is missing

Task 4—To emotionally relocate the deceased and move on with life.

Stress and coping model

Stroebe and Schut (1999), in their dual process model of coping with grief, suggested that bereaved people tend to oscillate between loss-oriented experiences and restoration-oriented activity and that both are necessary to successfully negotiate the bereavement journey.

Social and relationship-focused models

Walters (1996) and Klass et al. (1996) have explored continuing bonds, emphasizing the importance for the living of interpreting the memory of the dead into their ongoing lives, recognizing the enduring influence of the deceased.

Stress and coping

These ideas are based on an assumption that if certain things, called stressors, are present in sufficient amounts, they trigger a stress response which is both physical and psychological. Humans are able to adapt to most things but things that challenge the adaptation process are considered to be stressful. The transactional model (Lazarus and Folkman 1991) proposed that any event may be seen as threatening and that cognitive appraisal is undertaken to estimate the degree of threat needed to mobilize resources to cope with it. Coping may focus on dealing with the threat directly (problem-focused), or may emphasize the emotional response (emotion-focused). Stroebe and Schut (1999) developed this idea proposing that after death people oscillate between restoration-focused coping (dealing with everyday life) and grief-focused coping (e.g. expressing their distress). People move between these extremes but become more restoration-focused with time. This is known as the dual processing model.

Continuity theory

This is based on an assumption that people wish to maintain feelings of continuity and that even though physical relationships may end at the time of death, relationships become transformed but remain important within the memory of the individual. Walters (1996) explored continuing bonds, emphasizing the importance for the living of interpreting the memory of the dead into their ongoing lives, recognizing their enduring influence.

Bereavement support

In practice, bereavement support whether through GPs or formally trained counsellors helps clients to tell their story. Staged or phased models are recognized, the bereaved being given affirmation that they are progressing satisfactorily along a path over time, even though this progression may not be linear.

It is recognizsed that people may become 'stuck' and unable to move through grief satisfactorily. Various techniques are used to support and encourage people to move forward and to begin engaging in life again.

GPs may become involved in grief counselling, but their main rôle is to screen for people who may be most at risk (📖 see below) from a complicated bereavement.

Specialist palliative care and bereavement

The philosophy of the hospice movement encompasses the care of patients and their families after death and into the bereavement period. The provision of bereavement support is regarded as integral to their services. Most services are based on the assumption that bereavement is a major stressful life event but that a minority experience substantial disruption to physical, psychological and social functioning.

Some argue that offering support to those people who have adequate internal and external resources can be disempowering and detrimental to coping. Bereavement support may include a broad range of activities such as social evenings, befriending, one to one counselling and support groups.

A mutlidisciplinary team including social workers, nurses chaplains, counsellors and doctors are usually involved. Occasionally clients present such difficult and complex problems that psychiatrists, clinical psychologists or other specialist healthcare workers may be required.

Table 14.1 Types of hospice and palliative care bereavement support for adults

Social activities	Supportive activities	Therapeutic activities
Condolence cards	Drop-in centre/coffee mornings	One-to-one counselling with professional or trained volunteer
Anniversary (of death) Cards	Self-help groups	Therapeutic support groups
Bereavement information leaflets	Information support groups	Drama, music or art therapy
Bereavement information resources (videos/books)	Volunteer visiting or befriending	Relaxation classes
Staff attending the funeral		Complementary therapies
Social evenings	Psychotherapy	
Memorial service or other rituals		

From M. Lloyd-Williams (ed.) (2003) *Psychosocial Issues in Palliative Care*. Oxford: Oxford University Press.

Complicated grief

Normal and abnormal responses to bereavement cover a continuum in which intensity of reaction, presence of a range of related grief behaviours, and time course betray the presence of an abnormal grief response.

'Complicated grief involves the presentation of certain grief-related symptoms at a time beyond that which is considered adaptive. We hypothesize that the presence of these symptoms after approximately 6 months puts the bereaved individual at heightened risk for enduring social, psychological and medical impairment.'

Prigerson, et al., 1995

'Complicated mourning means that, given the amount of time since the death, there is some compromise, distortion or failure of one of more of the …processes of mourning.'

Full realization of the pain of living without the deceased is denied, repressed or avoided The deceased is held on to as though alive. Symptoms do not resolve spontaneously and need active intervention

Rando, 1993

'…is more related to the intensity of a reaction or the duration of a reaction rather than the presence or absence of a specific behavior.'

Worden, 1982

Risk factors for developing complicated grief

Personal
- Markedly angry, ambivalent or dependent relationship with the decesed
- History of multiple loss experiences
- Mental health problems
- Perceived lack of social support

Circumstantial
- Sudden, unexpected death, especially when violent, mutilating or random
- Death from an overly lengthy llness
- Loss of a child
- Mourner's perception of loss as preventable

Historical
- Previous experience with complicated grief
- Insecurity in childhood attachments

Personality
- Inability to tolerate extremes of emotional distress
- Inability to tolerate dependency feelings
- Self-concept, rôle and value of 'being strong'

Social
- Socially unspeakable loss (e.g. suicide)
- Socially negated loss (e.g. loss of ex-spouse)
- Absence of social support network

Complicated grief includes:
- Symptoms of depression
- Symptoms of anxiety

- Grief specific symptoms of extraordinary intensity and duration that include:
  - Preoccupation with thoughts of the deceased
  - Disbelief
  - Feelings of being stunned
- Lack of acceptance of the death
- Yearning for the deceased
- Searching for the deceased
- Crying

The common psychiatric disorders related to grief include:
- Clinical depression
- Anxiety disorders, alcohol abuse or other substance abuse and dependence
- Psychotic disorders
- Post-traumatic stress disorder (PTSD)

While frank psychiatric disorders following bereavement are reasonably straightforward to diagnose, it is more difficult to pick up complicated grief, in which the pathological nature of the grief response is only distinguishable from normal grief by its character.

Recognition of complicated bereavement calls for an experienced clinical judgement that does not 'rationalize' the distress as understandable.

Warning signs of complicated grief
- Long term functional impairment
- Exaggerated, prolonged and intense grief reactions
- Significant neglect of self-care
- Frequent themes of loss in conversation, activity, behavior
- Idealization of the deceased
- Impulsive decision making
- Mental disorders following loss
- PTSD-like symptoms

Ways of helping a bereaved person
- 'Being there' for them
- Non-judgemental listening
- Encouraging them to talk about the deceased
- Giving permission for the expression of feelings
- Offering reassurance about the normality of feelings and experiences
- Promoting coping with everyday life and self care (eg adequate food intake)
- Screening for damaging behaviours (eg increased alcohol use, smoking, etc)
- Providing information, when requested, about the illness and death of their loved ones—also about the range of grief responses
- Educating others (family members and other support networks) about how best to help the bereaved person
- Becoming familiar with your own feelings about loss and grief
- Offer information about local bereavement support services eg. Hospice services or Cruse

Table 14.2 Clinical presentations of complicated grief

Category	Features
Inhibited or delayed grief	Avoidance postpones expression
Chronic grief	Perpetuation of mourning long-term
Traumatic grief	Unexpected and shocking form of death
Depressive disorders	Both major and minor depressions
Anxiety disorders	Insecurity and relational problems
Alcohol and substance abuse/dependence	Excessive use of substances impairs adaptive coping
Post-traumatic stress disorder	Persistent, intrusive images with cues
Psychotic disorders	Manic, severe depressive states, and schizophrenia

From Doyle, D.H., Hanks, G., Cherny, N. (2004) *Oxford Textbook of Palliative Medicine*, 3rd edn, p. 1140. Oxford: Oxford University Press.

Bereavement involving children

One feature of the grief of most children is that they do not sustain grief over continuing periods of time, but tend rather to dip in and out of grief—jumping in and out of puddles, rather than wading through the river of grief.

Adults should be aware that children will learn what is 'acceptable grief' from the adults around them.

Allowing expression of feelings—children will be helped by knowing that the expression of feelings is acceptable. Children may express their emotions and grief in many ways e.g. through play, artwork, music, drama etc.

Children's understanding, responses and needs will be affected by many factors, including their previous experiences of loss and how these were handled. It is important also to consider the age and the developmental level of the child, although any attempt to consider responses according to age will require flexibility and there is considerable crossover between different children.

Children under the age of 2–3 years may have little concept of death, but will be aware of separation and may protest against this by detachment or regressive behaviour. Children of this age need a consistent caregiver, familiar routines and the meeting of their physical and emotional needs.

Children aged between 3 and 5 years do not see death as irreversible. Their concerns will relate to separation, abandonment and the physical aspects of death and dying. Their response may include aggressive and rejecting behaviour. They may also become withdrawn or demonstrate an increase in clinging or demanding behaviour. There may also be regression to infant needs. Routine, comfort, reassurance and a simple answering of their questions will help a child of this age. They should be allowed to participate in family rituals and to keep mementos of the deceased. Adults should be aware of the words they use since they can be misinterpreted (e.g. do not associate death with sleep or a long journey).

Children age between 6 and 8 years seek causal explanations. A whole range of behaviours may be evidence of their response to grief—withdrawal, sadness, loneliness, depression, acting-out behaviour or becoming a 'perfect' child. Short, honest, concrete explanations will help a child of this age, as will maintaining contact with friends and normal activities. Short-term regression may be allowed and they should be reassured that they will always be cared for. Involvement in the family's grief related rituals will also help.

Pre-teenage children appear to have a calmer, more accepting attitude to death. They often have a good factual understanding of what has happened. The child should be encouraged to talk about the deceased and provided with clear and truthful answers to their questions. The feelings of adults do not need to be hidden, allowing the child to provide mutual help and reassurance.

Teenage years—children of this age are engaged in a search for meaning and purpose in life and for identity. They feel that they have deep and powerful emotions that no one else has experienced. Teenagers may exhibit withdrawal, sadness, loneliness and depression, or they may act-out in an angry, hostile and rejecting way. They may seek to cover up fears with joking and sarcasm. Young people of this age need as much comfort as possible, involvement, boundaries, a sense that their feelings are being taken seriously and reassurance that their feelings are normal. Continuing

---

Risk factors for complicated grief in bereaved children
These may be divided into three groups:

Features of the loss
- Traumatic
- Unexpected

Features of the child
- History of psychiatric disorder
- Multiple losses
- Child less than 5 years old
- Adolescent

Features of the relationship
- Ambivalent/conflicted
- Unsupportive family
- Death of a father (adolescent boys)
- Death of a mother (very young children)
- Mental illness in surviving parent

---

contact with their peers should be encouraged. Young people will often identify for themselves someone with whom they feel comfortable to talk.

Bereavement due to death of a child

The death of a child is a devastating loss, particularly in times where most childhood illness can be prevented or cured. It profoundly affects all those involved—parents, siblings, grandparents, extended family, friends and others involved in caring for the child. As a community we rarely experience the death of a child, which makes it all the more difficult when we do. There is a sense that the natural order of things has been upset.

Principles for working with bereaved parents

1 Make early contact and assess the bereaved parents.
2 Provide assurance that they can survive their loss, but acknowledge the uniqueness of their pain.
3 Allow adequate time for parents to grieve.
4 Facilitate the identification and expression of feelings including negative feelings such as anger, and guilt.
5 Encourage recall of memories of the deceased child.
6 Maintain a professional and realistic perspective—not all pain can be 'fixed'.
7 Allow for individual differences in response relating to gender, age, culture, personality, religion and the characteristics of the death.
8 Assist in finding a source of continuing support.
9 Identify complicated grief reactions and refer to appropriate services.

Interpret recovery to parents, and that 'recovery' is not a betrayal of their child. Health professionals need to recognize the significance they may have in a family's life. Many children are treated over long periods of time and the hospital/hospice may become something of a second home. Health professionals also care for families during the intense highs and lows of serious illness, and may even be present at the time the child dies. The significance of this cannot be overstated. These relationships cannot be abruptly ended and many (but not all) families will want ongoing contact with people they feel truly understand what they have experienced. A follow-up appointment with the child's paediatrician should always be offered to discuss the child's illness and treatment, the results of any outstanding investigations including post-mortem examinations and how the family is coping.

Sibling grief

Siblings almost universally experience distress, but many feel unable to share this for fear of burdening their already fragile parents. One of the many factors which influence sibling grief is developmental level and the impact this has on the child's understanding of illness and death.

Most children learn to recognize when something is dead before they reach three years of age. However, at this early age, death, separation and sleep are almost synonymous in the child's mind. As children develop and experience life, their concept of death becomes more mature. Six sub-concepts are acquired during this process (average age of attainment in brackets):

Separation (age 5)	Dead people do not co-exist with the living
Causality (age 6)	Death is caused by something, be it trauma, disease, or old age
Irreversibility (age 6)	A dead person can not 'come alive' again
Cessation of bodily functions (age 6)	The dead person does not need to eat or breathe
Universality (age 7)	All living things will die
Insensitivity (age 8)	The dead can not feel fear or pain

Supporting bereaved children

- Adjusting to the loss of a loved person does not necessarily require 'letting go' of the relationship. Indeed, bereaved children (and adults) often maintain a connection to the dead person. The relationship is reconstructed over time and maintained by remembering the person, keeping their belongings and sometimes talking to them. Children spend most of their time in the care of their parents. It is therefore important to empower parents to support siblings by equipping them with knowledge and ideas. Staff can encourage the family to:
  - **Provide information** in simple, developmentally appropriate language
  - **Be alert to misunderstandings** which may arise as a consequence of an incomplete death concept
  - Set aside special **time** for the child/young person
  - Openly **express emotion**
  - Recruit family, friends and teachers to help
  - **Allow the child to play** with friends and reassure them that it is OK to have fun
  - Help the child **create memories** e.g. Stories, photos, drawings, memory books
  - **Maintain normal routines and discipline** as much as possible
  - Allow the child/young person opportunities to feel in control
  - Resist any temptation to 'fix their grief'
  - Encourage them to do what feels right for them
  - Be there—to provide love, reassurance and routine
  - **Allow the child time alone.** Private 'space' is important
  - Talk about the death
  - **Answer questions,** no matter how explicit
  - Not be surprised if children use symbolic play, stories and art to make sense of their experience.

School grief

The following is adapted from *A Practical Guide to Paediatric Oncology Palliative Care*, Royal Children's Hospital, Brisbane 1999.

After the family, the school community may contain the people most affected by the death of a child—friends, fellow students, teachers, administrative staff. Parents form part of a wider school community. It may well be the first bereavement experience for the child's peers, their parents and teachers. Close attachments are formed between children and their teachers, so that the death of a child may be a personal as well as a professional loss.

In a school, there will be a range of grief responses. It is anticipated that both staff and students will be vulnerable to stress and may express themselves differently. For the student, the closer they were to the child the more profound will be the consequences. Teachers may notice a change in the other student's behaviour, thought processes, concentration and academic performance. A greater level of support, monitoring and care may be warranted, even for those students who may not be expressing their grief in an obvious way.

People who may be at increased risk are:
- those who have already experienced significant loss in their lives
- those who have a close relationship with the child who has died or the child's siblings, and those who have similar health problems themselves or in their family

The school is in an ideal position to provide opportunities for students to be supported as well as to identify those who may be experiencing difficulty. The child's parents should always be consulted before any information is released so that their privacy and the best interests of any siblings are considered and respected.

Ways in which the school can help include:
- Informing staff and students of the child's death is a priority. Anxiety and misinformation are fuelled by uncertainty and delay
- Senior staff need to acknowledge the sadness of what has happened, perhaps by way of assemblies, class announcements and letters home
- Staff and children need the opportunity to talk about what has happened, to ask questions, and to express their feelings. This is best done in familiar small groups, though it may also be appropriate to set aside a time where people can come and talk together. Students can also be given opportunities to write farewell letters or tributes, and to create artwork as an expression of thoughts and feelings
- A sense of routine provides reassurance to staff and students who have experienced trauma. It is therefore important that the school continues to function as a supportive and stable part of the staff and student's environment
- Staff will need their own support. Staff meetings provide an opportunity to provide information, monitor the reactions of the children and discuss feelings. In some cases, it may be helpful to hold a special meeting facilitated by someone with expertise in this area. Senior staff are usually required to manage the immediate crisis and may experience a 'delayed reaction'
- There are a number of ways in which the school can maintain contact with the family. This may be through friends or formal rituals. Some families welcome the participation of the school in the funeral for example, and may wish to be involved in school memorial services. The child may also have expressed wishes regarding the involvement of their school friends

Assessment of bereavement risk
The assessment of bereavement risk presupposes that some individuals will display a grief reaction that does not fit a 'normal' or expected pattern or level of intensity. Factors that influence complicated bereavement are:
- stage of the life cycle particularly when:
  the bereaved parent is an adolescent and family support is perceived as inadequate. the surviving parent of a deceased child is a single mother/father as a result of divorce or being widowed
- a history of previous losses, particularly if unresolved. Losses may include:
  - loss of a pregnancy
  - loss of a job
  - divorce

- the presence of concurrent or additional stressors such as:
  - family tension
  - compromised financial status
  - dissatisfaction with caregiving
  - reliance on alcohol and psychotropic medications, pre-bereavement
- physical and mental illness particularly:
  - current/past history of mental health problems that have required psychiatric/psychological support
  - family history of psychiatric disorders
- high pre-death distress
- inability or restriction in use of coping strategies such as:
  - maintenance of physical self-care
  - identification of prominent themes of grief
  - attributing meaning to the loss
  - differentiation between letting go of grief and forgetting the bereaved
  - accessing available support
- isolated, alienated individuals
- low levels of internal control beliefs, such as:
  - feeling as if he/she has no control over life
- the availability of social support particularly if:
  - people in the immediate environment are, or are perceived to be, unsupportive
  - support from family and friends immediately prior to death was good and following death it subsided
- the bereaved lack a confidant with whom to share feelings, concerns, doubts, dreams and nightmares
- the bereaved is dissatisfied with the help available during their child's illness

Further Reading

Bowlby, J. (1969) *Attachment and loss: vol.* 1. Harmondsworth: Penguin.

Freud, S. (1961a) Mourning and melancholia. In J. Strachey (ed. and trans.) *The standard edition of the complete psychological works of Sigmund Freud*, vol. 14, pp. 243–58. London: Hogarth Press (original work published 1917).

Klass, D., Silverman, P., Nickman, S. (eds.) (1996) *Continuing bonds*. London: Taylor & Francis.

Kubler-Ross, E. (1969) *On death and dying*. London: Tavistock Publications.

Lazarus, R., Folkman, S. (1991) *Stress and coping*. 3rd edn. New York: Columbia University Press.

Parkes, C. M. (1996) *Bereavement*. 3rd edn. London: Routledge.

Prigerson, H. G., *et al.* (1995) Inventory of complicated grief. *Psychiatry research,* **59**: 65–79.

Rando, T. A. (1993) *Treatment of complicated mourning*. Champaign: Research Press.

Stroebe, M., Schut, H. (1999) The dual process model of coping with bereavement. *Death studies,* **23**: 197–224.

Walters, T. (1996) A new model of grief. *Mortality,* **1**: 7–25.

Winston's Wish. *www.winstonswish.org.uk.*

Worden, J. W. (1991) *Grief counselling and grief therapy*. 2nd edn. London: Routledge.

A Charter for Bereaved Children

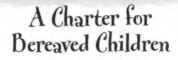

"A child can live through anything provided they are told the truth and allowed to share the natural feelings people have when they are suffering" Eda Le Shan

This Charter has been written following our conversations with over 2,000 bereaved children and their families since Winston's Wish began in 1992. Although supporting a bereaved child can seem a daunting challenge, we have found that there are simple and straightforward ways which can make a positive difference to a grieving child. If we live in a society that genuinely wants to enable children and young people to re-build their lives after the death of a family member, then we need to respect their rights to the following:

1. Adequate Information

Bereaved children are entitled to receive answers to their questions and information that clearly explains **what** has happened, **why** it has happened and **what** will happen **next**.

'Daddy died of a tumour, but I don't know what a tumour is.' Alice, age 6, whose father died of stomach cancer.

2. Being Involved

Bereaved children should be asked if they wish to be **involved** in important decisions that have an impact on their lives (such as planning the funeral, remembering anniversaries).

'I helped to choose mum's favourite music which they played at her funeral.' Kim, age 12.

3. Family Involvement

Bereaved children should receive support which **includes their parent(s)** and which also respects each child's confidentiality.

'Meeting other parents in exactly the same situation as me was so helpful.' John whose wife died from a brain haemorrhage.

4. Meeting Others

Bereaved children can benefit from the opportunity of **meeting other children** who have had similar experiences.

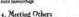

'Often I went to break down and cry but I can't do that in front of my school mates... meeting all the other kids who have been through the same thing – I don't feel alone any more.' Colin, age 12, whose mother died.

5. Telling the Story

Bereaved children have the right to **tell their story** in a variety of ways and for those stories to be heard, read or seen by those important to them. For example, through drawing, puppets, letters and words.

'My picture shows the car banged dad on the head, he fell off his bike, hit his head and died later in hospital.' Georgina, age 7, whose father died in a road accident.

6. Expressing Feelings

Bereaved children should feel comfortable expressing **all** feelings associated with grief such as anger, sadness, guilt and anxiety, and to be helped to find appropriate ways to do this.

'It's alright to cry and OK to be happy as well.' James, age 9, whose dad died from a heart attack.

7. Not to Blame

Bereaved children should be helped to understand that they are **not responsible and not to blame** for the death.

'I now understand it wasn't anyone's fault.' Chris, age 12, whose dad died by suicide.

8. Established Routines

Bereaved children should be able to choose to **continue** previously enjoyed activities and interests.

'I went to Brownies after Meg died. I wanted my friends to know.'

9. School Response

Bereaved children can benefit from receiving an appropriate and positive response from their **school or college**.

'My teacher remembers the days which are difficult, like Father's Day and dad's birthday.' Alex, age 9.

10. Remembering

Bereaved children have the right to remember the person who has died for the rest of their lives if they wish to do so. This may involve re-living memories (both good and difficult) so that the person becomes a comfortable part of the child's on-going life story.

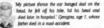

'I like to show my memory book to people who didn't have the chance to know my dad.' Bethany, age 8, whose father died from cancer.

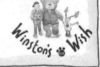

Winston's Wish

Fig. 14.1 A charter for bereaved children

Chapter 15

Emergencies in palliative care

While this chapter focuses on the common oncological emergencies in palliative practice, other emergencies include a wider range of issues such as:

- An emergency discharge so a patient's wish to die at home can be met
- Emotional emergencies, with high levels of expressed anxiety
- Spiritual/existential/social emergencies with pressure to 'sort things out' before it is too late

It is important to have a clear understanding of the management of emergencies in palliative care as clear thinking is crucial in handling such, thankfully rare, situations. Providing transparent decisiveness to the patient, family and staff can transform a crisis situation filled with anxiety.

> The time frame for normal hospice and palliative care interventions are modulated by the need for calmness and patient comfort. There are however several emergency situations which can occur for hospice patients requiring urgent and prompt diagnosis and management. This may create some dissonance among staff and other patients. It is vital that all staff appreciate the nature of these emergencies and the importance of an emergency response.

Sepsis in the neutropaenic patient

All clinical staff should be acutely aware of the serious risk and potential rapid fatality of patients who have become neutropaenic and febrile with oncological treatments.

Patients should be admitted to a unit where essential investigations can be carried out rapidly and where intravenous antibiotics can be given and suitable monitoring maintained. Appropriate facilities are not usually available within a hospice unit. Occasionally patients may develop neutropaenic sepsis while in a palliative care unit, which may create a dilemma. After full discussion of the seriousness of the situation and the high chance of a good response to optimal management in an acute unit, patients may still refuse ambulance transfer, preferring to stay in the hospice and to risk suboptimal care. This should be discussed with their oncologist if possible.

Empirical treatment of a febrile neutropaenic patient should be instigated and an appropriate antibiotic regime started, *with advice from the local bacteriologist since antibiotic regimes vary across the country.*

A regime currently being advocated at The Royal Marsden Hospital is outlined below as an example:

- Tazocin 4.5g q.d.s. + gentamicin 5mg/kg i/v o.d.
- Or, if allergic to penicillin
- Ceftazidime 2g i/v t.d.s. + gentamicin5mg/kg i/v o.d.
- If still febrile after 48 h:
- Add vancomycin 1g i/v b.d.

- If still febrile after 96–120 h:
- Stop tazocin + gentamicin
- Start ciprofloxacin 400mg i/v b.d.
- Add amphotericin 0.75mg/kg/day i/v (or 1mg/kg/day for haemato-oncology patients)
- Treat for a minimum of seven days and continue until neutrophil count >0.5 × 10^9/l.[1]

Signs of Spinal Cord Compression
- Back pain 90%
- Weak legs
- Increased reflexes
- Sensory level
- Urinary hesitancy (late feature)

Spinal cord compression

Spinal cord compression occurs in 3–5 per cent of patients with cancer, and 10% of patients with spinal metastases develop cord compression,[2] the frequency being highest in multiple myeloma and cancers of the prostate, breast and bronchus.
- Malignant causes:
  - intramedullary metastases
  - intradural metastases
  - extradural compression (80 per cent)—vertebral body metastasis
    - vertebral collapse
    - tumour spread
    - interruption of vascular supply

It is important to have a high index of suspicion for possible cord compression, because of the consequences of paraplegia and urine and faecal incontinence with a delay in diagnosis.

Symptoms and signs
- Back pain, a sensation of weakness in the legs and often vague sensory symptoms in the legs may be early manifestations. Patients may complain of a band-like pain, particularly on coughing or sneezing
- For those presenting with profound weakness, a sensory 'level' and sphincter disturbance, which are relatively late features, the outcome is poor and the compression is much less likely to be reversible

The site of compression is
- thoracic in 70%
- lumbosacral 20%
- cervical 10%

Lesions above L1 (lower end of spinal cord) will produce upper motor neurone signs and often a sensory level, whereas lesions below L1 will produce lower motor neurone signs and peri-anal numbness (cauda equina syndrome). Multiple sites of compression may produce different and confusing neurological signs.

Table 15.1 Neurological signs of upper and lower motor neurone lesions

	Upper motor neurone lesion	Lower motor neurone lesion
Power	Reduced/absent	Reduced/absent
Tone	Increased	Reduced
Sensation	Sensory loss	Sensory loss
Reflexes (plantars)	Increased (upgoing)	Absent/reduced (downgoing)

Management

High dose corticosteroids (dexamethasone 16 mg/day) to relieve peritumoural oedema; urgent referral to oncology centre.

Spinal cord compression is an EMERGENCY and two questions need to be answered urgently.

1 Does this patient have a reasonable likelihood of having spinal cord compression?
2 Would this patient benefit from instituting emergency investigation and treatment?

Does this patient have a reasonable likelihood of having spinal cord compression?

Even the most skilled clinician is unable to diagnose spinal cord compression with absolute certainty. Often by the time clinical signs are 'classic', it is too late for patients to benefit from treatment, as it has a limited rôle in reversing symptoms which are already established. Thus if intervention to prevent paraplegia is to be successful, potential compression needs to be diagnosed early.

The keys to diagnosing Spinal Cord Compression include:

- Having a high index of suspicion in patients with spinal metastases particularly in patients with breast, lung and prostate cancer and with pain and tenderness on palpation or percussion of the vertebra at the level of the suspected lesion
- Taking patients' complaints about back pain, odd sensations in the legs, and difficulties in passing urine seriously

Would this patient benefit from instituting emergency investigation and treatment?

The patient will need to be transferred to a specialized unit where an MRI scan can be carried out and treatment given. In the context of metastatic cancer, radiotherapy is often the most appropriate treatment, but surgery may need considering in specific circumstances.

Deciding whether the particular course of treatment is appropriate for a particular patient involves an overall assessment.

---

1 The Royal Marsden Drug and Therapeutics Advisory Committee Prescribing Guidelines, including symptom control guidelines, p. 110. London: Royal Marsden NHS Trust.

2 Kaye P. (1999) *Decision-making in Palliative Care*, p. 183. Northampton: EPL Publications.

Key questions in deciding on emergency investigations and management.
- Does the patient want emergency management?
- Is the patient still walking?
- Is the patient suffering from severe back pain?
- Has the patient already established cord compression?
- Has the patient a short prognosis (eg. week by week deterioration.)

Where suspicion of spinal cord compression is high, it is quickest to contact by telephone the oncological team in the cancer centre where the patient has been managed, who can then co-ordinate the necessary scan and appropriate emergency treatment.

Table 15.2 Definitive treatment of spinal cord compression

Indications for surgical decompression	Indications for radiotherapy
1 Uncertain cause—to obtain histology	1 Radiosensitive tumour
2 Radiotherapy has not been effective or symptoms persist despite maximum radiotherapy	2 Multiple levels of compression
3 Radio-resistant tumour e.g. melanoma, sarcoma	3 Unfit for major surgery
4 Unstable spine	4 Patient choice
5 Major structural compression	
6 Cervical cord lesion	
7 Solitary vertebral metastasis	

Patients with spinal cord compression provide great challenges to the multidisciplinary team. These challenges include:
- Mobility management (risk of venous thrombosis)
- Skin management in a patient confined to bed (risk of pressure sores)
- Bowel management
- Urinary system management
- Psychological management.

There is no consensus on the optimum time to start mobilizing patients diagnosed with cord compression. In general principles, if the spine is stable and the pain is relatively well controlled it would seem wise to introduce physiotherapy as soon as possible to maintain muscle tone and motor function as well as possible. The occupational therapist will be crucial in helping with goal-setting and rehabilitative techniques.

Steroids are usually continued at high dose to start with and then tailed off gradually and completely over a few weeks (4–6 weeks or so) or to the lowest dose that maintains stability. Radiation-induced oedema may exacerbate symptoms and the dose of steroids may need to increase temporarily during treatment.

Prognosis

Overall, 30 per cent of patients may survive for one year. A patient who is ambulant after treatment may survive 8–9 months, but the life expectancy for a patient who remains paraplegic is a few weeks only. Function will be retained in 70 per cent of patients who were ambulant prior to treatment but will return in only 5 per cent of those who were paraplegic at the outset. Return of motor function is better in those with incomplete spinal compression and particularly with partial lesions of the cauda equina. Loss of sphincter function is a bad prognostic sign.

In practice, most patients with an established diagnosis are relatively unwell and have multiple metastases, and will be referred for radiotherapy, achieving similar results to those of surgery.

Superior vena cava obstruction

Superior vena cava obstruction (SVCO) is due to external compression of and/or thrombosis of the SVC by mediastinal lymph nodes or tumour in the region of the right main bronchus. It is caused most commonly by carcinoma of the bronchus (75 per cent) and lymphomas (15 per cent). Cancers of the breast, colon, oesophagus and testis account for the remaining 10 per cent.

Symptoms and signs

Symptoms are those of venous hypertension and include breathlessness (laryngeal oedema or tracheal or bronchial obstruction/compression), headache (cerebral oedema), visual changes, dizziness and swelling of the face, neck and arms.

Signs include engorged conjunctivae, peri-orbital oedema, non-pulsatile dilated neck veins and dilated collateral veins (chest and arms). If the latter sign evolves, the symptoms of SVCO may stabilize. Papilloedema is a late feature.

Management

In the palliative care setting, the diagnosis (usually of carcinoma of the bronchus) is established already. SVCO can present acutely, resulting in very distressing symptoms. The patient should be referred to the oncology centre for urgent management.

- Dexamethasone 8–16mg p.o. or i/v. There is no good evidence for the efficacy of steroids but they may be helpful in reducing oedema (if there is associated stridor), or as an anti-tumour agent for lymphoma
- Frusemide 40mg p.o. or i/v
- Consider prophylactic anticonvulsant
- Treatment is the standard oncology treatment for the particular underlying cancer; for instance, chemotherapy for SCLC and lymphoma, radiotherapy for non-small cell carcinoma of the bronchus
- Intraluminal stents can be inserted via the femoral vein and is the treatment of choice for patients with severe symptoms
- Thrombolysis may be considered prior to stenting

Prognosis

Without treatment, SVCO can progress over several days leading to death. Prognosis is poor in a patient presenting with advanced SVCO unless the primary cancer is responsive to radiotherapy or chemotherapy. Generally, the prognosis is that of the underlying tumour.

Haemorrhage

Haemorrhage may be directly related to the underlying tumour or caused by treatments such as steroids or non steroidal anti-inflammatory drugs resulting in gastric/duodenal erosion. A generalized clotting deficiency, seen in thrombocytopaenia, hepatic insufficiency or anti-coagulation with warfarin, are also contributory factors in patients with cancer.

Treatments for *non-acute haemorrhage* include oncological, systemic and local measures. Palliative radiotherapy is very useful for superficial tumours and those of the bronchus and genito-urinary tract. If radiotherapy is not appropriate, coagulation should be enhanced with oral tranexamic acid 1 g t.d.s., but caution is necessary with haematuria since clots may form in the renal tract, resulting in further problems. Local measures for superficial tumours, such as topical tranexamic acid or adrenalin (1:1000) soaks, may be useful. Sucralfate may act as a local astringent to stop stomach mucosal bleeding in addition to a proton pump inhibitor such as lansoprazole.

Erosion of a major artery can cause *acute haemorrhage*, which may be a rapidly terminal event. It may be possible to anticipate such an occurrence, and appropriate medication and a red blanket to reduce the visual impact should be readily available. Relatives or others who witness such an event will need a great deal of support. If the haemorrhage is not immediately fatal, such as with a haematemesis or bleeding from the rectum, vagina or superficially ulcerated wound, the aim of treatment is local control if possible and sedation of a shocked, frightened patient. Rectal or sublingual diazepam (stesolid 10 mg) or midazolam 10 mg SC or buccally act quickly.

The palliative care team need to balance the anxiety of alerting and preparing the family for such an event against the likelihood of it occurring. If the patient chooses to be looked after at home, the issues of managing acute haemorrhage need to be discussed with the family and the home care team and a clear plan worked out.

It may be appropriate to have emergency medication in the home to sedate the acutely bleeding patient. Such a strategy needs lengthy discussion with the family, carers, and the patient's local GP, and clearly documented plans.

Convulsions 📖 see Chapter 6j

Hypercalcaemia

Hypercalcaemia occurs in 10 per cent of patients with cancer. The pathogenesis of hypercalcaemia includes increased bone resorption (osteolysis) and systemic release of humoral hypercalcaemic factors, with or without evidence of metastatic bone disease. Calcium is released from bone and in addition there may be a decrease in excretion of urinary calcium. Calcium release from bone is attributed to locally active substances produced by bone metastases (cytokines, particularly interleukins and tumour necrosis factor, and other factors which stimulate prostaglandin function), or by factors such as ectopic parathyroid hormone related protein (PTHrP). The tumours most commonly associated with hypercalcaemia include squamous cell carcinoma of the bronchus (and other squamous cell tumours), carcinoma of the breast and prostate and multiple myeloma.

A corrected plasma calcium concentration above 2.6 mmol/litre defines hypercalcaemia. It is often mild and asymptomatic and significant symptoms usually only develop with levels above 3.0 mmol/litre. Levels of 4.0 mmol/litre and above will cause death in a few days if left untreated.

Symptoms include drowsiness, confusion, nausea, vomiting, thirst, polyuria, weakness and constipation.

Management

Treatment is only necessary if there are symptoms and may be unnecessary if the patient is very near to death. Patients should be encouraged to mobilize if appropriate. Absorption of calcium from the gut is generally reduced, so patients may eat what they wish regardless of the calcium content of food.

Hypercalcaemia usually responds to specific antitumour therapy if appropriate.

Fluid replacement

Patients are usually dehydrated and need adequate fluid replacement. A high oral intake of fluid should be encouraged as appropriate for the individual clinical situation. Alternatively, extra fluid should be given intravenously. Fluid replacement alone improves symptoms but rarely achieves total control.

Bisphosphonates

Bisphosphonates inhibit osteoclast activity and thereby inhibit bone resorption. Because of poor alimentary absorption, they are usually given intravenously initially. Disodium pamidronate or sodium clodronate are effective in 70–80 per cent of patients for an average of two to three weeks. Zoledronic acid can be given over a shorter period and the effect lasts for longer. Patients receiving bisphoshonates may develop transient fever and bone pains; they may also become hypocalcaemic and need to be monitored.

Give:

- e.g. zoledronic acid 4 mg in 50 ml sodium chloride 0.9 per cent over 15 minutes
- disodium pamidronate 60–90 mg in sodium chloride 0.9 per cent, 500 ml over 2–4 h
- sodium clodronate 1.5 g in sodium chloride 0.9 per cent, 500 ml over 4 h
- Plasma calcium levels start to fall after 48 h and fall progressively for the next six days. Oral bisphosphonates have been reported to delay the recurrence of hypercalcaemia and may be important for maintenance

The introduction of once or twice daily oral bisphosphonates have made complying with the strictures to avoid eating for one hour before and after treatment easier.

Prognosis

Eighty per cent of cancer patients with hypercalcaemia survive less than one year.

Further reading

Books

Doyle D., Hanks G., Cherny N., Calman K. (2004) *Oxford Textbook of Palliative Medicine*, 3 rd edn. Oxford: Oxford University Press.

Regnard C., Tempest S. *A Guide to Symptom Relief in Advanced Disease.*

Twycross R., Wilcock A. (2001) *Symptom Management in Advanced Cancer*. 3rd edn. Oxford: Radcliffe Medical Press.

Handbooks

Back, I. (2001) *Palliative Medicine Handbook*. 3rd edn. Cardiff: BPM Books.

Kaye P. (1999) *Decision-Making in Palliative Care*, pp. 182–3. Northampton: EPL Publications.

The Royal Marsden Hospital (2000) *Prescribing Guidelines*, including symptom and control guidelines p. 110. London: Royal Marsden NHS Trust.

Articles

Falk S., Fallon M. (1997) ABC of palliative care. Emergencies. *BMJ*, **315**, 7121: 1525–8.

Kramer J. A. (1992) Spinal cord compression in malignancy. *Palliative Medicine*, **6**: 202–11.

Hillier R., Wee B. (1997) Palliative management of spinal cord compression. *European Journal of Palliative Care*, **4**: 189–92.

Smith A. M. (1994) Emergencies in palliative care. *Annals of Medicine*, **23**, 2: 186–90.

Chapter 16

Miscellaneous

Fitness to drive

In the interest of road safety those who suffer from a medical condition likely to cause a sudden disabling event at the wheel or inability to safely control their vehicle from any other cause should not drive.

Doctors have a duty to inform patients when they are prescribed medication which may impair their driving (GMC guidelines). Patients should be reminded that motor insurance may become invalid if there are changes in medical circumstances.

Many drugs used in palliative care may impair cognitive and motor skills including:-

1 Opioid analgesics
2 Benzodiazepines-e.g. diazepam, lorazepam
3 Antidepressants-e.g. amitriptyline
4 Phenothiazines-e.g. levomepromazine
5 Antihistamines-e.g. cyclizine

It is the duty of the **licence-holder** to notify the DVLA of any medical conditions which may affect safe driving. Most patients are sensible and responsible and with the support of family members are safe on the roads. They will avoid driving when their physical or mental condition begins to affect their judgement and ability to react quickly to unpredictable circumstances.

Driving is often seen as an important factor in maintaining the struggle for independence. It may be very hard for the patient, on both a practical and emotional level, to agree to letting go of the last vestiges of control over their lives. Very sensitive handling is needed.

If a patient is obviously unfit to drive for any reason and refuses to comply, the GMC issues the following guidelines:

1 The DVLA is legally responsible for deciding if a person is medically unfit to drive. They need to know when driving licence holders have a condition which may, now or in the future, affect their safety as a driver.
2 Therefore, where patients have such conditions, the doctor should:
   • Make sure that the patients understand that the condition may impair their ability to drive. If a patient is incapable of understanding this advice, for example because of dementia, you should inform the DVLA immediately.
3 Explain to patients that they have a legal duty to inform the DVLA about the condition. If the patient refuses to accept the diagnosis or the effect of the condition on his/her ability to drive, you can suggest that he/she seeks a second opinion, and make appropriate arrangements for

this. You should advise patients not to drive until the second opinion has been obtained.

4 If patients continue to drive when they are not fit to do so, you should make every reasonable effort to persuade them to stop. This may include telling their next of kin.

5 If you do not manage to persuade patients to stop driving, or you are given or find evidence that a patient is continuing to drive contrary to advice, you should disclose relevant medical information immediately, in confidence, to the medical adviser at DVLA.

6 Before giving information to the DVLA you should inform the patient of your decision to do so. Once the DVLA has been informed, you should also write to the patient, to confirm that a disclosure has been made.

Driving and opioid analgesia

Patients on longer term stable doses of opioids show only minor effects in terms of diminished cognition, perception, coordination or behaviour related to driving.

Patients, however, who are started on opioids or who are prescribed an increase above their 'normal' stable dose may show cognitive impairment for a few weeks or so. These patients should be advised not to drive during this period.

Driving and brain tumours

The diagnosis of a high grade primary or secondary brain tumour, whether or not a convulsion has occurred, must be notified to the DVLA. Patients will not be allowed to drive for at least two years after treatment.

Driving and seat belts

Exemption from having to wear a seat belt may be sought if it is thought to pose a danger to the patient's safety, such as in the situation of significant intra-abdominal disease.

Application forms for a Certificate of Exemption in the UK, may be obtained through the NHS Response telephone line.

Useful contact

The Medical Adviser
Drivers Medical Unit DVLA
Longview Road
Morriston
Swansea SA99 1TU
DVLA At A Glance—Current medical standards of fitness to drive—www.dvla.gov.uk

Tissue donation

The benefits offered by organ and tissue transplantation are now recognized by many, but demand continues to exceed supply. The majority of organs are donated by the relatives of patients who fulfil brainstem death criteria in intensive care units. There is evidence that donation, far from increasing relative's distress, may help in bereavement, families gaining comfort and meaning to the sudden death. Studies have shown that relatives are generally happy to talk about donation and to feel that some good has resulted from the death. Donation of tissues of patients dying from cancer, however, is relatively uncommon, possibly stemming from the relative lack of research in this group of patients.

Some professionals feel that there is a 'duty to ask' for tissue donation and indeed some families have felt cheated by not being given the opportunity to discuss the issue.

The subject of tissue donation may be straight forward if it has been discussed with the patient prior to death and if a donor card is available. Even in this situation, a lack of objection should always be sought from the next of kin.

In practice, it is easiest for corneas to be donated since this can be organized (it must be within 24 h) at the location of death without the need for transfer to a hospital pathologist. The transplant coordinator will arrange for the eyes to be removed. (The sockets are packed to ensure that the body does not appear to have been mutilated.)

A fear in popular culture that mutilation of the body, particularly the eyes, affects the deceased's beauty, identity or personhood and the idea that vision is necessary for the after-life, may be some of the reasons cited for families being reluctant to agree to donation.

Debate continues on presumed consent with an 'opt out' clause. There is evidence that those who consent to donation do so not out of social duty but out of altruism and generosity, with which they gain positive rewards. The subject of tissue donation remains a very individual and sensitive issue which needs careful handling in inevitably vulnerable families.

There are various practical considerations, some are outlined below.

	Cornea	Heart valves and trachea	Kidneys
Max. age of donor	Any age	60 years	70 years
Max. time from asystole to tissue removal	24h	72h	1hr

Contra-indications

The criteria for acceptability of tissues for donation are inevitably becoming more stringent. In the UK, a regional transplant coordinator is available 24 h a day and gives very helpful advice.

Follow up

The transplant team writes an acknowledgement letter to the family informing them of how the tissues have been used. Families usually find this very comforting.

Travelling abroad

It is not uncommon for terminally ill patients to want to travel abroad in order to see family or to die in their home country. A wish to travel by air needs to be balanced against the risk to the individual and the inconvenience and cost to fellow passengers and airlines in the event of unscheduled changes to flight plans. If there is any doubt, the airline medical officer, who will give the final authorization, should be contacted well in advance of travel.

In flight

During flight, changes in air pressure occur and p02 may be reduced. For this reason, patients with marked breathlessness (who are not able to walk more than 50 metres), with Hb less than 7.5g/l, ischaemic heart disease, cardiac failure or those who are oxygen-dependent may have difficulty.

In-flight cabin oxygen is inadequate for such patients. Extra supplies of oxygen may be made available as necessary if the airline is aware in advance.

At lower atmospheric pressures, air expands and for this reason patients with a pneumothorax, large bullae, ear/sinus disease and recent surgery or colonoscopy should not fly without advice. Other conditions to consider carefully are patients with intracranial tumours or confusion.

Patients will be at risk of thromboembolism on long haul flights, especially if they are not able to mobilize adequately; the use of support stockings or foot rocking devices may be appropriate.

Special arrangements

Transport to and from airports is arranged by the patient. If a stretcher is required, nine economy class seats are required, the cost of which is born by the patient.

Cabin staff are not authorized to look after personal care needs, medical treatment or specialized medical equipment.

An escort for a patient who is flying will be needed if:
- a patient is relatively dependent
- if a patient has a syringe driver
- if a patient has surgical drains
- if emergency management of symptoms may be needed
- if medication might need to be given by injection
- if the journey is long and interrupted by several transfers

It is important to remember that all medication or equipment that might be needed during the flight are kept in *hand* luggage. This includes all regular medication including analgesics, antiemetics, anticonvulsants, steroids, insulin, inhalers and any medication such as GTN which might be needed on an 'as required' basis. Syringes, needles, spare batteries and a sharps disposal box, if appropriate, should be remembered.

Medication

All drugs, particularly controlled drugs, should be contained in the original packaging, clearly labelled and in a sturdy shockproof container. A letter from the doctor outlining the medical condition and prescribed medication should also be carried for customs officers. Prior to travelling it is sensible to liaise with medical services in the area of destination, and to check that all medication, especially opioids, are available in that country.

Opioids to an equivalent total dose of morphine 1200mg may be taken abroad legally; however, a Home Office licence needs to be obtained for drugs taken out of the UK in excess of the following amounts:

Total dose allowed:

- Oral morphine 1200mg
- Diamorphine 1350mg
- Oxycodone 900mg
- Hydromorphone 360mg
- Fentanyl 45mg
- Methadone 500mg
- Benzodiazepine 900mg

Useful information address

Home Office Licensing Department
For taking opioids abroad
Tel: 020 7273 3806; 020 7217 8457

Further reading

Books

Doyle D., Hanks G., Cherny N., Calman, K. (2004) *Oxford Textbook of Palliative Medicine*. 3rd edn. Oxford: Oxford University Press.

The Liverpool integrated care pathway for the dying patient

What is an integrated care pathway?

Integrated care pathways (ICP) were originally developed in the North American healthcare system. More recently they have been introduced in Great Britain (1,2). An ICP provides a template of care which outlines best practice for a given clinical situation e.g. chest pain, breast cancer, leg ulceration, care of the dying. It incorporates guidelines and supporting documentation to facilitate the integration of evidence-based practice into care. The ICP is the central organizational tool for documenting patient care and is completed by all healthcare professionals. It replaces all other documentation. ICPs are widely seen as the precursor of the electronic patient record (3).

Developing an ICP

To develop integrated care pathways throughout an organization is an ambitious aim. The process is usually initiated by identifying a particular phase of care from which a pathway can be developed, for example in palliative care, the care of the dying. Following the development and implementation of a care pathway for one phase of care, subsequent ICPs can be developed to include the whole patient journey.

In order to develop an ICP, all professions involved in the care of the patient during the identified phase of care meet to review and identify the key goals of care. Key goals or outcomes of care reflect evidence-based practice and incorporate national and local guidelines. Having identified the key goals, prompts that enable the goal to be achieved or not achieved (i.e. a variance) are identified for each goal. Involvement and ownership of the pathway by all members of the team is crucial at this stage if the document is to be a true reflection of multidisciplinary working. It is therefore essential that when appropriate nurses, doctors, social workers, chaplains, occupational therapists and physiotherapists all participate in the development process and that the perspective of the user is sought.

The use and understanding of *variance* is critical to the success of integrated care pathways. When used in the context of integrated care pathways, a variance can be defined as a deviation from the identified plan of care. These variances should not be viewed as failures, but can be subdivided into those that are avoidable and those that are unavoidable. An example of an avoidable variance in the care of the dying would be an occasion when no member of the team had informed the relatives that the patient was dying. If the patient had no relatives, then this would be an unavoidable variance. By analysing the variance, it is possible to identify potential training and resource needs. In the example given above, a need for training in communication skills would be identified to improve communication with relatives regarding dying patients.

Further reading

Books

de Luc K. (2000) *Developing Care Pathways*. Oxford: Radcliffe Medical Press.

Department of Health (2000) *The NHS Cancer Plan—A plan for investment, A plan for reform*. London: DoH.

Ellershaw J. E., Wilkinson S. (eds) (2003) *Care of the Dying: A pathway to excellence*. Oxford: Oxford University Press.

Articles

Campbell H., Hotchkiss R., Bradshaw N., Porteous M. (1998) Integrated care pathways. *BMJ*, **316**: 133–7.

Elllershaw J. E., Smith, C., Overill S., et al. (2001) Care of the dying. *Journal of Pain & Symptom Management*, **21**: 12–17.

Elllershaw J. E., Ward C. (2003) Care of the dying patient: the last hours or days of life. *BMJ*, **326**: 30–4.

Death certification and referral to coroner

In the UK death certification has been a medical obligatory legal procedure since 1874, to provide proof of death and statistics of causes of death. A certificate must be issued by a medical practitioner who has been in attendance during the deceased's last illness. It states the cause of death to the best of the doctors' beliefs and knowledge.

The certificate should be filled in promptly to avoid further distress to the relatives, and clear statements of the disease process should be used, avoiding giving the mode of death as the only entry. Abbreviations should not be used.

The death must then be formally registered (within five days) at the Registration Office for Deaths, Births and Marriages, and arrangements can be made for disposal of the body. The doctor is legally responsible for the delivery of the death certificate but a family member can act as the doctor's agent, (which is usual practice).

It usually less complicated for families to register the death at the registration office in the area where the patient died, although it is possible to register at any registry. The registrar will exchange the doctor's certificate for a certificate for burial or cremation which must be handed to the funeral director involved. Copies of the entries made in the Register of Death by the registrar can be obtained and are needed for probate (wills) or letters of adminstration (if intestate), insurance claims and so on.

- Deaths that cannot be readily certified as due to natural causes should be referred to the coroner
- Once a death has been reported to the coroner, he or she has duty to investigate the cause of death
- The coroner may order a post-mortem to establish a cause of death
- If the family objects to this for religious or other reasons an appeal can be made, but this may delay the funeral
- There is no statutory duty to report any death to the coroner.
- Nevertheless doctors are encouraged to report voluntarily any death where it is judged that the Registrar should refer to the coroner. Such circumstances include:
- Death within 24 h of admission
- Death during detention under the Mental Health Act
- Death where there is a court case pending

In a hospice setting it is not uncommon for a patient to die with a pathological fracture or to die within a short time of arrival at the hospice. The coroner is very helpful in discussion of these cases.

A death should be referred to the coroner if:

- Cause Unknown
- Suspicious or violent circumstances
- Accidental injury
- Industrial diseases e.g. mesothelioma
- Abortion
- Anyone operated on with 48 h of death
- Suicide
- All drug deaths
- Operative or anaesthetic procedures
- Medical procedures/ treatment
- Self neglect/drug abuse
- Police/prison custody
- Septicaemia
- Doctor not attended within 14 days
- Poisoning
- Creutzfeldt Jakob Disease

If in doubt, discuss the situation with the coroner

Doctors have a legal duty to state all they know. However, it is relatively easy for any member of the public to obtain a copy of the death register entry which will include the cause of death. There is therefore the potential for a breach of confidence. The Office of Population Census and Surveys (OPCS) accepts that the present system is unsatisfactory.

The current practice of stating a superficial cause of death rather than the underlying disease process in such cases is widespread. Although it is technically illegal it is condoned by the OPCS—PROVIDED the box on the reverse side of the certificate is ticked stating that additional information may be forthcoming.

This point has yet to be tested in the courts. These comments often apply to patients dying with AIDS-related illnesses.

Cremation

If a body is to be cremated a certificate of medical attendant (Form B) and a confirmatory medical certificate (Form C) should be completed.

In **Form B**, if the doctor has not attended the deceased within 14 days of death, the coroner should be notified. The doctor must see the body after death.

Form C must be completed by a registered medical practitioner of not less than five years standing, who shall not be a relative of the deceased or a relative or partner of the doctor who has given the certificate in Form B.

The doctor must see and examine the body after death. In addition the doctor must have seen and questioned the medical practitioner who completed Form B.

Wills

- If there is a will, the executors named in the will (or if there is no will, the deceased person's representative) is responsible for arranging the funeral and looking after (and subsequently disposing of) the person's assets and property
- If there is a will, the executor should prove this to obtain probate
- If there is no will, the deceased's personal representative should apply for letters of administration

Funeral director

- The funeral director will need to know whether the body is to be buried or cremated (60 per cent of deaths in the UK are followed by cremation)
- They will need to know of any religious customs or rituals that might be necessary
- Bodies may be 'partially' embalmed routinely or this might be discussed with the family
- Traditionally, embalming involves draining blood from body and replacing it with formaldehyde plus a pinkish dye pumped under pressure, which has a hardening and disinfecting effect
- Nowadays the blood is not drained, but a small amount of embalming fluid is infused to help prevent the body smelling and to make the face more presentable
- This is particularly relevant either for hygienic reasons or if the families wish to view

Help and advice for patients

UK national resources

Macmillan Cancer Relief

Funds Macmillan nurses: referral via GP or hospital. Information line; financial help through patient grants. Applications for patient grants through hospital and hospice nurses, social workers and other healthcare professionals. (London)

☎ 0845 601 6161

Cancerline 0808 808 2020

🖳 http://www.macmillan.org.uk/

@ information_line@macmillan.org.uk

Marie Curie Cancer Care

Hands-on palliative nursing care, available through the local district nursing service. Also runs inpatient centres: admission by referral from GP or consultant. Both the services are free of charge. (London)

🖳 http://www.mariecurie.org.uk/

Tenovus Cancer Information Centre (Wales)

Information and support for patients, their families, carer. Helpline staffed by experienced cancer trained nurses, counsellors and social workers. Individual counselling service; free literature.

Velindre Hospital, Whitchurch, Cardiff CF14 2TL

☎ 0808 808 1010

🖳 http://www.tenovus.org.uk/

CancerBACUP

Helps people with cancer, their families and friends live with cancer. Cancer nurses provide information, emotional support and practical advice by telephone or letter. Booklets, factsheets, a newsletter, website and CD-ROM provide information. (London)

☎ 0808 800 1234

🖳 http://www.cancerbacup.org.uk/

Cancerlink

Provides emotional support and information. Register of over 600 cancer support and self-help groups nationwide. Free training and consultancy in setting up and running groups. (London)

Bereavement

Asian Family Counselling Service

Includes bereavement counselling.

☎ 020 8571 3933

CancerBACUP Counselling

☎ 020 7833 2451

🖳 http://www.cancerbacup.org.uk

Cruse

Bereavement counselling

☎ 0870 167 1677

🖳 http://www.crusebereavementcare.org.uk

The Compassionate Friends
A self-help group of parents whose son or daughter (of any age, including adults) has died from any cause.
🖳 http://www.compassionatefriends.org

Samaritans/Age Concern/Citizens Advice Bureaux
☎ From local directory

Carers
Carers National Association
Information and support to people caring for relatives and friends. Free leaflets and information sheets.
☎ 0345 573369 (Mon–Fri 10am–midday, 2pm–4pm)
☎ 029 2088 0176 (Cardiff)

Crossroads—Caring for Carers
Provide a range of services for carers, including care in the home to enable the carer to have a break.
☎ 0845 450 0350
🖳 http://www.crossroads.org.uk

Children
ACT—Association for Children with Life-threatening or Terminal Conditions and their Families
🖳 http://www.act.org.uk

Complementary therapies
Bristol Cancer Help Centre
☎ 0845 123 2310
🖳 http://www.bristolcancerhelp.org

British Acupuncture Council
☎ 020 8735 0400
🖳 http://www.acupuncture.org.uk

British Homoeopathic Association
☎ 0870 444 3950
🖳 http://www.trusthomeopathy.org

National Federation of Spiritual Healers
☎ 0845 123 2777
🖳 http://www.nfsh.org.uk

Institute for Complementary Medicine
☎ 020 7 237 5165
🖳 http://www.i-c-m.org.uk

Conditions other than cancer
Parkinson's Disease Society
☎ 020 7931 8080
🖳 http://www.parkinsons.org.uk

Stroke Association
☎ 0845 303 3100
🖳 http://www.stroke.org.uk

British Brain and Spine Foundation
Helpline provides information and support about neurological disorders for patients, carers and health professionals.
☎ 0808 808 1000
@ info@bbsf.org.uk
🖳 http://www.bbsf.org.uk/

Alzheimer's Disease Society
☎ 020 7306 0606
🖳 http://www.alzheimers.org.uk

Motor Neurone Disease Association
Professional and general enquiries: 0604 250505
Helpline: 0845 7626 262
🖳 http://www.mndassociation.org

Specific Cancers
Brain Tumour Foundation
☎ 020 8336 2020
🖳 http://www.patient.co.uk/showdoc/26739371

Breast Cancer Care
☎ 0808 800 600
@ information@breastcancercare.org.uk
🖳 http://www.breastcancercare.org.uk/

Lymphoma Association
☎ 0808 808 5555 (Mon–Fri 10am–8pm)
🖳 http://www.lymphoma.org.uk/

Oesophageal Patients' Association
☎ 0121 704 9860
🖳 http://www.opa.org.uk

Ovacome
A support organization for women with ovarian cancer.
☎ 020 7380 9589
@ ovacome@ovacome.org.uk
🖳 http://www.ovacome.org.uk/ovacome

Prostate Cancer Charity
☎ (Mon–Fri 10am–4pm) 0845 300 8383
🖳 http://www.prostate-cancer.org.uk/
@ info@prstate-cancer.org.uk

Prostate Cancer Support Association (PSA)
☎ 0845 601 0766 (10am–8pm)
🖳 http://www.prostatecancersupport.co.uk

The Roy Castle Lung Cancer Foundation
☎ 0800 358 7200
🖳 http://www.roycastle.org/

Specific health problems
Changing Faces
Offers information, social skills training and counselling for people with facial disfigurements.
☎ 0845 4500 275
🖳 http://www.changingfaces.co.uk/

British Colostomy Association
☎ 0118 939 1537
Freephone: 0800 32842 57
🖳 http://www.bcass.org.uk

Impotence Association
☎ 0870 774 3571
🖳 http://www.impotence.org.uk/

Let's Face It
A contact point for people of any age coping with facial disfigurement.
☎ 01843 833 724
Tel/Fax: 020 8 931 2829
🖳 http://www.Letsfaceit.force9.co.uk

Lymphoedema Support Network
☎ 020 7 351 4480
🖳 http://www.lymphoedema.org/
@ ADMINLSN@lymphoedema.freeserve.co.uk

National Association of Laryngectomy Clubs
☎ 020 7 381 9993
🖳 http://www.nalc.ik.com

Urostomy Association
☎ 0870 770 7931
🖳 http://www.uagbi.org

Specific patient groups
Chai
Lifeline Cancer Support and Centre for Health
Emotional, physical, practical and spiritual support to Jewish cancer patients, their families and friends.
🖳 http://www.chailifeline.org.uk
@ info@chai-lifeline.org.uk

Gayscan
Offers completely confidential help and support to gay men living with cancer, their partners and carers.
Helpline: 020 8 368 9027

National Network for Palliative Care of People with Learning Disability
☎ 01284 766 133

Investigations

Blood tests
- Blood tests should never be taken 'routinely'
- Blood tests may be taken to confirm or exclude a treatable/reversible diagnosis such as anaemia or hypercalcaemia
- Blood tests may also help assess disease progression **if** this will in turn:
  - help with management decisions (e.g. deteriorating renal function may make plans for discharge inappropriate), or
  - help the patient understand his/her disease (e.g. demonstrating deteriorating liver function tests may help in explaining to the patient why he/she is not getting better)

Microbiology investigations
Midstream specimen of urine (MSU)
Urinalysis checks will show a positive result to blood and/or protein (largely representing red and white cells in the urine) in >90 per cent of urinary tract infections (UTI). Generally speaking an MSU need only be sent if urinalysis is positive but this has to be judged in relation to the specific clinical situation of the patient.

Urinalysis may not be positive if:
- The patient is immunosuppressed (usually a diabetic/septicaemic patient (only true if neutropaenic ie no white cells), OR
- The UTI is present in an obstructed urinary tract, in which case the sample of urine will not be representative. For example, in a bladder tumour obstructing a ureter, infection can develop in the obstructed kidney, which is effectively isolated from the rest of the urinary tract

Catheter specimen of urine (CSU)
Up to 5 per cent of healthy people have bacteriuria (bacteria found in the urine) without symptoms of a UTI. In patients with a catheter this figure is very much higher.

Attempts to sterilize the urine in patients with catheters by treating with antibiotics are only successful as long as the patient continues to take the drug. Bacteriuria always returns on stopping.

In view of this, patients with urinary catheters are only investigated if they have **symptoms** that might relate to a UTI, and that warrant treatment e.g.
- dysuria, frequency or urgency
- suprapubic pains—'bladder spasms'
- loin pain
- toxic symptoms e.g. confusion, nausea and vomiting especially if associated with fever.
- sludging, bypassing and blocking catheter

Unpleasant-smelling urine indicates infection rather than simple bacteriuria, but does not by itself warrant investigation unless the patient considers it a problem.

Magnetic resonance imaging (MRI)

MRI cannot be performed on patients who have a cardiac pacemaker *or ferrous/magnetic* metal in their body since the magnetic field may interfere with function. This includes patients with:

- aneurysm clips in the brain
- cochlear implants
- metal fragments in the eye
- shrapnel

Hip replacements are made of non-ferrous metal and do not exclude an MRI.

Intravenous contrast studies

Radiological examinations requiring intravenous contrast to be given (IVP, CT scan etc.) can precipitate lactic acidosis in patients taking metformin. The metformin should be stopped well in advance of the investigation.

Influenza vaccination

Annual immunization with influenza vaccine is recommended for those of all ages with:
- immunosuppression due to disease or treatment
- chronic respiratory or heart disease
- chronic renal failure
- diabetes mellitus
- persons over the age of 65 years
- residents of nursing and residential homes

There is evidence that it is still effective in patients with cancer. The 'flu vaccine is a preparation of inactivated virus, and will not cause influenza in immunosuppressed patients. The main contra-indication is an allergy to eggs.

Needlestick injury and HIV
- The risk of HIV transmission following needlestick injury involving contaminated blood is about 0.4 per cent. Zidovudine treatment reduces the transmission rate by about 80 per cent
- Ideally treatment should start within 1–2h of such exposure
- All needlestick injuries should be reported and prompt advice sought from local infection control advisors

Falls

All patients who have had a fall should have a full history, examination and appropriate investigations looking for reversible causes whether or not they have terminal cancer. The consequences of the fall, e.g. hip fracture, subdural bleed etc. will need managing on an individual basis according to clinical frailty and patient's wishes.

Assessment should include:

Blood pressure

Postural hypotension should be assessed by measuring the blood pressure both lying and standing. If there is a significant blood pressure drop on standing, reversible possibilities should be sought such as medication (e.g. diuretics, antihypertensives, antimuscrinics, beta-blockers, phenothiazines, withdrawal of steroids), anaemia, dehydration, insufficient adreno-cortical function etc. Patients should be advised to rise slowly from a lying/sitting position, to sleep propped up with pillows and to consider support hosiery. If no obviously reversible cause is found, treatment with fludrocortisone 0.05–0.1mg o.d. may be appropriate.

Medication review

- Consider reducing or stopping:
  - Hypotensive drugs: antimuscarinics, beta-blockers, phenothiazines etc.
  - Sedative drugs: benzodiazepines, opioid analgesics etc.
  - Anticonvulsants (ataxia)
  - Corticosteroids (proximal myopathy)
- Neurological assessment for:
  - Spinal cord compression
  - Cerebellar dysfunction
  - Parkinson's disease or extrapyramidal symptoms
  - Long tract signs suggestive of hemiparesis etc.
  - History suggestive of a seizure, TIA etc.
- Physiotherapist assessment for:
  - Balance
  - Transfers
  - Gait

Legal standard of care

All doctors and other health professionals work in an increasingly litigious climate. In palliative medicine, a specialty where doctors are involved at a highly emotional time in patients' and families' lives, and in light of the aftermath of a number of high profile medicolegal/ethical cases, the importance of the shift from the traditional Bolam approach to a new more enquiring approach should be understood.

- In medical litigation, the central question that arises is whether or not a doctor has attained the standard of care that is required by law
- The standard expected is one of 'reasonable care'
- This is judged by taking into account all the circumstances surrounding a particular situation and by balancing the diversity inherent in medical practice against the interests of the patient
- In determining the standard, the court uses the Bolam test
- The Bolam principle, however, has been perceived as being excessively reliant upon medical testimony supporting the defendant
- The judgement given by the House of Lords in the recent case of Bolitho imposes a requirement that the standard proclaimed must be justified on a logical basis and the risks and benefits of competing options must have been considered
- The effect of this case is that the court will take a more enquiring stance to test the medical evidence offered by both parties in litigation in order to reach its conclusions

In 1954, Mr Bolam underwent electroconvulsive therapy (ECT) for clinical depression. At that time medical opinion differed on how best to minimise the risk of injuries possible from convulsions induced by ECT. In Mr Bolam's case the technique of manual restraint was ineffective and as a result he fractured his pelvis. He subsequently argued that the doctor had been in breach of the standard of care in providing treatment and that the hospital had been negligent. The judge in his direction to the jury said that a doctor is not guilty of negligence if he has acted in accordance with the practice accepted as proper by a responsible body of medical opinion skilled in that particular art. If therefore a medical practice is supported by a body of peers, then the Bolam test is satisfied and the practitioner has met the required standard of care in law. This test has been used on numerous occasions in cases of medical litigation.

Wills

- Palliative care involves looking after patients and families in the broadest sense
- Many people delay writing a will for a number of reasons, which often leaves families in a difficult situation, not knowing what the deceased would have wanted
- Palliative care teams are often in contact with patients for several months before death, and are in a good position to encourage the family to discuss important issues and the patient to consider making a will
- This is particularly important if the family dynamics are complicated
- The intestacy rules dictate not only who receives the estate but also who should manage the affairs of the estate
- Unmarried partners may have no claim on the estate unless they are dependent on the deceased
- If the deceased is divorced or separated, the rules will determine who the legal guardians of the children will be

It is not uncommon for patients to wish to make a will in the last few days of life, having not wanted to face up to it before this time. This is a time when patients may have episodes of being distressed or muddled, a situation which lends itself to the possibility of family members contesting what they attest to be an incompetently considered 'death bed' will. Although it is not absolutely necessary, it is best to advise that the will is drawn up by a qualified solicitor who will be in the best position to defend the will if it is ever contested. If a doctor is asked to witness a signature, it would be wise to confirm first that the patient is competent to do so.

Competency for drawing up a will

The legal test for Testamentary Capacity was described by Mr Justice Cockburn in the case of Banks v. Goodfellow in 1879:

> 'It is essential . . . that a testator shall understand the nature of the act and its effects; shall understand the extent of the property of which he is disposing; shall be able to comprehend and appreciate the claims to which he ought to give effect and, with a view to the latter object, that no disorder of the mind shall poison his affections, pervert his sense of right, or prevent the exercise of his natural faculties, that no insane delusion shall influence his will in disposing of his property and bring about a disposal of it which, if the mind had been sound, would not have been made.'

Following death:
- If a will has been written, the executors appointed in the will apply for a grant of probate
- If a will has not been written, the administrators apply for a grant of letters of administration
- When it comes to distributing the estate the nearest relatives in a fixed order are entitled to apply for the grant
- If the nearest relative does not wish to apply, he can renounce his right to do so in which case the next-nearest becomes entitled to be the administrator and so on down the line of kinship

- There is a hierarchy of those that are legally next of kin and as such entitled to apply for the grant
- The widow or widower is primarily entitled to be the administrator and if there is no surviving spouse or he/she does not apply for a grant, then any of the children can apply
- Grandchildren and other offspring may apply if their parents have died
- In-laws and people related by marriage do not count, only blood relations
- There is no distinction made between natural, adopted or illegitimate relationships
- An adopted child is deemed to be the legal child of his adoptive parents and has exactly the same inheritance right as the adoptive parents' other (natural) children, but loses any rights to his natural parents estate

Enduring Power of Attorney

An Enduring Power of Attorney can continue in force after the maker of the power (donor) becomes mentally incapable of handling his or her affairs. The donor must me competent at the time of appointing an attorney.

It may give:
- General power—which authorizes the attorney to carry out any transaction on behalf of the donor, or
- Specific power—which authorizes the attorney to deal only with those aspects of the donor's affairs which are specified in the power

When the donor becomes mentally incapable, the attorney must apply to register the Enduring Power of Attorney with the Court of Protection, before it can be undertaken.

The donor can revoke or cancel it at any time while she or he is mentally capable, but cannot revoke it once it has been registered unless the Court of Protection confirms the revocation.

Once registered, the attorney has the power to act on behalf of the donor, either in the general or specific way as outlined, but has no power over the 'person' of the donor and cannot make a will on behalf of the donor.

- Most attorneys are honest, decent people. Some, however, abuse their situation
- Financial abuse probably occurs in 10–15 per cent of cases involving registered Enduring Power of Attorney and more often when they are unregistered
- The powers of the Court of Protection and the Public Trust Office (a registration authority only) are limited where the donor is being financially abused
- The court can only intervene when the donor is, or is becoming, mentally incapable
- The court is generally not concerned with unregistered powers.
- The court can revoke the Enduring Power of Attorney (but this is often too late) and can appoint a receiver with authority to investigate but this is often not satisfactory
- Some people believe they have an indefeasible right to inherit another person's estate intact
- In a number of cases, attorneys have disposed of the donor's assets to secure entitlement to public funding for long term care

- The risk is greater if the attorney lives abroad
- Mutual dependency is also a problem, since the donor is dependent on the attorney as the principal or only carer but also the attorney is dependent on the donor, especially when they share living accommodation and financial arrangements
- In cases where a donor comes from an unreliable or dysfunctional family and has a relatively short life expectation, it may be prudent for solicitors to recommend that the donor appoints a receiver and not an attorney

Donors who are more at risk from abuse include those with no immediate family or only one child, those who are moderately affluent (but not extremely rich or extremely poor) and those who suddenly come into additional wealth through inheritance on the death of a relative. An aggravating factor is the expectation of inheritance and the desire to preserve and precipitate it.

Advance Directive (also known as Living Will)

> Where is the wisdom we have lost in Knowledge?
> Where is the knowledge we have lost in information?
>
> T. S. Eliot, *The Rock*, 1934

Medical advances such as cardiopulmonary resuscitation, renal dialysis, artificial ventilation and artificial hydration and nutrition may prolong life. The fear of being kept alive artificially, with no prospect of recovery and no perceived quality of life, has prompted society to discuss and to draw up guidance on the issue of end-of-life care. This is supported by health-care professionals who are concerned about providing non-beneficial, over-burdensome medical interventions to patients with a terminal illness.

> Advance Directives allow a competent patient to express their wishes about treatment decisions in the event of them becoming incompetent and unable to give consent.

The US was the first country to formalize the use of Advance Directives following a case in which a patient, whose previously held wishes for treatment and care and basic values were unknown, lapsed into a permanent vegetative state in 1976. A similar debate on the rôle of Advance Directives took place in the UK following the case of Tony Bland (1993).

A House of Lords select committee on medical ethics discussed the merits of Advance Directives, although it did not consider that legislation was necessary. It encouraged the development of a 'code of practice' which was produced by the British Medical Association in1995, outlining the inherent ethical and legal issues.

The UK government is satisfied for the time being that this BMA document, *Advance Statements about Medical Treatment*, together with case law, provides sufficient clarity and flexibility to enable the validity and applicability of Advance Directives to be decided on a case by case basis.

The idea of patients discussing their wishes is not new, but the aim of the Advance Directive is to provide a more formal, registered means for the patient to continue to exercise autonomy in the event of future mental incapacity.

Advance Directives can encompasses all type of anticipatory decision-making, including oral and written decisions and records of discussion in case notes, of advance refusals or authorisations of treatment. They can be specific, general or list the patient's fundamental values as a guide for others to decide. Legally, no person has a right to accept or decline treatment on behalf of another but a representative, nominated by the patient, may be helpful in communicating the patient's views.

Advance Directives of refusal are only of repute if the patient was;
- competent
- fully informed
- uncoerced at the time of drawing up the Advance Directive
- In addition, it must be valid and clearly applicable to this particular situation

The legality of non-documented verbal advance refusals is debatable.

There should be no reason to suggest that the patient might have changed his/her mind. Others should not be put at potentially serious harm by applying the Advance Directive. Patients are not able to authorize treatment that is not legal (e.g. euthanasia) nor are they able to refuse future basic care.

Any Advance Directive is superseded by a clear and competent contemporaneous decision. An Advance Directive of a patient under the age of 18 years should be taken into account and accommodated if possible but can be overruled by a court or a person with parental responsibility.

If the patient has been detained for compulsory treatment under mental health legislation, any advance refusal of treatment can be overruled.

Advising the person enquiring about creating an Advance Directive

- Ensure that the patient is competent. An Advance Directive should not be made under pressure, particularly if the patient has recently received a poor prognosis. The patient should not be unduly influenced in any way and there should be no question of clinical depression that might affect competence
- Provide the patient with information on Advance Directives (Patients Association 2000)
- Allow for dialogue and openness in discussion with relevant healthcare professionals including doctors and nurses. Patients must be able to make informed choices and will need to be aware of predictable phases of their disease and treatment options, diagnosis, prognosis and rehabilitation potential. They need to know the options considered to be in the patient's best interests although the patient will be the ultimate judge. They will also need to know what will be done if the treatment is not carried out. (Advance Directives are an aid to, and not a substitute for, discussion and communication.)
- Written statements, on firm decisions or general views, should use clear and unambiguous language. Oral statements are equally valid if supported by appropriate evidence
- Advance Directives should be signed by the individual and a witness. The witness should not be a family member since they may stand to gain from the death. If a healthcare professional witnesses, it is implied that assessment of competence has taken place
- Review the Advance Directive regularly
- Encourage the patient to store the document safely. It is the patient's responsibility to ensure its availability. A copy should be sent to the GP, specialist team and stored in the case notes
- In an emergency situation, health professionals should make all reasonable efforts to acquaint themselves with the contents of the Advance Directive if they know or have reason to believe that one is available but should not delay treatment in anticipation of finding one

A guide to core content of an Advance Directive

- Full name
- Address
- Name and address of GP

- Whether advice was sought from health professionals
- Signature of patient
- Date drafted and reviewed
- Witnessed
- Clear statement of the patient's wishes, either general or specific
- Name, address and telephone number of patient's nominated person, if one chosen
- Consider for inclusion:
  - List of the individual's values as a basis for others to reach appropriate decisions
  - Request for all medically reasonable efforts to be made to prolong life or expression of preferences for treatment options
  - Where the patient would like to be cared for
  - Contingency issues for pregnancy where appropriate

Further reading

Travis S., Mason J., Mallett J., Laverty D. (2001) Guidelines in respect of Advance Directives: the position in England. *International Journal of Palliative Nursing*, **7, 10**: 493–500.

BMA (1995) *Advance Statements about Medical Treatment. Code of practice with explanatory notes.* London: BMJ Publishing Group.

Luttrell S. (1996) Living wills do have legal effect provided certain criteria are met. *BMJ*, **313**: 1148.

Dermatomes

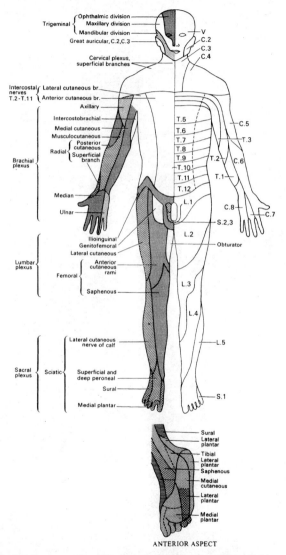

Fig. 16.1 Dermatomes. Reproduced from the *Oxford Handbook of Clinical Medicine*, 6th ed. M. Longmore *et al.* Oxford: Oxford University Press. With permission.

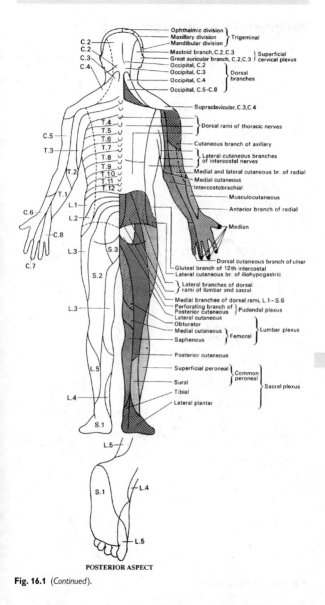

Fig. 16.1 (Continued).

Peripheral nerve assessment

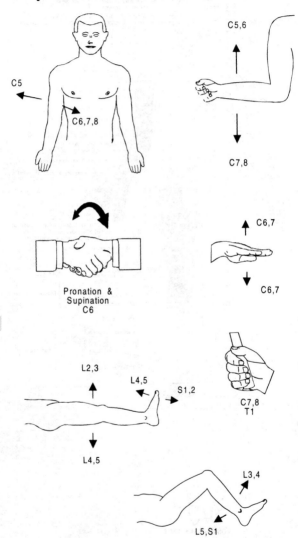

Fig. 16.2 Neurological diagrams.

Drawing a family tree (genogram)

Family Tree

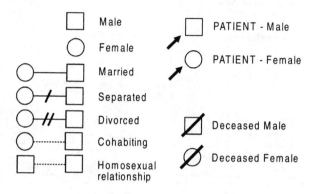

2nd AND 3rd MARRIAGES

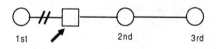

1st   2nd   3rd

PARENTS

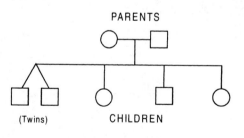

(Twins)   CHILDREN

NB Alternative system: $\otimes$ for the Patient and ● for Deceased

Fig. 16.3 How to draw up a family tree.

Emergency drug doses

Table 16.1 Emergency drug doses[1]

	Route	Adult	Child
Anaphylaxis/asthma			
Adrenaline 1:1,000			
(epinephrine)	i/m	0.5ml	0.1ml/yr
Aminophylline	i/v 20mins	250–500mg	5mg/kg
	infusion	0.5mg/kg/h	1mg/kg/h
Chlorphenamine			
(chlorpheniramine)	i/v	10mg	200 mcg/kg
Salbutamol	i/v slow	0.25mg	4 mcg/kg
	SC, i/m	0.5mg	
neb	5mg	2.5mg	
Hydrocortisone	i/v	100–300mg	
Fits/sedation			
Diazepam	i/v, PR	10mg	0.25–0.5mg/kg
Diabetes—hypoglycaemia			
Glucagon	i/m	1mg >12yrs	0.5mg <12yrs

1 Back I. (2001). *Palliative Medicine Handbook*. 3rd edn. BPM Books: Cardiff.

Laboratory reference values

These are guides only—different labs use different ranges. Pregnant women and children also have different normal ranges—consult the lab.

Haematology

Measurement	Reference interval
White cell count (WCC)	$4.0–11.0 \times 10^9$/l
Red cell count (RCC)	Men: $4.5–6.5 \times 10^{12}$/l
	Women: $3.9–5.6 \times 10^{12}$/l
Haemoglobin	Men: 13.5–18g/dl
	Women: 11.5–16.0g/dl
Packed cell volume (PCV) or	Men: 38.5–50.1%
haematocrit	Women: 36.0–44.5%
Mean cell volume (MCV)	76–97fl
Mean cell haemoglobin (MCHC)	32.7–34.6 g/dl
Neutrophils	$2.0–7.5 \times 10^9$/l _40–75% WCC_
Lymphocytes	$1.3–3.5 \times 10^9$/l _20–45% WCC_
Esoinophils	$0.04–0.44 \times 10^9$/l _1–6% WCC_
Basophils	$0.0–0.1 \times 10^9$/l _0–1% WCC_
Monocytes	$0.2–0.8 \times 10^9$/l _2–10% WCC_
Platelet count	$150–400 \times 10^9$/l
Reticulocyte count	$25–100 \times 10^9$/l _0.8–2% RCC*_
Erythrocyte sedimentation rate (ESR)	Depends on age
International normalized ratio (INR)	0.8–1.2
	Ranges for warfarin therapy depend on indication, 📖 Chapter 6c
Prothrombin time (PTT) Factors I, II, VII, X	12–17 sec.
Activated partial thromboplastin time Factors VIII, IX, XI, XII	28–40 sec.
Red cell folate	180–300 ng/ml

---

* Only use percentages as reference interval if red cell count is normal. Otherwise use absolute value.

Biochemistry

Substance		*Reference interval*
Adrenocorticotrophic hormone	P	<80ng/l
Alanine aminotransferase (ALT)	P	5–35iu/l
Albumin	P	35–50g/l
Alkaline phosphatase	P	30–150u/l
α-amylase	P	0–180u/dl
Aspartate transaminase (AST)	P	5–35iu/l
Bicarbonate	P	24–30mmol/l
Bilirubin	P	3–17μmol/l
Calcium (total)	P	2.12–2.65mmol/l
Creatinine kinase (CK)	P	Men: 25–195iu/l
		Women: 25–170iu/l
Creatinine	P	70–≤150μmol/l
Ferritin	P	12–200μg/l
Folate	S	2.1μg/l
Follicle stimulating hormone (FSH)	P/S	2–8u/l *>25u/l post menopause*
Gamma-glutamyl transpeptidase (GGT, γGT)	P	Men: 11–51iu/l
		Women: 7–33iu/l
Glucose (fasting)	P	3.5–5.5mmol/l
Iron	S	Men: 14–31μmol/l
		Women: 11–30μmol/l
Luteinizing hormone (LH)	P	3–16u/l
Osmolality	P	278–305mosmol/kg
Phosphate (inorganic)	P	0.8–1.45mmol/l
Potassium	P	3.5–5.0mmol/l
Prolactin	P	Men: <450u/l
		Women: <600u/l
Prostate specific antigen (PSA)	P	0–4ngrams/ml
Protein (total)	P	60–80g/l
Sodium	P	135–145mmol/l
Thyroxine (T_4)	P	70–140nmol/l
Total iron binding capacity	S	54–75μmol/l
Triglyceride	P	0.55–1.90mmol/l
Urate	P	Men: 210–480μmol/l
		Women: 150–390μmol/l
Urea	P	2.5–6.7mmol/l
Vitamin B_{12}	S	0.13–0.68nmol/l
		(>150ng/l)

P = plasma (e.g. heparin bottle); S = serum (clotted—no anticoagulant).

Index

Page numbers in *italics* indicate tables and figures.